PROGRESS IN BRAIN RESEARCH

VOLUME 83

UNDERSTANDING THE BRAIN THROUGH THE HIPPOCAMPUS

The Hippocampal Region as a Model for Studying Brain Structure and Function

PROGRESS IN BRAIN RESEARCH

VOLUME 83

UNDERSTANDING THE BRAIN THROUGH THE HIPPOCAMPUS

The Hippocampal Region as a Model for Studying Brain Structure and Function

EDITED BY

J. STORM-MATHISEN

Anatomical Institute, University of Oslo, Oslo, Norway

J. ZIMMER

Institute of Neurobiology, University of Aarhus, Aarhus, Denmark

and

O.P. OTTERSEN

Anatomical Institute, University of Oslo, Oslo, Norway

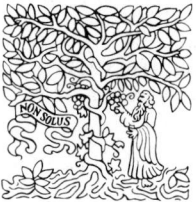

ELSEVIER

AMSTERDAM – NEW YORK – OXFORD

1990

ISBN 0-444-81149-4 (volume)
ISBN 0-444-80104-9 (series)

This book is printed on acid-free paper

Published by:
Elsevier Science Publishers B.V. (Biomedical Division)
P.O. Box 211
1000 AE Amsterdam
The Netherlands

Sole distributors for the USA and Canada:
Elsevier Science Publishing Company, Inc.
655 Avenue of the Americas
New York, NY 10010
USA

Library of Congress Cataloging-in-Publication Data

Understanding the brain through the hippocampus : the hippocampal
  region as a model for studying brain structure and function / edited
  by J. Storm-Mathisen, J. Zimmer, and O.P. Ottersen.
      p.   cm. -- (Progress in brain research ; v. 83)
    Includes bibliographical references.
    ISBN 0-444-81149-4 (U.S. : alk. paper)
    1. Hippocampus--Physiology. I. Storm-Mathisen, Jon. II. Zimmer,
J. (Jens) III. Ottersen, O. P. (Ole P.) IV. Series.
    [DNLM: 1. Brain--anatomy & histology. 2. Brain--physiology.
3. Hippocampus. W1 PR667J v. 83 / WL 314 U55]
QP376.P7   vol. 83
[QP383.25]
612′.82 s--dc20
[599′.0188]
DNLM/DLC
for Library of Congress   90-2864
                                                            CIP

Printed in the Netherlands

This volume is dedicated to
Professor Theodor W. Blackstad
on the occasion of his 65th
anniversary

List of Contributors

D.G. Amaral, The Salk Institute for Biological Studies, P.O. Box 85800, San Diego, CA 92138, U.S.A., p. 1

P. Andersen, Institute of Neurophysiology, University of Oslo, Karl Johans gate 47, N-0162 Oslo 1, Norway, p. 215

A. Arai, Bonney Center for the Neurobiology of Learning and Memory, University of California, Irvine, CA 92717, U.S.A., p. 233

D.M. Armstrong, Department of Neuroscience, M-024, University of California at San Diego, La Jolla, CA 92093, U.S.A., p. 357

K.G. Baimbridge, Department of Physiology, Faculty of Medicine, University of British Columbia, Vancouver, B.C., Canada, p. 85

C.A. Barnes, Department of Psychology, Campus Box 345, University of Colorado, Boulder, CO 80309, U.S.A., p. 287

J.M. Bekkers, Section of Molecular Neurobiology, Howard Hughes Medical Institute at Yale University School of Medicine, 333 Cedar Street, New Haven, CT 06510, U.S.A., p. 37

Y. Ben-Ari, INSERM U-29, 123 Boulevard de Port-Royal, F-75014, Paris, France, p. 313

A. Björklund, Department of Medical Cell Research, Section of Neurobiology, University of Lund, Biskopsgatan 5, S-223 62 Lund, Sweden, p. 411

T.V.P. Bliss, Division of Neurophysiology and Neuropharmacology, National Institute for Medical Research, Mill Hill, London NW7 1AA, U.K., p. 251

P. Bovolenta, Laboratorio de Plasticidad Neural, Instituto Cajal, Doctor Arce 37, 28002 Madrid, Spain, p. 341

M.A. Bowe, Departments of Pharmacology and Neurobiology, Duke University Medical Center, Durham, NC 27710, U.S.A., p. 115

C. Bramham, Department of Physiology, University of Bergen, N-5000 Bergen, Norway, p. 99

D.A. Brown, Department of Pharmacology, University College London, Gower Street, London WC1E 6BT, U.K., p. 141, p. 189

S.P. Burke, Departments of Pharmacology and Neurobiology, Duke University Medical Center, Durham, NC 27710, U.S.A., p. 115

G.A. Bustos, Laboratory of Biochemical Pharmacology, Faculty of Biological Sciences, Catholic University of Chile, Santiago, Chile, p. 115

G. Buzsáki, Department of Neurosciences, M-024, University of California at San Diego, La Jolla, CA 92093, U.S.A., p. 257, p. 357

S. Charpak, Brain Research Institute, University of Zürich, August Forel Strasse 1, CH-8029 Zürich, Switzerland, p. 189

L.S. Chen, Department of Neurosciences, M-024, University of California at San Diego, La Jolla, CA 92093, U.S.A., p. 257

E. Cherubini, INSERM U-29, 123 Boulevard de Port-Royal, F-75014 Paris, France, p. 313

B. Claiborne, Division of Life Sciences, University of Texas at San Antonio, San Antonio, TX 78285, U.S.A., p. 1

M.P. Clements, Division of Neurophysiology and Neuropharmacology, National Institute for Medical Research, Mill Hill, London NW7 1AA, U.K., p. 251

P.D. Coleman, Department of Neurobiology and Anatomy, School of Medicine and Dentistry, University of Rochester, 601 Elmwood Avenue, Rochester, NY 14642, U.S.A., p. 435

R. Corradetti, Department of Preclinical and Clinical Pharmacology, University of Florence, Viale G.B. Morgagni 65, 50134 Florence, Italy, p. 313

C.W. Cotman, Department of Psychobiology, Room 249, Steinhaus Hall, University of California, Irvine, CA 92717, U.S.A., p. 427

G. Danscher, Institute of Neurobiology, University of Aarhus, DK-8000 Aarhus C, Denmark, p. 71

M.L. Errington, Division of Neurophysiology and Neuropharmacology, National Institute for Medical Research, Mill Hill, London NW7 1AA, U.K., p. 251

D.G. Flood, Department of Neurology, School of Medicine and Dentistry, University of Rochester, Box 673, 601 Elmwood Avenue, Rochester, NY 14642, U.S.A., p. 435

C.J. Frederickson, Laboratory for Neurobiology, University of Texas at Dallas, Richardson, TX 75083, U.S.A., p. 71

M. Frotscher, Institute of Anatomy, University of Freiburg, Albertstr. 17, D-7800 Freiburg, F.R.G., p. 323

F.H. Gage, Department of Neurosciences, M-024, University of California at San Diego, La Jolla, CA 92093, U.S.A., p. 257, p. 357

B.H. Gähwiler, Brain Research Institute, University of Zürich, CH-8029 Zürich, Switzerland, p. 141, p. 189

J.L. Gaiarsa, INSERM U-29, 123 Boulevard de Port-Royal, F-75014 Paris, France, p. 313

C. Gall, Department of Anatomy and Neurobiology, University of California, Irvine, CA 92717, U.S.A., p. 371

J.W. Geddes, Department of Neurosurgery, University of California, Irvine, CA 92717, U.S.A., p. 427

F.A. Geneser, Institute of Neurobiology, University of Aarhus, DK-8000 Aarhus C, Denmark, p. 85

W.H. Griffith, Department of Medical Pharmacology, Texas A & M University, College Station, TX 77077, U.S.A., p. 141

H.J. Groenewegen, Department of Anatomy and Embryology, Vrije Universiteit, van der Boechorststraat 7, 1081 BT Amsterdam, The Netherlands, p. 47

V. Gundersen, Anatomical Institute, University of Oslo, Karl Johans gate 47, N-0162 Oslo 1, Norway, p. 99

B. Gustafsson, Department of Physiology, University of Göteborg, Box 33031, S-400 33 Göteborg, Sweden, p. 223

J.V. Halliwell, Department of Physiology, Royal Free Hospital School of Medicine, University of London, London NW3 2PF, U.K., p. 141

B. Heimrich, Institute of Anatomy, University of Freiburg, Albertstr. 17, D-7800 Freiburg, F.R.G., p. 323

U. Heinemann, Institut für Neurophysiologie, Zentrum Physiologie und Pathophysiologie, Universität zu Köln, Robert Kochstrasse 39, D-5000 Köln 41, F.R.G., p. 197

I.E. Holm, Institute of Neurobiology, University of Aarhus, DK-8000 Aarhus C, Denmark, p. 85

Ø. Hvalby, Institute of Neurophysiology, University of Oslo, Karl Johans gate 47, N-0162 Oslo 1, Norway, p. 131

B.T. Hyman, Neurology Service, Harvard Medical School, Massachusetts General Hospital, Fruit Street, Boston, MA 02114, U.S.A., p. 445

P. Isackson, Department of Anatomy and Neurobiology, University of California, Irvine, CA 92717, U.S.A., p. 371

N. Ishizuka, Department of Neuroanatomy, Institute of Brain Research, Faculty of Medicine, University of Tokyo, 7-3-1 Hongo, Bunkyo-ku, Tokyo 113, Japan, p. 1

J.S. Kahle, Department of Psychobiology, University of California, Irvine, CA 92717, U.S.A., p. 427

P. Kalén, Department of Medical Cell Research, Section of Neurobiology, University of Lund, Biskopsgatan 5, S-223 62 Lund, Sweden, p. 411

M. Kessler, Bonney Center for the Neurobiology of Learning and Memory, University of California, Irvine, CA 92717, U.S.A., p. 233

T. Knöpfel, Brain Research Institute, University of Zürich, August Forel Strasse 1, CH-8029 Zürich, Switzerland, p. 189

C. Köhler, Department of Neuropharmacology, Astra Research Centre AB, S-151 85 Södertälje, Sweden, p. 59

J. Laake, Anatomical Institute, University of Oslo, Karl Johans gate 47, N-0162 Oslo 1, Norway, p. 99

S. Laroche, Département de Psychophysiologie, LPN2, Centre National de la Recherche Scientifique, F-91198 Gif-sur-Yvette, France, p. 251

J. Larson, Bonney Center for the Neurobiology of Learning and Memory, University of California, Irvine, CA 92717, U.S.A., p. 233

J. Lauterborn, Department of Anatomy and Neurobiology, University of Irvine, Irvine, CA 92717, U.S.A., p. 371

B.W. Leonard, Department of Psychology, Campus Box 345, University of Colorado, Boulder, CO 80309, U.S.A., p. 287

L.-H. Lin, Department of Psychology, Campus Box 345, University of Colorado, Boulder, CO 80309, U.S.A., p. 287

G. Lynch, Bonney Center for the Neurobiology of Learning and Memory, University of California, Irvine, CA 92717, U.S.A., p. 233

M.A. Lynch, Division of Neurophysiology and Neuropharmacology, National Institute for Medical Research, Mill Hill, London NW7 1AA, U.K., p. 251

D. Martin, Departments of Pharmacology and Neurobiology, Duke University Medical Center, Durham, NC 27710, U.S.A., p. 115

B.L. McNaughton, Department of Psychology, Campus Box 345, University of Colorado, Boulder, CO 80309, U.S.A., p. 287

S.J.Y. Mizumori, Department of Psychology, Campus Box 345, University of Colorado, Boulder, CO 80309, U.S.A., p. 287

J.V. Nadler, Department of Pharmacology, Room 325, Building MSIA, Duke University Medical Center, Durham, NC 27710, U.S.A., p. 115

M. Nieto-Sampedro, Laboratorio de Plasticidad Neural, Instituto Cajal, Doctor Arce 37, 28002 Madrid, Spain, p. 341

O.G. Nilsson, Department of Medical Cell Research, Section of Neurobiology, University of Lund, Biskopsgatan 5, S-223 62 Lund, Sweden, p. 411

J. O'Keefe, Department of Anatomy and Developmental Biology, University College London, Gower Street, London WC1E 6BT, U.K., p. 301

O.P. Ottersen, Anatomical Institute, University of Oslo, Karl Johans gate 47, N-0162 Oslo 1, Norway, p. 99

G. Rausche, Institut für Neurophysiologie, Zentrum Physiologie und Pathophysiologie, Universität zu Köln, Robert Kochstrasse 39, D-5000 Köln 41, F.R.G., p. 197

C. Rédini-Del Negro, Département de Psychophysiologie, LPN2, Centre National de la Recherche Scientifique, F-91198 Gif-sur-Yvette, France, p. 251

O. Robain, INSERM U-29, 123 Boulevard de Port-Royal, F-75014 Paris, France, p. 313

C. Rovira, INSERM U-29, 123 Boulevard de Port-Royal, F-75014 Paris, France, p. 313

H.E. Scharfman, Howard Hughes Medical Institute and Department of Neurobiology and Behavior, State University of New York at Stony Brook, Stony Brook, NY 11794, U.S.A., p. 269

P.A. Schwartzkroin, Departments of Neurological Surgery, Physiology and Biophysics, University of Washington, Seattle, WA 98195, U.S.A., p. 269

H. Schwegler, Institute of Anatomy, University of Freiburg, Albertstr. 17, D-7800 Freiburg, F.R.G., p. 323

R.S. Sloviter, Neurology Research Center, Helen Hayes Hospital, New York State Department of Health, West Haverstraw, NY 10993, U.S.A. and Departments of Pharmacology and Neurology, Columbia University, New York, NY 10032, U.S.A., p. 269

T. Sørensen, PharmaBiotec Research Center, Institute of Neurobiology, University of Aarhus, DK-8000 Aarhus C, Denmark, p. 391

J. Stabel, Institut für Neurophysiologie, Zentrum Physiologie und Pathophysiologie, Universität zu Köln, Robert Kochstrasse 39, D-5000 Köln 41, F.R.G., p. 197

C.F. Stevens, The Salk Institute, 10010 North Torrey Pines Road, La Jolla, CA 92037, U.S.A., p. 37

J.F. Storm, Institute of Neurophysiology, University of Oslo, Karl Johans gate 47, N-0162 Oslo 1, Norway, p. 161

J. Storm-Mathisen, Anatomical Institute, University of Oslo, Karl Johans gate 47, N-0162 Oslo 1, Norway, p. 99

N. Tønder, PharmaBiotec Research Center, Institute of Neurobiology, University of Aarhus, DK-8000 Aarhus C, Denmark, p. 391

R. Torp, Anatomical Institute, University of Oslo, Karl Johans gate 47, N-0162 Oslo 1, Norway, p. 99

G.W. Van Hoesen, Department of Anatomy, University of Iowa College of Medicine, 51 Newton Road, Iowa City, IA 52242, U.S.A., p. 445

M.J. West, Stereological Research Laboratory, Bartholin Building, University of Aarhus, DK-8000 Aarhus C, Denmark, p. 37

J. White, Division of Endocrinology, Department of Medicine, State University of New York, Stony Brook, NY 11794, U.S.A., p. 371

H. Wigström, Department of Medical Physics, University of Göteborg, Box 33031, S-400 33 Göteborg, Sweden, p. 223

M.P. Witter, Department of Anatomy, Vrije Universiteit, van der Boechorststraat 7, 1081 BT Amsterdam, The Netherlands, p. 47

J. Zimmer, Institute of Neurobiology, University of Aarhus, DK-8000 Aarhus C, Denmark, p. 85, p. 391

Preface

The present volume has been compiled as a tribute to Professor Theodor W. Blackstad and his pioneering work on the anatomy of the hippocampal region. Our ambition has been to make this 'Festschrift' a high quality reference volume on contemporary hippocampal research.

To this end, and to achieve a result in accordance with the 'Blackstad Spirit', the contributors were selected strictly on the basis of scientific criteria and were asked to adhere to the following guidelines when writing their papers: 1. Emphasis should be put on results that can increase our understanding of the structure and function of the CNS in general, and whenever appropriate the discussion should focus on the extent to which the findings in the hippocampus can be extrapolated to other brain regions. 2. The contributions should be up to date and preferably focussed on the current interests of the authors. 3. The chapters should be prepared with the understanding that the book is intended to be of interest to neuroscientists in general. We feel that the authors have complied with these requirements and we would like to thank everyone for fruitful collaboration on the project. We are also grateful to Ms Tove Eliassen and Ms Karin Wiedemann for excellent secretarial assistance.

Theodor's contribution has undoubtedly influenced most neuroscientists who today use the hippocampal region as a research model. Accordingly, the response to our invitations to contribute to the present volume was overwhelmingly positive. Several authors expressed their great respect for Theodor as a scientist and as a human being. Their views are epitomized by the following quotation from a letter from Professor Gary Van Hoesen: ' . . . Blackstad . . . a wonderful individual who, as you know, is the gene for all modern investigations on the hippocampal formation'.

Oslo and Aarhus, 1st March 1990

Jon Storm-Mathisen   Jens Zimmer   Ole Petter Ottersen

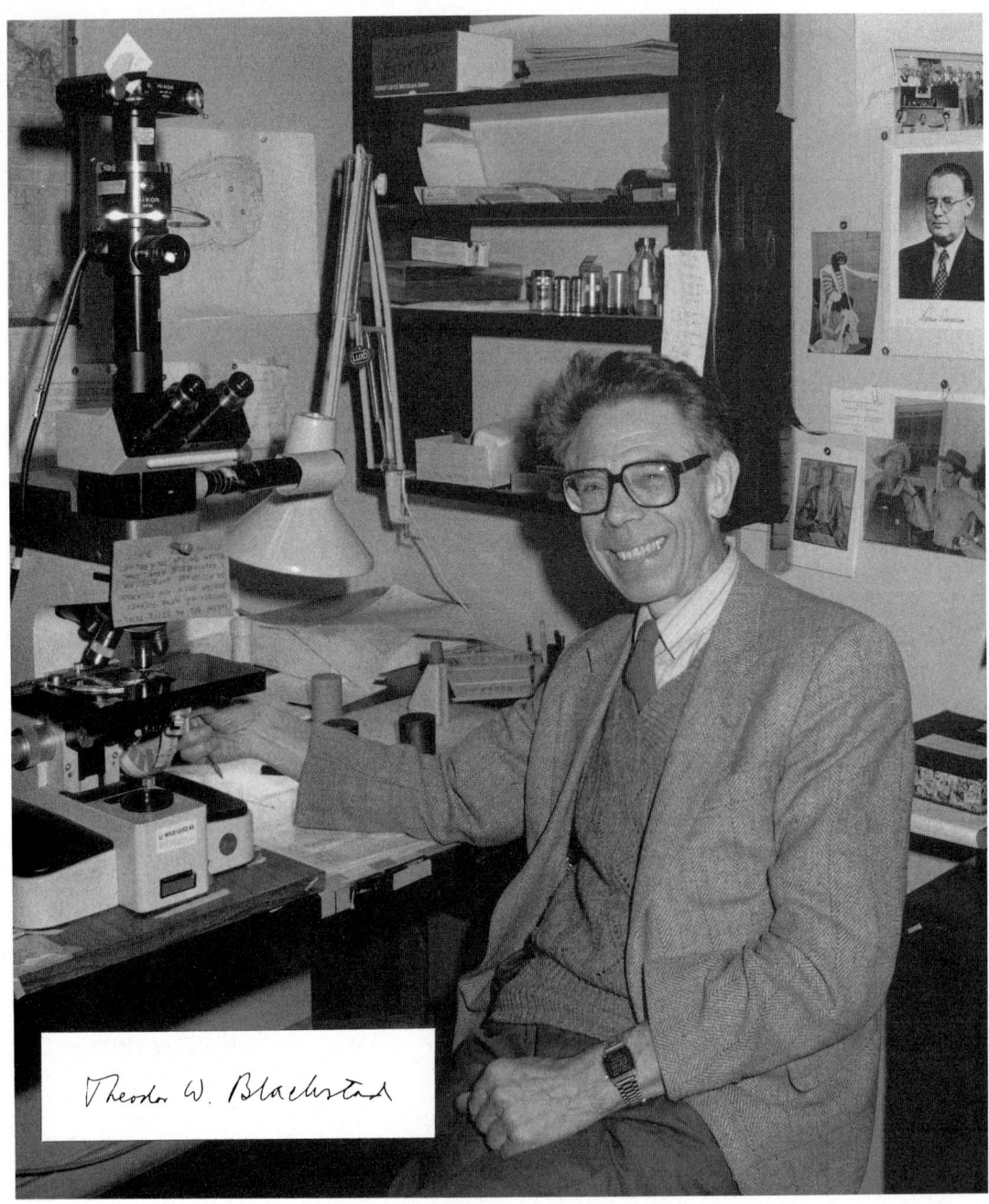

Professor Theodor W. Blackstad at work, 1989.

(Photograph by G.F. Lothe)

THEODOR WILHELM BLACKSTAD

A Unique Neuroanatomist and Human Being

Theodor Wilhelm Blackstad celebrates his 65th birthday on July 29th, 1990. With the present collection of papers, his colleagues, students and friends wish to pay tribute to his inspiring search for ways to obtain exact knowledge on the structure of the brain.

Theodor has been associated with the Medical Faculty, University of Oslo, for most of his professional life, apart from 10 important years when he served at the Medical Faculty, University of Aarhus. He was appointed prosector (assistant professor) of Anatomy in Oslo in 1953 and obtained the degree of doctor medicinae in 1958. In 1964 he was appointed docent (associate professor). From 1967 to 1977 he was professor of Anatomy in Aarhus and from 1977 again in Oslo.

His main scientific goal through these years has been to unravel the structure, circuitry and chemical anatomy of the hippocampus. Together with students and colleagues, he has applied a broad spectrum of tools and approaches to this end, pushing methods to and beyond existing limits.

Theodor's comprehensive and careful work on commissural connections of the rat hippocampal region, published as his doctoral thesis in 1956, was among the first studies to probe and prove the usefulness of Nauta's revolutionary method for impregnating degenerating boutons and preterminal axons. In this and other early studies he uncovered the precise laminar distribution of terminal fields in the hippocampal region, opening up the field of hippocampal circuitry and synaptology to concerted study by morphologists, physiologists and neurochemists. His meticulous style of work set a standard of exactitude for others to follow.

Recognizing the fundamental limitation of light microscopy for investigating synaptic connections (and cell structure in general), Theodor in 1956 took upon himself the task of creating an electron microscopical laboratory at the Anatomical Institute in Oslo, a project in which he was aided by repeated generous grants from the NIH, US Public Health Service. As this in effect became Norway's first operative laboratory for biological electron microscopy, his undertaking meant getting intimately involved with technical details at all levels of the nascent technology. It was fortunate to have a person with the technical bent, patience and resoluteness required to create an effective laboratory in less than five years. At that time, primarily through the work of Jan Jansen and Alf Brodal, the Anatomical Institute already offered an established neuroanatomical research environment. Theodor contributed greatly to this by introducing new technology and ideas. From an early time, in increasing numbers, students and visitors from Norway and abroad came to learn from him and contribute to the combination of neuroanatomical and ultrastructural research. Several important contributions to the ultrastructure and synaptology of the nervous system, with and without his co-authorship, resulted from this period of work. They are all characterized by close correlation of electron microscopy with previous and parallel light microscopical investigations.

While the emphasis was on neurobiological studies, research into the ultrastructure of the eye, the ear, muscles and connective tissue, as well as into molecular biology, was also started in the laboratory under Theodor's guidance and was allowed to evolve according to the specific interests of the young persons involved.

Having set up electron microscopy as a routine method in the institute by the early 1960s, Theodor was ready to take the step that he had previously planned into neuro-histochemistry, another nascent field. Again, his goal was the closest possible correlation of histochemistry with existing knowledge on the structure and connections of the central nervous system. A logical starting point was to survey the normal staining of regions, fields and laminae of the hippocampal region to establish a base for further, more experimentally orientated, studies. Detailed maps of the distribution of, e.g., acetylcholinesterase, oxidative enzymes and the sulphide silver staining pattern of the hippocampal region in the rat and several other species have come out of this approach, initially as collaborations between Theodor and his students in Oslo and Aarhus. Finally, Theodor left it to his students, collaborators and independent colleagues to develop experimental approaches from this base of descriptive neurohistochemistry. This has resulted in a variety of surgical, microchemical, neuropharmacological and im-munohistochemical approaches to the chemistry of hippocampal fiber systems and synapses in normal, developing and regenerating brains.

Then he turned to three other dominant threads in his scientific activities, which more than anything else illustrate his uncompromising efforts to base morphology on exact data.

In 1965 he published his first attempts at combining Golgi impregnation with electron microscopy and axonal degeneration as a general and powerful means to identify precisely the pre- and postsynaptic components of a given synapse. The traditional Golgi-impregnation will destroy or hide the ultrastructural features that are wanted in this kind of work. Through an elaborate series of trials and errors, supplemented with systematic investigation into the nature of the Golgi precipitate Theodor, and others building on his work, have succeeded in establishing combined Golgi-EM as a practical method.

Two other main goals of Theodor's later methodological work have been to develop computerized methods for constructing three-dimensional models of neural structures, ranging from whole brains to subcellular profiles, and for collecting quantitative estimates of simple and complex neuromorphological parameters. In this effort he has once more placed himself at the front of an emerging technology. Assuming the dual roles of biologist and programmer/computer-technician obviously carries significant risks of being diverted by methodological problems and accidents. Although this certainly happened to him as to most of his fellow anatomists engaging in similar ventures, Theodor always manages to stay close to the biological problems he sets out to solve and sees to it that his systems are put to immediate use in collaboration with colleagues already engaged in various neuromorphological projects.

Some of his recent approaches, which are being put to extensive use, involve systems for reconstructing and visualizing dendritic trees, quantitating particle densities over immunogold-labelled profiles in electron micrographs, and analyzing the distribution of large numbers of retrogradely labelled cell somata. As the field of quantitative and reconstructive morphology now develops rapidly, the needs and possibilities for systematic collaboration are becoming evident. In this perspective, Theodor in 1989 ran a very successful European Neuroscience Association workshop on computer-aided three-dimensional reconstruction in morphology.

The meticulous investigations into the Golgi method, and the time-consuming project of assembling computer equipment and personally developing programs for quantitative and reconstructive morphology, were carried out concurrently with high teaching and administrative loads particularly at The Anatomical Institute in Aarhus. In 1967, that 30-year-old institute of medical anatomy was overloaded with students and greatly needed to expand and develop its staff and research. Having accepted the chair of the first of two new institutes created to alleviate this situation, Theodor was extremely active in setting up a new curriculum for the preclinical part of the medical school and in planning and implementing a new building for teaching purposes.

His major obligation, however, which he managed to fulfil, was to revive and modernize neuroanatomical research in Aarhus. Bringing new techniques, the new research field of hippocampal anatomy, and his efficient and pleasant style, he immediately attracted young doctors and medical students. Inviting medical students into research was a novelty in Denmark at the time. By setting standards for scientific curiosity and rigor, hard work and personal integrity, he was able to lead by example. Constantly accessible for free discussions and personal contact, rarely interfering with the design or experimental phases of his apprentices' work, he dealt efficiently and constructively with any draft that was placed on his desk.

The expansion of the institute was expected and supported by the university. In addition, Theodor continued to secure a considerable support through grants from the US Public Health Service. When he returned to Oslo in 1977, to take over Alf Brodal's chair as professor of anatomy, he had raised a new generation of Danish neuroscientists and placed Aarhus on the international map of brain research. Through continued collaboration and frequent visits, his 'Danish pupils' and their students continue to benefit from his never failing enthusiasm and interest.

Theodor has recruited an impressive array of young neuroscientists. His enthusiasm over an intriguing biological problem, his broad knowledge and his never failing quest for new methods, have created around him groups of excited and devoted colleagues wherever he has worked. At the same time, he has set an example of personal integrity and honesty. Characteristically, Theodor is much more interested in solving the problem than in receiving the associated publicity. In many a case, his name is absent on the title page of papers that would not have existed without his efforts. His apprentices have been greatly inspired by the remarkable blend of enthusiasm, support and complete freedom to design one's own work, which is part of the essence of Theodor's great success as a mentor. The number of students, graduates and mature biologists that have worked with him, or have been influenced by his research, is remarkably large and the present volume is a token of their gratitude.

Per Andersen   Jan G. Bjaalie   Hans A. Dahl
Finn-Mogens Haug   Kirsten K. Osen   Ole Petter Ottersen
Eric Rinvik   Jon Storm-Mathisen   Fred Walberg
                      Jens Zimmer

Contents

J. Storm-Mathisen, J. Zimmer and O.P. Ottersen (Eds.)
Progress in Brain Research, Vol. 83
© 1990 Elsevier Science Publishers B.V. (Biomedical Division)

1

CHAPTER 1

Neurons, numbers and the hippocampal network

David G. Amaral[1], Norio Ishizuka[2] and Brenda Claiborne[3]

[1]*The Salk Institute for Biological Studies, San Diego, CA 92138, U.S.A.,* [2]*Department of Neuroanatomy, Institute of Brain Research, Faculty of Medicine, University of Tokyo, 7-3-1 Hongo, Bunkyo-ku, Tokyo, 113, Japan and* [3]*Division of Life Sciences, University of Texas at San Antonio, San Antonio, TX 78285, U.S.A.*

Anatomists involved with studies of the hippocampal formation are being prodded by computational modelers and physiologists who demand detailed and quantitative information concerning hippocampal neurons and circuits. The beautiful camera lucida drawings of old, and the elegant descriptions of dendritic form that accompanied them are giving way to computer-reconstructed and three-dimensionally analyzed cells with rigorous determination of dendritic lengths and volumes, branching pattern and spine distribution. We will review certain quantitative aspects of hippocampal organization in the rat based on a survey of available literature and on our own intracellular labeling studies of granule cells of the dentate gyrus and pyramidal cells of the hippocampus. Some of the potential implications of these data for hippocampal information processing will be discussed.

Introduction

Most of us are guilty of it. Hippocampologists have preached for decades that the hippocampus[a] is a relatively simple structure and thus an ideal region for studying the relationships between structure and function. And it is! But one potentially misleading implication of the "hippocampus is simple" message, is that the anatomical organization of the structure is thoroughly understood. It is certainly true that the basic organizational scheme of hippocampal anatomy has been well established through the classical Golgi studies of Ramón y Cajal (1893), and Lorente de Nó (1934), and the more recent experimental studies, such as those conducted for the last 40 years by Blackstad

and his colleagues, (e.g. Blackstad, 1956). However, as the computational modelers and physiologists ask the anatomists for detailed information concerning the network characteristics of the hippocampal formation, it becomes painfully apparent that there are still gaping holes in our understanding of hippocampal circuitry, even at a descriptive level. And when quantitative questions are raised concerning hippocampal neurons or circuitry, they are more often met with shrugs than with answers.

Perhaps a few examples might emphasize the gap between where we are and where we would like to be. It is well established that the layer II cells of the entorhinal cortex provide the main input to the outer portion of the molecular layer of the dentate gyrus. Yet, it is still not particularly clear which specific cells in the entorhinal cortex project to a specific septotemporal level of the dentate gyrus. Moreover, there is no direct anatomical evidence regarding the total number of synapses that each entorhinal neuron contributes to the dentate gyrus or whether an entorhinal cell makes 1, 100, or

---

[a] We consider the hippocampal formation to comprise several distinct regions including: the dentate gyrus; the hippocampus proper (which can be divided into CA3, CA2 and CA1 fields); the subicular complex (which itself can be divided into the subiculum, presubiculum and parasubiculum); and the entorhinal cortex (which in the rat is generally divided into medial and lateral divisions).

1000 synapses on a single dentate granule cell. Similarly, there is little or no information concerning the total number of inputs to a single hippocampal neuron. The lack of this type of information, while regrettable, is nonetheless understandable given the high level of difficulty associated with obtaining it.

One way of collecting information about the number of inputs to a single neuron necessitates accurate three-dimensional reconstruction of the dendritic tree and subsequent determination of the total number of dendritic spines. These are technically demanding enterprises. Yet when completed, they would provide a reasonably accurate estimate of the amount of excitatory input to the neuron. Even these efforts, however, do not produce the whole picture of neuronal innervation since the inhibitory inputs, most of which end on the neuronal cell body or dendritic shafts, would not be appreciated. The definitive establishment of the total amount of input to a single hippocampal cell, through the serial electron microscopic analysis of a single labeled neuron is, while technically possible, probably prohibitively time-consuming. The intracellular labeling studies that we have conducted over the last several years and that we shall briefly describe in this chapter are considered to be first steps down the path of realistically defining the number and types of inputs to identified hippocampal neurons.

The point of these opening paragraphs is that the hippocampal neuroanatomist is faced with a challenge. The computational modelers and physiologists are attempting to construct realistic simulations of hippocampal structure and function. The short-term goals might be to model the establishment of long-term potentiation or the selective responsivity of a CA1 place field. The long-term goal might be to model the role of the hippocampal formation in human memory function. If the silicon hippocampus is to faithfully represent the mechanisms employed in the biological hippocampus, it is important that the modelers be provided with an accurate summary of hippocampal circuitry. There are many exciting new anatomical techniques that can potentially provide the kinds of quantitative data needed for accurate simulation of the hippocampal formation. The challenge for the neuroanatomist is to use these techniques to uncover the fundamental organizational principles of the hippocampal network. Rather than completed, the effort to establish a quantitative, functional neuroanatomy of the hippocampal formation has just gotten underway.

In the remaining sections of this chapter, we will review some of the quantitative aspects of hippocampal neuroanatomy. We will also briefly summarize our own studies of the dendritic and axonal organization of neurons intracellularly filled with horseradish peroxidase (HRP) in the in vitro slice preparation. We will combine these two bodies of data to discuss the pattern of interconnectivity between the various fields of the hippocampal formation.

Neuronal numbers in the hippocampal formation

A reasonable starting point for discussing the quantitative aspects of the rat hippocampal formation is a summary of the numbers of neurons in each of its fields (Fig. 1). Substantial work has been conducted to determine the number of cells in the dentate gyrus and hippocampus but unfortunately there is little or no information on the number of cells in much of the subicular complex and entorhinal cortex.

To our knowledge, there has been no attempt to count the number of layer II entorhinal cells that project to the rat dentate gyrus. We have arrived at a rough estimate of this number by first estimating the surface area of layer II in a flattened entorhinal cortex preparation. For a mature rat we have estimated that the surface area of layer II is something in the order of 26 mm^2 though this number might be inflated somewhat due to the flattening procedure. The depth of layer II, while variable, is around 75 μm yielding a volume of about 1.95×10^9 μm^3. The average volume of a layer II cell is approximately 3500 μm^3. If the

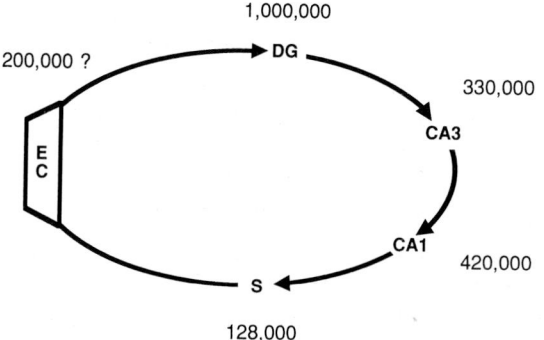

Fig. 1. Schematic diagram of the major excitatory connections in the hippocampal formation. The number of principal neurons in each of the cytoarchitectonic subdivisions is also indicated. The number of layer II cells in the rat entorhinal cortex (EC) that project to the dentate gyrus is estimated to be approximately 200,000. There are about 1,000,000 granule cells in the dentate gyrus (DG), 330,000 pyramidal cells in the CA3 and CA2 fields of the hippocampus, 420,000 pyramidal cells in the CA1 field and about 128,000 pyramidal cells in the subiculum. No counts are available for the presubiculum or parasubiculum.

volume of the layer were totally accounted for by the cell bodies, then approximately 560,000 cells could be packed into layer II. However, the cell bodies occupy only about 40% of the volume of the cell layer and thus the total number of layer II cells might be something closer to 225,000 cells. Since these values are only approximate, in the calculations presented in the following sections we will use a value of 200,000 for the number of entorhinal cells that project to the dentate gyrus. This should only be considered a rough approximation to the real value, however, which ultimately must be determined by rigorous morphometric methods.

There has been substantially more work done to establish the number of granule cells in the rat dentate gyrus. As indicated in Table I, the number of granule cells counted in one hemisphere appears to depend somewhat on the strain and age of the animal studied. One reason for this is that there is a continual increase in the number of granule cells in the juvenile and adult rat brain (Bayer, 1982; Bayer et al., 1982), and the age at which the cells are counted, therefore, can be influential on the number obtained. The range of granule cell counts is from approximately 0.6×10^6 to 2.2×10^6.

The Sprague–Dawley rat, which we have used for the dendritic analyses described below, has approximately 1×10^6 granule cells in the dentate gyrus (Boss et al., 1985), and we shall use this number in our subsequent calculations. Seress and Pokorny (1981) also noted that there were about 3500 pyramidal basket cells in the dentate gyrus for an average ratio of 1 basket cell for every 180 granule cells (as indicated in Table I, they counted approximately 0.63×10^6 granule cells in the dentate gyrus). These basket cells, which are situated at the interface of the granule cell and polymorphic layers, are predominantly GABAergic and supply an inhibitory input to the granule cells. Seress and Pokorny (1981) made the important point that these inhibitory interneurons are not homogeneously distributed throughout the septotemporal extent of the hippocampal formation. They found that the ratio of basket cells to granule cells was highest septally (1 : 100 in the suprapyramidal blade of the dentate gyrus and 1: 180 in the infrapyramidal blade) and lowest at the temporal pole (1 : 150 in the suprapyramidal blade and 1 : 300 in the infrapyramidal blade). Seress (1988) also established that there are approximately 32,500 cells in the polymorphic layer of the dentate gyrus. Of these, approximately 30%, or about 10,000 cells, are immunoreactive for somatostatin and GAD (Kosaka et al., 1988; Amaral, unpublished observations). The remaining 20,000 hilar neurons are heterogeneous but many are presumably the mossy cells that originate in the associational and commissural projections of the dentate gyrus.

Cell counts in the CA fields of the hippocampus also appear to be somewhat strain-dependent (Table I). Boss et al. (1987) found that in the Sprague–Dawley rat, there were approximately 3.3×10^5 neurons in the CA3/CA2 field and 4.2×10^5 cells in CA1. In the Wistar rat, they found 2.1×10^5 cells in CA3/CA2 and 3.2×10^5 in CA1. For the discussions of interconnectivity below, we will use the data obtained by Boss et al. (1987) for Sprague–Dawley rats since these can be used in conjunction with their similarly derived

TABLE I

Neuronal numbers in rat hippocampal formation

Field	Strain	Age	Sex	Number	Authors
GCL	Wistar	adult	M	0.998×10^6	Gaarskjaer (1978)
GCL	Wistar	adult	M	2.17×10^6	West and Andersen (1980)
GCL	Wistar	adult	M, F	0.635×10^6	Seress and Pokorny (1981)
GCL	Wistar	30 days	M	0.894×10^6	Bayer (1982)
GCL	Wistar	120 days	M	0.978×10^6	Bayer (1982)
GCL	Wistar	200 days	M	1.107×10^6	Bayer (1982)
GCL	Wistar	365 days	M	1.276×10^6	Bayer (1982)
GCL	Wistar	30 days	F	0.71×10^6	Boss et al. (1985)
GCL	Wistar	120 days	F	1.02×10^6	Boss et al. (1985)
GCL	Wistar	365 days	F	0.81×10^6	Boss et al. (1985)
GCL	SD	30 days	F	1.03×10^6	Boss et al. (1985)
GCL	SD	120 days	F	0.99×10^6	Boss et al. (1985)
GCL	SD	365 days	F	1.04×10^6	Boss et al. (1985)
GCL	Holtzman	28 days	?	0.63×10^6	Schlessinger et al. (1975)
GCL	Long – Evans	3 – 4 months	?	0.656×10^6	Seress (1988)
GCL	CFY	3 – 4 months	?	0.892×10^6	Seress (1988)
CA3/CA2	Wistar	adult	M	0.19×10^6 (0.143×10^6)[a]	Gaarskjaer (1978)
CA3/CA2	Wistar	adult	M	0.157×10^6	Cassell (1980)
CA3/CA2	SD	1 month	F	0.33×10^6	Boss et al. (1987)
CA3/CA2	Long – Evans	3 – 4 months	?	0.184×10^6	Seress (1988)
CA3/CA2	CFY	3 – 4 months	?	0.170×10^6	Seress (1988)
CA1	Wistar	adult	F	0.213×10^6	Cassell (1980)
CA1	SD	1 month	F	0.42×10^6	Boss et al. (1987)
Subiculum	Wistar	adult	F	0.128×10^6	Cassell (1980)

[a] This number resulted when a correction for partial neurons was employed.

data for the dentate gyrus of the same rat strain. Cassell (1980) found that the CA2 field contained approximately 7.9% of the cells in the CA3/CA2 region or about 12,390 in his studies. He also reported that there are about 1.28×10^5 neurons in the subiculum.

Neurons and connections of the dentate gyrus

In the last several years we have developed a means of labeling and quantitatively analyzing the dendritic and local axonal plexus of neurons in the hippocampal formation (Claiborne et al., 1986, 1990; Ishizuka et al., in preparation). The procedure we have adopted involves the intracellular injection of HRP into neurons in the in vitro hippocampal slice preparation. After an appropriate survival period, the 400-μm-thick slice is fixed by immersion in aldehydes and ultimately processed without sectioning for the visualization of the HRP. The neurons are initially analyzed for the completeness of staining and the occurrence of cut dendrites at the surfaces of the slice. Neurons that meet a set of stringent selection criteria are then analyzed using a three-dimensional computer digitizing system and various parameters of dendritic and axonal organization are quantitatively evaluated.

We have analyzed the organization of dendrites of the dentate granule cells located at a mid-septotemporal level and within the supra- and infrapyramidal blades of the granule cell layer. The mean total dendritic length for the population of 48 granule cells that we have systematically studied was approximately 3200 μm with individual values ranging from 2324 μm to 4582 μm (Claiborne et al., 1990). The mean value in our study compares favorably with the value of about 3600 μm obtained by Desmond and Levy (1982) who used the Golgi technique and probabilistic mathematical corrections for cut dendrites based on serial section reconstruction of a small number of labeled cells. Caceres and Steward (1983) using similar methods arrived at an average granule cell dendritic length of 2986 μm. We found that the size and shape of the dendritic trees of the granule cells varied in a consistent fashion dependent on the position of the cell in the granule cell layer and in the transverse axis of the dentate gyrus (Fig. 2). The dendritic trees of granule cells in the suprapyramidal blade, for example, were significantly larger than those in the infrapyramidal blade (3478 ± 88 μm versus 2793 ± 74 μm; mean ± S.E.M.). We also found that about 23% of the total dendritic length was located in the granule cell layer and the inner fourth of the molecular layer. The next fourth of the molecular layer contained about 21%, the third fourth contained about 25% and the superficial fourth contained 31%. Thus, the outer three-fourths of the layer, where the fibers of the entorhinal cortex terminate, contain approximately 77% of the total dendritic length of the granule cells.

It is notoriously difficult to obtain total spine counts for individual neurons. With the Golgi method, which is commonly used for studies of spine density, spines on the deep surface of visualized dendrites are obscured by the dense precipitate of the dendritic shaft. A number of correction procedures have been developed, however, in order to achieve realistic estimates of the total number of spines (e.g. Stirling and Bliss, 1978; Feldman and Peters, 1979). Desmond and Levy (1985) used the correction procedure of Stirling and Bliss (1979), and arrived at spine densities of

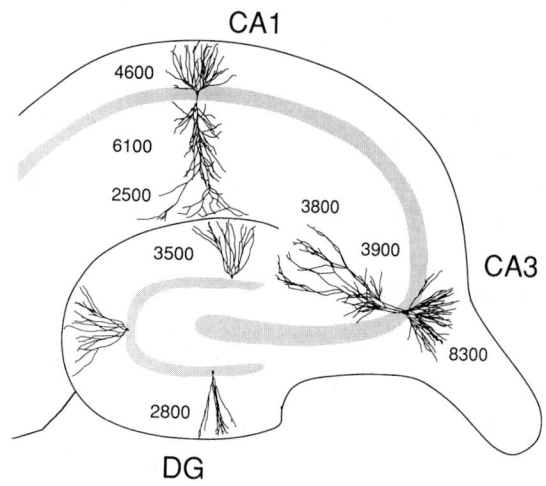

Fig. 2. Diagram of the rat hippocampus with computer-generated drawings of dentate granule cells and hippocampal pyramidal cells. In the dentate gyrus (DG) 3 cells are drawn. The average total dendritic length for cells in the suprapyramidal blade (3500 μm) is significantly larger than for cells in the infrapyramidal blade (2800 μm). For the CA3 and CA1 cells, the dendritic lengths indicated are the averages for the population of neurons described in the text. In the population of CA3 neurons, about 8300 μm of dendrite were located in stratum oriens, 3900 μm in stratum radiatum and approximately 3800 μm in stratum lacunosum-moleculare. For the population of CA1 cells, approximately 4600 μm of dendrite were located in stratum oriens, 6100 μm in stratum radiatum and 2500 μm in stratum lacunosum-moleculare.

1.6 spines/μm for cells in the suprapyramidal blade and 1.3 spines/μm for cells in the infrapyramidal blade. Given the average total dendritic lengths we found for granule cells, cells in the suprapyramidal blade would have about 5600 spines while cells in the infrapyramidal blade would have about 3600 spines. If we divide the total number of granule cells between these two categories, there would be approximately ((500,000 × 5600) + (500,000 × 3600)) or 4.6 × 10⁹ total spines on the population of dentate granule cells.

Matthews et al. (1976) found that unilateral removal of the entorhinal cortex resulted in a loss of at least 86% of the synapses in the outer three-fourths of the molecular layer. Something between 1% (Matthews et al., 1976) and 10% (Crain et al., 1973), of the synapses in the molecular layer demonstrate symmetric contacts and are presumably formed on the dendritic shaft rather than on spines. Thus, it is not unreasonable to make the simplifying assumption that entorhinal terminals occupy most, if not all, of the spines in the outer three-fourths of the molecular layer. Since the entorhinal termination zone of the molecular layer contains about 77% of the total granule cell dendritic length, we would expect that approximately 3.542×10^9 spines would be available for perforant path termination. If this number is divided by the total number of layer II entorhinal cells, then each entorhinal cell could be expected to terminate on approximately 17,710 spines in the molecular layer of the dentate gyrus[b]. If each entorhinal cell makes only one contact per granule cell, then a layer II cell would terminate on 17,710 granule cells or approximately 2% of the total population. Of course, if each entorhinal cell makes 10 contacts per granule cell dendritic tree, then these numbers would be reduced to 1771 and 0.2%. Conversely, each granule cell in the suprapyramidal blade has about (0.77×5600) or 4312 spines in the entorhinal termination zone and thus can receive input from a maximum of (4312/200,000) or 2.2% of the layer II entorhinal cells; granule cells in the infrapyramidal blade would be innervated by approximately $(0.77 \times 3600)/200,000$ or 1.4% of the entorhinal cells. While the absolute parameters of the entorhinal to dentate projection are not yet certain, it appears that this projection provides for relatively widespread distribution of entorhinal influence on the dentate gyrus.

The dentate granule cells give rise to distinctive axons, the mossy fibers, that collateralize in the

polymorphic layer of the dentate gyrus before entering the CA3 field of the hippocampus. Within the polymorphic layer, the mossy fiber collaterals bear two types of varicosities. Numerous small ($\simeq 2$ μm) varicosities are distributed unevenly along the collaterals. The collateral plexus of a single granule cell contains, on average, 160 of these varicosities which electron microscopic analysis confirmed to be presynaptic boutons. Each collateral (there are 7 collaterals, on average, arising from each mossy fiber as it traverses the polymorphic layer) also generally bears one larger, irregularly shaped varicosity that resembles a smaller version of the mossy fiber expansions that contact the CA3 pyramidal cells.

The mossy fiber collaterals terminate on many cells in the polymorphic layer including basket cells and the mossy cells (Ribak et al., 1985). The proximal dendrites of the mossy cells are heavily encrusted with thorny excrescences (the postsynaptic spine-like specialization that is characteristic of mossy fiber contact). Unfortunately, it is difficult to predict how many granule cells innervate an individual mossy cell. Similarly, while the mossy cell axon is known to provide the major input to the deep quarter of the molecular layer, this projection overlaps partially with the projection from the supramammillary area of the hypothalamus. However, the hypothalamic projection terminates preferentially on dendritic shafts rather than on spines (Dent et al., 1983). The inner fourth of the molecular layer contains approximately $((0.23 \times 5600 \times 500,000) + (0.23 \times 3600 \times 500,000))$ or 1.058×10^9 spines. If we assume that the mossy cell axons terminate on most of the spines in the inner fourth of the molecular layer and that the inputs are about equally divided from ipsilateral and contralateral mossy cells (Fricke and Cowan, 1978; Kishi et al., 1980), then each mossy cell would be expected to terminate on approximately $((1.058 \times 10^9/20,000)/2) = 26,450$ spines in the molecular layer. (Note that this calculation assumes that the mossy cells make up the major portion of the non GABAergic cells located in the polymorphic layer.) As with the entorhinal projection to the dentate

---

[b] One assumption in these discussions of connectivity is that each spine receives only 1 asymmetric contact. Westrum and Blackstad, 1962, have demonstrated by three-dimensional reconstruction of electron micrographs of spines in stratum radiatum of CA1, that a spine was almost never in contact with more than one presynaptic varicosity. A similar situation appears to be the case for the molecular layer of the dentate gyrus (Laatsch and Cowan, 1966).

gyrus, it is not known how many contacts each mossy cell makes with each granule cell and thus the total number of granule cells influenced by one mossy cell is presently unknown.

The principal output of the dentate gyrus is to the CA3 field of the hippocampus. Mossy fibers make several en passant synapses on the proximal dendrites of the CA3 cells. The presynaptic expansion is unusually large ($\simeq 3 - 6 \ \mu m$) and irregular in shape with several fine filipodial extensions (Amaral, 1979). We found that the mossy fiber expansions were spaced approximately 140 μm apart along the trajectory of individual mossy fibers. Thus, each mossy fiber contains approximately 14 expansions along its trajectory. Assuming that each presynaptic expansion terminates on only one pyramidal cell (there is no evidence that this is, or is not, the case) each granule cell would then contact approximately 14 pyramidal cells. Mossy fibers do not contact the pyramidal cells of the CA2 region. Thus, if we correct the figure of CA3/CA2 pyramidal cells provided by Boss et al. (1987) by subtracting 7.9% of the cells (this is the figure that Cassell (1980) found for the number of CA2 cells), then the CA3 field alone would contain $(330,000 \times 0.921) = 303,930$ pyramidal cells. Each CA3 cell, then, could be expected to be innervated by approximately $((1 \times 10^6 \times 14)/303,930) = 46$ granule cells. In contrast to the apparently widespread entorhino-dentate projection, the mossy fiber projection to the CA3 field appears to be both spatially and numerically limited. If the calculations given above prove to be accurate, then each granule cell would contact only $(14/303,930)$ or 0.0046% of the pyramidal cells and each CA3 pyramidal cell would be influenced by only $(46/1,000,000)$ or 0.0046% of the granule cells.

Neurons and connections in the hippocampus

We have conducted intracellular HRP investigations of the pyramidal cells of the hippocampus similar to those described above for the dentate gyrus (Ishizuka et al., in preparation). In general,

we have found that the dendritic trees of hippocampal pyramidal cells are substantially longer than previously published reports have indicated. Moreover, we found that the size and shape of dendritic trees of the CA3 cells vary in a consistent manner depending on the transverse location of the cell in the pyramidal cell layer. In contrast, the pyramidal cells of the CA1 field demonstrate a striking homogeneity in total dendritic length despite differences in the number and distribution of dendritic branches. While it is beyond the scope of this chapter to fully describe these findings, we will briefly summarize some of them to provide the basis for comments on the connectivity of the hippocampal fields.

The CA3 neurons with the largest dendritic trees are located distally in the field, i.e. close to CA2. In our population of labeled cells there were 4 neurons in this region that had complete or nearly complete dendritic trees: 3 of the cells had no cut dendrites and 1 cell had 1 cut distal apical branch (Fig. 2). The total dendritic length of these neurons averaged 16,146 μm with a range of 15,243 μm to 17,492 μm. In these distally located cells, the largest component of the dendritic tree was located in stratum oriens. The average total dendritic length in stratum oriens was approximately 8281 μm or 51% of the total dendritic length. The next highest amount was found in stratum radiatum with approximately 3896 μm (or 24% of the total dendritic length) followed by stratum lacunosum-moleculare with 3742 μm (or 23% of the total dendritic length). The pyramidal cell layer and stratum lucidum contained about 352 μm (or 2%).

The dendritic trees of the CA1 pyramidal cells show a fair amount of variability in overall organization. Some, for example, have one principal apical dendritic shaft while others have two. The total dendritic lengths, however, were quite similar across the population of sampled pyramidal cells. A description of 8 CA1 pyramidal cells with no cut dendrites located in the mid-transverse position of the CA1 field will serve to summarize their dendritic patterns (Fig. 2). The average total dendritic length for this group of

CA1 neurons was 13,265 μm with a range of 11,127 μm to 14,472 μm. In contrast to the CA3 cells, the largest single component of the dendritic tree was located in stratum radiatum which contained, on average, 6125 μm (or 46% of the total dendritic length). Stratum oriens contained an average of 4644 μm (or 35% of the total dendritic length) and stratum lacunosum-moleculare contained an average of 2475 μm (or 19% of the total).

As noted above, the total dendritic lengths of CA1 and CA3 cells observed using the in vitro, intracellular staining procedures were substantially higher than those typically published from Golgi studies. Englisch et al. (1974), for example, found that the total dendritic length of CA1 cells from mature rats was approximately 4359 μm and Pokorny and Yamamoto (1981) found a total dendritic length of about 4886 μm. Minkwitz (1976) found a slightly higher total dendritic length (5613 μm) in the 20-day-old rat. Even the latter figure, however, is roughly 40% of the length we observed in our cells. Seress and Pokorny (1981) found that cells located in the proximal part of CA3 had a total dendritic length of 4450 μm which was well below the smallest dendritic tree we observed in this area (7569 μm). More recently, Fitch et al. (1989) quantitatively examined CA3 pyramidal cells located about midway along the transverse axis of the CA3 field. The largest of the cells investigated in their study had an average total dendritic length of approximately 5115 μm. The average length of the intracellularly labeled cells in this region in our in vitro studies, however, was approximately 12,213 μm. It would appear, therefore, that while the Golgi method is ideal for qualitative examinations of neuronal form and connectivity, substantial caution must be exercised in using it for quantitative investigations of neuronal size and connectivity. The numerous technical limitations of the Golgi method can certainly be overcome using strategies such as those developed by Desmond and Levy (1982), yet, if uncorrected, estimates of dendritic lengths using the Golgi method probably greatly underestimate the true lengths of neurons.

A number of studies have investigated the distribution and density of spines on the pyramidal cells of the hippocampus. Most of these studies were conducted, however, in the context of developmental analyses or investigations of environmental modifications of dendritic form. Wenzel et al. (1972) estimated the number of spines on the main apical shafts of CA1 pyramidal cells. They found that the density of spines was not uniform along the dendrite and peaked at approximately 1 spine/μm in the superficial portion of stratum radiatum and the deep portion of stratum lacunosum-moleculare. The overall spine density was approximately 0.5 spines/μm. These figures were uncorrected for unseen spines as are all available spine counts conducted in the hippocampal fields. When counts of spines were made on the lateral side-branches of the apical and basal dendrites of CA1 pyramidal cells, the average density of visible spines was approximately 0.78 spines/μm (Englisch et al., 1974). Lacey (1985) reported a spine density of approximately 1 spine/μm on secondary dendrites of CA1 cells and slightly lower numbers on CA3 cells. Meyer et al. (1978) found a slightly higher density of spines (1.5/μm) along the higher order apical dendrites of CA1 pyramidal cells of the albino mouse. Meyer and Ferres-Torres (1978) analyzed several portions of the dendritic trees of pyramidal cells in the developing mouse hippocampus and, in mature animals, found that the distal apical dendrites on CA1 cells contained approximately 1.5 spines/μm; basal dendrites contained slightly lower densities. Distal CA3 apical dendrites also contained approximately the same density. Muma and Rowell (1988) found a spine density of 0.825/μm for mice aged 20 – 24 months. Because of the 400 μm thickness of the in vitro hippocampal slices with the resulting limited resolution, we have not attempted to count spines on the intracellularly labeled neurons. It is clear, however, that a refined analysis of the inputs to hippocampal pyramidal cells will necessitate a realistic estimate of spine density.

From the data reviewed above, it would seem reasonable to use a value of 1 spine/μm of dendritic length as a conservative estimate of spine density in the CA1 and CA3 pyramidal cells. Thus, within stratum radiatum and stratum oriens, the larger CA3 cells would have something in the order of 12,000 spines. The dendrites in the same regions of CA1 cells would have about 11,000 spines. We can make the simplifying assumption that most of these spines receive inputs from CA3 cells (either through the longitudinal associational connections in CA3 or through the Schaffer collateral system in CA1) and that the inputs arise equally from the ipsilateral and contralateral sides. Thus, a single CA3 pyramidal cell would be innervated by approximately 6000 other CA3 pyramidal cells or about (6000/303,930) or 1.9% of the CA3 cell population. Similarly, a CA1 pyramidal cell might receive input from 5500 CA3 cells or about 1.8% of the CA3 pyramidal cell population. Thus, like the entorhinal cortex to dentate gyrus projection, the CA3 projections to CA3 and CA1 appear to be divergent and organized for fairly extensive intercommunication.

It is also interesting to point out that the distal dendrites of the larger CA3 cells may have as many as 3742 spines in stratum lacunosum-moleculare (a CA1 cell would have about 2475 spines in this layer) which is innervated heavily, though not exclusively, by fibers of the perforant path. Since the average dentate granule cell has something in the order of 3600 spines in the entorhinal zone of the molecular layer, it is conceivable that the larger hippocampal pyramidal cells may receive direct synaptic innervation from the entorhinal cortex that is quantitatively similar to that directed to the average dentate granule cell.

Conclusions

The numerical conclusions described in this chapter are preliminary attempts at demonstrating the potential power of a quantitative functional neuroanatomy of the hippocampus. Many of the calculations were derived from imperfect data or fairly crude approximations of neuronal numbers or spine densities. Moreover, many of the projec-

tions discussed in this chapter are organized in a highly topographic fashion and the probability of cell interactions, therefore, would be dependent not only on cell and synapse number but on the three-dimensional position of the cells in the hippocampal formation (Amaral and Witter, 1989). We have also highlighted the interconnectivity of the major excitatory projections of the hippocampal formation and ignored, for the most part, characteristics of inhibitory local circuits. However, the intention of this chapter has been to show that quantitative assessment of the hippocampal neuronal machinery is tractable. We have also pointed out that much of the fundamental data needed as a basis for a functional neuroanatomy of the hippocampus has yet to be accumulated. We are optimistic, however, that as these data are acquired, they will be increasingly useful to those who are endeavoring to build models of hippocampal function. The emergence of a quantitative neuroanatomy of the hippocampal formation will forge a symbiotic relationship between the anatomist, the physiologist and the computational modeler that should quicken the pace of efforts to understand the structural basis of hippocampal function.

Acknowledgements

Original work described in this chapter was supported by NIH Grant NS-16980.

References

Amaral, D.G. (1979) Synaptic extensions from the mossy fibers of the fascia dentata. *Anat. Embryol.,* 155: 241 – 251.

Amaral, D.G. and Witter, M.P. (1989) The three dimensional organization of the hippocampal formation: a review of anatomical data. *Neuroscience,* 31: 571 – 591.

Bayer, S.A. (1982) Changes in the total number of dentate granule cells in juvenile and adult rats: a correlated volumetric and ^{3}H-thymidine autoradiographic study. *Exp. Brain Res.,* 46: 315 – 323.

Bayer, S.A., Yackel, J.W. and Puri, P.S. (1982) Neurons in the rat dentate gyrus granular layer substantially increase during juvenile and adult life. *Science,* 216: 890 – 892.

Blackstad, T.W. (1956) Commissural connections of the hip-

10

pocampal region in the rat, with special reference to their mode of termination. *J. Comp. Neurol.*, 105: 417–537.

Boss, B.D., Peterson, G.M. and Cowan, W.M. (1985) On the number of neurons in the dentate gyrus of the rat. *Brain Res.*, 338: 144–150.

Boss, B.D., Turlejski, K., Stanfield, B.B. and Cowan, W.M. (1987) On the numbers of neurons in fields CA1 and CA3 of the hippocampus of Sprague–Dawley and Wistar rats. *Brain Res.*, 406: 280–287.

Caceres, A. and Steward, O. (1983) Dendritic reorganization in the denervated dentate gyrus of the rat following entorhinal cortical lesions: a Golgi and electron microscopic analysis. *J. Comp. Neurol.*, 214: 387–403.

Cassell, M.D. (1980) *The Numbers of Cells in the Stratum Pyramidal of the Rat and Human Hippocampal Formation*. Ph.D. Thesis, University of Bristol, UK.

Claiborne, B.J., Amaral, D.G. and Cowan, W.M. (1986) A light and electron microscopic analysis of the mossy fibers of the rat dentate gyrus. *J. Comp. Neurol.*, 246: 435–458.

Claiborne, B.J., Amaral, D.G. and Cowan, W.M. (1990) A quantitative, three-dimensional analysis of HRP-labeled granule cell dendrites in the rat dentate gyrus. *J. Comp. Neurol.*, in press.

Crain, B., Cotman, C., Taylor, D. and Lynch, G. (1973) A quantitative electron microscopic study of synaptogenesis in the dentate gyrus of the rat. *Brain Res.*, 63: 195–204.

Dent, J.A., Galvin, N.J., Stanfield, B.B. and Cowan, W.M. (1983) The mode of termination of the hypothalamic projection to the dentate gyrus: an EM autoradiographic study. *Brain Res.*, 258: 1–10.

Desmond, N.L. and Levy, W.B. (1982) A quantitative anatomical study of the granule cell dendritic fields of the rat dentate gyrus using a novel probabilistic method. *J. Comp. Neurol.*, 212: 131–145.

Desmond, N.L. and Levy, W.B. (1985) Granule cell dendritic spine density in the rat hippocampus varies with spine shape and location. *Neurosci. Lett.*, 54: 219–224.

Englisch, H.-J., Kunz, G. and Wenzel, J. (1974) Zur Spinesverteilung an Pyramidenneuronen der CA-1-region des Hippocampus der Ratte. *Z. Mikrosk. Anat. Forsch.*, 88: 85–102.

Feldman, M.L. and Peters, A. (1979) A technique for estimating total spine numbers on Golgi-impregnated dendrites. *J. Comp. Neurol.*, 188: 527–542.

Fitch, J.M., Juraska, J.M. and Washington, L.W. (1989) The dendritic morphology of pyramidal neurons in the rat hippocampal CA3 area. I. Cell types. *Brain Res.*, 479: 105–114.

Fricke, R. and Cowan, W.M. (1978) An autoradiographic study of the commissural and ipsilateral hippocampo-dentate projections in the adult rat. *J. Comp. Neurol.*, 181: 253–269.

Gaarskjaer, F.B. (1978) Organization of the mossy fiber system of the rat studied in extended hippocampi. I. Terminal area related to number of granule and pyramidal cells. *J. Comp. Neurol.*, 178: 49–72.

Kishi, K., Stanfield, B.B. and Cowan, W.M. (1980) A quan-

titative EM autoradiographic study of the commissural and associational connections of the dentate gyrus in the rat. *Anat. Embryol.*, 160: 173–186.

Kosaka, T., Wu, J.-Y. and Benoit, R. (1988) GABAergic neurons containing somatostatin-like immunoreactivity in the rat hippocampus and dentate gyrus. *Exp. Brain Res.*, 71: 388–398.

Laatsch, R.H. and Cowan, W.M. (1966) Electron microscopic studies of the dentate gyrus of the rat. I. Normal structure with special reference to synaptic organization. *J. Comp. Neurol.*, 128: 359–396.

Lacey, D.J. (1985) Normalization of dendritic spine numbers in rat hippocampus after termination of phenylacetate injections (PKU model). *Brain Res.*, 329: 354–355.

Lorente de Nó, R. (1934) Studies on the structure of the cerebral cortex II. Continuation of the study of the ammonic system. *J. Psychol. Neurol.*, 46: 113–117.

Matthews, D., Cotman, C. and Lynch, G. (1976) An electron microscopic study of lesion-induced synaptogenesis in the dentate gyrus of the adult rat. I. Magnitude and time course of degeneration. *Brain Res.*, 115: 1–21.

Meyer, G. and Ferres-Torres, R. (1978) Quantitative altersasabhängige Variationen der Dendritenspines im Hippocampus (CA1, CA3 und Fascia dentata) der Albinomaus. *J. Hirnforsch.*, 19: 371–378.

Meyer, G., Ferres-Torres, R. and Feo-Ramos, J.J. (1978) Quantitative Auswertung der spontanen Entwicklung der Dendritendornen im Hippocampus. *Verh. Anat. Ges.*, 72: 735–738.

Minkwitz, H.-G. (1976) Zur Entwicklung der Neuronenstruktur des Hippocampus während der prä- und postnatalen Ontogenese der Albinoratte. III. Mitteilung: morphometrische Erfassung der ontogenetischen Veränderungen in Dendritenstruktur und Spinebesatz an Pyramidenneuronen (CA1) des Hippocampus. *J. Hirnforsch.*, 17: 255–275.

Muma, N.A. and Rowell, P.P. (1988) Effects of chronic choline and lecithin on mouse hippocampal dendritic spine density. *Exp. Aging Res.*, 14: 137–141.

Pokorny, J. and Yamamoto, T. (1981) Postnatal ontogenesis of hippocampal CA1 area in rats. I. Development of dendritic arborisation in pyramidal neurons. *Brain Res. Bull.*, 7: 113–120.

Ramón y Cajal, S. (1893) Estructura del asta de Ammon y fascia dentata. *Ann. Soc. Esp. Hist. Nat.*, 22.

Ribak, C.E., Seress, L. and Amaral, D.G. (1985) The development, ultrastructure and synaptic connections of the mossy cells of the dentate gyrus. *J. Neurocytol.*, 14: 835–857.

Schlessinger, A.R., Cowan, W.M. and Gottlieb, D.I. (1975) An autoradiographic study of the time of origin and the pattern of granule cell migration in the dentate gyrus of the rat. *J. Comp. Neurol.*, 159: 149–176.

Seress, L. (1988) Interspecies comparison of the hippocampal formation shows increased emphasis on the regio superior in the Ammon's horn of the human brain. *J. Hirnforsch.*, 29:

335 – 340.

Seress, L. and Pokorny, J. (1981) Structure of the granular layer of the rat dentate gyrus: a light microscopic and Golgi study. *J. Anat.,* 133: 181 – 195.

Stirling, R.V. and Bliss, T.V.P. (1978) Observations on the commissural projection to the dentate gyrus in the reeler mutant mouse. *Brain Res.,* 150: 447 – 465.

Wenzel, J., Wenzel, M., Kirsche, W., Kunz, G. and Neumann, H. (1972) Quantitative Untersuchungen über die Verteilung der Dendritenspines an Pyramidenneuronen des Hippocampus (CA1). *Z. Mikrosk. Anat. Forsch.,* 85: 23 – 34.

West, M.J. and Andersen, A.H. (1980) An allometric study of the area dentata in the rat and mouse. *Brain Res. Rev.,* 2: 317 – 348.

Westrum, L.E. and Blackstad, T.W. (1962) An electron microscopic study of the stratum radiatum of the rat hippocampus (regio superior, CA1) with particular emphasis on synaptology. *J. Comp. Neurol.,* 119: 281 – 309.

J. Storm-Mathisen, J. Zimmer and O.P. Ottersen (Eds.)
Progress in Brain Research, Vol. 83
© 1990 Elsevier Science Publishers B.V. (Biomedical Division)

CHAPTER 2

Stereological studies of the hippocampus: a comparison of the hippocampal subdivisions of diverse species including hedgehogs, laboratory rodents, wild mice and men

Mark J. West

Stereological Research Laboratory, University Institute of Pathology and Second University Clinic of Internal Medicine, Institute of Experimental Clinical Research, and Department of Neurobiology, University of Aarhus, DK-8000 Aarhus C, Denmark

The volumes of the fascia dentata, hilus, regio inferior, regio superior and subiculum of 9 species that differ significantly in size and degree of forebrain evolution have been compared with the intent of identifying phylogenetic trends in the internal organization of the mammalian hippocampus. The study includes data from the hippocampi of a basal insectivore, 2 species of wild mice, 3 commonly used laboratory rodents and 3 species (including man) that resemble an ascending primate series. In addition to comparisons of the absolute and relative volumes, an allometric approach is used to identify "progressive" size differences not related to body size. Both regio superior and hilus become larger during evolution, while fascia dentata and regio inferior maintain a relationship to body size that is similar to that for the hippocampus in basal insectivores. The inter-species differences are discussed in terms of neuron number and size, for which data are presented from two species, and with reference to a neural model of the cognitive map theory for hippocampal function. Special emphasis is placed on the unique aspects of the human hippocampus. The data represents a quantitative morphological framework within which the observations from physiological, biochemical and behavioral studies in laboratory animals can be related to studies of the human hippocampus.

Introduction

Although the volume of the hippocampus can vary by a factor of 400 in different mammals, it is possible to unambiguously identify the subdivisions of the hippocampus due to the remarkable inter-specific stability of the cytoarchitecture, histochemistry and connectivity of the region. Each subdivision (fascia dentata, hilus, regio inferior, regio superior, and subiculum) is characterized by a relatively small number of unique types of neurons organized in a characteristic manner and, in a variety of histological preparations, it is possible to identify laminae that correspond to the cellular layers and the terminal fields of the various intrinsic and extrinsic fiber systems. Because the borders of the components of each subdivision can be readily defined along the entire length of the hippocampus, it is possible with simple stereological techniques, to estimate the absolute volumes of the subdivisions and total numbers of neurons within them.

These features of the hippocampus have prompted a number of quantitative studies in our laboratory aimed at investigating various morphometric aspects of development (Poulsen et al., 1990), aging (Coleman et al., 1987), toxicology (Ryngby et al., 1987; Slomianka et al., 1989) and evolution (West and Andersen, 1980; West and Schwerdtfeger, 1985; Slomianka and West, 1989). In the course of these studies, volumetric data have been collected from a variety of species that vary significantly in size and degree of forebrain evolution. The previously published data and data from additional species, including man, will be presented together here with the aim of identifying the trends in the size of the major subdivisions of the mammalian hippocampus during evolution. This will be accomplished through comparisons of the absolute and relative sizes of the subdivisions of the individual species and through allometric comparisons, in which scaling due to body size will be taken into account. Additional data describing the number and size of neurons in the subdivisions of the hippocampus of rats and humans will be presented to provide additional information about the functional implications of the observed volumetric differences.

When volume is viewed as a statistic for functional entities such as neurons and synapses, the relative proportions of the hippocampal subdivisions can provide a basis for comparing the relative weights of the different types of information-processing carried out by the subdivisions in different species. Similarly, comparisons of the absolute size can provide a means for comparing the information-processing capacities of homologous subdivisions. However, neither absolute size nor relative size can be used for criteria for phylogenetic change unless body size is taken into account. Large animals have large brains, small animals small brains. Small animals have large brain – body weight ratios, large animals have small ratios. The brain – body relationship is often described as a power function in which brain weight or volume E is directly proportional to body weight P raised to some power (b), $E \sim P^b$. Estimates of b range from 0.66 to 0.75 (Jerison, 1973; Gould, 1975; Hofman, 1982). In spite of the strength of this correlation over wide ranging taxonomic groups, there is little evidence that this relationship represents one basic interaction between brain size and body size (Mann et al., 1988). A similar power function describes the relationship between hippocampus volume and body weight. Based on the data of Stephan et al. (1981) from 75 species of insectivores, prosimians and simians, b has a value of 0.65. Body size must therefore also be taken into account when attempting to evaluate

phylogenetic changes in the size of the hippocampus and its subdivisions.

The strategy for identifying evolutionary changes used here involves the idenfication of differences in the size of hippocampal components not related to body weight, that is identifying deviations from an ancestral relationship between the size of hippocampal subdivisions and body size. The hippocampus – body size relationship of ancestral mammals, Gould's "criteria for subtraction", could be deduced from values observed in modern species to identify and quantify deviations. The major problem with this approach is that the brains of ancestral mammals are not available for histological analysis. Although macroscopic parameters such as total brain volume may be estimated for ancestral forms from fossil data, information regarding regional differentiations are not preserved in this material.

However, Stephan (1967) identified a group of extant species, the basal insectivores, which on the basis of the organization of the cerebrum can be considered to have changed least during evolution and can function as "representatives" of archetypical forms. He introduced an allometric approach in which the relationships between specific brain components and body size in this "basal" group is used as the criterion for subtraction (Stephan and Andy, 1969). Within this group there is close to the requisite 2/3 power relationship between brain and body size and an extrapolation of the regression line of a log-log plot of brain weight versus body weight passes through the values predicted from the fossil remains of archaic animals (see Gould, 1975). Stephan and co-workers have used the brain – body relationship of the basal insectivores as the basis for an extensive series of comparative studies aimed at identifying evolutionary changes in wide ranges of brain structures and species (Stephan et al., 1970; Stephan, 1983). Observed values, in excess of those predicted from the relationships in basal insectivores, have been termed "progressive changes". In the present study, the hippocampus – body size relationship of the basal insectivores and the volumes of the subdivisions of one of the members of the group, the European hedgehog, serve as the criteria for subtraction.

One of the most important considerations in comparisons of the type presented here is the degree to which the subdivisions of the different species are functionally comparable. This issue can be addressed at two levels: (1) in terms of the intrinsic organization of the subdivisions, i.e. how the hippocampal region processes information, and (2) in terms of the extrinsic connections of the components, i.e. what kind of information the region receives and where the hippocampal output is sent. Since the pioneering work of Blackstad (1956) on the experimental examination of the hippocampal fiber connections, a myriad of studies involving reduced silver, degeneration and retrograde-anterograde tracing techniques have provided a wealth of information about hippocampal connections. Much of this work, with emphasis on the findings in rodents and primates, has recently been reviewed by Rosene and Van Hoesen (1987). Comparative aspects of the connections in *Callithrix* and *Tupaia* have been dealt with by Schwerdtfeger (1984). Additional comments on the comparative aspects of the subiculum can be found in Sørensen (1985).

A number of points made by these authors are pertinent to the comparisons made here. (1) The unidirectional chain of intrinsic connections (mossy fiber axons of dentate granule cells to CA3 pyramids, Schaffer collaterals from CA3 to CA1, and the ammonic-subicular-system from CA1 to subiculum) is a constant feature of the mammalian hippocampus. (2) The organization of the intrinsic associational systems is similar in different species (e.g. dentate associational, Schaffer collateral, and longitudinal associational systems). (3) A major system of afferents from the entorhinal cortex reach the molecular layer of all subdivisions in species in which it has been studied. (4) In primates, unlike rodents, there are cortical afferents from outside the perirhinal cortex (neocortical input to the molecular layer of CA1, prosubiculum, and presubiculum) and there is

evidence that the molecular layer of CA1 becomes dominated by telencephalic input rather than diencephalic input. (5) The subiculum gives rise to more diverse complex cortical and subcortical projections in primates than it does in rodents. (6) Amygdaloid afferents innervate the entire longitudinal extent of the hippocampal formation of monkeys and only the deep subiculum in rats. The conclusions that can be drawn from these differences and similarities are that the intrinsic circuitry of the hippocampus is preserved to a high degree and the extrinsic connections become more related to neocortical and telencephalic regions during mammalian evolution.

The increasing neocorticalization of the extrinsic connections of the hippocampus can be considered to be a progressive change (Rosene and Van Hoesen, 1987). There are also qualitative interspecies differences in the cytological organization of the subdivisions, some of which can be considered progressive in that they are most pronounced in primates and represent changes that enhance performance. In regio superior of primates, for example, the cell bodies of the pyramidal cells are distributed over various positions on the radial axis, opposed to being confined to a single heavily packed layer (Stephan, 1975; Rosene and Van Hoesen, 1987), with the consequence that there is an increase in the variation of the biases of adjacent neurons to the laminated efferents to this region, an obvious asset for neural structures involved in associative functions. In the hilus there is also a diversity of lamination patterns (Amaral, 1978; Geneser, 1987) suggesting a differentiation of functional neuronal types, though a correlation with more evolved forms is less clear. The designation progressive in these cases is at best a semi-quantitative distinction due to the complexity of the described features. In contrast, allometric comparisons are quantitative and permit more rigorous comparisons. Together they indicate that the hippocampus has expanded its role in central nervous system activities during evolution.

The hippocampus is an allometrically progressive brain region in that there is an increase in its size relative to body weight during evolution (Stephan, 1983). This relationship is not readily apparent because the neocortex is even more progressive in the allometric sense, with the consequence that the hippocampus occupies a smaller proportion of the forebrain in more evolved forms (Fig. 1). Within the hippocampus itself there is evidence for differential progression in the subdivisions. On the basis of lengths of the cellular layers of the various subdivisions of the hippocampi of a wide range of species, Stephan and Monolescu (1980) concluded that CA1 contributed most to

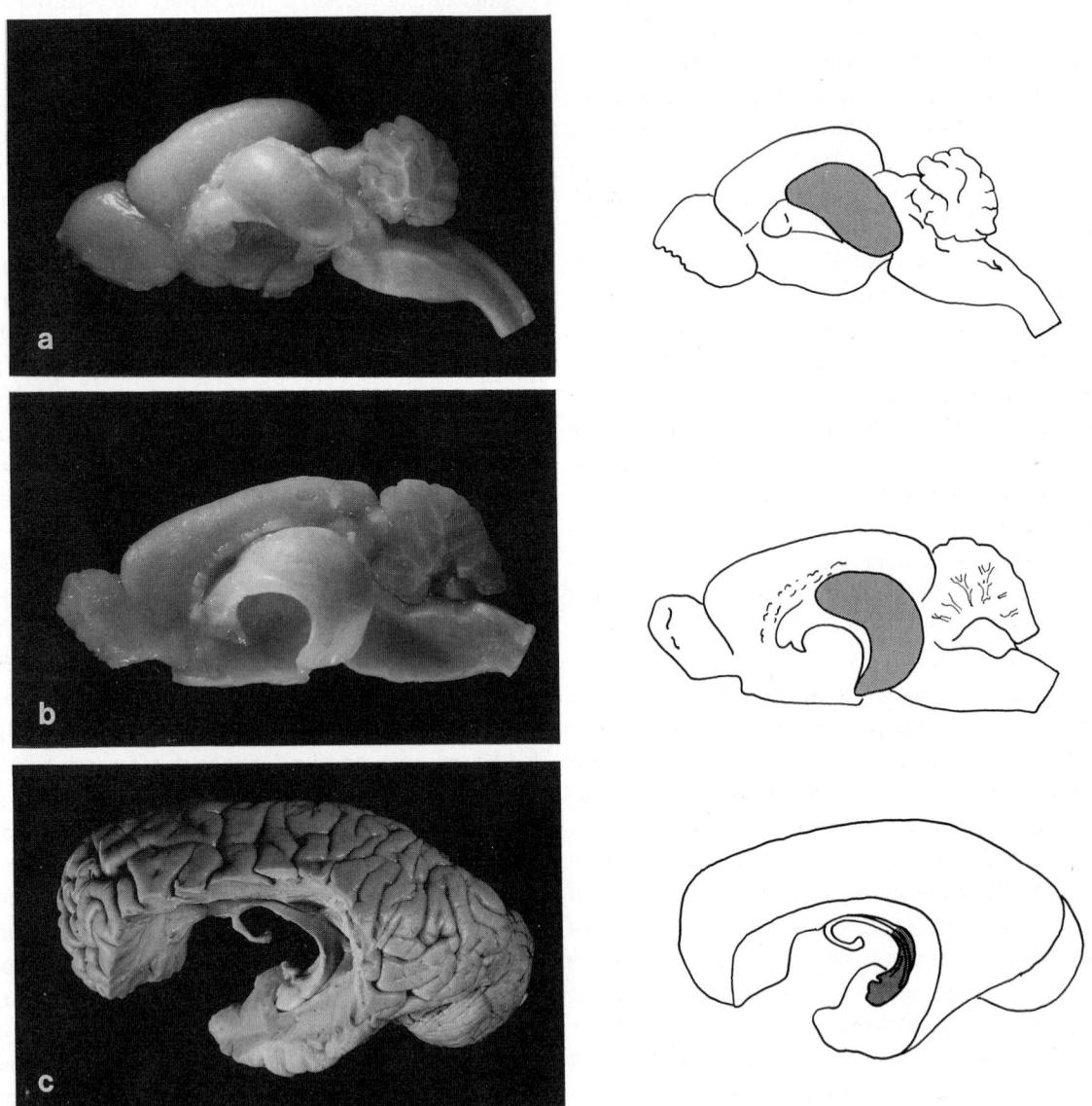

Fig. 1. a: hippocampus of the European hedgehog after removal of overlying cortex. ×2; b: hippocampus of the Wistar albino rat after removal of overlying cortex. ×3; c: hippocampus of man after removal of overlying cortex. ×0.3. To the right of each figure is a diagram showing the hippocampal region (shaded). Note the dorsal, occipital, and temporal placement of the hippocampus within the respective hemispheres corresponding to the clockwise phylogenetic displacement related to the development of the temporal lobe.

progression of the hippocampus. Similar conclusions were drawn by West and Schwerdtfeger (1985) on the basis of a more rigorous volumetric study of a smaller number of species and by Seress (1988) on the basis of differences in the relative numbers of neurons in the different subdivisions of 4 species. In the present study the volumetric comparisons are extended to a larger number of species that include extreme forms with respect to absolute brain size and telencephalic evolution, and includes data on the hippocampi of commonly used laboratory rodents and humans.

In view of the phylogenetic stability of the internal organization of the hippocampus, the functional consequences of the interspecific differences in the sizes of the subdivisions will be discussed within the framework of the cognitive map theory of O'Keefe and Nadel (1978) (see also O'Keefe, 1989). This theory is a particularly attractive basis for the discussion of the interspecific comparisons made in the present chapter because it is built on the premise that differences of large magnitude do not exist between mammalian species in regard to the function of specific brain areas. It is based on data obtained primarily from experimental animals but is consonant with observations made in humans. Most importantly, the authors of the theory have attempted to relate the components of a proposed neural model for spatial memory to subdivisions of the hippocampus that are comparable to those quantified in the present chapter. Although this attempt may admittedly be premature, such a discussion can serve as an example of how quantitative data of the type presented here can be related to models of hippocampal function. Since all of the requirements posed on the different hippocampal subdivisions by the model can be realized by parallel distributed processing, PDP (O'Keefe, 1989), and the intrinsic organization of the subdivisions is compatible with PDP (Marr, 1971; Braitenberg and Schüz, 1983; McNaughton and Morris, 1987; McNaughton, 1989) the discussion of the functional consequences of differences in the size of the hippocampal components will focus on features of hippocampal anatomy that can be related to this type of information-processing.

Materials and methods

Histological material from different species

Among the species included in this study are the European hedgehog *(Erinaceus europaeus),* a basal insectivore which shares many of the characteristics of the early insectivorous mammals that comprised the stock from which the mammalian orders evolved (Romer, 1966; Starck, 1978). The volumetric data for the subdivisions of the hippocampus of the hedgehog serve as a basis for allometric comparisons of the hippocampal components of the other species. These include 4 murine species that differ significantly in size: two species of wild mice, *Micromys minutus* and *Apodemus flavicollis,* and 3 strains of laboratory rodents that include DBA/2J mice and Fisher-344 and Wistar rats. In addition, data has been included from 3 species that resemble an ascending primate series on the basis of neocortical development (Stephan and Andy, 1969). These are the common tree shrew *(Tupaia glis),* which is believed to share a common pool of ancestors with primative prosimian species (Starck, 1965) but has recently been placed in a separate order, *Scandentia* (Corbet and Hill, 1980; Luckett, 1980), and two simians: the common marmoset monkey, which has one of the least evolved simian brains (Thinius, 1967) and man, who has the most progressive mammalian brain (Stephan and Andy, 1969). The ordering of this series is based on neocortical progression and does not represent a direct evolutionary line along which the respective higher forms have passed.

With the exception of the human material, the estimates of the volumes of the hippocampal subdivisions were made from sections stained with the Timm technique for visualization of heavy metals. The estimation of the volumes of the subdivisions of the human hippocampus were made on glycolmethacrylate sections stained with the Giemsa stain. The estimates of neuron number in the subdivisions of the human hippocampus and of Wistar rats were made in methacrylate-embedded, Giemsa-stained material. The macroscopic appearance of hippocampi from representatives of the species included in this study are shown in Fig. 1. The materials used in this study, along with references to studies in which the species have been dealt with in detail, are summarized in Table I.

Allometric comparisons based on a representative basal insectivore

The allometric analysis involves comparing the volume of a specific hippocampal component of a particular species (γ) with that of a hypothetical hedgehog of the same body weight. This is accomplished by calculating the volume of a subdivi-

TABLE I

List of species included in the present study, showing the number of individuals (V_n) used in the estimates of the volumes of the subdivisions and the number of individuals (N_n) used in the estimates of neuron numbers

Species	Estimates	Histology	Reference
1. European hedgehog *(Erinaceus europaeus)*	V_n, 5 adult males	Timm	West et al., 1984 West and Schwerdtfeger, 1985
2. Harvest mouse *(Micromys minutus)*	V_n, 5 adult males	Timm	
3. DBA/2J laboratory mouse *(Mus musculus)*	V_n, 5 adult males	Timm	
4. Yellow-necked wood mouse *(Apodemus flavicollis)*	V_n, 5 adult males	Timm	Slomianka and West, 1989
5. Wistar strain albino laboratory rat *(Mus norvegicus albinus)*	V_n, 5 males 28 days N_n, 5 males 28 days	Timm Giemsa	Slomianka et al., 1989
6. Fisher-344 albino laboratory rat *(Mus norvegicus albinus)*	V_n, 6 males 365 days	Timm	Coleman et al., 1987
7. Tree shrew *(Tupaia glis)*	V_n, 2 adults males	Timm	West and Schwerdtfeger, 1985
8. Marmoset monkey *(Callithrix jacchus)*	V_n, 2 adult males	Timm	West and Schwerdtfeger, 1985
9. Man *(Homo sapiens)*	V_n, 5 adult males N_n, 5 adult males 47 – 85 years	Giemsa Giemsa	West and Gundersen (1990)

The histological preparations used for the individual estimates of neuron number and subdivision volume are shown in the third column. References to earlier work that describe in detail the histological material and techniques used for the estimates in different species are given in the column to the right.

sion expected in an isoponderous hedgehog, from the allometric relationship between hippocampal volume and body size observed in basal insectivores, with the allometric equation:

$$y = bx^a \qquad (1)$$

$$\log y = a \cdot \log x + \log b \qquad (2)$$

$$\begin{aligned}\log\,(&\text{expected volume of a subdivision,}\\ &\text{isoponderous hedgehog})\\ &= 0.57 \log\,(\text{b.wt, species } \gamma) + \log b \qquad (3)\end{aligned}$$

in which a, the slope of the regression line of a log–log plot of hippocampal volume versus body weight for basal insectivores, is 0.57 (Stephan and Andy, 1969), and log b, the y intercept of that regression line, is calculated for each subdivision with the following equation:

$$\begin{aligned}\log b = &\log\,(\text{volume of subdivision, hedgehog})\\ &- 0.57 \log\,(\text{b.wt, hedgehog}) \qquad (4)\end{aligned}$$

The observed volume for the hippocampal component of an individual is divided by the volume expected in a hypothetical isoponderous hedgehog to produce a progression index (PI). For example, if the observed volume in an individual is twice that expected in an isoponderous hedgehog, the PI would be 2.

The approach used here is a slight departure from that used by Stephan in which the regression line for a particular brain structure is calculated from measures of that structure made in members of the basal group. In the approach used here, the specific values for the subdivisions of the hedgehog are extrapolated along a line with a slope defined by the relationship, in the basal group, between the volume of the entire hippocampus and body weight. Implicit in the approach used here is the assumption that in basal insectivores the allometric relationship between the size of the subdivisions and the size of the body is the same as that between the size of the entire hippocampus and body size, that is the relative volumes of the subdivisions are

the same in the different members of the group. This seems reasonable in view of the stability of the relative proportions of components of the brain in individuals in a related group (see Stephan et al., 1970 and "Geometrical Scaling" in Gould, 1975). The hedgehog has a body weight that lies close to the middle of the range of the body weights of the basal insectivores. The progression index for the brain is 1.15, also in the middle of the range for basal insectivores.

Estimating the volumes of the subdivisions

In all of the species studied, with the exception of man, the estimates of the volumes of the major subdivisions were made with a technique that has been described in detail previously (West et al., 1978). Briefly, a series of 20–30 sections from each specimen, with a known intersection distance, are selected systematically along the entire length of the hippocampus. The areas of the profiles of the subdivisions on each of these sections are computed from digitized representations of the boundaries of the subdivisions and multiplied by the distance to the next section in the series. The estimate of the volume is the sum of the volumes calculated between each pair of sections in the series.

In the human hippocampus a similar technique was used except that the areas of the subdivisions were estimated by point-counting performed directly on the slide while it was being viewed under a dissection microscope. Each section was separated by 3 mm and the points in the counting grid separated by 1 mm. Additional details are described in West and Gundersen (1990).

Delineation of the subdivisions for volumetric estimates in Timm-stained material

The following subdivisions were delineated in the Timm-stained preparations. They are illustrated in Fig. 2 for representatives of the species included in this study. The terminology adopted here is based on that used by Blackstad (1956). Details regarding

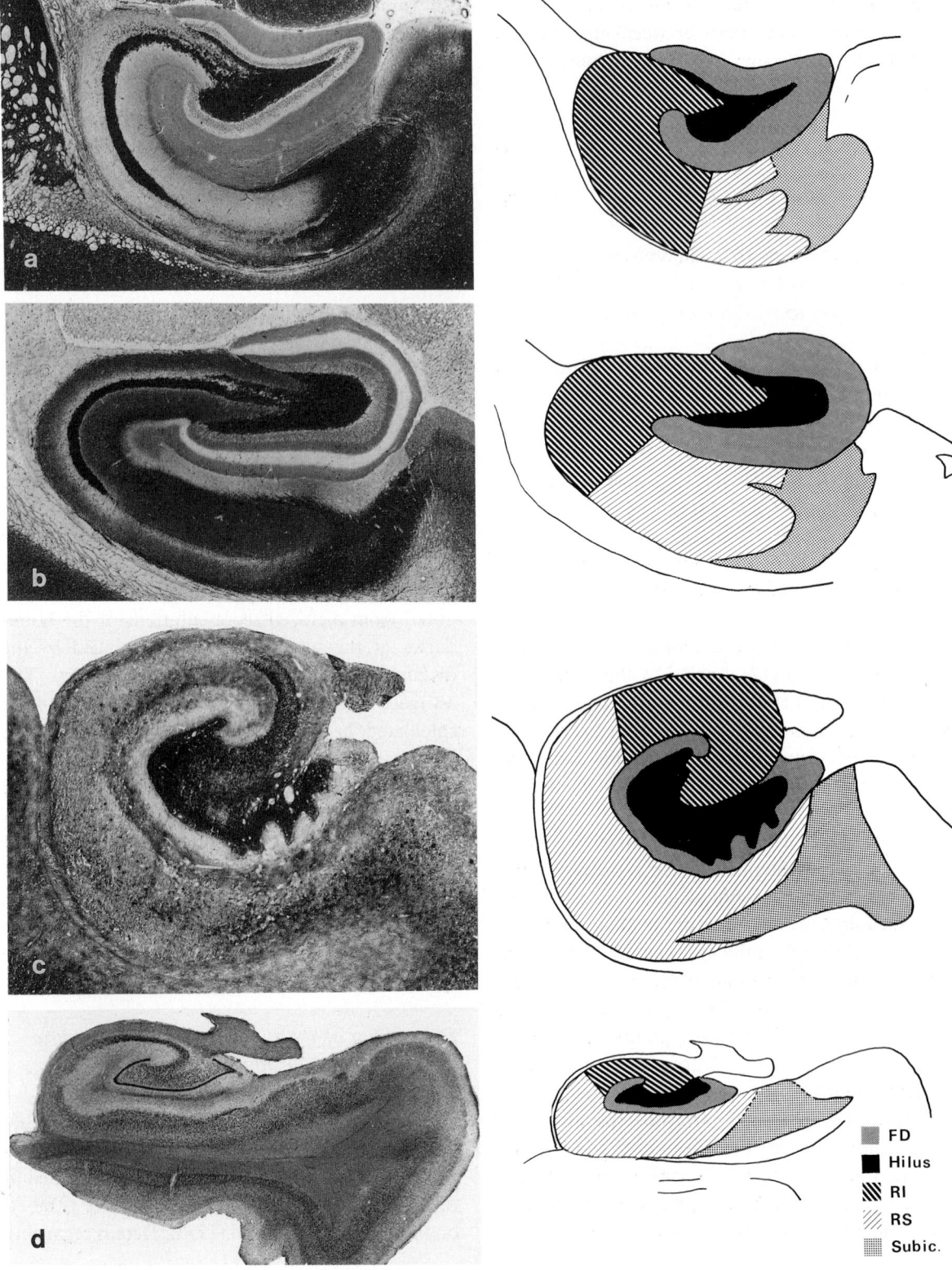

FD
Hilus
RI
RS
Subic.

the definition of the subdivisions can be found in the references listed in Table I. Details of the correlation between the architectonically and histochemically defined subdivisions can be found in Haug (1974) and Zimmer and Haug (1978) for the rat and in Casell and Brown (1984) for the human hippocampus. Additional details regarding the histochemical staining of the hippocampal region of the European hedgehog can be found in West et al. (1984) and Crutcher et al. (1988).

Fascia dentata. The molecular and granule cell layers of the fascia dentata are readily identified at all septotemporal levels by the laminated staining pattern of the molecular layer.

Hilus of the fascia dentata. The hilus is defined as the intensely stained crescent-shaped region between the blades of the fascia dentata which has a concave border with regio inferior.

Regio inferior. This region includes the mossy fiber zone and the segments of the stratum oriens, stratum pyramidale, and stratum moleculare that lie deep and superficial to the intensely stained mossy fiber zone. The regio inferior is limited along the dentato-subicular axis by the hilus and a line drawn along the radial axis at the tip of the mossy fiber zone.

Regio superior. This region includes the segments of strata oriens, pyramidale, radiatum and moleculare not associated with the mossy fiber zone. Medially it is bound by the subiculum described below.

Subiculum. The deep zone of the subiculum, which in most species stains darkly and is homogeneous in appearance, has a well defined convex border with the presubiculum and a concave border with regio superior that in most species includes triangular projections that point back toward the regio inferior and are insinuated between some of the layers of the latter. This component is readily defined at all septo-temporal levels of the species included here. There is, however, no well defined change in the appearance of the staining of the molecular layer at the transition between regio superior and subiculum. As a consequence, the volumes of the molecular layers of these two subdivisions were estimated initially as a single entity and then distributed between the two subdivisions on the basis of the relative volumes of the subdivisions minus the molecular layer.

Delineation of the subdivisions of the human hippocampus used for volume estimates

The delineations in the human hippocampus were based on cytoarchitectonic information present in the Giemsa-stained methacrylate sections (Fig. 2d). Difficulties encountered when staining postmortem material with the Timm stain precluded the use of this stain for delineating the subdivisions. The few cases in which it was possible to obtain an acceptable Timm staining pattern (Fig. 2c) were used to confirm the correspondence between the definitions of the subdivisions made on the basis of the cytoarchitectonics in the human material and those made on the basis of histochemistry in other species. This was particularly important for the

Fig. 2. Histological sections from representatives of the species used in the study. To the right of each section is a diagram showing the borders of the subdivisions that were quantified. See text for additional details. a: Timm-stained transverse section through the hippocampus of the hedgehog. ×15. b: Timm-stained transverse section through the hippocampus of the Wistar rat. ×26. c: Timm-stained transverse section through the hippocampus of man used to determine the correlation between Timm-stained subdivisions and architectonic subdivisions defined in Giemsa-stained sections. ×5. d: Giemsa-stained transverse section through the hippocampus of man. The borders depicted on the right were used for the volumetric estimates. ×3.5. FD, fascia dentata; Hilus, hilus of the fascia dentata; RI, regio inferior; RS, regio superior; Subic, subiculum (see text for additional details about the definitions of the subdivisions).

definitions of hilus and regio inferior. The Timm-stained hilus in the human hippocampus corresponds to the inner and outer plexiform and cellular layers (Fig. 2c, see also Casell and Brown, 1984; West and Gundersen, 1990). Regio inferior, delineated on the basis of the larger more densely packed cells in this region when compared to those in regio superior, corresponded to the region associated with the darkly stained mossy fiber layer plus a small variable transition zone CA2 which has large pyramidal cells but no mossy fibers. The boundaries of the sectional profiles of the fascia dentata were readily defined by free surfaces, the hippocampal fissure and the deep border of the granule cell layer. The part of the molecular layer associated with the subiculum was defined by continuing the lateral and medial borders of the subiculum toward the surface (Fig. 2d, dashed lines). Islands of presubicular neurons were often observed within these borders, but points hitting them were not used in the volume estimates.

Revised volumetric data for hedgehog, Tupaia and marmoset

The volumetric data for hedgehog, *Tupaia* and marmoset, which have in part been published previously (West and Schwerdtfeger, 1985), are revised with regard to the definition of the layers included in regio inferior, regio superior and subiculum. In the present chapter these subdivisions include the molecular layer. In the data published previously, the molecular layer was excluded from the definition of the subdivisions used in the comparisons because natural borders corresponding to the borders of the subdivisions could not be identified within this layer (see the dashed portion of the border of subiculum, Fig. 2a and b). The inclusion of data from the human hippocampus has necessitated this revision in that it was not possible in the Giemsa-stained human material to rigorously define a separate molecular layer in Ammon's horn and subiculum. In an attempt to have the hippocampal subdivisions of the various species correspond as much as possible with regard to the

layers that were included in their boundaries, the molecular layers of Ammon's horn and subiculum, which were initially estimated as a single entity in the Timm-stained preparations, have been distributed between the subdivisions on the basis of the relative volumes of the other layers in the subdivisions.

Definition of telencephalon

With the exception of the human material, the estimates of the volume of the telencephalon were made on one side of the brain using the technique described above for estimating the volumes of the Timm-stained hippocampal subdivisions. The telencephalic borders encompassed the corpus callosum, striatum and amygdala and excluded the septum, the alveus, the fornix, the hippocampal commissures, and the internal capsule.

The volume of the telencephalon of the human brains was estimated with point counting techniques similar to those used for estimating the volumes of the subdivisions of the hippocampus, which are described above. The point counting was performed with a grid placed directly on the cut surface of 6-mm-thick slabs cut in the frontal plane of the right hemisphere. The area corresponding to each point was 210 mm^2. Only points falling on regions corresponding to those included in the definition of telencephalon of the other species (see above) were counted. The number of points counted was multiplied by the area represented by each point and the slab thickness to obtain an estimate of volume.

Estimating the number of neurons in the hippocampus

Wistar rats

The numbers of neurons in each of the 5 hippocampal subdivisions of 5 Wistar rats were estimated with a modified fractionator (Gundersen, 1986) in which optical disectors were used (Gundersen et al., 1988; West and Gundersen, 1990). Briefly, this consisted of counting, in each animal, the neurons in a known fraction of the volume of the layers of a subdivision that contained neurons. That is, the hippocampus is sectioned exhaustively and the number of sections containing profiles of the neuron containing layers of the various subdivisions determined, *(S)*. For each hippocampus, 20 – 30 equally spaced sections *(s)* were selected for further analysis. The fraction of the total number of sections that is sampled is consequently known, *s/S* (e.g. 23/150 or 15.3%). Each of these sections is scanned by moving it systematically with a motor-driven microscope stage in a raster pattern with *x,y* steps of known dimensions. Each time a sampling frame superimposed on the microscope field fell within the boundaries of the neuron containing layers of a subdivision, neuronal nuclei were counted *(n)* with an optical disector. The area of the sample frame of the optical "disector" (*f*) was known relative to the area corresponding to a raster movement (*r*). The height of the disector (*h*) is known relative to the thickness of the section *(t)* from measurements made with a microcator. The total number of neurons *(N)* is then

$$N = \Sigma n \cdot S/s \cdot r/f \cdot t/h$$

in which Σn is the number of neuronal nuclei counted, *s/S* the fraction of sections analyzed, *f/r* the fraction of the area of the section analyzed, and *h/t* the fraction of the thickness of the sections analyzed.

The sample frame was dimensioned so that approximately 1 – 2 nuclei were counted in each disector. The *x,y* stage movement was dimensioned so that approximately 100 systematic samples would be made on the selected sections.

Human

The number of neurons *(N)* in each of the 5 subdivisions of each hippocampus was calculated from estimates of the numerical density (N_V) of the neuronal nuclei and the volumes of the neuron containing layers *Vref* of each subdivision.

$$N = N_V \cdot Vref$$

The *Vref* values were estimated by point counting on the same sections used to estimate N_V. The estimates of N_V were made with optical disectors. The numerical data and details of this procedure have been published previously (West and Gundersen, 1990).

Unbiased and biased stereological estimates

The estimates of neuron number, *N*, presented here are all truly unbiased in that they have been obtained with a three-dimensional probe, the disector (Sterio, 1984; see also West and Gundersen, 1990), involve no assumptions about size, shape, or orientation of neuronal nuclei, and approach the true value of the parameter being estimated as the sample size is increased. The absolute values of the estimates of *N* and N_V for granule cells presented in an earlier study (West and Andersen, 1980) have not been included here because of the biased technique (Weibel and Gomez, 1962) used in that study.

There are two theoretical sources of bias in the estimates of the volumes of the Timm-stained subdivisions obtained with the described technique (West et al., 1978). These are only now apparent after recent essays on systematic sampling and the popularization of Cavalieri's principles for obtaining unbiased estimates of volume (Cruz-Orive, 1985, 1987; Mattfeldt, 1987; Gundersen and Jensen, 1987). The first is that the sections used in the estimates were not systematically chosen with a regular intersection interval. That is, the distance between sections was less in the regions where the areas of the profiles of the subdivisions changed most from section to section. In effect the shape of the region was taken into account when selecting the sections, creating a bias. The other theoretical source of bias in these estimates is the non-random selection of the first section in the series. In these studies the first section analyzed was the first section that passed through the subdivision being analyzed, rather than a random section within the first interval as required for truly unbiased estimates. While it is difficult, if not impossible, to estimate the biases introduced by these two aspects of the methodology, they are most likely negligible due to the large number of sections (20 – 30) used in the estimates. It has been shown by Gundersen and Jensen (1987) that typically about 10 systematic random sections are required for accurate estimates of volumes of objects with shapes similar to those encountered in the hippocampus. The unnecessarily large number of sections used in these studies results in a reduction in the bias introduced by the non-random systematic sampling that was performed.

The estimates of volumes of the subdivisions of the human hippocampus (i.e. all layers including the cell body containing layer, as seen in Fig. 2d) are free of biases of the type mentioned above in that the sections used in the analysis were selected in a systematic random manner. There is however another source of bias in these estimates related to uncertainties as to the degrees to which stratum moleculare, stratum radiatum, and stratum oriens in the rostral parts of the hippocampus, where the section plane deviates from the transverse axis of the hippocampus, belong to regio inferior, regio superior and subiculum. In the Giemsa-stained sections used for the volumetric analysis of the subdivisions of the human hippocampus, unlike in the Timm-stained sections used in the other species, there is little differential staining in the perikarya-free layers that can be used to identify the layers with certainty. These biases are negligible for fascia dentata and hilus because the boundaries of these subdivisions are readily apparent on all sections cut in the frontal plane. The estimates of V_{ref} for regio superior, regio inferior, and subiculum are another matter. Unfortunately it is virtually impossible to quantify these biases. However, in view of the numbers and the shapes of the sections on which this is a problem, the bias is unlikely to be more than 5 – 10%.

Results

Volumetric data

The mean body weights, telencephalic volumes, and volumes of the hippocampal subdivisions of the species included in this study are presented in Table II.

Percentage of telencephalon

The percentage of the telencephalic volume occupied by the hippocampus in each of the species is presented in Fig. 3. Of note is the relatively small percentage of the telencephalon occupied by the hippocampus in man and the decreasing proportion of the telencephalon occupied by the hippocampus in the primate line (i.e. *Tupaia*, marmoset, man). The largest percentage of the telencephalon occupied by hippocampus is found in *Micromys*, the species with the smallest telencephalon and body weight. There is, however, no clear interspecies relationship between this percentage and the absolute size of the telencephalon or body.

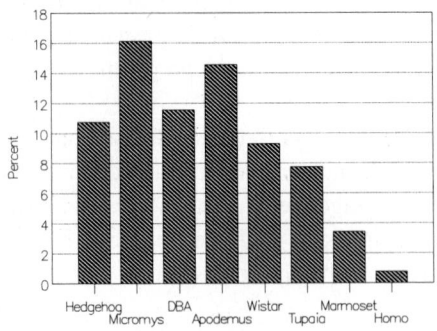

Fig. 3. The percent of the volume of the telencephalon occupied by the hippocampus. See text for definition of telencephalon. The ordering of species, with the exception of the hedgehog, has been made on the basis of body weight.

TABLE II

Mean volumes of the hippocampal subdivisions in mm³ (bilateral values)

	N	Hippo.	FD	Hilus	AH	RI	RS	Sub.	Telen.	Body (g)
Erinaceus europaeus	4	197 (0.11)	44.8 (0.13)	9.22 (0.14)	109 (0.16)	76.9 (0.11)	32.5 (0.28)	33.7 (0.13)	917 (0.16)	860 (*)
Micromys minutus	5	18.1 (0.05)	3.99 (0.07)	0.70 (0.14)	10.4 (0.05)	5.10 (0.04)	5.31 (0.06)	3.08 (0.06)	112 (0.02)	5.75 (0.08)
DBA/2J mouse	5	21.3 (0.08)	4.16 (0.08)	0.65 (0.04)	12.9 (0.08)	5.40 (0.12)	7.52 (0.06)	3.61 (0.10)	184 (0.05)	28.0 (0.10)
Apodemus flavicollis	5	54.0 (0.09)	11.1 (0.12)	2.28 (0.10)	30.3 (0.07)	–	–	10.4 (0.13)	371 (0.10)	24.8 (0.04)
Wistar rat	6	79.7 (0.03)	15.6 (0.04)	3.71 (0.03)	44.4 (0.03)	19.7 (0.04)	24.8 (0.02)	15.9 (0.02)	–	84.2 (0.05)
Fisher 344 rat	6	119 (0.04)	29.1 (0.04)	5.95 (0.04)	–	–	–	–	616 (0.09)	401 (0.05)
Tupaia glis	2	145 (0.08)	32.6 (0.02)	7.33 (0.01)	85.4 (0.20)	41.4 (0.25)	43.9 (0.14)	20.2 (0.18)	1703 (0.11)	170 (*)
Callithrix jacchus	2	183 (0.02)	35.7 (0.13)	11.9 (0.08)	119 (0.07)	54.6 (0.10)	64.0 (0.04)	17.0 (0.04)	4944 (0.06)	280 (*)
Homo sapiens	5	7718 (0.10)	768 (0.10)	712 (0.21)	4795 (0.06)	984 (0.21)	3811 (0.07)	1444 (0.16)	1,040,000 (0.10)	70.000 (0.17)

N, number of specimens; Hippo, sum of the volumes of the subdivisions; FD, fascia dentata; RI, regio inferior; RS, regio superior; Sub, subiculum; AH (Ammon's horn), RI plus RS; Telen, telencephalon; Body, body weight (g). The coefficient of variation, CV, (S.D./mean) is shown beside each estimate. –, the unavailability of volumetric data. Asterix (*) indicates that the subdivisions of a species have been "standardized", i.e. adjusted for deviations in body size from that descriptive of a larger sample (see West and Schwerdtfeger, 1985).

Relative proportions of subdivisions

The relative proportions of the major subdivisions of the hippocampus of each species are shown in Fig. 4, as percentages of the total volume of the hippocampus. For each species the percentages were based on the mean volumes of the subdivisions. (In *Apodemus,* regio superior and regio inferior are dealt with as one entity. In the F344 rat, regio inferior, regio superior, and subiculum are dealt with as one entity.) Noteworthy are: (1) the relatively constant contributions made to the total hippocampal volume by the fascia dentata, the major exception being that of humans which is about half the relative size of the fascia dentata of the other species; (2) the relatively large percentages of the hippocampi of marmosets and men occupied by the hilus. The largest hilus is found in man and is twice the relative size of that of any of the other species studied; (3) the relatively large regio inferior and small regio superior in the hedgehog, the relatively small regio inferior and large regio superior in man, and the roughly equal sizes of these two subdivisions in the other species; and (4) the constant proportion of the volume of the hippocampus occupied by the subiculum, the exceptions being the subiculum of *Tupaia* and marmoset which are relatively small.

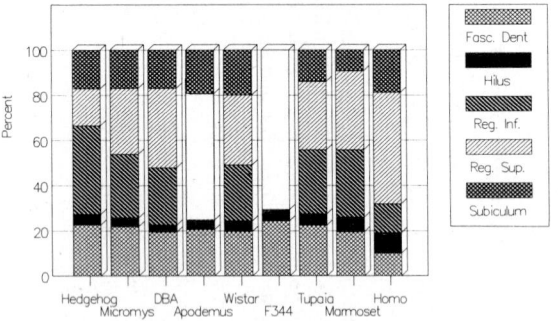

Fig. 4. The percent of the hippocampus occupied by the different subdivisions. Separate estimates of regio inferior and regio superior were not made in *Apodemus,* the clear zone represents these subdivisions. In the F-344 rat, regio inferior, regio superior and subiculum were not estimated separately. In this case the clear zone collectively represents these subdivisions.

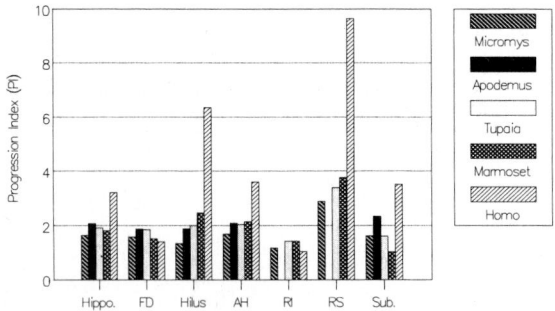

Fig. 5. The progression indices for 5 of the species presented in Table III. The progression index, PI, is the observed volume of a specific subdivision divided by the volume expected in an isoponderous hedgehog. RI and RS data were not available for *Apodemus.* Hippo, all subdivisions; FD, fascia dentata; Hilus, hilus of the fascia dentata; AH, Ammon's horn (i.e. regio inferior plus regio superior); RI, regio inferior; RS, regio superior; Sub., subiculum.

Allometric comparisons

The progression indices (PIs) of the various components of the species studied are presented in Table III, along with the logs of the *b* values for the different components that were used in the allometric equation (equation 3). The PIs for the major subdivisions of 5 species are presented graphically in Fig. 5. Noteworthy points follow below.

The progressive human hippocampus

There is a large amount of progression in the hippocampus of humans. While fascia dentata and regio inferior show the least amount of progression (with PIs comparable to the other species studied, i.e. under 2), dramatic progression is observed in regio superior and hilus which, respectively, have volumes that are roughly 10 and 6 times those expected in hedgehogs of equal body weight (PIs of 9.65 and 6.35, respectively). The volume of the human subiculum is between 3 and 4 times that expected in an isoponderous hedgehog (PI of 3.51) and has progressed to the same degree as Ammon's horn (i.e. regio superior and regio inferior combined, PI of 3.60). The net effect of the differential progression in the various subdivisions is that the human hippocampus has a PI of 3.21.

TABLE III

Progression indices (PIs) for the hippocampal subdivisons of the species studied

	Hippo.	FD	Hilus	AH	RI	RS	Subic.
Micromys	1.63	1.58	1.34	1.68	1.17	2.89	1.62
DBA	0.76	0.65	0.49	0.82	0.49	1.62	0.75
Apodemus	2.07	1.86	1.87	2.09	–	–	2.34
Wistar	1.52	1.32	1.52	1.53	0.96	2.87	1.77
F-344	0.94	1.00	1.00	–	–	–	–
Tupaia	1.91	1.84	2.00	2.03	1.42	3.39	1.61
Marmoset	1.81	1.51	2.46	2.14	1.42	3.76	1.03
Homo	3.21	1.40	6.35	3.60	1.04	9.65	3.51
log *b*	0.62	−0.02	−0.71	0.37	0.21	−0.16	−0.15

The PI for each subdivision of each species is calculated as the group mean of the ratio of the volume estimated in an individual to the volume expected in an isoponderous hedgehog (equation 3). The log of the *b* value used in equation 3 for each subdivision was calculated from equation 4 and is shown in the bottom row. A PI of 2 indicates that the subdivision is 2 times larger than that expected in a hedgehog of equal body weight. Blank values indicate the unavailability of volumetric data necessary for the calculation of the PI.

PIs of laboratory animals

The hippocampi of two of the laboratory rodents (DBA mice, F344 rats) have PIs that are less than 1, Table III. That is, they have hippocampi that are smaller than expected in isoponderous hedgehogs. Because this is most likely related to the variable body weights of mature laboratory animals (Coleman et al., 1987) and selection pressures generated during domestication and breeding (Ebinger, 1974; Kruska and Röhrs, 1974; Kruska, 1987), these two species and the Wistar rat have not been included in the graphic presentation of the PIs of the major subdivisions (Fig. 5) and are excluded from the discussion of allometric trends.

Trends in the primate series

There are increasing degrees of progression in both the regio superior and hilus of the "primate series" (i.e. *Tupaia,* marmoset, and man), and slightly decreasing degrees of progression in fascia dentata and regio inferior in this series. No consistent trend in the progression of the subiculum in these species was observed. In both *Tupaia* and marmoset, the progression of the subiculum does not keep pace with that of the entire hippocampus

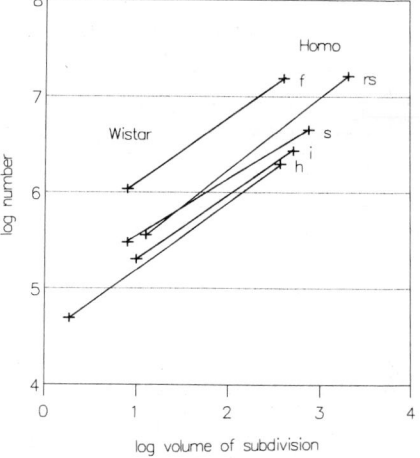

Fig. 6. The relationship between the volume of the individual hippocampal subdivisions, in Wistar rats and humans, and the number of neurons in the respective subdivisions. The log of *N* (neuron number) is plotted against the log of *V* (volume in mm³) for each subdivision (+). f, fascia dentata; h, hilus; i, regio inferior; rs, regio superior; s, subiculum. Lines connect the values for homologous subdivisions in man and Wistar rats. The upper right +s represent the values in man. Each point represents the mean of estimates of *N* and *V* in the same 5 individuals. In the rats, *N* and *V* were estimated in two separate groups of 5 individuals. The slopes of the lines are presented in Table V (average, 0.68). See text for additional details.

TABLE IV

Estimates of N, number of neurons, and V, volume of the subdivisions (mm^3) for each of the subdivisions of the hippocampus of humans and Wistar rats (unilateral values)

	Humans		Wistar		Humans/Wistar
FD					
N	1.54×10^7	(0.28)	1.08×10^6	(0.15)	14.3
V	3.84×10^2	(0.24)	7.88	(0.04)	48.7
T	2.49×10^4		7.30×10^3		3.4
Hilus					
N	1.98×10^6	(0.16)	4.91×10^4	(0.14)	40.4
V	3.56×10^2	(0.21)	1.85	(0.03)	192.4
T	1.80×10^5		3.77×10^4		4.8
RI					
N	2.70×10^6	(0.21)	2.02×10^5	(0.17)	13.4
V	4.92×10^2	(0.21)	9.83	(0.04)	50.1
T	1.82×10^5		4.87×10^4		3.7
RS					
N	1.64×10^7	(0.32)	3.61×10^5	(0.09)	45.5
V	1.90×10^3	(0.07)	1.24×10	(0.02)	154
T	1.16×10^5		3.43×10^4		3.4
Subic.					
N	4.51×10^6	(0.20)	3.03×10^5	(0.10)	14.9
V	7.22×10^2	(0.16)	7.93	(0.02)	91
T	1.60×10^5		2.62×10^4		6.1

Beside each estimate can be seen the coefficient of variation (S.D./mean). The neuron territory, T, or volume of the subdivision per neuron V/N (μm^3/neuron) is also shown for each subdivision. The individual estimates of N and V were made in the same 5 human hippocampi. The individual estimates of N and V in Wistar rats were made in two separate groups of 5 specimens each. The ratios of N, V, and T in man to N, V, and T in rats, respectively, are shown in the right column.

TABLE V

Difference in logs (δ log) of V (mm^3), N, T (μm^3/neuron) in *Homo* and Wistar rats shown in Table III

	δ log V	δ log N	δ log T	δ log N/δ log V	δ log T/δ log V
FD	1.69	1.15	0.53	0.68	0.32
Hilus	2.28	1.61	0.58	0.70	0.30
RI	1.70	1.13	0.57	0.66	0.34
RS	2.19	1.66	0.53	0.76	0.24
Subic.	1.96	1.17	0.79	0.60	0.40
			Mean =	0.68	0.32

The two columns on the right show the ratios of the differences in the log values for N to the differences in the log values for V, (i.e. δ log N/δ log V, the slope of the lines plotted in Fig. 6, mean = 0.68) and the ratio of the differences in the log values for T to the difference in the log values for V, (i.e. δ log T/δ log N, the slope of the lines plotted in Fig. 7, mean = 0.32).

and is less than that seen in one of the murine species *(Apodemus)*.

The number and size of neurons in the subdivisions of rats and men

Estimates of the number of neurons N in each of the subdivisions of the hippocampus of Wistar rats and humans are shown in Table IV, along with the estimates of the volumes of the subdivisions V and the neuron territories T. The neuron territories represent the volume of the neuropil associated with each neuron V/N (i.e. the reciprocal of the neuron density).

Neuron number

The relationship between neuron number and the volume of the subdivisions is shown in Fig. 6. The log of the number of neurons in specific subdivisions is plotted against the log of the volume of that subdivision in both rats and humans. The values for the subdivisions in humans are located at the + signs at the upper right, reflecting the larger number of neurons and the larger volumes relative to those in rats. The values of the homologous subdivisions in humans and rats (+ signs lower left) are connected by lines, the slopes of which are given in Table V ($\delta \log N/\delta \log V$). The slopes of these lines indicate that the relationship between the volume and the number of neurons in each subdivision is similar. The larger homologues have more neurons and the relationship is non-linear. On the average, the difference in the number of neurons in homologous subdivisions is proportional to the 0.68 power of the difference in volume. $N \sim V^{0.68}$.

Neuron territory

The relationship between neuron territory T and volume V is shown in a similar manner in Fig. 7. The logs of the volumes and cell territories of the individual subdivisions are plotted against each other. Again the values from the subdivisions of the rat fall to the lower left reflecting the smaller volumes and neuron territories in the rat. The

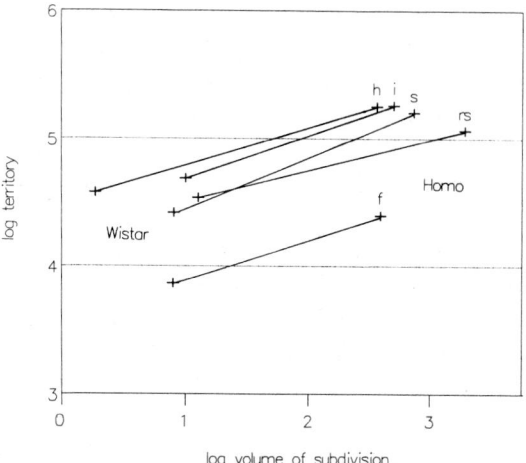

Fig. 7. The relationship between the volume of the individual subdivisions, in Wistar rats and humans, and neuron territory, T (V/N, see text) in the respective subdivisions. The log of T (territory in μm^3) is plotted against the log of V (volume in mm³) for each subdivision (+). The slopes of the lines are presented in Table V (average, 0.32). f, fascia dentata; h, hilus; i, regio inferior; rs, regio superior; s, subiculum.

points representing values in homologous subdivisions (+) are connected by lines, the slopes of which are also given in Table V. The mean slope is 0.32. These data indicate that the relationship between neuron territory and the volume of the subdivision is similar in the different subdivisions. On the average, the difference in neuron number is proportional to the 0.32 power of the volume difference. $T \sim V^{0.32}$.

Discussion

The similarities in the organization of the intrinsic connections of the hippocampi of the different species and the roles of the subdivisions in processing different aspects of the spatial environment proposed in the cognitive map theory of O'Keefe and Nadel (1978), (see also O'Keefe, 1989) will be used as a basis for the discussion of the functional consequences of the interspecies differences in the size of the hippocampal components. Three different aspects of size will be considered: (1) absolute size, (2) allometric progression and (3) the relative proportions of the subdivisions. The latter two will be dealt with first and the issue of absolute size will be dealt with below in the discussion of the relationship between subdivision volume and neuron number.

Fascia dentata and regio inferior

The fascia dentata and regio inferior are progressive structures in that they are larger than expected in basal insectivores. However, they do not display marked differences in the degree of progression in the species studied. That is, the amount of hippocampal tissue, relative to body weight, involved with the processes associated with the fascia dentata and regio inferior does not appear to be altered during phylogeny once it has progressed to a level slightly less than twice that seen in basal insectivores. In the ascending series of primates included here there is even a tendency toward a slight decrease in the progression.

In the spatial map model, the fascia dentata is involved in the formation of simple representations from complex combinations of polysensory input coming from entorhinal cortex, and regio inferior is involved in the formation and maintenance of a map of compound stimuli in which spatial relationships such as direction and contiguity are represented. In the updated version of the theory (O'Keefe, 1989), fascia dentata is also involved in "translocation" of spatial information. Regio inferior, in addition to containing the "current location matrix" is also involved in the transformation started in fascia dentata and acts as a search funnel for map retrieval. In view of the evidence that the main extrinsic input to these subdivisions is a transform of the polysensory information contained in the entorhinal area, it is tempting to suggest that the phylogenetically stable relationship between the size of these subdivisions and body size is related to the scaling of internal representations of sensory information. The examination of this proposition awaits quantitative comparative studies of sensory systems.

Another noteworthy aspect of the scaling of these two subdivisions is that they maintain roughly the same relative sizes in all of the species studied in spite of dramatic changes in the relative proportions of other hippocampal subdivisions. This suggests that both maintain the same quantitative relationship to some external factor, such as sensory input, or that their functional relationship is so tightly linked (as suggested in the updated theory referred to above) that there is a strong tendency for co-evolution of these two subdivisions in quantitative terms.

Hilus

In view of the relative conservatism in the evolution of the fascia dentata and regio inferior it is somewhat unexpected that the hilus, which is positioned between these two subdivisions, is characterized by varying degrees of progression. It is the second most progressive subdivision of the human hippocampus and shows a trend toward increasing progression in the series of ascending primates. Because the hilus has not been appropriated a specific role in the original spatial map model, the size differences in this subdivision will be discussed in terms of a proposed role that is consistent with the anatomical connections of this region and the spatial map model.

The polymorphic cells of the hilus are known to receive efferents from the granule cells (Claiborne et al., 1986) and to project back to the dendrites of the granule cells (Zimmer, 1971; J.R. West et al., 1979; Berger et al., 1980) and are therefore admirably designed to serve as a recurrent autoassociative input to the fascia dentata and be involved in the coding of the information sent to regio inferior. In closely related species there is a strong correlation between the size of the hilus and the size of the terminal field of the association projection to fascia dentata (West and Andersen, 1980; Slomianka and West, 1989). If an increase in the relative size of the hilus is interpreted as an increase in its involvement in coding in fascia dentata, the advantages of a larger hilus can be understood in terms of the importance of efficient coding in the fascia dentata to the functional capacity of regio inferior. The degradation of information in an associative network, like that proposed for regio inferior, can be dealt with in 3 ways (McNaughton and Morris, 1987): (1) expansion of the network, which does not appear to be the case above a certain limit as discussed above; (2) erasure of the network, which has certain temporal constraints related to movement in the environment which must be similar for most animals; and (3) increased efficiency in the coding of input. A proportionally larger hilus could enhance the performance of the regio inferior by increasing the efficiency of the coding that takes place in the fascia dentata while preserving the volumetric parity of regio inferior and fascia dentata described above. The relatively large progression of the hilus and the low constant progression in regio inferior observed here is consistent with the idea that the performance of regio inferior of primates is enhanced by increasing the efficiency of the coding that takes place in fascia dentata rather than by network expansion, a mechanism which does appear to have been adopted in the adjacent regio superior, however, as discussed below. The phylogenetic "dynamics" of the hilus underlined the priority given to the preservation of the relative proportions of fascia dentata and regio inferior during phylogenesis. Even in closely related species, the hilus can differ significantly in size, while the fascia dentata remains unchanged (Slomianka and West, 1989).

Regio superior

Regio superior is clearly the subdivision of the hippocampus in which the most dramatic changes take place during mammalian evolution. In an allometric sense it is the most progressive subdivision in all of the species compared here. In humans it reaches its height of progression, is roughly 10 times the size expected in an isoponderous hedgehog, and occupies more than half the volume of the hippocampal region (compared to about 15% in the hedgehog and about 25% in rodents). In view of the position of regio superior in the unidirectional chain of intrinsic connections, it can be concluded that the processing of the higher levels of transformations of the spatial information presented to the hippocampus has become a proportionately larger part of the hippocampal activities in man. In terms of the spatial map hypothesis this would represent an increase in size, relative to both the other hippocampal subdivisions and to body weight, of the component in which mismatch signals are generated, i.e. signals indicating that representations in the spatial map (in regio inferior) do not match experienced stimuli and where the transform matrix required to take the animal from its present location to the location of the incentive is computed. The high levels of progression in regio superior and the constant levels of progression in regio inferior indicate that there has been a relative increase in the associative functions of regio superior that has been achieved through network expansion in the latter. The progression in the regio superior is most pronounced in man but increases in progression can be traced back to prosimian and simian forms.

Subiculum

It is clear from recent anatomical studies (see Rosene and Van Hoesen, 1987) that the bulk of output from regio superior will be transferred through the subiculum, which has the appropriate paucity of intrinsic connections and wealth of extrinsic connections, to regions involved in the behavioral responses to mismatches (i.e. in general terms, exploration or withdrawal). In view of the dramatic increase in the size of the regio superior, it is surprising that the subiculum, which is the primary recipient of regio superior efferents and distributor of information processed in the hippocampal formation (Van Hoesen, 1982), progresses to a significantly lesser degree than regio superior and that it does not reflect more of the progression seen in the telencephalon to which it becomes more intimately related. In man, the relative contribution of the subiculum to the volume of the hippocampus is similar to that observed in the hedgehog and rodents. In *Tupaia* and the marmoset monkey it is even relatively smaller. One explanation is that while the associative capacity of regio superior has increased, the output requirements of this region have not increased, that is, more things can be associated but the number of responses is not altered proportionately. Another explanation, which is less speculative, is that an increasing proportion of the output from regio superior does not proceed through the subiculum. In Rosene and Van Hoesen's studies of monkey hippocampal efferents (Rosene and Van Hoesen, 1977), significant numbers were observed to originate from the pro-subiculum, which is included in the human regio superior in the data presented here, and from CA1 itself (here referred to as regio superior). Part of the dramatic progression of regio superior may be a reflection of a relative increase in hippocampal output that does not involve subiculum.

Relationship between the number and size of neurons and the volumes of the subdivisions

The functional implications of the observed differences in the volumes of the subdivisions can be more completely understood by considering the relationship between neuron number and the volume of the hippocampal subdivisions. In homologous subdivisions, the number of neurons appears to scale in a non-linear fashion with the volume of the subdivision $N \sim V^{0.68}$ (Fig. 6, Table V). This relationship is similar to the scaling relationship observed between surface and volume of isomorphic (similarly shaped) objects of different sizes. A number of other structural features of the hippocampal subdivisions suggest that homologues in different species are isomorphic forms, such as the consistent appearance of the neuron types and the similar architectonics of homologous regions in different species. The geometrical relationship between surface and volume in isomorphs has important implications for the number and size of neurons that are organized in a two-dimensional sheet. One is that

in differently sized homologues the number of neurons per unit area of the plane of the sheet would be constant, i.e. the number of neurons would be directly proportional to the area of the plane of the layer. The other is that the numerical density of the neurons would be inversely proportional to the height of the region along the radial axis, i.e. that which lies perpendicular to the plane of the layer. Since the cell territory T is the reciprocal of the numerical density, the cell territory would be directly proportional to the thickness of the subdivision and proportional to the 1/3 power of the volume of the subdivision. In summary, in isomorphic forms in which neurons are organized in a two-dimensional plane (layer), neuron number scales as a surface function and neuron territory (size) scales as a linear function of the volume. There is evidence that the fascia dentata of rats and mice are isomorphs (West and Andersen, 1980). The inverse relationship between neuron number and cerebral cortical volume (Tower, 1954; Bok, 1959) and the constancy of neuron number under equal areas of cortical surface in neocortex (Rockel et al., 1980) is evidence that many homologous cortical regions are isomorphs, though this relationship may be most common in closely related species (Haug, 1987).

Another functional parameter for which volume can be considered a statistic is neuronal connectivity. Studies of numerical densities of synapses in various parts of the hippocampus of rats and mice and specific layers of neocortical areas indicate that synaptic densities are similar in the cortical regions of different species (Table VI). This uniformity implies that the number of synapses made in a cortical region is directly proportional to the volume of the region, with the consequence that cell territory $T(V/N)$ would be proportional to the number of synapses made on an average neuron in that region.

The consequences of size scaling in homologous subdivisions in terms of the information-processing capacity of the entire region and the individual neurons would be the following. First, the total number of synaptic contacts made in the

TABLE VI

List of previous publications in which the numerical density (N_V or number per mm^3) of synaptic contacts has been estimated with stereological techniques showing the similarity of the N_V in different cortical regions of different species

Area, species	N_V	Reference
Parietal cortex, Wistar rat	2.16×10^9	Caverley et al., 1988
CA3 molecular l., Wistar rat	2.7×10^9	de Groot and Bierman, 1986
Fascia dentata, Sprague – Dawley rat	2.22×10^9	Desmond and Levy, 1986
Fascia dentata, F-344 rat	0.85×10^9	Geinisman et al., 1986
Visual cortex II – IV, Lister rat	1×10^9	Warren and Bedi, 1981
Fascia dentata, DBA/2J	2.58×10^9	West and Andersen, 1980
Fascia dentata, Wistar rat	2.44×10^9	West and Andersen, 1980

region will be increased in direct proportion to the volume increase. Second, the number of discrete output chanels (neurons) will increase by a factor proportional to the 2/3 power of the volume difference. Third, the individual neurons will receive input from an increased number of synapses (in proportion to the 1/3 power of the volume difference), with the functional consequence that random variation in the threshold of the neurons will be reduced and that there will be an increased probability that what is on the output corresponds to something on the input (McCulloch, 1951).

Isomorphic forms are well suited for scaling in that the numerical relationships between neurons of two subdivisions can be maintained when connected regions progress in parallel. The fascia dentata and regio inferior have roughly the same sizes relative to each other in the species studied. In both rats and humans, the ratio of granule cells to regio inferior pyramids is essentially the same (5.7, 5.4) and the relationship between neuron number and volume in both regions is close to that expected in isomorphic transformations (0.68 and 0.66, Table V).

Although thinking of homologous subdivisions as isomorphs provides a simple rule of thumb for evaluating the relationship between absolute volume and total numbers of neurons, this rule should be applied with reservation when the architectonic organization of the homologues differ. Both the histological appearance and the neuron density data presented here suggest that the regio

superior of man is not a simple isomorphic transform of its homologue in rats. The regio superior of man, for example, contains more and smaller neurons than expected from a strict isomorphic transformation. This deviation, although small, is in a direction that further enhances the divergence in the connections from regio inferior that results from a disproportionate increase in the relative size of regio superior in man. The opposite trend is observed in the subiculum in that the neurons are fewer and larger than expected if the subiculum of humans were a simple isomorphic transform of that of the rat. In this case the deviation from isomorphy tends to increase the convergence resulting from the differential progression of these two regions. These observations indicate that mechanisms other than isomorphic network expansion can be involved in progressive changes. Clearly more data on neuron territory and number is needed to determine the degree to which isomorphism is characteristic of hippocampal scaling.

There has been shown to be an age-related loss of neurons in regio superior in the human hippocampal material described here (West and Gundersen, 1990) in that in the younger hippocampi there are about twice the number of neurons in regio superior as there are in the older hippocampi. There are no aged-related differences in the number of neurons in the other subdivisions. The question then arises as to the appropriate age of the human hippocampal material to be used in a comparative study of the type presented here. The number of neurons in each of the different subdivisions of the human hippocampus used in this study is the mean of the estimates made in 5 brains from patients that ranged from 47 to 85 years of age. It therefore represents an underestimation of the number of neurons found in regio superior at the time when the brain reaches maturity. This underestimation does not alter the conclusions drawn with regard to the divergent and convergent relationships described above. If data from the younger hippocampi were used exclusively in the comparisons made here, these relationships would have been even more pronounced.

Comments on the human hippocampus

The human hippocampus is progressive in the sense that it is larger than that expected in primative mammals of the same body weight. Almost all of this progression can be attributed to increases in the size of regio superior and the hilus. The subiculum occupies a somewhat constant proportion of the hippocampus in a number of species including man and neither the fascia dentata nor the regio inferior of humans have progressed beyond the levels observed in *Micromys, Apodemus, Tupaia* and marmoset. The similar, low, levels of progression in fascia dentata and regio inferior in all of the species studied, including man, indicates that once the fascia dentata and regio inferior attain a certain volume relative to body size, this relationship is maintained over a wide range of body sizes and varying degrees of progression in other hippocampal components and in other telencephalic structures. The human hippocampus is unique in terms of the large absolute size of all of its components and progressive changes in the size of regio superior and hilus. However, the large absolute sizes of the fascia dentata and regio inferior are related to the large bodies of humans. In relation to body size, these two subdivisions are of the same size in mice and men.

Acknowledgements

The author thanks Albert Meier for assistance with the photographic illustrations, Thorkild Nielsen for assistance with the disections. This work has been supported in part by Aarhus University Research Fund and Fonden til Forskning af Sindslidelser.

References

Amaral, D.G. (1978) A Golgi study of cell types in the hilar region of the hippocampus in the rat. *J. Comp. Neurol.,* 182: 851 – 914.

Berger, T.W., Semple-Rowland, S. and Basset, J.L. (1980) Hippocampal polymorph neurons are the cells of origin for ipsilateral association and commissural afferents to the dentate gyrus. *Brain Res.,* 215: 329 – 336.

Blackstad, T.W. (1956) Commissural connections of the hippocampal region in the rat, with special reference to their mode of termination. *J. Comp. Neurol.,* 105: 417 – 537.

Bok, S.T. (1959) *Histonomy of the Cerebral Cortex,* Elsevier, Amsterdam.

Braitenberg, V. and Schüz, A. (1983) Some anatomical comments on the hippocampus. In W. Seifert (Ed.), *Neurobiology of the Hippocampus,* Academic Press, London, pp. 39 – 64.

Casell, M.D. and Brown, M.W. (1984) The distribution of Timm's stain in nonsulphide-perfused human hippocampal formation. *J. Comp. Neurol.,* 222: 461 – 471.

Calverley, R.K.S., Bedi, K.S. and Jones, D.G. (1988) Estimation of the numerical density of synapses in rat neocortex. Comparison of the "disector" with an "unfolding" method. *J. Neurosci. Methods,* 23: 195 – 205.

Claiborne, B.J., Amaral, D.G. and Cowan, W.M. (1986) A light and electron microscopic analysis of the mossy fibers of the rat dentate gyrus. *J. Comp. Neurol.,* 246: 435 – 458.

Coleman, P.D., Flood, D.G. and West, M.J. (1987) Volumes of the components of the hippocampus in the aging F344 rat. *J. Comp. Neurol.,* 266: 300 – 306.

Corbet, G.B. and Hill, J.E. (1980) *A World List of Mammalian Species,* Br. Mus. Nat. Hist., London.

Crutcher, K.A., Danscher, G. and Geneser, F.A. (1988) Hippocampus and dentate area of the European hedgehog. *Brain Behav. Evol.,* 32: 269 – 276.

Cruz-Orive, L.M. (1985) Estimating volumes from systematic hyperplane sections. *J. Appl. Prob.,* 2: 518 – 530.

Cruz-Orive, L.M. (1987) Precision of stereological estimators from systematic probes. *Acta Stereol.,* 6: 153 – 158.

de Groot, D.M.G. and Bierman, E.P.B. (1986) A critical evaluation of methods for estimating numerical density of synapses. *J. Neurosci. Methods,* 18: 79 – 101.

Desmond, N.L. and Levy, W.B. (1986) Changes in the numerical density of synaptic contacts with long-term potentiation in the hippocampal dentate gyrus. *J. Comp. Neurol.,* 253: 466 – 475.

Ebinger, P. (1974) A cytoarchitectonic volumetric comparison of brains in wild and domestic sheep. *Z. Anat. Entwickl.-Gesch.,* 144: 267 – 302.

Geinisman, Y., de Toledo-Morell, L. and Morrell, F. (1986) Aged rats need a preserved compliment of perforated axospinous synapses per hippocampal neuron to maintain good spatial memory. *Brain Res.,* 398: 266 – 275.

Geneser, F.A. (1987) Distribution of acetylcholinesterase in the hippocampal region of the rat. *J. Comp. Neurol.,* 262: 594 – 606.

Gould, S.J. (1975) Allometry in primates, with emphasis on scaling and evolution of the brain. *Contrib. Primat.,* 5: 244 – 292.

Gundersen, H.J.G. (1986) Stereology of arbitrary particles. *J. Microsc.,* 143: 3 – 45.

Gundersen, H.J.G. and Jensen, E.B. (1987) The efficiency of systematic sampling in stereology and its prediction. *J. Microsc.,* 17: 229 – 263.

Gundersen, H.J.G., Bagger, P., Bentsen, T.F., Evans, S.M., Korbo, L., Marcussen, N., Møller, A., Nielsen, K., Nyengaard, J.R., Pakkenberg, B., Sørensen, F.B., Vesterby, A. and West, M.J. (1988) The new stereological tools: disector, fractionator, nucleator and point sampled intercepts and their use in pathological research and diagnosis, *APMIS,* 96: 857 – 881.

Haug, F.-M. (1974) Light microscopical mapping of the hippocampal region, the pyriform cortex and the corticomedial amygdaloid nuclei of the rat with Timm's sulfide silver method. *Z. Anat. Entwickl.-Gesch.,* 145: 1 – 27.

Haug, H. (1987) Brain sizes, surfaces, and neuronal sizes of the cortex cerebri: a stereological investigation of man and his variability and a comparison with some mammals (primates, whales, marsupials, insectivores, and one elephant). *Am. J. Anat.,* 180: 126 – 142.

Hofman, M.A. (1982) Encephalization in mammals in relation to the size of the cerebral cortex. *Brain Behav. Evol.,* 20: 84 – 96.

Jerison, H.J. (1973) *Evolution of the Brain and Intelligence,* Academic, New York.

Kruska, D. (1987) How fast can total brain size change in mammals? *J. Hirnforsch.,* 28: 59 – 70.

Kruska, D. and Röhrs, M. (1974) Comparative-quantitative investigations on brains of feral pigs from the Galapagos Islands and of European domestic pigs. *Z. Anat. Entwickl.-Gesch.,* 144: 61 – 73.

Luckett, W.P. (1980) *Comparative Biology and Evolutionary Relationships of Tree Shrews,* Plenum, New York.

Mann, M.D., Glickman, S.E. and Towe, A.L. (1988) Brain/body relations among Myomorph rodents. *Brain Behav. Evol.,* 31: 111 – 124.

Marr, D. (1971) Simple memory: a theory for archicortex. *Phil. Trans. R. Soc. Lond. B,* 262: 23 – 81.

Mattfeldt, T. (1987) Volume estimation of biological objects by systematic sections. *J. Math. Biol.,* 25: 685 – 695.

McCulloch, W.S. (1951) Why the mind is in the head. In L.A. Jeffress (Ed.), *Cerebral Mechanisms in Behavior,* John Wiley and Sons, New York, pp. 42 – 57.

McNaughton, B.L. (1989) Neuronal mechanisms for spatial computation and information storage. In L. Nadel, L.A. Cooper, P. Culicover and R.M. Harish (Eds.), *Neural Connections, Mental Computations,* MIT Press, Cambridge, MA, pp. 225 – 284.

McNaughton, B.L. and Morris, R.G.M. (1987) Hippocampal synaptic enhancement and information storage within a distributed memory system. *Trends Neurosci.,* 10: 408 – 415.

O'Keefe, J. (1989) Computations the hippocampus might perform. In L. Nadel, L.A. Cooper, P. Culicover and R.M. Harish (Eds.), *Neural Connections, Mental Computations,* MIT Press, Cambridge, MA, pp. 225 – 284.

O'Keefe, J. and Nadel, L. (1978) *The Hippocampus as a Cognitive Map,* Clarendon Press, Oxford.

Poulsen, P., West, M.J., Blackstad, Th.W. and Zimmer, J. (1990) Compensatory changes in dentate and hippocampal terminal fields after radiation damage to the fascia dentata of the newborn rat. *Restor. Neurol. Neurosci.,* submitted.

Rockel, A.J., Hiorns, R.W. and Powell, T.P.S. (1980) The basic uniformity in structure of the neocortex. *Brain,* 103: 221 – 244.

Romer, A.S. (1966) *Vergleichende Anatomie der Wirbeltiere,* 2nd edn., Parey, Hamburg.

Rosene, D.L. and Van Hoesen, G.W. (1977) Hippocampal efferents reach widespread areas of cerebral cortex and amygdala in the Rhesus monkey. *Science,* 198: 315 – 317.

Rosene, D.L. and Van Hoesen, G.W. (1987) The hippocampal formation of the primate brain. A review of some comparative aspects of cytoarchitecture and connections. In E.G. Jones and A. Peters (Eds.), *Cerebral Cortex Vol. 6, Further Aspects of Cortical Function, Including Hippocampus,* Plenum, New York, pp. 345 – 356.

Ryngby, J., Slomianka, L., Danscher, G., Holst Andersen, A. and West, M.J. (1987) A quantitative evaluation of the neurotoxic effect of silver on the volumes of the components of the developing rat hippocampus. *Toxicology,* 43: 261 – 268.

Schwerdtfeger, W.K. (1984) Structure and fiber connections of the hippocampus. A comparative study. *Adv. Anat. Embryol. Cell Biol.,* 83: 1 – 74.

Seress, L. (1988) Interspecies comparison of the hippocampal formation shows increased emphasis on the regio superior in the Ammon's horn of the human brain. *J. Hirnforsch.,* 29: 335 – 340.

Slomianka, L., Rungby, J., West, M., Danscher, G. and Andersen, A.H. (1989) Dose-dependent bimodal effect of low-lead exposure on the developing hippocampal region of the rat: a volumetric study. *Neurotoxicology,* 10: 185 – 198.

Slomianka, L. and West, M.J. (1989) Comparative quantitative study of the hippocampal region of two closely related species of wild mice: interspecific and intraspecific variations in volumes of hippocampal components. *J. Comp. Neurol.,* 280: 544 – 552.

Sørensen, K.E. (1985) The connections of the hippocampal region. New observations on efferent connections in the guinea pig, and their functional implications. *Acta Neurol. Scand.,* 72: 550 – 560.

Stark, D. (1965) Die Neencephalisation, In A. Heberer (Ed.), *Menschliche Abstammungslehre,* Fisher, Stuttgart, pp. 103 – 144.

Stark, D. (1978) *Vergleichende Anatomie der Wirbeltiere uf evolutionsbiologischer Grundlag. 1. Theoretische Grundlagen: Stammesgeschichte und Systematik unter Berücksichtigung die niederen Chordata,* Springer, Berlin.

Stephan, H. (1967) Zur entwicklungshöhe der Insektivoren nach Merkmalen des Gehirns und die Definition der "Basalen Insektivoren". *Zool. Anz.,* 179: 177 – 199.

Stephan, H. (1975) Allocortex. In W. Bargmann (Ed.) *Handbuch der mikroskopischen Anatomie des Menschen, Band 4, Teil 9: Nervensystem,* Springer, Berlin, pp. 1 – 998.

Stephan, H. (1983) Evolutionary trends in limbic structures. *Neurosci. Biobehav. Rev.,* 7: 367 – 374.

Stephan, H. and Andy, O.J. (1969) Quantitative comparative neuroanatomy of primates: an attempt at a phylogenetic interpretation. *Ann. N.Y. Acad. Sci.,* 167: 370 – 387.

Stephan, H. and Manolescu, J. (1980) Comparative investigations on hippocampus in insectivores and primates. *Z. Mikrosk.-Anat. Forsch.,* 94: 1025 – 1050.

Stephan, H., Bauchot, R. and Andy, O.J. (1970) Data on size of the brain and of various brain parts in insectivores and primates. In C.A. Noback and W. Montagna (Eds.) *Advances in Primatology. Vol. 1: The Primate Brain,* Appleton Century Crofts, New York, pp. 289 – 297.

Stephan, H., Frahm, H. and Baron, G. (1981) New and revised data on volumes of brain structures in insectivores and primates. *Folia primatol.,* 35: 1 – 29.

Sterio, D.C. (1984) The unbiased estimation of number and sizes of arbitrary particles using the disector. *J. Microsc.,* 134: 127 – 136.

Thenius, E. (1967) Stammengeschichte der Affen. In A. Grzimek (Ed.), *Saugetiere 1, Grzimeks Tierleben, Vol. 10,* Kindler, Zürich.

Tower, D.B. (1954) Structural and functional organization of mammalian cerebral cortex: the correlation of neuron density with brain size. *J. Comp. Neurol.,* 101: 19 – 52.

Van Hoesen, G. (1982) The parahippocampal gyrus, new observations regarding its cortical connections in the monkey. *Trends Neurosci.,* 5: 345 – 350.

Warren, M.A. and Bedi, K.S. (1981) A quantitative assessment of the development of synapses and neurons in the visual cortex of control and undernourished rats. *J. Comp. Neurol.,* 227: 104 – 108.

Weibel, E.R. and Gomez, D.M. (1962) A principle for counting tissue structures on random sections. *J. Appl. Physiol.,* 17: 343 – 348.

West, J.R., Nornes, H.O., Barnes, C.L. and Bronfenbrenner, M. (1979) The cells of origin of the commissural afferents to the area dentata in the mouse. *Brain Res.,* 160: 202 – 215.

West, M.J. and Andersen, A.H. (1980) An allometric study of the area dentata in the rat and mouse. *Brain Res. Rev.,* 2: 317 – 348.

West, M.J. and Gundersen, H.J.G. (1990) Unbiased stereological estimation of the number of neurons in the human hippocampus. *J. Comp. Neurol.,* in press.

West, M.J. and Schwerdtfeger, W. (1985) An allometric study of hippocampal components. A comparative study of the brains of the European Hedgehog *(Erinaceus europaeus),* the tree shrew *(Tupaia glis),* and the Marmoset Monkey *(Callithrix jacchus). Brain Behav. Evol.,* 27: 93 – 105.

West, M.J., Danscher, G. and Gydesen, H. (1978) A determination of the volumes of the layers of the rat hippocampal region. *Cell Tissue Res.,* 188: 345 – 359.

West, M.J., Gaarskjaer, F.B. and Danscher, G. (1984) The Timm-stained hippocampus of the European hedgehog: a basal mammalian form. *J. Comp. Neurol.,* 226: 477 – 488.

Zimmer, J. (1971) Ipsilateral afferents to the commissural zone of the fascia dentata, demonstrated in decommissurated rats by silver impregnation. *J. Comp. Neurol.,* 142: 393 – 416.

Zimmer, J. and Haug, F.-M. (1978) Laminar differentiation of the hippocampus, fascia dentata and subiculum in developing rats, observed with Timm sulfide silver method. *J. Comp. Neurol.,* 179: 581 – 617.

J. Storm-Mathisen, J. Zimmer and O.P. Ottersen (Eds.)
Progress in Brain Research, Vol. 83
© 1990 Elsevier Science Publishers B.V. (Biomedical Division)

CHAPTER 3

Two different ways evolution makes neurons larger

John M. Bekkers and Charles F. Stevens*

Section of Molecular Neurobiology, Howard Hughes Medical Institute at Yale University School of Medicine, 333 Cedar Street, New Haven, CT 06510, U.S.A.

As evolution makes larger brains it also increases the size of many of the individual neurons that make up the brain. How neurons are made larger can give clues about design principles of the brain's circuits. One way of making a larger neuron is called *conservative scaling*. If evolution magnifies a particular type of neuron by a factor of two − that is, each dendrite is made twice as long − then the neuron is scaled conservatively if the magnified neuron has dendrites with 4 times the diameter of their unscaled counterparts. This type of scaling leaves the passive cable properties of the neuron unchanged and so maintains a balance in effectiveness between proximal and distal dendritic inputs. One might imagine that, for some types of circuits, maintaining such a balance would be necessary to use just the same neuronal interconnections in both large and small brains. We have compared dentate granule cells and CA1 pyramidal neurons in cat and human to establish how these cell types are, in fact, scaled. Both cell types are larger in human than in cat, even though their general form is conserved. Pyramidal neurons scale conservatively, but dentate granule cells do not. The CA1 circuits seem, then, to require conservation of the passive cable properties of their elements, whereas dentate does not. We suggest that the reason CA1 neurons scale conservatively is that, for this region, each individual synaptic input exerts a significant effect on the cell's output, whereas in dentate the neuronal output represents the average of a large number of anonymous individual inputs.

Introduction

The brains of mammals, from pigmy tree shrew to man, range in size over about 4 orders of magnitude. Although the various mammalian brains have greatly different capabilities, most workers nevertheless believe they all conform to a generally uniform design; this belief is the basis for comparative neuroanatomy, and provides the justification for using, for example, rat or cat brains as models in neurobiological experiments intended to enlighten us about the workings of the human nervous system. To make any computational machine, including a brain, a thousand times larger is a difficult task, and the way this magnification is achieved can give some clues about the underlying principles used for designing

the computing circuitry. The goal of this chapter is to explore one aspect of this scaling problem related to altered cable properties in neurons that are magnified. Some background information will be necessary before we can give a precise statement of the problem we wish to investigate.

As brains grow in size, so do the nerve cells of which they are composed (Hardesty, 1902; Bok, 1959). The brain is unusual in this regard because the cells used to construct other organs − liver or gut, for example − do no differ very much in size between small and large animals (Teissier, 1939; Altman and Dittmer, 1961). The cell bodies of spinal motoneurons have about half the diameter in a small animal like a mouse than they have in man, and cortical neurons generally differ by about the same amount. In fact, the thickness of the cerebral cortex varies approximately as the 0.1 power of the cortical surface area (Stevens, 1989) so that if one brain is a thousand times larger than

* Present address: C.F. Stevens, The Salk Institute, 10010 North Torrey Pines Road, La Jolla, CA 92037, U.S.A.

another (mouse to man), its cortex is twice as thick and the corresponding neurons have dendritic trees that are double in length. Why do large brains have larger neurons? One likely explanation is that the increase in cell body size reflects the need for a larger biosynthetic capacity to maintain the larger axonal tree that must reach over longer distances. This presumably is at least part of the reason why spinal motoneurons and Betz cells are so large compared to other neurons in the same brain. Why then must cortical neurons have longer dendritic trees? The answer here is perhaps that the cortex must be thicker to accommodate larger and more rapidly conducting axons that communicate over greater distances in the large brain.

Different parts of a neuron's dendritic tree commonly have quite specific inputs (see, for example: Blackstad, 1956; Andersen et al., 1966; Blackstad et al., 1970; Blackstad, 1975). The most distal part, for example, might receive information from one brain region and the more proximal parts from another. The distal information is somewhat more attenuated by the neuron's cable properties than that arriving over proximal inputs. A particular distal synapse might, for example, have half the effect at the soma of a proximal synapse. In this case, if one neuron has a dendritic tree that is twice as long as that of another, and if the dendrites had the same diameters in both cases, then the distal input in the larger neuron would have only one fourth the effect of a proximal synapse. The relative influence of proximal and distal synapses, then, might be quite different for large and small neurons, and this difference could be of great functional significance if the circuitry assumed a particular balance between the influences of nearby and distant synapses. Thus larger brains must, whenever inputs are stratified as they generally are in cortex, deal with the problem of maintaining a constant balance between distal and proximal inputs. We wish to investigate theoretically and experimentally this scaling problem. Our goal, then, is to ask how neurons differ between small and large brains, to estimate how significant cable at-

tenuation of distal signals is likely to be in particular classes of neuron, to propose several ways the brain might deal with the problem of keeping proximal and distal inputs in balance, and to ask which methods are used in fact. Our preliminary observations suggest that different classes of neurons deal with the size problem in different ways, and this in turn indicates that the various parts of the brain may not have just the same organizational principles.

The following discussion is organized in 4 parts. In the first part we present experimental data, gathered in a new way, that provides estimates of the cable characteristics of hippocampal neurons, and also presents measurements on the magnitude of depolarization produced by a single quantum of neurotransmitter. These data will highlight the implications of dendritic cable properties for neuronal function and provide the physiological basis for the consideration of morphological features that follows. The second part presents a theoretical analysis of the functional implications of making a neuron larger and develops the concept of "conservative scaling", a set of rules according to which a larger neuron would be electrically equivalent to a smaller one of the same shape. This section is needed to indicate what morphological features of a dendritic tree must be measured to gain insight into the functional implications of neuronal size changes. The third section gives some preliminary measurements that indicate what rules neurons actually follow when they are enlarged by evolution. We will conclude that not all neurons follow the same rules. In the final section we speculate on the implication of our observations for neuronal function. We shall suggest that the rules a neuron follows in being evolutionarily enlarged may give clues to differences in function.

We have chosen the hippocampus as a model system in which to investigate these questions because of its importance and simple structure. We shall consider neuronal properties in the dentate granule cells and pyramidal cells of the CA1 region in cat and human.

Attenuation of synaptic signals by dendrites

This section will present some preliminary data on the cable properties of hippocampal pyramidal cells in tissue culture. These results were obtained using a technique that should make immediately clear the issues in cable attenuation of synaptic signals. In particular, we will show directly the dramatic effect of cable filtering when a synaptic current is injected far out on the dendritic tree.

Briefly, the experimental procedure was as follows. Pyramidal cells from the CA1 and CA3 fields of the hippocampi of neonatal rats were maintained in culture for up to 3 weeks using the methods described by Jahr and Stevens (1987). The cell density was sufficiently low that the dendritic field of each cell could be traced without much ambiguity, i.e. cells were separated, on average, by several hundred microns. Membrane currents were measured from a cell via a patch electrode, sealed onto the cell body, in the whole-cell configuration as described by Bekkers and Stevens (1989). The objective was to inject a known current at different places on the dendritic tree and measure the cable-distorted form of it that reached the soma. This was done using a trick suggested by a finding made at the neuromuscular junction: Fatt and Katz (1952) showed that applying hypertonic solutions increased the frequency of miniature endplate potentials, an effect possibly due to osmotic shrinkage causing asynchronous exocytosis of presynaptic, neurotransmitter-loaded vesicles. We found that a similar process occurred in our culture system. When we applied a narrow stream of hypertonic solution to a place close to the voltage-clamped soma of a pyramidal cell, we usually observed a sudden increase in small, rapid currents. We have shown elsewhere that these currents are evoked local to the flow of solution, and have all the features of miniature excitatory postsynaptic currents ("mini EPSCs") (Bekkers and Stevens, 1989).

Use can be made of these solution-evoked currents to study cable properties if one makes the following assumption: that the currents have a constant mean size, as seen at their site of origin, no matter where on the dendritic tree they are elicited. This is equivalent to supposing that all excitatory synapses, wherever they are located, possess similar amounts of the same kind of receptor. This seems reasonable, and is also supported by studies of synaptic currents in these cultures (Bekkers and Stevens, unpublished). Local solution application now becomes equivalent to the local injection of a known current, equal to the mean mini EPSC amplitude, at known places on the cell, allowing direct estimation of dendritic cable properties.

Examples of hypertonic solution-evoked mini EPSCs are shown in Fig. 1. Panel A shows a train of mini EPSCs recorded at the soma when applying the solution close to the soma, i.e. when cable distortion is minimal. The currents vary markedly in size − we think this is mainly due to a distribu-

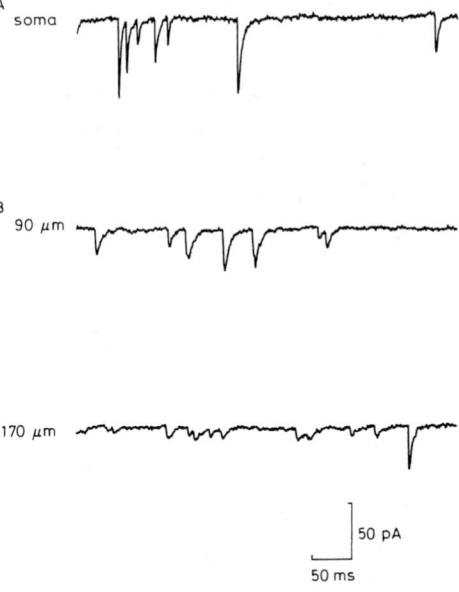

Fig. 1. Miniature EPSCs elicited by the application of hypertonic solution at the soma (A) and at the indicated distances from the soma down a dendrite (B,C). The soma was voltage clamped at − 70 mV; the patch electrode contained CsCl. The hypertonic solution was bath solution (standard mammalian Ringers) plus 0.5 M sucrose, and was applied in short bursts from a puffer pipette and removed via a nearby suction pipette, localizing its flow to a narrow (20 − 30 μm) plume.

tion in the sizes of presynaptic vesicles at one or a few synapses — but their shapes are similar. Panels B and C show mini EPSCs recorded when the solution is applied on the same dendrite but at 90 μm and 170 μm, respectively, from the soma. The currents now look much smaller and slower, and this is, by the above assumption, entirely due to the cable distortion of the dendrite. The traces in Fig. 1 thus show directly what current the cell body "sees" when a presynaptic impulse arrives at a synapse located proximally (panel A) or increasingly distally (panels B and C).

A preliminary analysis of data like these was done as follows. The patch pipette contained, in addition to the usual electrolyte solution, a fluorescent dye (Lucifer yellow) that allowed us to measure accurately the lengths and diameters of all the dendrites of the cell. Usually we applied the hypertonic solution to a dendrite that extended for a couple of hundred microns from the soma without branching or tapering significantly (total dendritic length was typically 300 – 600 μm); thus, to a first approximation the dendrite could be treated as a semi-infinite cable with the diameter we measured (Rall, 1962). The decrement of voltage (DC) along such a cable, when a constant voltage V_0 is applied at the sealed end, is given by $V(x) = V_0 \exp(-x/\lambda)$ where x is distance and λ is the DC length constant. It can be shown that the time integral of current reaching the sealed end (or soma) from distance x (i.e. the charge transfer) behaves the same as $V(x)$. Thus, the DC length constant can be extracted from our voltage clamp data by integrating the currents evoked at different distances along the dendrite and fitting an exponential to a plot of this charge versus distance.

Results are shown in Fig. 2A for 3 different cells. The vertical axis is charge transfer to the soma normalized to the mean charge measured from synapses located on the soma. (Each open symbol represents an average of 60 – 100 individual integrated currents.) Note the logarithmic scale. The horizontal axis is distance from the soma at which the minis were elicited, normalized to a dendrite diameter of 1 μm (because λ depends

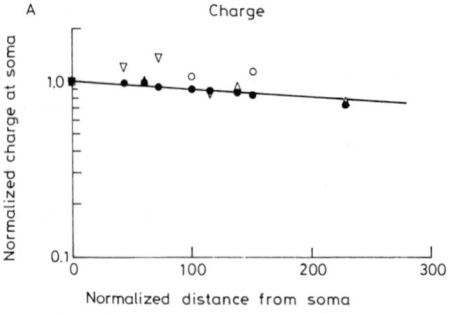

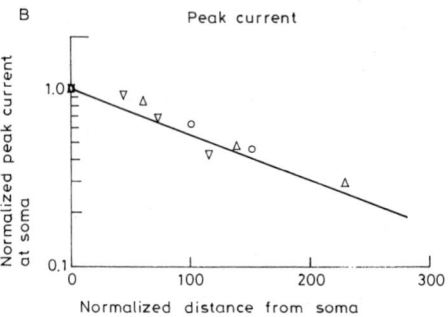

Fig. 2. Dependence of charge transfer to the soma (A) and peak current at the soma (B) on distance between the soma and the point on the dendrite at which current was injected using the hypertonic solution technique described in the text. Actual distances have been normalized to equivalent distances for a 1-μm-diameter dendrite. Data are from 3 different cells and each of the 3 symbol types refers to one of the 3 neurons.

on diameter; see later on). Data from 3 cells are shown, with actual dendrite diameters of 0.5 μm, 1 μm and 1.9 μm. The straight line is fitted by eye and gives $\lambda = 1000$ μm for a 1 μm diameter dendrite. Also shown in the figure (filled symbols) are the same data analyzed in a slightly different way: the transfer function for a semi-infinite cable was used to calculate the expected distortion of mini EPSCs elicited at different distances, and λ was varied for each cell until the calculated and measured currents looked similar. The agreement between the two methods was good, supporting the validity of the semi-infinite cable approximation.

Fig. 2B shows data from the same 3 cells as in Fig. 2A except that instead of charge transfer, the peak mini current is plotted against normalized distance to the injection site. It can immediately be noted that the peak of the current seen at the soma falls off much more rapidly with distance than does the charge transfer. The *transient length constant* estimated from these data (from the slope of the straight line in the figure) is about 170 μm for the unit diameter dendrite. Note that the transient length constant, although a useful descriptive term, is not a true constant. It depends on the temporal form of the input signal, and changes (becomes smaller) as distance from the synapse is increased.

The technique used above causes single quanta of neurotransmitter to be released and permits us to produce releases close to the recording site. This means that we can, in the same experiments, measure the depolarization produced by a single quantum of transmitter, the smallest effect that a synapse can have on its target neuron. We find that the mean mini EPSP amplitude is about 2 mV for releases induced close to the soma although mini amplitudes can sometimes exceed 10 mV. Since the average number of quanta released at hippocampal synapses is unknown, we cannot estimate the effect of a single impulse arrival on a hippocampal pyramidal cell. Nevertheless, we note that the depolarization caused by a single quantum is at least an order of magnitude larger than reported in spinal motoneurons (Kuno, 1964; Edwards et al., 1976; Jack et al., 1981), and that the coincident release of only a few quanta would be sufficient to cause the cell to fire. We also note that our minis are somewhat larger than those reported by Sayer et al. (1989); this discrepancy may result from differences between cultured neurons and those in slices, or from the fact that the intracellular electrodes cause a larger shunt conductance than do patch electrodes.

In summary, these results show directly the effects of cable distortion on physiological inputs at varying distances out on a dendrite. In particular, they emphasize that different features of synaptic transmission are affected differently by this distortion: charge transfer to the soma is attenuated much less significantly than is peak current.

How might a neuron scale?

For convenience in discussion, we will take the neurons in an animal with a particular size as a reference, and refer to these neurons as "standard"; we take the cat as our reference and will compare human neurons to this standard. Thus, we will note, for example, that human dentate granule cells have dendrites that are about three and a half times the standard length, and that mouse granule cells would be smaller than standard.

As discussed in the preceding section, distal inputs into a cortical neuron's dendritic tree can be quite strikingly attenuated. If the length of a standard dendrite were doubled, the effect on inputs to the distal third, say, would be comparatively smaller than in the standard dendrite if the dendritic diameter were unchanged. In order to have some guidance as to what morphological characteristics to examine in neurons of different sizes, we start with a theoretical treatment of how a neuron might be scaled up in such a way as to preserve its passive electrical properties. We assume for simplicity that the neuron's dendritic tree can be treated as being constructed of nontapering cylinders with uniform membrane properties and intracellular resistivity, and that the resistance of the extracellular space can be neglected.

The obvious way to keep peripheral and distal inputs in balance as a neuron is made larger is to increase the dendritic diameter so that the length of the neuron's dendritic cable remains the same as the standard. The DC length constant for a cable is (see Rall, 1962):

$$\lambda = \sqrt{\frac{Rd}{4r}} \tag{1}$$

where R is the membrane resistance ($\Omega \cdot cm^2$), d is the dendrite diameter, and r is the resistivity of the dendritic cytoplasm ($\Omega \cdot cm$). In our cultured neurons, we found the length constant to be about

1 mm for $d = 1$ μm. If a neuron is magnified from the standard by a factor m, the length constant must also be magnified by m to keep the electrotonic length of the dendrites unchanged. The new length constant is related to the standard one by

$$\lambda = m \lambda_s \qquad (2)$$

The new dendritic diameter d must then be related to the standard diameter d_s by the relation (which arises by substituting equation 1 for 2 with the appropriate subscripts)

$$\sqrt{d} = m\sqrt{d_s} \text{ or } d = m^2 d_s \qquad (3)$$

Thus, dendritic diameters must scale like the square of the magnification factor. For example, if a particular neuron is twice as large as the standard, it must have dendrites that have 4 times the standard diameter (not twice) for the entire neuron to have the same electrotonic length and thus achieve the same balance between distal and proximal inputs.

When a neuron has dendrites with increased diameter, however, it has a much greater surface area, and a correspondingly lower input resistance. This means that each synapse providing a standard amount of current would have a smaller effect on a magnified neuron than it would on the standard neuron.

More specifically, the input resistance of a cable varies in proportion to the length constant and inversely as the dendritic diameter squared (see equation 3.06 of Rall, 1977). When a neuron's linear dimensions are magnified by a factor m and the dendritic diameters by m^2, the input resistance therefore varies inversely with m^3. For a particular synapse to have the same effect in the magnified neuron, then, it must provide current that is m^3 times larger than the standard. For example, a neuron that has twice the linear dimensions as standard with 4 times the dendritic diameter (to have a standard electrotonic length for its dendritic

tree) would require 8 times the strength of each synapse in order for the synapses to cause a standard depolarization.

The required m^3-fold increase in effectiveness could be achieved in two ways. First, each synapse could have a sufficiently increased conductance to provide the required current. Since the synapses in large and small brains seem about the same size, this possibility seems unlikely. Alternatively, each synapse could be functionally duplicated m^3-fold times. In the example given above where $m = 2$, each synaptic type could be represented 8 times as often on the cell dendrites. When a neuron's linear dimensions are increased by m and its dendritic diameters increased by m^2, the surface area increases by the product m^3. Thus, if dendrites had a constant number of synapses per unit surface area, the required functional increase in synaptic current could be achieved by appropriate reduplication of contacts.

We shall term magnification of this sort – longitudinal dimensions (that is, dendritic lengths) magnified by m and dendritic diameters by m^2 – *conservative scaling* because the dendritic cable properties and receptive surface area vary jointly in a way that could leave the neuron's integrative electrical properties unchanged. Note that, because the cable equation can be written in terms of length constant and time constant units, all passive electrical properties of a neuron are unchanged by conservative scaling.

One way a brain could increase the size of its neurons and leave them functionally unchanged, then, is by conservative scaling. Other alternatives are more difficult to evaluate. For example, membrane properties could in principle be altered, or synaptic patterns on a neuron's dendrites could perhaps be rearranged in a way to achieve the same end.

The preceding theory has indicated one way a neuron can deal with the problems that arise when it is magnified, and we now know which morphological characteristic to measure to determine the extent to which conservative scaling is used.

How do neurons scale?

The human hippocampus has about 5 times as many neurons as the cat's (Seress, 1988). Are hippocampal neurons magnified when the hippocampal size is increased? Measurements of cat dentate gyrus show that the dendritic layer is about 155 μm thick whereas comparable measurements on human hippocampus give a value of 540 μm; the dendritic layer in human is thus about 3.5 times thicker, suggesting that the dendrites are 3–4 times longer in humans.

For the CA1 region, the cat dendritic layer averaged about 440 μm while that for the human, in a comparable region, was about 610 μm, a ratio of about one and a third.

Clearly, then, human hippocampal neurons are larger than those in cat with the disparity being considerably greater for dentate granule cells than for CA1 pyramidal neurons.

The magnification factor m used in the preceding section cannot, however, be estimated simply from the dendritic layer thickness. Because dendrites do not run normal to the cortical surface but rather at an angle, a dendrite that traversed the entire dendritic layer of a cortex would have a length increased by a further factor of $1/\cos(A)$ where A is the angle relative to the surface. We therefore have compared the longitudinal and lateral extent of cat and human dendritic trees in Golgi – Cox preparations. The forms of dentate granule cells are strikingly similar in the two species and, in fact, the human cells are, in terms of dendritic length, simply magnified versions of the cat neurons so that the magnification factor, in fact, can be obtained directly from the dendritic layer thickness. For the dentate, the dendrites of both species fit in a cone with an angle at its apex of approximately 90°. The similarity of granule cell forms in cat and human is well illustrated by the very typical examples shown superimposed in Fig. 3.

Pyramidal cells have dendritic trees with more complex forms, but here again one is struck by the great similarity in shapes. For both species, the

apical dendrites mostly fit in a cone with an apical angle of about 65°, and most basal dendrites are contained in a cone characterized by a 75° angle (although a few dendrites stray outside their cones in both cases). In summary, then, both human dentate granule cells and pyramidal neurons have the same form as the corresponding cells in the cat but are magnified 3.5 and 1.4 times respectively.

Because dendrites vary considerably in diameter, a complete comparison of the diameters between cat and human is quite difficult. If the neurons investigated here scaled conservatively, the human granule cells should have dendritic diameters $3.5^2 = 12.3$ times larger than the cat, and the human pyramidal neurons should have dendritic diameters $1.4^2 = 2$ times larger than the cat. Since the expected effects are rather large, we adopted a simpler approach: for all of the cell types, the diameters of a population of dendrites were measured at a point in the dendritic layer that is one half the entire extent of the dendritic length. This approach avoids the complete reconstruction of a large number of neurons and provides a preliminary quantitative test of the hypothesis that

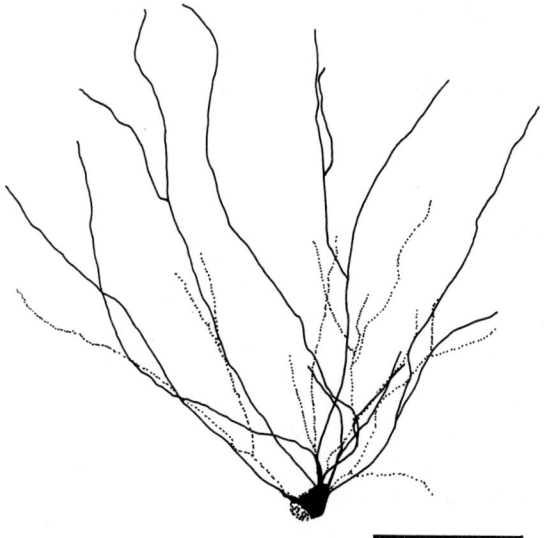

Fig. 3. A typical cat dentate granule cell drawn (dotted) superimposed on a corresponding human neuron. Note that many of the human neuron dendrites are truncated because they have left the plane of the section. Scale bar = 0.1 mm.

a particular neuronal class scales conservatively.

For the human granule cells the dendritic diameter at half tree averaged 0.89 μm $\pm$ 0.06 μm (mean $\pm$ S.E.M.) whereas for the cat it was 0.79 μm $\pm$ 0.05 μm. Although these measurements are subject to many errors, the human dendritic diameters clearly were not appreciably different from those in the cat, and certainly nothing like the twelve-fold ratio of diameters required by conservative scaling. We conclude, then, that dentate granule cells have much longer dendrites in the large human brain than in the small cat brain, but that the dendritic diameters are not different in the two cases. This conclusion is immediately obvious from an examination of the Golgi – Cox preparations.

Although the human CA1 pyramids had (in the areas compared) dendrites that were only 40% longer than those in the cat, the dendritic diameters at half tree were very different in the two cases: 1.6 μm $\pm$ 0.17 μm (mean $\pm$ S.E.M.) for human and 0.64 μm $\pm$ 0.02 μm for cat. If these neurons scaled conservatively the cat neurons should have half the diameter of the human neurons as indicated above. Thus conservative scaling predicts the cat dendritic diameter half way out the dendritic tree should be 0.78 μm $\pm$ 0.12 μm whereas the observed diameter is 0.64 μm $\pm$ 0.02 μm; clearly the observed dendritic diameters are not significantly different from the conservation scaling predictions. Again, the human/cat difference is immediately apparent from the histological sections. CA1 pyramids seem, then, to conform to the expectations of conservative scaling. Although we have not made measurements on CA3 pyramids or on the pyramidal neurons of the subiculum, they appear, on inspection, to follow conservative scaling.

Functional implications

To summarize briefly: hippocampal pyramidal cells (in culture) have a DC length constant of about 1 mm for a 1-μm-diameter dendrite, but a transient length constant about 5 times smaller. A single quantum of transmitter produces a mean depolarization, at the site of origin, of about 2 mV, a value more than an order of magnitude greater than that reported for spinal motoneurons. The hippocampal pyramidal neurons scale conservatively, but neighboring dentate granule cells do not. What can these observations mean?

If synaptic inputs to a neuron are unstratified, or if the stratification of inputs is of no particular functional importance (although it may have developmental significance, for example), then maintaining the precise balance between inputs that are proximal and those that are distal on the dendritic tree may not be necessary for the circuits to function properly. Here, simply the net input may be what is significant, so conservative scaling would not be needed. Dentate granule cells perhaps are of this type.

Alternatively, if keeping the various proximal and distal inputs equivalent in their influence on the neuron's output is required for the circuits to function properly, then conservative scaling would be appropriate. An interesting feature of hippocampal neuronal function is that a single quantum of transmitter can have such a large effect on the membrane potential. As noted above, quantal size in the central nervous system seems to vary quite considerably, so that some individual quanta can approach the size necessary to fire a neuron single-handedly. In cases where the weights of specific inputs can be so important – in contradistinction to spinal motoneurons where individual synaptic events play little role in determining neuronal firing – keeping a balance between the various inputs assumes increased importance. Since our hippocampal pyramidal neurons seem to have outputs that can be determined by only a few inputs, we suggest that they must scale conservatively for just this reason.

Thus, hippocampal pyramidal cells may well need to use conservative scaling to maintain the effectiveness of distal inputs since each individual synapse can be significant in determining the neuron's output. We would suggest, then, that neurons like the dentate granule cells, which do not scale conservatively, effectively integrate synaptic currents and depend less on the synchronous activation of spike generation by only a few inputs. It will be interesting to investigate the electrophysiological properties of dentate neurons.

We propose that conservative scaling is used by neurons in which a balance between distal and proximal inputs must be maintained as neuronal size is altered and particularly when neuronal output is determined by the synchronous activation of only a few inputs. Alternatively, neurons whose outputs depend just on the net synaptic activation with little importance attached to the source of individual inputs need not scale conservatively. Hippocampal pyramidal neurons in the CA1 field would be an example in the first category and dentate granule cells in the second. If this proposal is correct, then considerable information about how a neuron behaves can be deduced from how evolution changes its size.

References

Altman, P.L. and Dittmer, D.S. (Eds.) (1961) *Blood and Other Body Fluids.* Federation of American Societies for Experimental Biology, Bethesda, MD.

Andersen, P., Blackstad, T.W. and Lomo, T. (1966) Location and identification of excitatory synapses on hippocampal pyramidal cells. *Exp. Brain Res.,* 1: 236–248.

Bekkers, J.M. and Stevens, C.F. (1989) NMDA and non-NMDA receptors are colocalized at individual excitatory synapses in cultured rat hippocampus. *Nature (Lond.),* 341: 230–233.

Blackstad, T.W. (1956) Commissural connections of the hippocampus of the rat, with special reference to their mode of termination. *J. Comp. Neurol.,* 105: 417–538.

Blackstad, T.W. (1975) Electron microscopy of experimental axonal degeneration in photochemically modified Golgi preparations: a procedure for precise mapping of nervous connections. *Brain Res.,* 95: 191–210.

Blackstad, T.W., Brink, K., Hem, J. and Jeune, B. (1970) Distribution of hippocampal mossy fibers in the rat. An experimental study with silver impregnation methods. *J. Comp. Neurol.,* 138: 433–449.

Bok, S.T. (1959) *Histonomy of the Cerebral Cortex.* Elsevier, Amsterdam.

Edwards, F.R., Redman, S.J. and Walmsley, B. (1976) Statistical fluctuations in charge transfer at Ia synapses on spinal motoneurones. *J. Physiol. (Lond.),* 259: 665–688.

Fatt, P. and Katz, B. (1952) Spontaneous subthreshold activity at motor nerve endings. *J. Physiol. (Lond.),* 117: 109–128.

Hardesty, I. (1902) Observations on the medulla spinalis of the elephant with some comparative studies of the intumescentia cervicalis and the neurones of the columna anterior. *J. Comp. Neurol.,* 12: 125–182.

Jack, J.J.B., Redman, S.J. and Wong, K. (1981) The components of synaptic potentials evoked in cat spinal motoneurones by impulses in single group Ia fibres. *J. Physiol. (Lond.),* 321: 65–96.

Jahr, C.E. and Stevens, C.F. (1987) Glutamate activates multiple single channel conductances in hippocampal neurons. *Nature (Lond.),* 325: No. 6104, 522–525.

Kuno, M. (1964) Quantal components of excitatory potentials in spinal motoneurones. *J. Physiol. (Lond.),* 175: 81–99.

Rall, W. (1962) Theory of physiological properties of dendrites. *Ann. N.Y. Acad. Sci.,* 96: 1071–1092.

Rall, W. (1977) Core conductor theory and cable properties of neurons. In J.M. Brookhart and V.B. Mountcastle (Eds.), *Handbook of Physiology. The Nervous System, Cellular Biology of Neurons, Vol. 1, Part 1,* Am. Physiol. Soc., Bethesda, MD, pp. 39–97.

Sayer, R.J., Redman, S.J. and Andersen, P. (1989) Amplitude fluctuations in small EPSPs recorded from CA1 pyramidal cells in the guinea pig hippocampal slice. *J. Neurosci.,* 9: 840–850.

Seress, L. (1988) Interspecies comparison of the hippocampal formation shows increased emphasis on the Regio superior in the Ammon's horn of the human brain. *J. Hirnforsch.,* 29: 335–340.

Stevens, C.F. (1989) How cortical interconnectedness varies with network size. *Neural Computation,* 1: 473–479.

Teissier, G. (1939) Biometrie de la cellule. *Tabulae Biol.,* 19: 1–64.

J. Storm-Mathisen, J. Zimmer and O.P. Ottersen (Eds.)
Progress in Brain Research, Vol. 83
© 1990 Elsevier Science Publishers B.V. (Biomedical Division)

CHAPTER 4

The subiculum: cytoarchitectonically a simple structure, but hodologically complex

Menno P. Witter and Henk J. Groenewegen

Department of Anatomy and Embryology, Vrije Universiteit, van der Boechorststraat 7, 1081 BT Amsterdam, The Netherlands

The subiculum gives rise to the majority of hippocampal projections to various telencephalic and diencephalic structures. Previously, these projections have been described using anterograde tracing with radioactively labeled amino acids. As part of an ongoing detailed analysis of the connectivity of the hippocampal region in the rat, we studied the projections of the subiculum by means of the recently introduced sensitive anterograde tracer *Phaseolus vulgaris*-leukoagglutinin (PHA-L) and double-labeling protocols with retrogradely transported fluorescent tracers. Within the subiculum, populations of neurons can be differentiated that each give rise to projections to a unique set of target structures. These populations of neurons, characterized according to common efferent connectivity, are differentially positioned along the transverse axis of the subiculum. Thus, subicular cells near the border with the CA1 field project to targets different from those reached by projections from subicular cells situated close to the border with the presubiculum. We further observed that major afferents of the subiculum, i.e. those arising from field CA1 and from the entorhinal cortex, are also organized along the transverse axis of the subiculum. We suggest that within the subiculum, that appears homogeneous with respect to both cytoarchitectonic and chemoarchitectonic characteristics, a differentiation can be made with respect to its major connections. Whether this differentiation takes the form of a "columnar organization" as known for the neocortex, or a "compartmentation" as shown for the striatum is not yet clear.

Introduction

The subiculum is considered to constitute the major output structure of the hippocampus (see Köhler, this volume). It gives rise to fibers that travel through the fornix to, among others, the mammillary bodies, the ventral hypothalamus, the midline nuclei of the thalamus, the septal complex and the nucleus accumbens. Other, extra-fornical projections reach the infralimbic, entorhinal, and perirhinal cortices, and the presubiculum and parasubiculum (Swanson and Cowan, 1977; Swanson et al., 1978). Within the circuitry of the hippocampus, the subiculum is the final waystation in what is generally considered a largely unidirectional sequence of projections that link the various subdivisions of the hippocampus (Fig. 1). The above-mentioned subicular projections exhibit a differential distribution that appears strongly related to the site of origin of these projections along the longitudinal axis of the hippocampus (Swanson and Cowan, 1977; see also Witter, 1986). For example, the dorsal portion of the subiculum (dorsal subiculum) distributes its efferents predominantly to the mammillary bodies and the presubiculum. By contrast, the ventral part of the subiculum (ventral subiculum) sends fibers to the ventral hypothalamus, the amygdaloid complex, and the parasubiculum. Likewise, the topographical organization of the projections to the septal complex is related to a dorsoventral axis in the subiculum (Meibach and Siegel, 1977a; Swanson and Cowan, 1979). The same holds for the reciprocal connections between the subiculum and the entorhinal cortex in the cat (Van Groen et al., 1986).

Apart from this dorsoventral differentiation within the subiculum, a few reports indicate the presence of mediolateral or transverse differences with respect to the origin of its efferent connections. Meibach and Siegel (1977a, b) described that in the rat the projections to the septal region originate predominantly from cells in that part of the subiculum that borders CA1 (the proximal part of the subiculum). In contrast, the projections to the anterior thalamus arise mainly from subiculum neurons adjacent to the presubiculum (the distal part of the subiculum). The projections to the

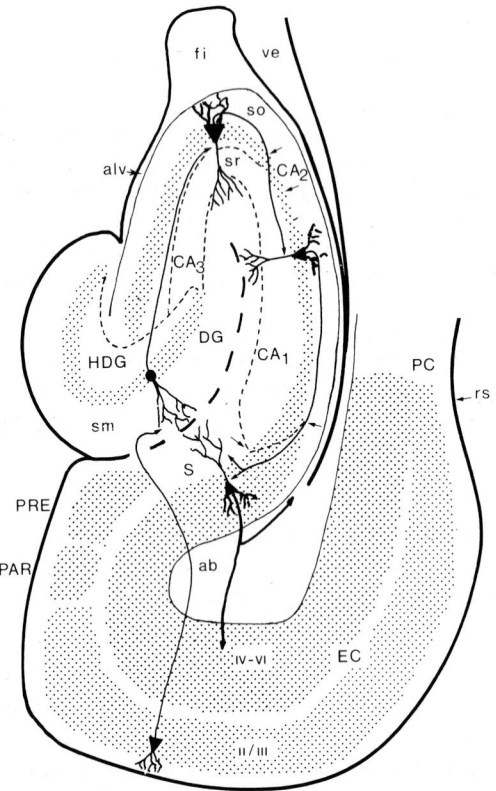

Fig. 1. Schematic representation of a horizontal section through the hippocampal region of the rat brain. The various subdivisions and their interconnecting pathways are indicated. Note that the projections of the entorhinal cortex to the Ammon's horn and the subiculum are not indicated (modified after Witter, 1989). Abbreviations: ab, angular bundle; alv, alveus; CA1 – 3, subdivisions of the Ammon's horn; DG, dentate gyrus; EC, entorhinal cortex; fi, fimbria; HDG, hilus of the dentate gyrus; PAR, parasubiculum; PC, perirhinal cortex; PRE, presubiculum; rs, rhinal sulcus; S, subiculum; sm, stratum moleculare; so, stratum oriens; sr, stratum radiatum; ve, lateral ventricle.

mammillary complex show a topographical organization, such that the proximal part of the subiculum projects to medial parts of the mammillary nuclei and the distal part of the subiculum projects to the lateral parts of this complex. Similar findings have been reported in the squirrel monkey (Krayniak et al., 1979). Furthermore, projections from the dorsal subiculum to the entorhinal cortex and the septal complex (Swanson et al., 1981), and those to the entorhinal cortex and the mammillary complex (Donovan and Wyss, 1983) arise, at least in part, as collaterals from single subicular neurons.

The level of precision with which connections in the brain, the hippocampal region not excepted, have been described, is largely dependent on the sensitivity and reliability of the available tracing techniques. The recently introduced technique, using the anterograde tracer *Phaseolus vulgaris* leukoagglutinin (PHA-L; Gerfen and Sawchenko, 1984) has several advantages over older anterograde tracing techniques. The iontophoretic application of PHA-L results in small, restricted injections that can be precisely delineated. The resulting labeling of fibers and of terminal ramifications as well as terminal specializations enables us to analyze a certain projection in far greater detail than with the older tracing methods (cf. Groenewegen and Wouterlood, 1990). In the course of our recent studies in the rat on the organization of the perforant pathway and the projections from the subiculum to the nucleus accumbens, we noted that with respect to these connections there are differences between the dorsal and ventral subiculum as well as between its proximal and distal parts (Groenewegen et al., 1987; Witter et al., 1989a). In the present account it is explored whether these and other efferent and afferent connections of the subiculum are similarly organized.

Materials and methods

The material on which the present observations are based, consists of a large collection of rat brains in which anterograde and/or retrograde tracers were injected in the hippocampal and parahippocampal areas or in one or several of the target structures of the subiculum. Injections of the anterograde tracer PHA-L were placed in the parahippocampal cortex in order to label the parahippocampal-hippocampal system, and in the subiculum to mark its efferent projections. The injection procedure and the subsequent histological and immunohistochemical treatments have been described in extenso previously (Gerfen and Sawchenko, 1984; Groenewegen et al., 1987; Groenewegen and Wouterlood, 1990). In order to determine the precise relationships of populations of subicular neurons projecting to different targets, two or three different fluorescent retrograde tracers were injected in target areas of the subiculum. These areas include the prefrontal, infralimbic, and retrosplenial cortices, the parahippocampal region, the ventral striatum, the septum, the anterior thalamic nuclei, the ventral hypothalamus, and the mammillary and supramammillary nuclei. The following fluorescent tracers were used: Fast blue (FB; Kuypers et al., 1977), Fluoro-Gold (FG; Schmued and Fallon, 1986) and Diamidino yellow (DY; Kuypers et al., 1977). These tracers can be easily distinguished from each other in the fluorescence microscope using a single filter combination. Detailed data on the injection- and histological procedures used in our laboratory have been given elsewhere (Groenewegen, 1988; Groenewegen and Wouterlood, 1990; Witter et al., 1990).

The three-dimensional shape of the rodent hippocampus is relatively complex. Its long axis is curved in a C-shaped manner from the septal complex rostrodorsally to the amygdaloid complex ventrally. As a result, routine frontal sectioning of the entire rat forebrain results in truly transverse sections of the hippocampus of only a very restricted dorsal part, where its longitudinal axis parallels the long axis of the brain. However, sections cut in the same manner through the caudal and ventral portions of the hippocampus, are not in the transverse plane. To facilitate the interpretation of the arrangement of the anterogradely labeled afferent fibers or the retrogradely labeled efferent neurons in the subiculum, in several cases the hippocampal region was dissected out of the perfused brain prior to sectioning and the hippocampus was flattened between two microscope slides as described by Gaarskjaer (1978). The longitudinal axis of this so-called "extended hippocampus" approaches a straight line and transverse sections over its entire longitudinal extent can be cut.

Results

Nomenclature and architectonics of the hippocampal region

The hippocampal region consists of the hippocampal formation and the parahippocampal region (Fig. 1). The hippocampal formation can be further subdivided into the dentate gyrus, the Ammon's horn, and the subiculum. As described above, the hippocampal formation is an elongated, C-shaped structure of which the long axis will be referred to as the dorsoventral axis, and the orthogonal dentate-to-subicular axis as the transverse or proximodistal axis. The constituent fields of the hippocampus have been further subdivided in various ways. Within the dentate gyrus the hilar region is generally distinguished from the cortical layers. The Ammon's horn is subdivided into at least two fields that differ with respect to the size of their pyramidal cells. The regio inferior (nomenclature according to Ramón y Cajal, 1911) or fields CA3/CA2 (nomenclature according to Lorente de Nó, 1934) contains large pyramidal cells, whereas the regio superior, or field CA1, is characterized by the presence of small pyramidal cells, that are more densely packed than in the region inferior (for a more detailed description of the dentate gyrus and Ammon's horn and for further references, see Swanson et al., 1987; Lopes da Silva et al., 1990). There are different opinions as to whether there exists a distinguishable field, the prosubiculum, between CA1 and the subiculum. This term was used by Lorente de Nó (1934) for a field that directly borders the CA1 field and shares some cytoarchitectonic characteristics with both CA1 and the subiculum. However, most contemporary authors consider the prosubiculum as an area where the fields CA1 and the subiculum overlap. As a consequence, the border between the CA1 field and the subiculum is markedly oblique. In the present paper, we will follow this usage and will not distinguish a prosubiculum (Fig. 1).

In essence, the architecture of all hippocampal subfields is remarkably similar. They consist of a single layer of neurons of which the apical dendrites extend in a cell-poor zone, i.e. the stratum moleculare of the dentate gyrus and the subiculum and the stratum lacunosum-moleculare and stratum radiatum of the Ammon's horn. Underneath the cell layer lies the polymorph layer which in turn is bordered by a fiber layer.

The subiculum is bordered distally by the presubiculum which, in turn, is bounded at its distal side by the parasubiculum. The latter area adjoins the entorhinal cortex. The entorhinal cortex, particularly in rodents, is generally divided into medial and lateral subdivisions. The lateral border of the entorhinal cortex coincides with the posterior rhinal sulcus where the perirhinal cortex is located (Fig. 1).

Outline of intrinsic organization of the hippocampal region

The generally accepted circuitry of the hippocampal region has been studied and described by numerous authors (Fig. 1). The most prominent projection from the entorhinal cortex is the so-called perforant pathway to the dentate gyrus (Steward, 1976; Wyss, 1981). Additional projections to CA3, CA1 and the subiculum have been noted. The numerical and possible functional importance of these latter projections have only recently been stressed (cf. Witter, 1989; Witter et al., 1989a and references therein). The granule cells of the dentate gyrus project through their mossy fibers to CA3. Pyramidal cells in CA3 give rise to collateralized axons of which the so-called

Schaffer-collaterals provide the major input to CA1. Finally, pyramidal cells in CA1 project to the subiculum. It should be pointed out that from recent anatomical studies a far more complex organizational pattern of the intrinsic connectivity has emerged which will not be discussed in the present context (for an overview see Amaral and Witter, 1989; Witter, 1989).

Efferents of the subiculum

Injections of PHA-L in the dorsal subiculum

Following an injection that labels subicular neurons in the dorsal subiculum, close to the border with CA1, i.e. in its proximal part (Fig. 2A), labeled fibers and terminals (not illustrated) are present in the infralimbic cortex, the perirhinal

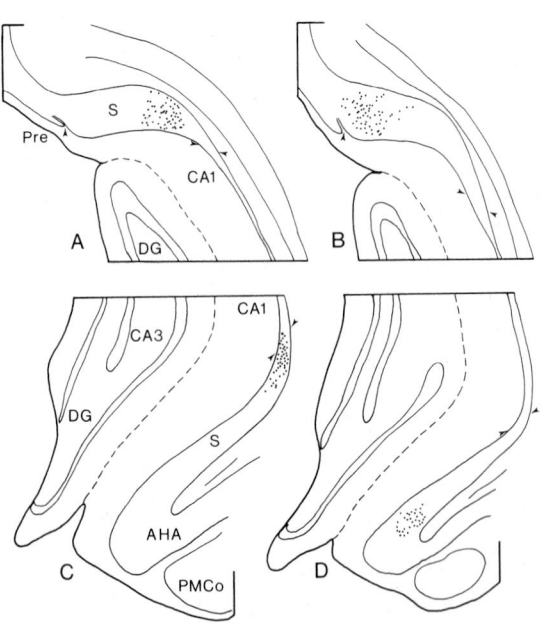

Fig. 2. Camera lucida drawings of representative frontal sections through the injection sites of PHA-L in the subiculum. Proximal (A) and distal (B) injections in the dorsal subiculum. Proximal (C) and distal (D) injections in the ventral subiculum. Neurons that incorporated the tracer and are thus considered to give rise to anterogradely labeled projections are indicated by small dots. Abbreviations: AHA, amygdalo-hippocampal area; CA1/3, subfields of the Ammon's horn; DG, dentate gyrus; PMCo, posteromedial nucleus of the amygdala; Pre, presubiculum; S, subiculum.

cortex and the adjacent lateral part of the entorhinal cortex, and, though weakly, dorsally in the presubiculum. Labeling is also visible rostrolaterally in the nucleus accumbens, in dorsal parts of the lateral septum, mainly in the dorsal and intermediate nuclei (nomenclature according to Swanson and Cowan, 1979), and in the interanteromedial nucleus of the thalamus.

In contrast, an injection of PHA-L located more distally in the dorsal subiculum, resulting in uptake by neurons located close to the border with the presubiculum (Fig. 2B), does not result in marked labeling in any of the structures that are labeled following the proximal injection. Only in the dorsal and intermediate nuclei of the septum and in the midline thalamus were a few labeled fibers observed. However, this injection results in marked labeling in the retrosplenial cortex, mainly in its ventral part directly bordering the presubiculum. Also this latter structure contains dense labeling. Furthermore, dense labeling is present in the anterodorsal and anteroventral nuclei of the thalamus.

Both injections in the dorsal subiculum result in clear labeling in the medial nuclei of the mammillary complex. However, the proximal part of the subiculum projects to medial parts of the medial mammillary nucleus, whereas its distal part projects to lateral parts of this nucleus. These observations confirm the earlier findings of Meibach and Siegel (1977a, b).

Injections of PHA-L in the ventral subiculum

Injections that involve the ventral subiculum result in labeling in a set of structures that only in part overlaps with the collection of structures that were labeled following dorsal subicular injections. Irrespective of the proximodistal location of the ventral injections, anterograde labeling in the anterior nuclei of the thalamus or in the interanteromedial nucleus is extremely weak or absent. Also the mammillary bodies and the perirhinal cortex contain little or no labeling. Following injections involving cells proximally in the ventral subiculum (Fig. 2C), the densest label-

ing is present medially in the entorhinal cortex, in the dorsal nucleus of the lateral septal complex, in the caudomedial part of the nucleus accumbens, and in the basolateral nucleus of the amygdaloid complex. Weaker labeling is present in the infralimbic cortex and the anterior olfactory nucleus.

In the amygdala, the nucleus accumbens, and the infralimbic cortex, a similar, though much weaker pattern of labeling results from an injection in the distal part of the ventral subiculum (Fig. 2D). In this case, no labeling is present in the dorsal nucleus of the lateral septal complex, but dense labeling can be observed in its intermediate and ventral subdivisions. Furthermore, in the hypothalamus a densely labeled plexus surrounds the ventromedial nucleus. Labeled fibers are also present in the nucleus reuniens and the paraventricular nucleus of the thalamus.

Injections of retrograde tracers in target areas of the subiculum

In these experiments we injected two or three different fluorescent retrograde tracers in various areas that contained labeled fibers after PHA-L injections in the dorsal or ventral subiculum. The injection sites for the retrograde tracers were chosen such that in each animal we aimed to inject at least one of the targets of the proximal and the distal parts of the subiculum. In general, the results from the retrograde tracing experiments confirm the anterograde findings and clearly indicate that within the subiculum at least two different compartments should be distinguished. A detailed analysis of these experiments is given elsewhere (Witter et al., 1990). In the present account, first a few representative cases with retrograde injections will be discussed. In one animal we injected the lateral part of the nucleus accumbens (FG) and the retrosplenial cortex (DY). As is illustrated in Fig. 3A, both FG- and DY-positive cells are present in the dorsal subiculum. In the ventral subiculum, only a few FG-labeled cells, but no DY-positive cells were observed (not illustrated). The distribution of the two types of labeled cells is

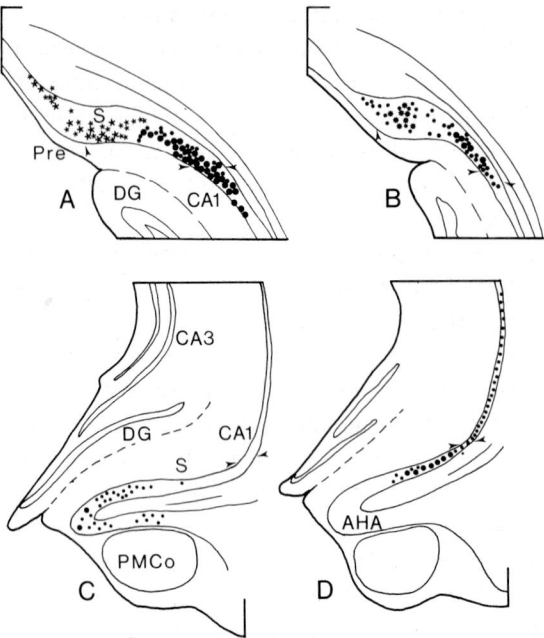

Fig. 3. Camera lucida drawings of representative frontal sections through the dorsal (A, B) and ventral (C, D) subiculum illustrating the distribution of retrogradely labeled cells following injections in various target areas of subicular projections: A: the retrosplenial cortex (cells represented by stars) and entorhinal cortex (cells represented by dots). B: the retrosplenial cortex (stars) and the nucleus accumbens (dots). C: the ventromedial hypothalamic area. D: the dorsal subdivision of the lateral septal nucleus. Small stars/dots represent 1 retrogradely labeled cell, large ones represent 5 marked cells. Abbreviations: see legend of Fig. 2.

are found only in the proximal part of the dorsal subiculum and in the adjacent part of CA1. In both experiments (Fig. 3A,B) there is very little overlap between the two populations of labeled cells, and no double-labeled cells are present.

In a separate series of experiments injections of retrograde tracers were placed in targets of the ventral subiculum. For example, in one animal we successfully injected Fluoro-Gold (FG) in the ventromedial hypothalamic area. This injection resulted in retrogradely labeled cells in the ventral subiculum, confined to its distal part (Fig. 3C). It should be noted that at more caudal levels, where the ventral part of the subiculum merges with the dorsal part, the number of labeled cells rapidly decreases. In Fig. 3D, the distribution of labeled cells following an FG-injection in the dorsal subdivision of the lateral septum is illustrated in a section that is taken at a level comparable to that of Fig. 3C. In this case, the retrogradely labeled cells are almost exclusively located in the proximal part of the ventral subiculum and the adjacent part of CA1. No FG-positive cells were observed in the distal part of the ventral subiculum or in its dorsal portion. Similar to what we described for the dorsal subiculum, in each experiment, the position of labeled neurons in the ventral subiculum is remarkably constant in sections taken from different rostrocaudal levels.

Afferents of the subiculum

In the course of an ongoing study of the precise organization of the major connections of the hippocampal formation in the rat, we analyzed the projections from the entorhinal cortex and field CA1 to the subiculum. Following injections of PHA-L in the superficial layers of the entorhinal cortex both fiber and dense terminal labeling was observed in the subiculum. The projections from the entorhinal cortex to the subiculum appear to be topographically organized along the dorsoventral axis of the subiculum, such that lateral parts of the entorhinal cortex, i.e. parts adjacent to the rhinal sulcus project preferentially to the dorsal

similar at all levels of the dorsal subiculum. The DY-labeled cells, that result from the injection in the retrosplenial cortex are virtually confined to the distal half of the dorsal subiculum. In contrast, the cells that project to the lateral nucleus accumbens (FG-positive) are present only in the proximal half of the dorsal subiculum. Also, the adjacent part of the CA1-field contains FG-labeled cells. A remarkably comparable pattern of cell labeling was observed following injections in the retrosplenial cortex (FB) and laterally in the entorhinal cortex (DY; Fig. 3B). Also in this case, the FB-labeled cells are confined to the distal part of the dorsal subiculum, whereas DY-positive cells subiculum, and medial parts of the entorhinal cortex project to the ventral subiculum. A similar topography is present in the projections to all other subfields of the hippocampal formation, i.e. the dentate gyrus and the Ammon's horn (Witter, 1989; Witter et al., 1989a). Also in the cat and the monkey such a topography has been observed (Witter and Groenewegen, 1984; Van Groen et al., 1986; Witter et al., 1989b).

It has been well established that the projections from the entorhinal cortex to the hippocampal formation terminate in the dentate gyrus in the molecular layer. The two, cytoarchitectonically defined, subdivisions of the entorhinal cortex, the lateral (LEA) and medial area (MEA) give rise to fibers that exhibit a different terminal distribution along the dendrites of the dentate granule cells. Fibers that originate in LEA, the so-called lateral perforant pathway, terminate in the outer one-third of the molecular layer, whereas those from the MEA distribute to the middle one-third (Steward, 1976; Wyss, 1981; Witter, 1989). A similar terminal differentiation has been noted with respect to the fibers that distribute to CA3. In contrast, the projections to CA1 are differentially organized. Steward (1976) reported that the medial perforant pathway preferentially terminates in the proximal part of CA1, whereas the lateral component distributes to the distal part of CA1. Using PHA-L as an anterograde tracer, in combination with the "extended preparation" of the hippocampal formation, we were recently able to confirm these observations (Fig. 4A,B). Moreover, a detailed analysis of the projections from the entorhinal cortex to the subiculum (cf. Witter, 1989) has revealed that these projections, like those to CA1, are also organized along the transverse axis. Injections of PHA-L that involve the lateral subdivision of the entorhinal cortex (LEA) preferentially label a terminal field in the molecular layer of the subiculum with a proximal position, whereas injections in the medial subdivision (MEA) result in a distally positioned terminal field. It should be stressed that the two terminal fields to some extent appear to overlap (compare Fig. 4A,B).

Following injections in the CA1 field, we observed that injections that have different positions along its transverse or proximal-to-distal axis, label projections that show a different terminal distribution along the transverse axis of the subiculum. Two representative cases are illustrated in Fig. 5. An injection in the distal part of CA1 (Fig. 5A) labels a terminal field in the pyramidal layer and the inner half of the molecular layer of the proximal part of the subiculum, close to the border with CA1 (Fig. 5B). In contrast, following an injection proximally in CA1, involving cells close to the border with field CA3 (Fig. 5C), a densely labeled terminal plexus is present in the distal part of the subiculum (Fig. 5D).

Discussion

The present results of both the anterograde and retrograde tracing experiments indicate that the subiculum is a heterogeneous structure with respect to its efferent and afferent connectivity. This heterogeneity occurs along both the longitudinal and transverse axes of the subiculum. The dif-

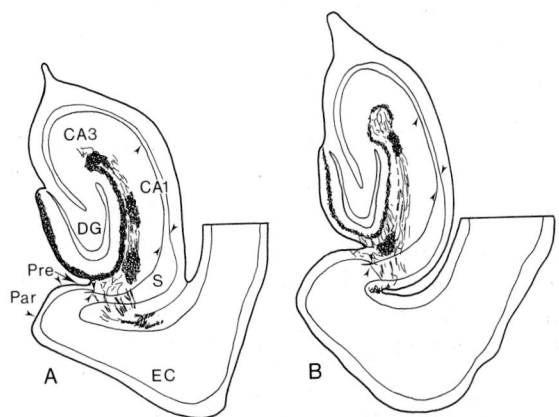

Fig. 4. Camera lucida drawings of sections cut transversely to the long axis of the hippocampus ("extended preparation" according to the protocol of Gaarskjaer, 1978) illustrating the distribution of PHA-L positive fibers and terminals following injections in the lateral (A) and medial subdivisions (B) of the entorhinal cortex. Note the different position of the terminal fields in the subiculum in relation to its borders with CA1 and the presubiculum. Abbreviations: see legend of Fig. 1.

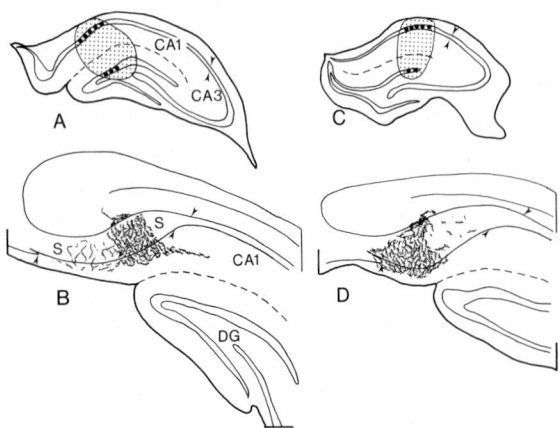

Fig. 5. Camera lucida drawings of frontal sections through PHA-L injection sites in the dorsal part of CA1 (A, C) and of representative frontal sections through the dorsal subiculum illustrating the resulting anterograde labeling (B, D). Following an injection in the distal part of CA1 (A), the labeled terminal field in the subiculum is located in the proximal half of the subiculum (B). In contrast, the injection in the proximal part of CA1 (C) labels a distally positioned terminal field in the subiculum (D). Abbreviations: see legend of Fig. 1.

ferential origin of a number of the efferent projections along the longitudinal axis of the subiculum have previously been published. Swanson and Cowan (1977) reported that the dorsal subiculum gives rise to dense projections to the mammillary complex and the anterior nuclei of the thalamus, but not to the ventral hypothalamus. In contrast, the ventral subiculum projects almost exclusively to a shell that surrounds the ventromedial hypothalamic nucleus and to the amygdaloid complex, but not to the mammillary nuclei or the anterior thalamic nuclei. Our data not only confirm these findings, but indicate that the ventral subiculum projects in addition to the nucleus reuniens and the paraventricular nucleus of the thalamus.

Also differentiation along the transverse axis of the subiculum has been observed previously (Meibach and Siegel, 1977a, b). These authors described that projections to the septal region originate predominantly from cells in the proximal part of the dorsal subiculum, whereas the projec-

tions to the anterior thalamus arise mainly from its distal part. Furthermore, the projections to the mammillary bodies are topographically organized, such that the proximal part of the dorsal subiculum projects to medial parts of the mammillary nuclei and the distal part of the dorsal subiculum projects to the lateral parts of this complex (Meibach and Siegel, 1977a, b). Our present results are in agreement with these findings, but extend them in a sense that projections which arise from the ventral subiculum show a comparable differentiation along the transverse axis. Projections to the ventromedial hypothalamic area, the paraventricular and reuniens nuclei arise mainly from the distal part of the ventral subiculum, whereas those to the entorhinal cortex, nucleus accumbens and dorsal subdivision of the lateral septal complex originate predominantly in the proximal part.

The projections to the entorhinal cortex, the septal complex, and the mammillary complex all appear to originate in the proximal half of the subiculum. These projections have been reported to arise, at least in part, as collaterals from single subicular neurons (Swanson et al., 1981; Donovan and Wyss, 1983). Since our retrograde tracing experiments were primarily designed to differentiate between populations of subicular projection neurons not necessarily located in the same part of the subiculum, our present material is not suited for an analysis of the degree of collateralization of subicular efferents.

With respect to the afferents of the subiculum, originating in the entorhinal cortex and CA1, it is important to note that both exhibit a terminal distribution that respects the transverse axis of the subiculum. Depending on the site of origin in CA1, distally or proximally in this hippocampal field, the terminal fields occupy the proximal or distal half of the subiculum, respectively. Therefore, they appear to differentiate between two components of the subiculum that are also recognized on the basis of the origin of subicular efferents as described above. However, other possibilities must be taken into account. Intracellular injections have indicated that the axonal distribution in the subiculum of the CA1-pyramidal cells resembles a very narrow column (Tamamaki et al., 1987). The authors also described a proximal-to-distal relation between origin and termination of the CA1 projection to the subiculum, similar to the organization we encountered. Therefore, the organization of the CA1-to-subiculum pathway may be more gradual, such that a shift in origin along the proximal-to-distal axis in CA1 results in a distal-to-proximal shift of the terminal field in the subiculum. With respect to the projections from the entorhinal cortex to the subiculum, comparable organizational schemes may apply. The lateral and medial subdivisions of the entorhinal cortex may give rise to two terminal fields, that are differently located along the transverse axis of the subiculum. As an alternative, a more gradual shift from a proximal to a distal position of the terminal field may be proposed. Clearly, more detailed data are required before the validity of either of the alternatives becomes clear. Finally, the question whether the terminal distributions in the subiculum of the projections from the entorhinal cortex and from field CA1 are organized according to the same set of principles can, as yet, not be answered.

The major novel finding of the present study is the hodological heterogeneity along the transverse axis of the subiculum. This heterogeneity is not reflected in any way in cytoarchitectonic or chemoarchitectonic differences. The results indicate that within the subiculum different populations of cells exist, each projecting to or receiving inputs from different brain areas or from different subdivisions within these areas. However, as outlined in the previous paragraph, it is not yet clear whether these connections are all organized according to the same principle(s), and thus characterize similar subdivisions of the subiculum. For example, is the population of neurons in the dorsal subiculum that project to the entorhinal cortex (i.e. the proximally located cells) the same group that receives inputs from the lateral part of the entorhinal cortex (LEA)? Alternatively, is each of the afferents and efferents of the subiculum

organized according to a specific set of rules, such that the resulting organizational pattern within the subiculum is a complex mosaic-like pattern? A third alternative is that some of the connections may actually divide the subiculum into two populations of neurons, each of which projects to a highly specific combination of targets, whereas others, like the projections to the mammillary complex, are arranged according to a gradient-like pattern with respect to their origin; still other connections, like the inputs from CA1 and the entorhinal cortex may have a columnar type of organization. As yet, there are no data that specifically single out one of these alternatives.

Are the presently described hodological differences within the subiculum reminiscent of a "columnar organization" as known for the neocortex, or a "compartmentation" as shown in the striatum? Both organizational principles probably reflect functional subunits in parts of the cortex and of a subcortical structure, respectively, that appear homogeneous in cytoarchitectonic respect. The cortical columnar organization has been demonstrated most elegantly, both anatomically and physiologically, for the primary visual cortex (cf. Braitenberg, 1985 and references therein), but appears to be a rather general organizational principle for other neocortical areas (cf. Eccles, 1984). However, it is not clear whether the functional columns in the visual cortex, that have been described with electrophysiological techniques and with the deoxyglucose method (Sokoloff et al., 1977), are similar to the patterns described with histochemical staining for the activity of cytochrome oxidase. The use of the latter marker leads to the definition of cortical units (so-called blobs and interblobs) that show a constant organization of their interconnections. In contrast, some of the characteristics of the columns that are defined by their metabolic activities (deoxyglucose patterns) are highly variable. For example, in the visual cortex, the location of columns is strongly related to the type of visual stimulus that is presented to identify them (Crawford, 1985). On the other hand, columns in the association cortex that are defined on the basis of corticocortical connections appear to be divided into at least two columns that are defined on the basis of their specific thalamic inputs (Eccles, 1984, and references therein).

The recognition of the compartmental structure of the striatum is of recent date, and, similar to the situation in the cortex, the relationship between the morphological/immunohistochemical and functional compartmentation is not yet clear (e.g. Graybiel, 1983; Alexander and DeLong, 1985a, b; Gerfen et al., 1987; Groenewegen et al., 1989; Voorn et al., 1989). However, recent evidence suggests that there is a morphological basis for the striatal compartments, in that the dendritic arbors of the most common striatal neuronal type, the medium-sized spiny cell, are confined to the borders of the compartments (Penny et al., 1988).

Before we can conclude that the organization of the subiculum exhibits columnar or compartmental characteristics, it will be necessary to gain more data. The results of present experiments indicate that this cytoarchitectonically homogeneous structure is not homogeneous with respect to its inputs and outputs. How these inputs and outputs are exactly arranged, along a transverse and a dorsal-to-ventral coordinate, and how the inputs and outputs are interrelated is not yet clear. In this respect the development of anatomical tracing techniques in which anterograde and retrograde tracers, and two anterograde tracers can be combined in one and the same tissue section (for review see Groenewegen and Wouterlood, 1990) appears to be very promising.

Acknowledgements

We gratefully acknowledge the help of Ms. Barbara Jorritsma-Byham, Ms. Andrea de Gier, and Mr. Robert Ostendorf with the preparation of the experimental material. We also thank Drs. Vera Fernandes de Lima and Hester Daelmans for letting us use part of their experimental material on the projections of CA1, and Dr. Anthony Lohman for critically reading the manuscript and providing helpful suggestions.

References

Alexander, G.E. and DeLong, M.R. (1985a) Microstimulation of the primate neostriatum. I. Physiological properties of striatal microexcitable zones. *J. Neurophysiol.,* 53: 1401 – 1416.

Alexander, G.E. and DeLong, M.R. (1985b) Microstimulation of the primate neostriatum. II. Somatotopic organization of striatal microexcitable zones and their relation to neuronal response properties. *J. Neurophysiol.,* 53: 1417 – 1430.

Amaral, D.G. and Witter, M.P. (1989) The three dimensional organization of the hippocampal formation: a review of anatomical data. *Neuroscience,* 31: 571 – 591.

Braitenberg, V. (1985) Charting the visual cortex. In E.G. Jones and A. Peters (Eds.), *Cerebral Cortex, Vol. 3, Visual Cortex,* Plenum Press, New York, pp. 379 – 414.

Crawford, M.L.J. (1985) Stimulus-specific columns in monkey visual cortex as revealed by the (14C)-2-deoxyglucose method. In E.G. Jones and A. Peters (Eds.), *Cerebral Cortex, Vol. 3, Visual Cortex,* Plenum Press, New York. pp. 331 – 350.

Donovan, M.K. and Wyss, J.M. (1983) Evidence for some collateralization between cortical and diencephalic efferent axons of the rat subicular cortex. *Brain Res.,* 259: 181 – 192.

Eccles, J.C. (1984) The cerebral cortex: a theory of its operation. In E.G. Jones and A. Peters (Eds.), *Cerebral Cortex, Vol. 2, Functional Properties of Cortical Cells,* Plenum Press, New York, pp. 1 – 38.

Gaarskjaer, F.B. (1978) Organization of the mossy fiber system of the rat studied in extended hippocampi. I. Terminal area related to number of granule and pyramidal cells. *J. Comp. Neurol.,* 178: 49 – 72.

Gerfen, C.R. and Sawchenko, P.E. (1984) An anterograde neuroanatomical method that shows the detailed morphology of neurons, their axons and terminals. Immunohistochemical localization of an axonally transported plant lectin *Phaseolus vulgaris* leucoagglutinin (PHA-L). *Brain Res.,* 290: 219 – 238.

Gerfen, C.R., Herkenham, M. and Thibault, J. (1987) The neostriatal mosaic. II. Compartmental organization of mesostriatal dopaminergic and non-dopaminergic systems. *J. Neurosci.,* 7: 3915 – 3934.

Graybiel, A.M. (1983) Compartmental organization of the mammalian striatum. In J.-P. Changeux, M. Imbert and F.E. Bloom (Eds.), *Molecular and Cellular Mechanisms Underlying Higher Brain Functions, Progress in Brain Research, Vol. 58,* Elsevier, Amsterdam, pp. 247 – 256.

Groenewegen, H.J. (1988) Organization of the afferent connections of the mediodorsal thalamic nucleus in the rat, related to the mediodorsal prefrontal topography. *Neuroscience,* 24: 379 – 431.

Groenewegen, H.J. and Wouterlood, F.G. (1990) Light and electron microscopic tracing of neuronal connections with *Phaseolus vulgaris*-leucoagglutinin (PHA-L), and combinations with other neuroanatomical techniques. In F.G.

Wouterlood, A.N. vandenPol, A. Björklund and T. Hökfelt (Eds.), *Handbook of Chemical Neuroanatomy, Vol. 8, Approaches to the Analysis of Neuronal Microcircuits and Synaptic Interactions,* Elsevier, Amsterdam, pp. 47 – 124.

Groenewegen, H.J., Vermeulen-Van der Zee, E., Te Kortschot, A. and Witter, M.P. (1987) Organization of the projections from the subiculum to the striatum in the rat. A study using anterograde transport of *Phaseolus vulgaris* leucoagglutinin (PHA-L). *Neuroscience,* 23: 103 – 120.

Groenewegen, H.J., Meredith, G.E., Berendse, H.W., Voorn, P. and Wolters, J.G. (1989) The compartmental organization of the ventral striatum in the rat. In A.R. Crossman and M.A. Sambrook (Eds.), *Current Problems in Neurology, Vol. 9, Neural Mechanisms in Disorders of Movement,* John Libbey, London, pp. 45 – 54.

Krayniak, P.F., Siegel, A., Meibach, R.C., Fruchtman, D. and Scrimenti, M. (1979) Origin of the fornix system in the squirrel monkey. *Brain Res.,* 160: 401 – 411.

Kuypers, H.G.J.M., Catsman-Berrevoets, C.E. and Padt, R.E. (1977) Retrograde axonal transport of fluorescent substances in the rat's forebrain. *Neurosci. Lett.,* 6: 127 – 135.

Lopes da Silva, F.H., Witter, M.P., Boeijinga, P.H. and Lohman, A.H.M. (1990) Anatomical organization and physiology of the limbic cortex. *Physiol. Rev.,* 70: 1 – 59.

Lorente de Nó, R. (1934) Studies on the structure of the cerebral cortex. II. Continuation of the study of the ammonic system. *J. Psychol. Neurol.,* 46: 113 – 177.

Meibach, R.C. and Siegel, A. (1977a) Efferent connections of the hippocampal formation in the rat. *Brain Res.,* 124: 197 – 224.

Meibach, R.C. and Siegel, A. (1977b) Thalamic projections of the hippocampal formation: evidence for an alternate pathway involving the internal capsule. *Brain Res.,* 134: 1 – 12.

Penny, G.R., Wilson, C.J. and Kitai, S.T. (1988) Relationship of the axonal and dendritic geometry of spiny projection neurons to the compartmental organization of the neostriatum. *J. Comp. Neurol.,* 269: 275 – 289.

Ramón y Cajal, S. (1911) *Histologie du Système Nerveux de l'Homme et des Vertebrés,* Maloine, Paris.

Schmued, L.C. and Fallon, J.H. (1986) Fluoro-Gold: a new fluorescent retrograde axonal tracer with numerous unique properties. *Brain Res.,* 377: 147 – 154.

Sokoloff, L., Reivich, M., Kennedy, C., Des Rosiers, M.H., Patlak, C.S., Pettigrew, K.D., Sakurada, O. and Shinohara, M. (1977) The C-14-deoxyglucose method for the measurement of local cerebral glucose utilization: theory, procedure, and normal values in the conscious and anaesthetized rat. *J. Neurochem.,* 28: 897 – 916.

Steward, O. (1976) Topographic organization of the projections from the entorhinal area to the hippocampal formation of the rat. *J. Comp. Neurol.,* 167: 285 – 314.

Swanson, L.W. and Cowan, W.M. (1977) An autoradiographic study of the organization of the efferent connections of the hippocampal formation in the rat. *J. Comp. Neurol.,* 172: 49 – 84.

Swanson, L.W. and Cowan, W.M. (1979) The connections of the septal region in the rat. *J. Comp. Neurol.,* 186: 621 – 656.

Swanson, L.W., Wyss, J.M. and Cowan, W.M. (1978) An autoradiography study of the organization of intrahippocampal association pathways in the rat. *J. Comp. Neurol.,* 181: 681 – 716.

Swanson, L.W., Sawchenko, P.E. and Cowan, W.M. (1981) Evidence for collateral projections by neurons in Ammon's horn, the dentate gyrus, and the subiculum: a multiple retrograde labeling study in the rat. *J. Neurosci.,* 1: 548 – 559.

Swanson, L.W., Köhler, C. and Björklund, A. (1987) The limbic region. I. The septohippocampal system. In A. Björklund, T. Hökfelt and L.W. Swanson (Eds.), *Handbook of Chemical Neuroanatomy, Vol. 5, Integrated Systems of the CNS, Part 1,* Elsevier, Amsterdam, pp. 125 – 227.

Tamamaki, N., Abe, K. and Nojyo, Y. (1987) Columnar organization in the subiculum formed by axon branches originating from single CA1 pyramidal neurons in the rat hippocampus. *Brain Res.,* 412: 156 – 160.

Van Groen, Th., Van Haren, F.J., Witter, M.P. and Groenewegen, H.J. (1986) The organization of the reciprocal connections between the subiculum and the entorhinal cortex in the cat. I. A neuroanatomical tracing study. *J. Comp. Neurol.,* 250: 485 – 497.

Voorn, P., Gerfen, C.R. and Groenewegen, H.J. (1989) The compartmentalized organization of the ventral striatum of the rat: immunohistochemical distribution of enkephalin, substance P, dopamine, and calcium-binding protein. *J. Comp. Neurol.,* 289: 189 – 201.

Witter, M.P. (1986) A survey of the anatomy of the hippocampal formation, with emphasis on the septotemporal organization of its intrinsic and extrinsic connections. In R. Schwarz and Y. Ben-Ari (Eds.), *Excitatory Amino Acids and Epilepsy, Advances in Experimental Medicine and Biology, Vol. 203,* Plenum Press, New York, pp. 67 – 82.

Witter, M.P. (1989) Connectivity of the rat hippocampus. In V. Chan-Palay and C. Köhler (Eds.), *The Hippocampus – New Vistas, Neurology and Neurobiology, Vol. 52,* Alan Liss Inc., New York, pp. 53 – 69.

Witter, M.P. and Groenewegen, H.J. (1984) Laminar origin and septotemporal distribution of entorhinal and perirhinal projections to the hippocampus in the cat. *J. Comp. Neurol.,* 224: 371 – 385.

Witter, M.P., Groenewegen, H.J., Lopes da Silva, F.H. and Lohman, A.H.M. (1989a) Functional organization of the extrinsic and intrinsic circuitry of the parahippocampal region. *Prog. Neurobiol.,* 33: 161 – 253.

Witter, M.P., Van Hoesen, G.W. and Amaral, D.G. (1989b) Topographical organization of the entorhinal projection to the dentate gyrus of the monkey. *J. Neurosci.*, 9: 216 – 228.

Witter, M.P., Ostendorf, R.H. and Groenewegen, H.J. (1989c) Heterogeneity in the dorsal subiculum of the rat. Distinct neuronal columns project to different cortical and subcor-

tical targets. *Eur. J. Neurosci.*, submitted.

Wyss, J.M. (1981) An autoradiographic study of the efferent connections of the entorhinal cortex in the rat. *J. Comp. Neurol.*, 199: 495 – 512.

J. Storm-Mathisen, J. Zimmer and O.P. Ottersen (Eds.)
Progress in Brain Research, Vol. 83
© 1990 Elsevier Science Publishers B.V. (Biomedical Division)

CHAPTER 5

Subicular projections to the hypothalamus and brainstem: some novel aspects revealed in the rat by the anterograde *Phaseolus vulgaris* leukoagglutinin (PHA-L) tracing method

Christer Köhler

Department of Neuropharmacology, Astra Research Centre AB, S-151 85 Södertälje, Sweden

The efferent projections from the subiculum to the hypothalamus were examined in the rat by using the anterograde PHA-L tract-tracing method. The density of the subicular projections to the hypothalamus increases at successively more ventral levels of the subiculum. The ventral tip of the region projects to the hypothalamus via 3 different routes: the postcommissural fornix, the medial corticohypothalamic tract (*mht*) and a ventral pathway running via the amygdala. The fibers in the fornix innervate the median subgroup of the mammillary bodies and, through collaterals, also the lateral hypothalamus. Axons innervating the medial preoptic area, anterior hypothalamus, ventromedial and dorsomedial nuclei as well as the median part of the mammillary nucleus run in the *mht*. The ventral pathway innervates the supraoptic and medial preoptic nuclei as well as the lateral hypothalamus. Taken together, efferents of the ventral subiculum reach most major areas situated along the longitudinal axis of the hypothalamus. Importantly, however, subicular efferents reach beyond the hypothalamus: PHA-L immunoreactive axons were traced into the mesencephalic central gray and medulla. These anatomical findings show that highly processed cortical information may reach hypothalamic and brainstem areas involved in the integration of endocrine and autonomic functions as well as motivated behaviors.

Introduction

The hippocampal region is composed of serially arranged cortical fields, interconnected by association pathways which form the morphological substrate for a more or less unidirectional flow of neurotransmission through the structure (Swanson et al., 1988). Anatomical findings suggest that information processed along the so-called intrahippocampal trisynaptic circuit[a] may be relayed back to the entorhinal cortex and/or transmitted out from the hippocampus to a large number of subcortical or cortical areas (Shipley and Sörensen, 1975; Swanson and Cowan, 1977; Hjorth-Simonsen, 1981; Swanson et al., 1988). Thus, each hippocampal subfield gives rise to efferent projections with terminal fields in a wide range of extrahippocampal areas.

The subiculum occupies the final position in the trisynaptic circuit. Through its projections to the deep layers of the entorhinal cortex (Shipley and Sörensen, 1975; Köhler 1985), it closes this circuit. In addition to this feedback (Bantesaghi et al., 1989) to the entorhinal cortex, the subiculum has probably the most massive and divergent efferent projections of all hippocampal subfields. The most prominent of all subicular efferent projections terminates in the mammillary bodies (Swanson and

---

[a] The term *trisynaptic circuit* has been used to describe the projection (perforant path) from the entorhinal cortex to the area dentata, the projection (mossy fibers) from the area dentata to CA3 of Ammon's horn and the projection (Schaffer collaterals) from subfield CA3 to CA1. Stimulation of the perforant path has been shown to activate these associational pathways in a sequential manner (Andersen et al., 1971).

Cowan, 1975, 1977; Meibach and Siegel, 1975). Partly due to the existence of this connection, the subiculum has gained special attention as a link in the circuit connecting the mammillary bodies with the anterior thalamus and the hippocampus, proposed by Papez (1937) as a neural substrate of emotion. Furthermore, the existence of this pathway linked the subiculum also to memory functions. Since the important observation (Swanson and Cowan, 1975) was made that the subiculum, and not the Ammon's horn, is the origin of the hippocampal projection to the mammillary bodies, it has been shown to send projections to several other brain areas. Thus, the subiculum reaches, through monosynaptic projections, the lateral septum, nucleus accumbens, bed nucleus of stria terminalis, several thalamic and hypothalamic nuclei, including the mammillary bodies (see Swanson et al., 1988, for review). In the light of the central position occupied by the subiculum in hippocampal communication with other brain areas, it was decided to examine its efferent projections using the anterograde PHA-L tracing method (for additional data on the subiculum and its projections, see the chapter by Witter and Groenewegen, this volume).

Preparation of tissue

The lectin *Phaseolus vulgaris* leukoagglutinin was injected by iontophoresis through a thin glass capillary into different parts of the subiculum in deeply anesthetized male Sprague – Dawley rats. Since the dorsal and ventral parts of the subiculum are known to have partly different projections (Swanson and Cowan, 1977; Groenewegen et al., 1987), injections were placed at dorsal, midtemporal and ventral levels.

A total of 11 rats with PHA-L injections into different parts of the subiculum were included in the analysis. Of these, 4 animals with PHA-L injections in the ventral one-third of the subiculum were analyzed in detail for this report. The rats were sacrificed and their brains fixed by transcardial perfusion as previously described (Gerfen and Sawchenko, 1984; Köhler, 1985).

The fixed brains were cut on a freezing microtome and horizontal sections were incubated floating free in anti-PHA-L antibody (Vector Laboratories, Burlingame, CA, U.S.A.) for a period of 5 days. The antigen – antibody complex was made visible through the biotin avidin complex method of Hsu et al. (1981), using a commercially available kit (Vector Laboratories, Burlingame, CA, U.S.A.). Some sections in every series were osmium-treated in order to enhance the visibility of the reaction product while other sections were stained with thionine in order to visualize cytoarchitectonic landmarks.

Results

Differences in the efferent projection patterns have been described previously for the dorsal and ventral subiculum (Swanson and Cowan, 1977; Groenewegen et al., 1987). In the present paper the analysis has been focused on projections of the ventral one-third of the subiculum. The subicular efferents leave the structure by two major routes: a dorsal route via the fimbria-fornix system and a ventral route via the angular bundle and entorhinal cortex. Axons leaving the subiculum via these two routes innervate partly different structures, although certain overlap does exist. Through the findings from previous studies using anterograde autoradiographic and retrograde tracing methods, the most prominent targets of the subicular efferent projections have been identified (see Swan-

Fig. 1. A: photomicrograph showing an injection of PHA-L into the ventral subiculum (horizontal section). The injection was made in stratum radiatum and spread into the stratum pyramidale. This injection did not involve the most ventral aspect of the subiculum. Arrows delimit the subiculum. Axons descended to innervate pyramidal cells in the subiculum ventral to the injection site (B). Photomicrograph in C shows numerous PHA-L-stained axons in all layers of the infralimbic cortex. The axons from the injection shown in A run primarily in the medial cortico-hypothalamic tract (arrow) (D). Scale bars: A, 1 mm; B, 25 μm; C and D, 100 μm.

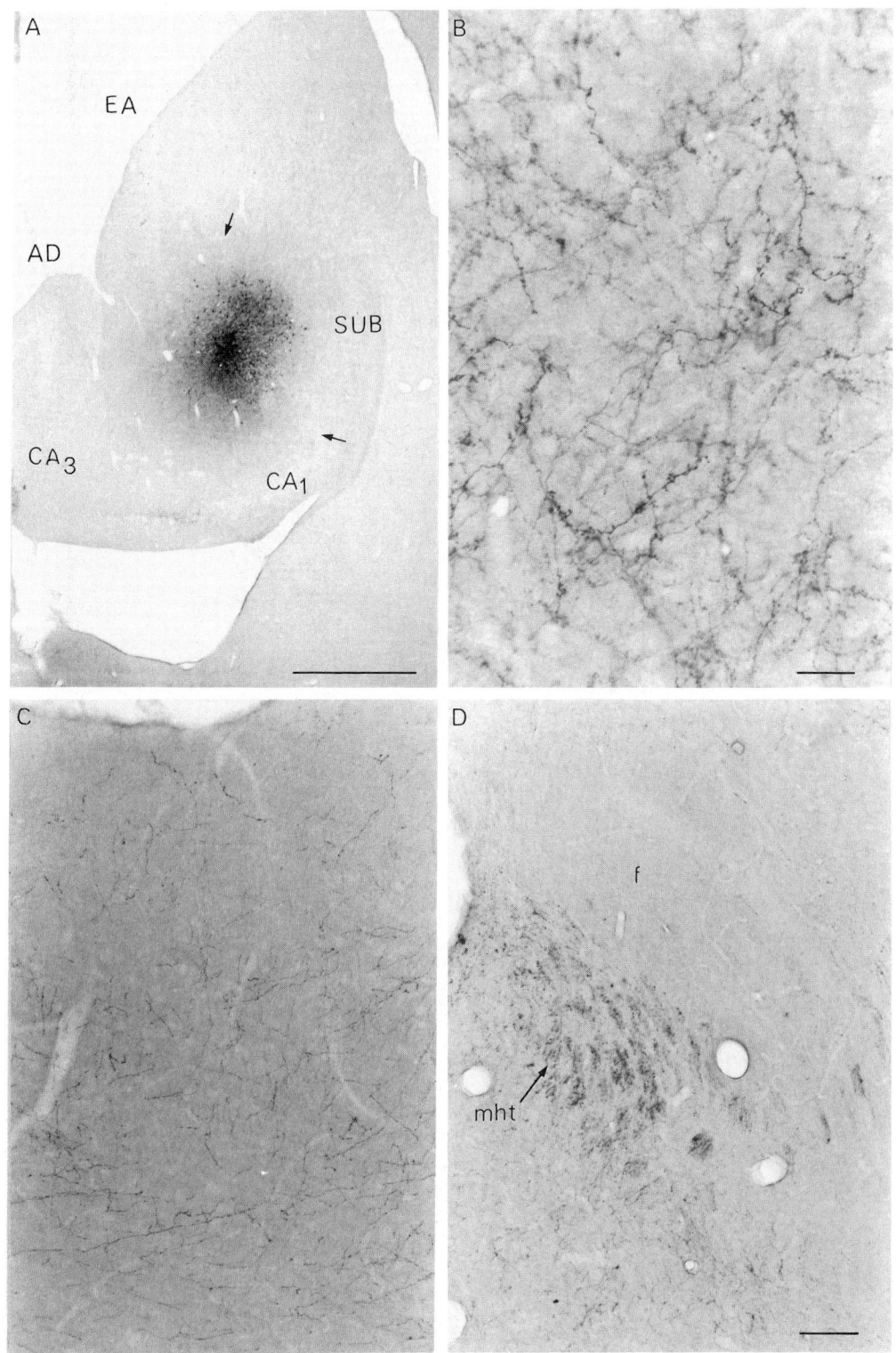

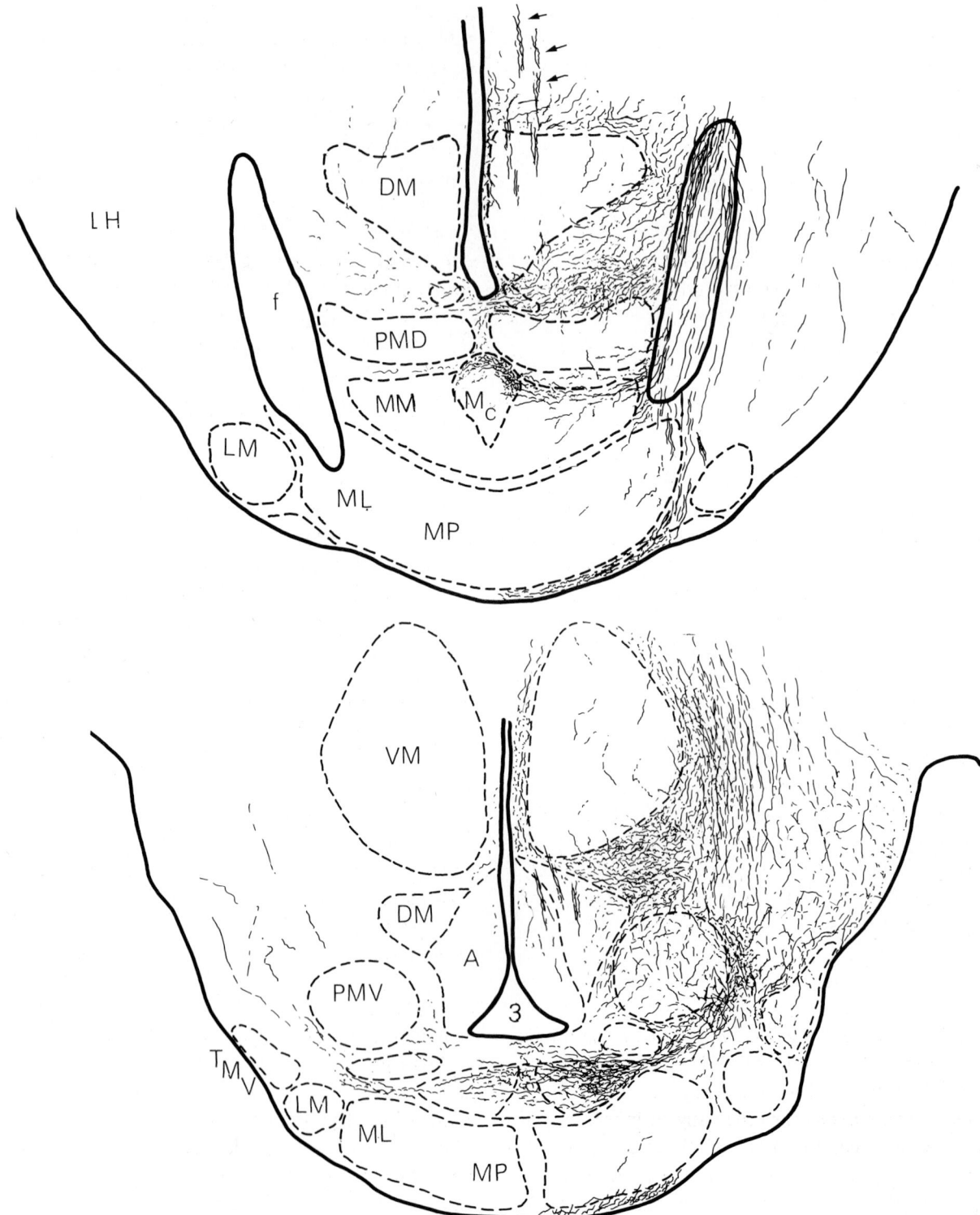

Fig. 2. Schematic drawings of horizontal sections through the ventral hypothalamus showing the principal pattern of ventral subicular efferents to this region. Arrows in the upper drawing (dorsal level) show fascicles of PHA-L stained axons running in the medial cortico-hypothalamic tract.

son et al. 1988, for review). Thus, after injections of PHA-L into the ventral subiculum (Fig. 1A), PHA-L immunostained axons could be followed into the fimbria and running towards the septum. As they enter the caudal septum, they divide and run in the pre- and postcommissural fornix. The precommissural fibers fan out rostrally to innervate the intermediate and lateral nuclei of the septum. Some fibers continue further rostrally into the deep layers of the infralimbic cortex (Fig. 1C), while another component provides a massive input to the nucleus accumbens and the rostromedial part of the caudate nucleus. The fibers in the postcommissural component of the fornix are destined for nuclei in the rostral and caudal hypothalamus. Importantly however, after PHA-L injections into the midtemporal and dorsal parts of the subiculum, PHA-L stained axons are running primarily in the columns of the fornix (Swanson and Cowand, 1977), while after deep ventral subicular injections immunostained axons run primarily in the medial cortico-hypothalamic tract (*mht*) (Fig. 1D). Thus, subicular efferents reach the hypothalamus by 3 different routes: the postcommissural fornix, the *mht* and a ventral pathway via the amygdala. The fibers of the well known subiculo-mammillary projection which originate primarily in the dorsal two-thirds of the subiculum, run on the other hand exclusively in the fornix. As the fibers in the fornix descend through the hypothalamus towards the mammillary bodies, axon-collaterals diverge to innervate the medially situated structures (Fig. 2). Together with fibers running in the *mht* they form a dense innervation of the anterior hypothalamic area and the ring structure of the ventromedial hypothalamus as well as the peripheral parts of the dorsomedial nucleus (Fig. 2). The central cores of these nuclei are essentially devoid of PHA-L stained axons (Fig. 2). As the fornix reaches the mammillary bodies some axons turn medially to innervate the medial and central parts of the median mammillary bodies. Some axons enter the dorsal premammillary nucleus while others continue in the fornix to the lateral part of the median mammillary bodies and to the ventral tuberomammillary nucleus (Figs. 2, 4D). Some axons can also be followed as they leave the fornix to innervate the lateral hypothalamic area.

The axons of the *mht* run in several distinct fascicles through the medial part of the hypothalamus (Fig. 2). The organization of these efferents has been described earlier, but the terminal fields of the *mht* have remained unknown. One component of this projection innervates the medial preoptic nucleus while the other runs as several distinct fascicles medial to the fornix. The *mht* innervates the medial zone of the hypothalamus along its entire rostro-caudal axis. Thus, these axons contribute major inputs to the anterior hypothalamic area, the ventomedial and dorsomedial nucleus (the ring structures around both nuclei), the paraventricular zone, the arcuate nucleus as well as the median part of the mamilllary nucleus (Fig. 2). A dense terminal field is surrounding the paraventricular nucleus, but no axons enter the nucleus (Fig. 4A).

After deep ventral PHA-L injections the innervation of the lateral hypothalamic area is quite prominent. The majority of the fibers enter the lateral hypothalamic area via the ventral route (Fig. 3D). This pathway passes through the entorhinal cortex and the amygdala. At the level of the optic tract it innervates the supraoptic nucleus (Fig. 4B) en route to its major terminal fields in the medial preoptic area, the ventral nucleus accumbens, and, after turning caudally, the lateral hypothalamic area.

It has been generally believed that efferents from the hippocampal region do not reach beyond the posterior hypothalamus. After ventral subicular PHA-L injections, however, numerous immunostained axons were found to leave the fornix at the level where it enters the mammillary bodies. These axons entered the mesencephalon and continue caudally as a distinct fiber bundle, which could be followed into the medulla. Scattered PHA-L-immunostained axons were found along the fourth ventricle all the way to the area postrema. Some of these axons appeared to fuse with the ependymal

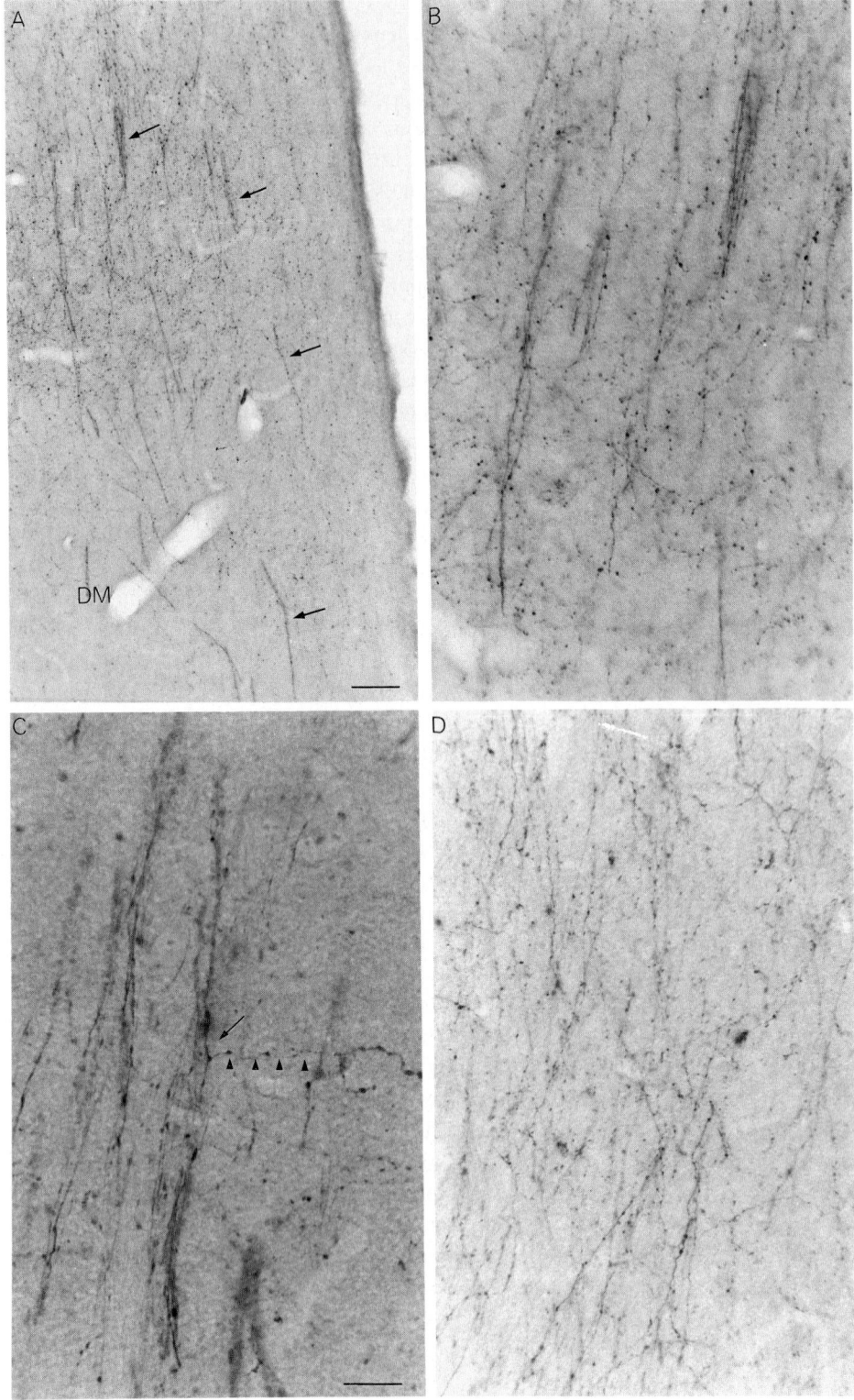

lining of the ventricular wall while others appeared slightly deeper in the brain (Fig. 5A – D).

PHA-L axons were also detected in the dorsal part of the central gray substance after the ventral subicular injections (Fig. 5B). These axons reach their targets via the thalamus and PHA-L-stained fibers could be followed as they radiated from the paraventricular nucleus of the thalamus all the way to the central gray substance. Scattered PHA-L axons were also found on the midline and ventricular surface of the dorsal raphe nucleus (Fig. 5D).

Discussion

Anatomical studies during the last 10 years position the subiculum as an important output station from the hippocampal region. It is becoming increasingly clear that the subiculum, through its divergent efferent projections, serves as an important link in the communication between the hippocampus and the rest of the brain. Thus, the processing of information along the intrahippocampal trisynaptic circuit is relayed via the subiculum to a wide range of cortical and subcortical areas, including the feedback to the entorhinal cortex. It is apparent from several detailed studies (Swanson and Cowan, 1977; Groenewegen et al., 1987) that the dorsal and ventral parts of the subiculum have different projection patterns. This topography displays a gradient along the dorso-ventral axis of the subiculum and it is only the ventral tip of the subiculum that shows exclusive projections.

The ventral subiculum was found, in agreement with previous studies, to project massively to the hypothalamus. In contrast to the findings of earlier studies which were based on the autoradiographic technique and which emphasized that the ventral subiculum projects primarily to the rostral hypothalamus, the present study shows that the ventral subiculum innervates, in principle, the medio-basal hypothalamus along its entire rostro-caudal axis.

The present findings are based on the PHA-L tracing technique (Gerfen and Sawchenko, 1984). This method is unsurpassed as an anterograde tracing method, due in principle to two features. First, it produces small, well restricted injection-sites and it is sensitive enough to detect long projections after labelling of only a small number of cells. Second, the staining of the axons in toto permits the visualization of morphological features such as varicosities and axon collaterals. The visualization of such morphological details aids in the analysis of projection patterns and terminal fields. These features of the PHA-L method make it suitable for the analysis of efferent projections of small cortical fields and even of individual cortical laminae (Köhler, 1985; 1988).

The connections between the subiculum and the mammillary bodies have been known for a long time and it is clear that the dorsal subiculum provides a more prominent input to this nucleus than the midtemporal and ventral parts. In fact, the ventral tip of the subiculum innervates only the median part of the nucleus. The prominent innervation by the ventral subiculum of the other hypothalamic nuclei such as the medial preoptic nucleus, the anterior hypothalamic area, ventromedial and dorsomedial hypothalamus as well as the entire lateral hypothalamus puts this cortical structure in a unique position to influence a wide range of hypothalamic functions. Of particular interest are the observations that ventral subicular afferents innervate the supraoptic and arcuate nuclei, and that a large number of fibers project up to the border of the paraventricular nucleus. It is thus possible that subicular efferents influence activity in the hypothalamo-pituitary axis. These

---

Fig. 3. Photomicrographs showing PHA-L immunoreactive axons in the hypothalamus after a ventral subicular PHA-L injection. Horizontal sections. A: axons running in the medial cortico-hypothalamic tract (arrows); the 3rd ventricle is on the left. A dense terminal field is present just rostral to the dorsomedial nucleus (A and B). Axon collaterals (arrowheads) from the axons in the medial cortico-hypothalamic tract (arrow) innervate medially situated areas (C). A prominent input to the preoptic area and lateral hypothalamic area enters the hypothalamus via the ventral pathway (D). Scale bars: A and B, 100 μm; C and D, 25 μm.

66

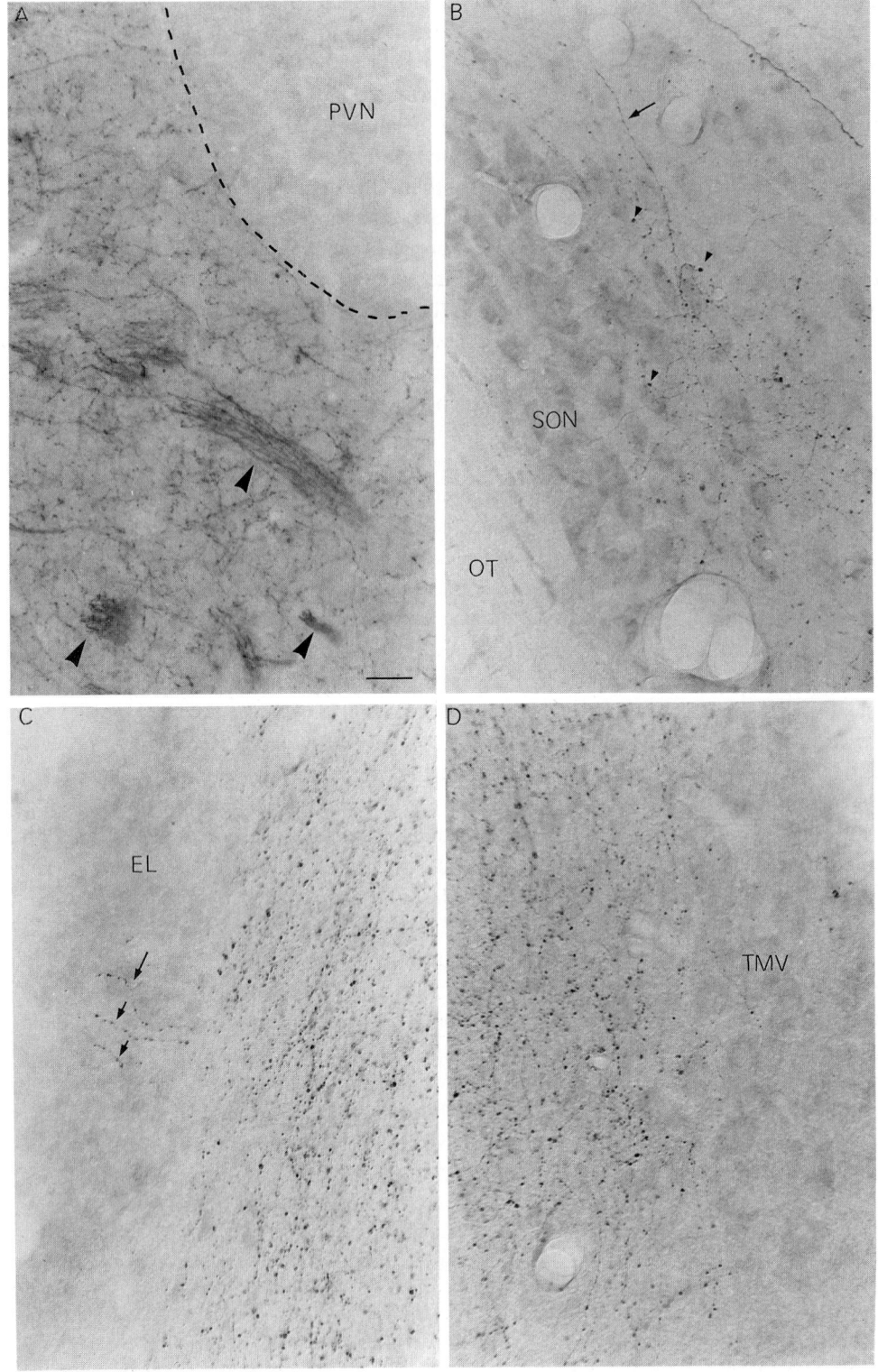

massive inputs to the hypothalamus from the ventral subiculum suggest that the hippocampus has closer connections with the hypothalamic structures than has been previously recognized.

The ventral subiculum is innervated not only by the other subfields of the Ammon's horn at the same level, but is also innervated from the subiculum at more dorsal levels. In addition to these intrinsic hippocampal afferents, the subiculum also receives afferent projections from the caudal parts of the basolateral amygdala (Krettek and Price, 1977). This finding is interesting in light of the suggestion (Van Hoesen, 1981) that afferents mediating most sensory modalities innervate this nucleus. Multisensory information may then be conveyed into the ventral subiculum. In addition the endopiriform component of the claustrum projects to the ventral subiculum (Krettek and Price, 1977). Thus, inputs from areas involved in the multisensory processing of information converge upon the ventral subiculum together with information processed in the hippocampal formation. In this manner highly processed sensory information may reach areas of the hypothalamus involved in the regulation of endocrine functions and of motivated behaviors. Other areas innervating the subiculum, including its ventral parts, are the septum, nucleus reuniens, lateral hypothalamus, premammillary and tuberomammillary nuclei in addition to the brainstem dorsal and median raphe nuclei and locus coeruleus.

It has been known for a long time that the hippocampal region receives afferent inputs from different brainstem areas. While efferent projections from the hippocampus have been demonstrated to most brain regions that provide input to the hippocampus, it has generally been assumed that the brainstem is excluded from this principal organizational pattern. However, using the sensitive PHA-L method, the present study has shown that a small component of the ventral subicular projections enter the central gray of the mesencephalon as well as regions situated as caudal as the medulla. These fibers constitute a small component of the total number of ventral subicular projections and they were detected after small injections involving relatively few cells. It is quite likely that other, less sensitive, tracing methods would not have detected this relatively modest projection. The innervation of the dorsal mesencephalic central gray is from fibers running in the thalamic radiation. The innervation of the caudal medulla is via axons which take off from the postcommissural fornix at the level of the mammillary bodies. The axons course in the brainstem as a distinct bundle while the terminals are scattered along the floor of the fourth ventricle all the way to the area postrema. In fact, numerous varicose fibers are present in the lateral parts of the area postrema. The function(s) of this pathway to the brainstem is not known but its existence raises the possibility that information processed in the hippocampus may be transmitted to the brainstem where it may influence the integration of sensory-motor as well as autonomic functions.

References

Andersen, P., Bliss, T.V.P. and Skrede, K.K. (1971) Lamellar organization of hippocampal excitatory pathways. *Exp. Brain Res.,* 13: 222–238.

Fig. 4. A: axons of the medial cortico-hypothalamic tract (arrowheads) and terminals in the hypothalamus. A dense terminal network is present around the paraventricular nucleus (dotted line). No innervation of the central parts of this nucleus. B: photomicrograph showing an innervation of the supraoptic nucleus from axons running in the ventral pathway (arrow). Small arrowheads show varicose fibers innervating the cells of the supraoptic nucleus. C: axons innervating the ependymal lining of the third ventricle. These axons are collaterals from axons innervating the zone between the central part of the median mammillary nucleus. D: a dense plexus of PHA-L-stained fibers in the ventral part of the lateral hypothalamic area. Numerous stained axons enter the ventral tuberomammillary nucleus. Scale bar: A–D, 50 μm.

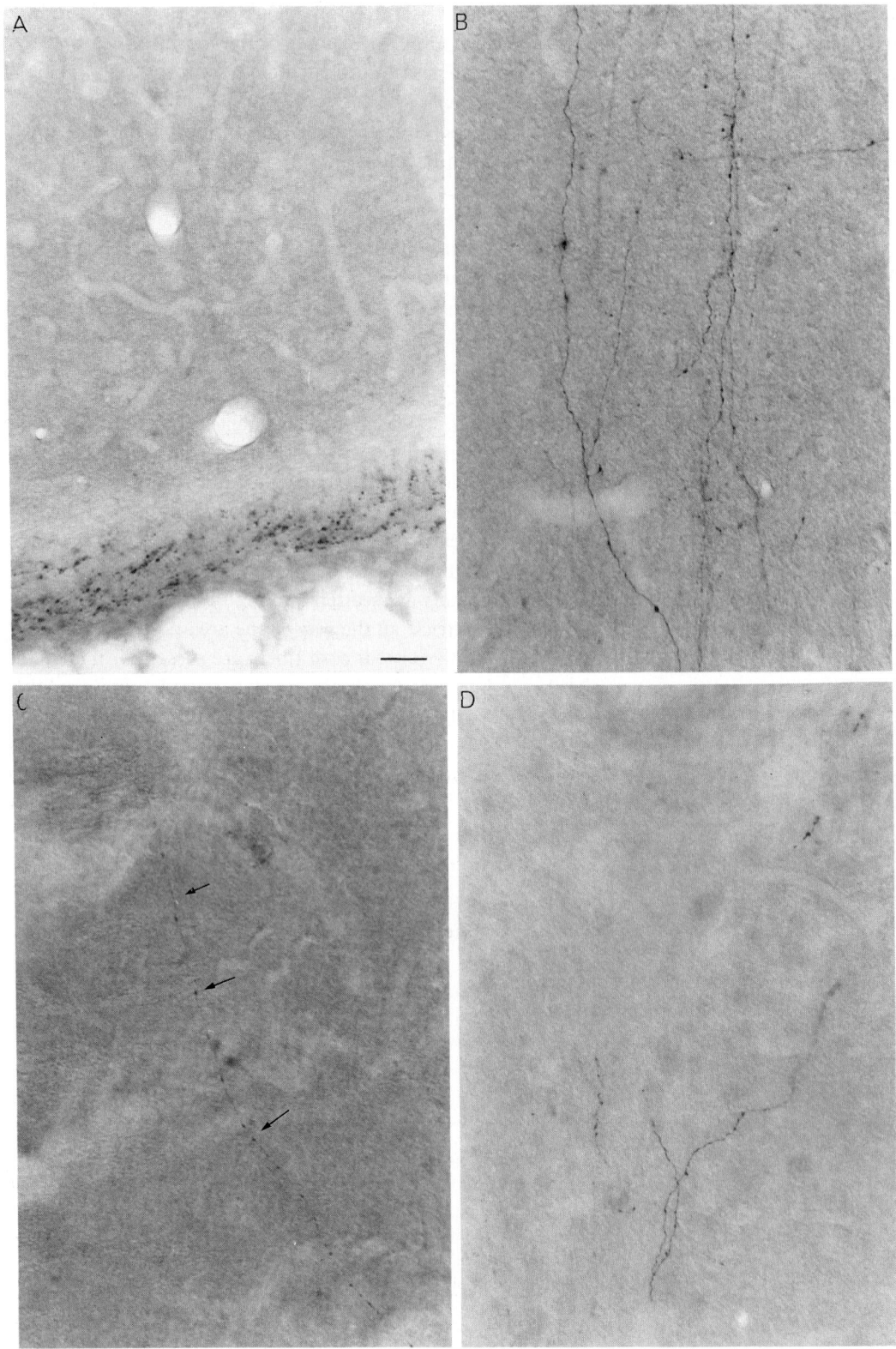

Fig. 5. A: photomicrograph showing PHA-L-stained axons between the mammillary bodies and the glia limitans. These axons run in rostro-caudal direction beneath the mammillary bodies. B: PHA-L-stained axons in the dorsal mesencephalic central gray substance. C: photomicrograph showing a solitary varicose PHA-L axon in the medulla en route towards the fourth ventricle. D: PHA-L-immunostained axons in the midline part of the dorsal raphe nucleus. Scale bar: A – D, 50 μm.

Bantesaghi, R., Gessi, T. and Sperti, L. (1989) Electrophysiological analysis of the hippocampal projections to the entorhinal area. *Neuroscience,* 30: 51 – 62.

Gerfen, C.R. and Sawchenko, P.E. (1984) An anterograde neuroanatomical tracing method that shows the detailed morphology of neurons, their axons and terminals: immunohistochemical localization of an axonally transported plant lectin, *Phaseolus vulgaris* leucoagglutinin. *Brain Res.* 290: 219 – 238.

Groenewegen, H.J., Vermeulen-van der Zee, E., te KortSchot, A. and Witter, M.P. (1987) Organization of the projections from the subiculum to the ventral striatum in the rat. A study using anterograde transport of *Phaseolus vulgaris* leucoagglutinin. *Neuroscience,* 23: 103 – 120.

Hjort-Simonsen, A. (1971) Hippocampal efferents to the ipsilateral entorhinal area: an experimental study in the rat. *J. Comp. Neurol.,* 142: 417 – 438.

Hsu, S.M., Raine, L. and Fanger, H. (1981) The use of avidin – biotin peroxidase complex in immunohistochemical techniques: a comparison between ABC and unlabelled antibody (PAP) procedures. *J. Histochem. Cytochem.,* 29: 577 – 580.

Krettek, J.E. and Price, J.L. (1977) Projections from the amygdaloid complex and adjacent olfactory structures to the entorhinal cortex and to the subiculum in rat and cat. *J. Comp. Neurol.,* 172: 732 – 752.

Köhler, C. (1985) Intrinsic projections of the retrohippocampal region in the rat brain. I. The subicular complex. *J. Comp. Neurol.,* 236: 504 – 522.

Köhler, C. (1988) Intrinsic connections of the retrohippocampal region in the rat brain: III. The lateral entorhinal area. *J. Comp. Neurol.,* 272: 208 – 228.

Meibach, R.C. and Siegel, A. (1975) The origin of the fornix fibers which project to the mammillary bodies in the rat: a horseradish peroxidase study. *Brain Res.,* 88: 508 – 512.

Meibach, R.C. and Siegel, A. (1977a) Subicular projections to the posterior cingulate cortex in rats. *Exp. Neurol.,* 57: 264 – 274.

Meibach, R.C. and Siegel, A. (1977b) Efferent connections of the hippocampal formation in the rat. *Brain Res.,* 124: 197 – 224.

Papez, J.W. (1937) A proposed mechanism of emotion. *Arch. Neurol. Psychiatry,* 38: 725 – 743.

Shipley, M.T. and Sörensen, K.E. (1975) Some afferent and intrinsic connections in the guinea pig hippocampal region and a new pathway from subiculum feeding back to para hippocampal cortex. *Exp. Brain Res.,* 1: 188 – 190.

Swanson, L.W. and Cowan, W.M. (1975) Hippocampo-hypothalamic connections: origin in subicular cortex not in Ammon's horn. *Science,* 189: 303 – 304.

Swanson, L.W. and Cowan, W.M. (1977) An autoradiographic study of the organization of the efferent connections of the hippocampal formation in the rat. *J. Comp. Neurol.,* 172: 49 – 84.

Swanson, L.W., Köhler, C. and Björklund, A. (1988) The limbic system: I. The septohippocampal system. In: A. Björklund, T. Hökfelt and L.W. Swanson (Eds.), *Handbook of Chemical Neuroanatomy, Vol. 5. Integrated Systems of the CNS, Part 1: Hypothalamus, Hippocampus, Amygdala, Retina,* Elsevier, Amsterdam, pp. 125 – 255.

Van Hoesen, G.W. (1981) The differential distribution, diversity and sprouting of cortical projections to the amygdala in the Rhesus monkey. In: Y. Ben-Ari (Ed.), *The Amygdaloid Complex,* Elsevier/North-Holland Biomedical Press, Amsterdam, pp. 77 – 90.

J. Storm-Mathisen, J. Zimmer and O.P. Ottersen (Eds.)
Progress in Brain Research, Vol. 83
© 1990 Elsevier Science Publishers B.V. (Biomedical Division)

CHAPTER 6

Zinc-containing neurons in hippocampus and related CNS structures

C.J. Frederickson[1] and G. Danscher[2]

[1] *Laboratory for Neurobiology, University of Texas at Dallas, Richardson, TX 75083 and* [2] *Institute of Neurobiology, University of Aarhus, DK-8000 Aarhus C, Denmark*

Recent advances in metallohistochemistry have substantiated the identification of a distinct class of neurons in the brain, the zinc-containing neurons. These neurons sequester peculiar amounts of zinc in their presynaptic boutons and show both high-affinity uptake and calcium- and impulse-dependent release of the cation. It is thought that the zinc may act to stabilize the storage of certain macromolecules in presynaptic vesicles, but there is also mounting evidence that zinc released from vesicles can produce a broad spectrum of neuromodulatory effects upon target cells. Zinc-containing neurons are found predominantly in limbic and cerebrocortical regions, and a possible role of these neurons in the modification of synaptic strength is considered.

Introduction

It has been just over 30 years since Maske (1955) developed his dithizone stain and used it to describe the first zinc-containing system in the brain. The question of the function of zinc in specific neural pathways has intrigued and challenged investigators from several disciplines ever since.

Identification of zinc-containing neurons

Paradoxically, it now appears that the real significance of Maske's seminal contribution was not that his stain labeled zinc, but quite the opposite. Zinc is an essential trace element and is a constituent of over 50 enzymes from among all 6 classes of enzyme function, occurring within virtually all cell compartments and organelles (Vallee and Galdes, 1984). The element is fairly evenly distributed throughout most soft tissue, including the gray matter of the brain (Hu and Friede, 1968), and a histological stain for "zinc" would therefore produce a rather even, diffuse coloring of tissue, rather like dipping the material in pale ink.

As it turns out, the real importance of Maske's pioneering work is that he was actually staining only a small, specific fraction or "pool" of the zinc in the brain, probably representing no more than about 10 – 20% of total brain zinc (Assaf and Chung, 1984; Crawford, 1983; Frederickson et al., 1983). That is why his procedure selectively stained only certain cytoarchitectonic regions even though zinc per se is fairly evenly spread throughout the brain.

Three new zinc histochemical methods have been developed since Maske's work, Timm – Danscher sulphide (Danscher, 1981), selenium (Danscher, 1982), and TSQ fluorescence (Frederickson et al., 1987a), and all 3 label the same brain regions originally identified with the dithizone methods as well as showing additional zinc-containing CNS regions that could not be seen with the rather insensitive dithizone method. Moreover, because prior treatment of brains with dithizone blocks staining with the new methods (neo-Timm, selenium, TSQ (Danscher, 1981, 1982; Frederickson et al., 1987a)) and prior treatment with sulphide or selenium blocks subsequent zinc:

TSQ fluorescent staining (Frederickson et al., 1987a), there can be little doubt that the metal in brain regions that stain with dithizone and/or TSQ as well as neo-Timm and selenium is, in fact, zinc (Danscher and Fredens, 1972; Danscher, 1984c; Danscher et al., 1985; Frederickson, 1989 for further discussion).

It is this special pool of histochemically reactive zinc, found only in certain brain regions, that identifies zinc-containing neurons. For the histochemically reactive zinc is located almost exclusively in the axonal boutons of specific groups of CNS neurons — the zinc-containing neurons (Fig. 1).

Definitive proof is still lacking, but it is reasonably certain at this point that the difference between the zinc which can be stained (histochemically reactive zinc) and that which cannot is that the latter is effectively "hidden" from histochemical reagents by virtue of its position within the quaternary structure of the zinc metalloenzymes. Metalloenzymes typically surround their zinc ions in a stable tri- or tetradentate proteinaceous claw (Vallee and Galdes, 1984) and would not be likely to yield those ions for full coordination or covalent bonding with histochemical reagents. Empirically, we have found (unpublished) that cells rich in such zinc metalloenzymes (e.g. erythrocytes and duodenal parietal cells, both rich in carbonic anhydrase) in fact do not stain with any of the zinc histochemical methods. Neither do

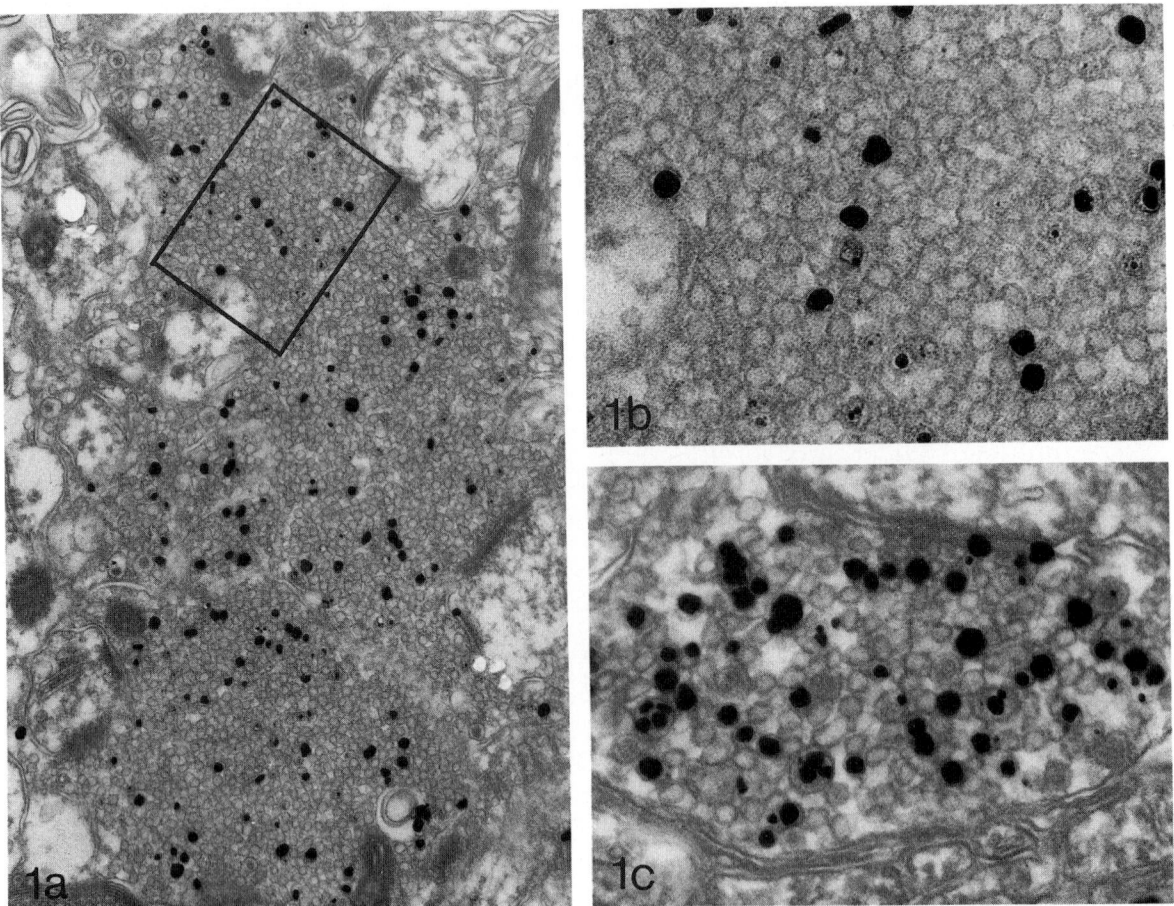

Fig. 1. a: mossy fiber bouton from rat hippocampus stained for zinc by the intravital selenium methods. ×28,000. b: frame in (a). ×80,000. c: bouton from olfactory tubercle of lizards stained for zinc by the Timm/Danscher procedure. ×58,000.

mitochondria, which are rich in zinc metalloenzymes, stain for zinc (e.g. Haug, 1967; Szerdahelyi and Kasa, 1984). Thus, we may presume that brain regions which have zinc but do not stain for zinc (such as the cerebellar cortex, containing about 60 p.p.m. of zinc (Hu and Friede, 1968) (Fig. 6)) have only metalloenzymatic zinc whereas regions which do stain (such as the hippocampus, containing about 72 p.p.m. of zinc (Hu and Friede, 1968; Frederickson et al., 1983)) have both enzymatic and "non-enzymatic" (weakly bound, histochemically reactive) zinc.

Nature of the zinc-containing neuron

Like the "glutamatergic" neuron, the "zinc-containing" neuron is defined by the fact that it sequesters a specific neuroactive substance (zinc) in its axon boutons and releases that substance in an impulse- and calcium-dependent fashion. The first such neuron discovered was the granule neuron of the fascia dentata, the giant "mossy" boutons of which are especially rich in zinc. Maske first found this zinc in the mossy fiber neuropil in 1955, and McLardy (1960) was the first to suggest that the metal might be concentrated in the mossy fiber axons per se. However, credit for the actual identification of the first zinc-containing neuron must go to Haug (1967) whose electronmicroscopic study showed convincingly that the histochemically reactive metal is selectively concentrated in the giant boutons of the granule cells' mossy fiber axons.

The picture emerging currently suggests that the zinc in the mossy boutons is actually embedded in the vesicles and behaves like other components of the intravesicular matrix (Fig. 2). Thus, in tissue where zinc deposits have been lightly labeled with small silver grains, these grains are typically found in the cores of small, clear, round vesicles (Danscher, 1984a; Pérez-Clausell and Danscher, 1985) (Figs. 1, 4); labeling in mitochondria and bouton cytoplasm is not above background levels (Pérez-Clausell and Danscher, 1985). The same pattern is found whether the zinc is precipitated as

a sulphide, by perfusion of the brain with a sulphide solution, or as a selenide, by intravital administration of selenium (Fig. 1). The latter results support the idea that the endogenous location of the zinc is, indeed, within the vesicles. Nonetheless it would be desirable to corroborate the apparent localization of zinc in the vesicles by analysis of the zinc content, uptake, and zinc staining of vesicles that have been isolated by tissue homogenization and fractionation methods.

Interestingly, in any given zinc-containing bouton it is only a small fraction ($< 10\%$) of the vesicles that stain for zinc (Pérez-Clausell and Danscher, 1985). Whether this is due to some probabilistic variation in the staining reaction, or instead reflects a true difference in the zinc content of individual vesicles cannot be resolved with present methods. However, the possibility that zinc may be present in only a specific subset of the vesicles is an intriguing one.

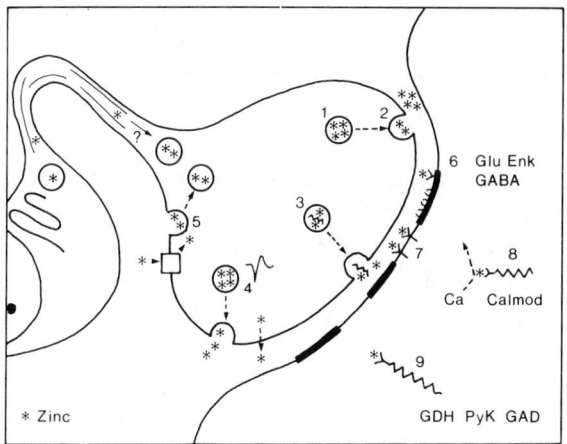

Fig. 2. Cartoon of terminal. Schematic summary of the histophysiology and possible roles of zinc in axon boutons. (1) Zinc is apparently in the vesicles. (2) Zinc-rich vesicles move to the presynaptic specializations and the clefts in vivo. (3) Zinc in vesicles may stabilize stored macromolecules (wavy lines). (4) Zinc is released from the neuropil in an impulse- and calcium-dependent fashion, possibly by exocytosis. (5) High-affinity uptake brings zinc into the neuropil. (6) Zinc modulates transmitter receptor binding, (7) membrane fluidity, (8) calcium-dependent calmodulin activities, and (9) enzyme activity levels. Zinc may be incorporated into secretory complexes in the Golgi cisternae and may be transported to boutons along the axon.

Like other substances in vesicles, zinc shows impulse- and calcium-dependent changes in turnover rate. In hippocampal slices, for example, the high-affinity uptake of ^{65}Zn into the mossy fiber neuropil is selectively accelerated by electrical stimulation of the cells of origin, the granule neurons (Howell et al., 1984). Similarly, depolarization of slices accelerates the efflux of both previously incorporated ^{65}Zn (Howell et al., 1984) and endogenous zinc (Assaf and Chung, 1984), a response which is suppressed in low Ca^{2+}/high Mg^{2+} media. Recent in vivo studies have produced parallel findings, indicating a rapid mobilization of zinc from the mossy fiber boutons during sustained paroxysmal activity (Sloviter, 1985; Aniksztejn et al., 1987; Frederickson et al., 1988a). It is not yet certain how zinc is released from the mossy fiber tissue during electrophysiologic activity, but one line of evidence suggests that it is by exocytosis of the zinc-rich vesicles. In the latter work, vesicular zinc was "tagged" in vivo by intracerebral infusion of sulphide ions, which precipitate the zinc in situ. In material obtained 1 h after the sulphide treatment, labeled vesicles were found distributed evenly throughout the boutons. However, when animals were allowed to survive for 24 h after the sulphide infusion, it was found that the labeled elements were dispersed from the interiors of the boutons, and typically lay poised at the presynaptic specializations or even embedded in the clefts (Danscher, 1984a; Pérez-Clausell and Danscher, 1986).

One of the major unanswered questions is how zinc might get into vesicles, i.e., whether it is linked to secretory products at the point of synthesis in the Golgi apparatus or whether it might be incorporated during endocytotic recycling of membranes at the bouton.

There is some evidence for both processes. Thus, fiber systems that interconnect zinc-rich brain structures, such as the posterior division of the anterior commissure and the fimbria of the hippocampus, show a pale, but definite, staining with neo-Timm and selenium methods (Fig. 3). This staining (which is almost completely absent in fibers interconnecting the zinc-poor olfactory bulbs) is plausibly due to the labeling of zinc in transit from somata to boutons. However, it should be noted that the standard procedure for "trapping" secretory products in somata for histochemical visualization, i.e., intraventricular treatment with colchicine, does not work with zinc. Prior colchicine treatment (150 µg i.v.; 24–36 h delay) does not produce any detectable staining for zinc (Timm–Danscher method) in the somata of zinc-containing neurons (Frederickson and

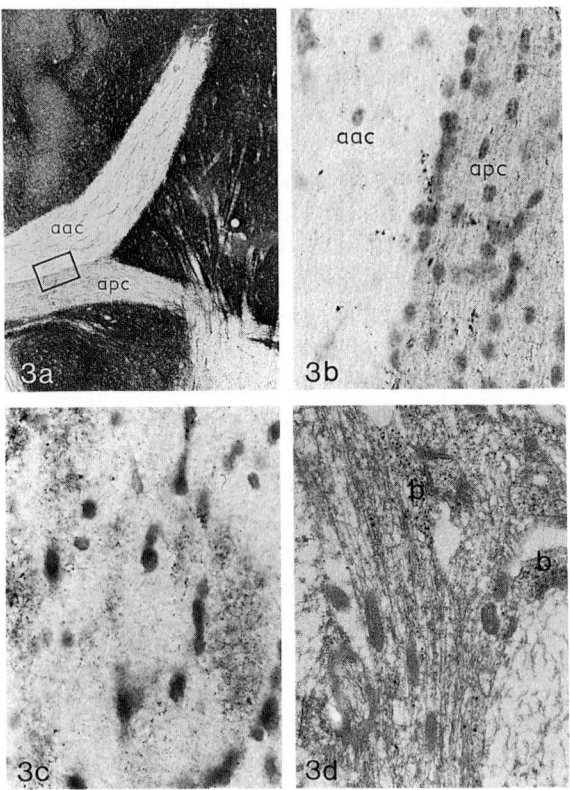

Fig. 3. a: 30-µm-thick horizontal brain cryostat section from selenium-treated mouse, autometallographically (AMG) developed. Note that the anterior parts of commissura anterior (ac) is almost devoid of staining as opposed to pars temporalis. ×30. b: the frame in (a). ×408. c: the animal was treated with sodium selenite 1 hour prior to being killed; 30-µm sagittal section counterstained with toluidine. ×408. d: zinc containing mossy fiber axons from Timm/Danscher stained Epon section. b: mossy fiber bouton. ×31,280.

Danscher, unpublished). Conceivably, zinc is incorporated into complexes of secretory material gradually, during the course of orthograde transport down the zinc-containing axons.

In addition to the possible orthograde transport of zinc to boutons, there is also good evidence for local recycling of zinc at the boutons. As mentioned above, within the zinc-rich mossy fiber neuropil of the hippocampus, there is preferential high-affinity uptake of zinc that is accelerated by electrical stimulation of the granule neurons (Howell et al., 1984).

Beyond the mossy fibers: other zinc-containing pathways in the brain

The granule cell/mossy fiber system is by far the most thoroughly studied zinc-containing neuron, but it is by no means the only zinc-containing pathway in the brain. Indeed, many specific limbic and cerebrocortical regions are densely innervated with zinc-containing boutons, and this pattern of zinc-rich innervation is relatively consistent in homologous brain areas throughout the vertebrate phyla from reptiles to man (Fleischhauer and Horstman, 1957; Lopez-Garcia et al., 1983; Chafetz, 1986). Until recently, the identification of zinc in these latter regions rested chiefly on the silver-based histochemical methods, but the advent of the TSQ quinoline fluorescence method has provided independent corroboration of the identity of the metal in the boutons (Frederickson et al., 1987a).

Fig. 6a shows the intense innervation of zinc-containing boutons in the telencephalic structures as opposed to the rest of the brain. An interesting exception to this pattern is the molecular zone of the dorsal cochlear nucleus, which alone in the entire brainstem receives a moderately heavy zinc-containing innervation (Haug, 1973; Frederickson et al., 1988a).

In the early 1970s Haug, Zimmer, and others (Haug et al., 1971; Zimmer, 1973, 1974; Haug, 1976, 1984) used lesion-degeneration methods coupled with Timm – Haug sulphide staining methods to map some of the fiber systems giving rise to "Timm-positive" axonal boutons. We have recently taken up that same problem, using neo-Timm, selenium, and TSQ methods to identify zinc-containing boutons.

The method of destroying cells of origin or efferent pathways and then searching for a loss of zinc staining in a given terminal field is complicated by two factors, both indirectly alluded to in the early reports of Haug, Zimmer and co-workers. Specifically, it is now clear that if one damages postsynaptic neurons that are innervated by zinc-containing boutons without damaging the zinc-containing boutons or their cells of origin (for example by ibotenic acid lesions of the dentate gyrus), then the normal staining for zinc (Timm – Danscher, selenium, TSQ) in the neuropil of the damaged region (e.g. in the lateral perforant path zone) can be markedly intensified for a period of some days after the insult. Conversely, prolonged paroxysmal activation of zinc-containing fiber systems can almost completely deplete the boutons of histochemically reactive zinc (Sloviter, 1985; Frederickson et al., 1988a). Thus there is always a possibility that a lesion can cause loss of zinc staining in a given region indirectly (e.g. by inducing local electrophysiologic firing or depolarization) without actual damage to the zinc-containing fiber system.

Fortunately, there is a method to supplement the lesion-degeneration technique for mapping zinc-containing pathways. Danscher (1984a) showed some years ago that local intracerebral infusions of selenium ions into the brain causes precipitates (presumably ZnSe) to form in zinc-containing axonal boutons and that the brains of animals allowed to survive for a period after the infusion showed reaction product in the somata of the cells of origin of the labeled boutons. Pérez-Clausell (unpublished) subsequently showed that infusion of S^{2-} into zinc-containing neuropil of the lizard brain resulted in a delayed, robust labeling to the cells of origin, suggesting that this method could be used as a zinc-specific retrograde labeling technique.

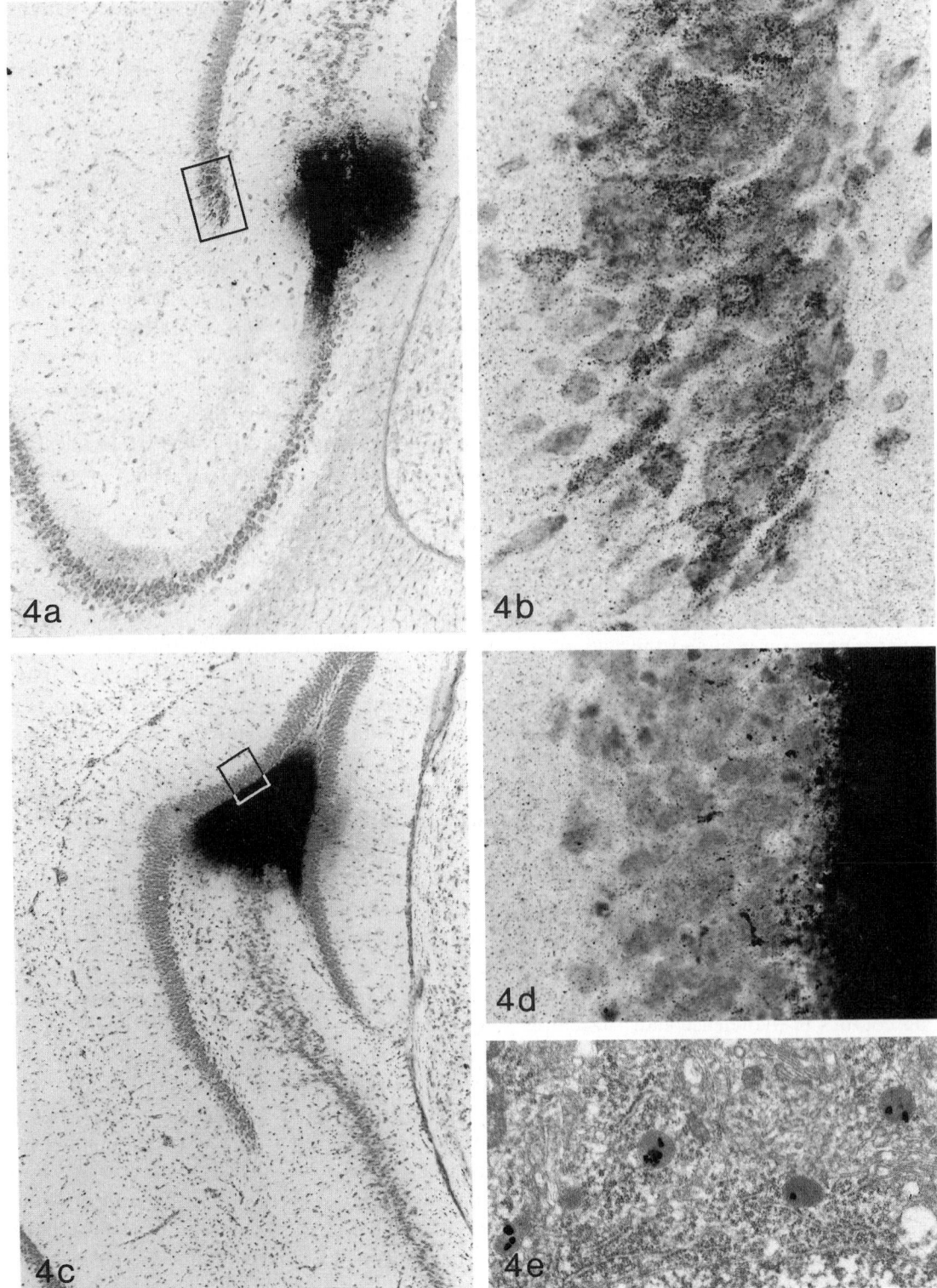

We now know that the retrograde transport of ZnS that occurs in lizard brains cannot be demonstrated in rats (Howell and Frederickson, 1988, 1989; Pérez-Clausell, unpublished) presumably due to dissolution of the reaction product within lysosomes. However, when selenium anions are used instead, the zinc-selenium reaction product is transported vigorously to somata and can be rendered visible for the light- and electron-microscope by silver enhancement (Danscher, 1984a; Howell and Frederickson, 1989) (Fig. 4). Interestingly, the same retrograde transport can be demonstrated when selenium is introduced into the entire brain by intraperitoneal (i.p.) administration. When animals are sacrificed 1 – 2 h after i.p. administration of selenium, the resulting staining is found in the boutons of zinc-containing fiber systems; after 24 h however (Fig. 5), the labeling has been translocated by (colchicine-sensitive) retrograde transport to the certain populations of neurons throughout the brain (Slomianka et al., in preparation). Potentially, this latter method can show all of the zinc-containing cells of origin in the brain simultaneously.

Thus far, the results from retrograde ZnSe transport and from lesion studies are complementary. That is, retrograde labeling after local selenium infusion into a particular brain region is found only in efferent systems, the removal of which causes the loss of zinc staining from that same brain region. For example, infusions of selenium into the caudate – putamen label cells in the cerebral cortex, but do not label cells in the midline thalamus or substantia nigra (Howell and Frederickson, 1988, 1989; Frederickson et al., 1989). Correspondingly, lesions interrupting the corticostriatal fibers cause loss of the zinc staining in the caudate – putamen, whereas cutting nigro-

and thalamo-striatal fibers do not (Frederickson et al., in preparation). The specificity of the selenide retrograde method is presumably due to the fact that the initial reaction product (probably ZnSe) can only form where zinc is available, that is, in zinc-containing axonal boutons. Some of the zinc-containing fiber systems identified by these methods and by earlier work are summarized in Fig. 6b.

The anatomical organization of the zinc-containing pathways in the hippocampal formation has not been systematically investigated with the contemporary methods. Still, from the combination of earlier data from others and recent preliminary results, some informed speculations are possible. The granule neurons, of course, are identified as the source of the major zinc staining in the mossy fiber neuropil: morphologic data (Haug, 1967), lesions (Haug et al., 1971) and retrograde transport (Fig. 4) methods show this to be true. Other zinc-containing pathways that have been tentatively identified on the basis of lesion data have included the lateral perforant path (Zimmer, 1973, 1974; Haug, 1976, 1984), the Schäffer collaterals (Haug, 1984), the projection from CA1 to subiculum (Haug, 1984), and the hippocamposeptal projection (Pérez-Clausell et al., 1986), amygdalo-hypothalamic projections through stria terminals (Pérez-Clausell et al., 1989) and the zinc-containing fiber systems in the cochlear nuclei (Frederickson et al., 1988b). Our preliminary findings with retrograde transport supplement the prior suggestions. For example, in the entorhinal cortex of brains prepared by the i.p. selenium retrograde method, neurons are conspicuously labeled in laminae II and III of the lateral, but not the medial entorhinal cortex (Slomianka et al., in preparation). Similarly, the heavy labeling of

Fig. 4 – e. Local retrograde transport in mossy fibers. a and b-frame in (a) show that ionophoresis of Se^{2-} (1 μA, 120 s) 24 h prior to sacrifice produces labeling of zinc-containing boutons, including mossy fiber boutons, and labeling of granule cell somata. a, $\times 57$; b, $\times 600$. c and d-frame in (c) are taken from a different rat; intraventricular treatment with colchicine, 12 h before iontophoresis leaves the bouton, prevents the subsequent labeling of the granule neurons. c $\times 42$, d $\times 600$. e: EM of CA1 neuron. Neuron at the CA1/subiculum transition retrogradely labeled by Na_2Se microinfusion into the ipsilateral CA1. Note the accumulation of the catalyst (silver grains) in apparent lysosomes. $\times 28,000$.

pyramids in distal CA1 that occurs with the i.p. selenium retrograde method (Fig. 5) favors the hypothesis that those cells supply a major portion of the dense zinc-containing afference to the subiculum. Because the CA1 pyramids also label intensely after iontophoresis of selenide into ipsilateral CA1 (Howell and Frederickson, 1989), their collaterals terminating within CA1 may also be presumed to be zinc-containing. Interestingly, both retrograde methods (i.p. and local infusions) label CA3 pyramids rather lightly, suggesting that the Schäffer and commissural systems arising from those neurons may contribute less extensively to the zinc-containing innervation of the hippocampal formation than do the fibers from CA1 neurons.

Possible functions of zinc within boutons

Most theories of zinc's role vis à vis presynaptic vesicles can be placed in one of two categories: metalloenzymatic theories and storage co-factor

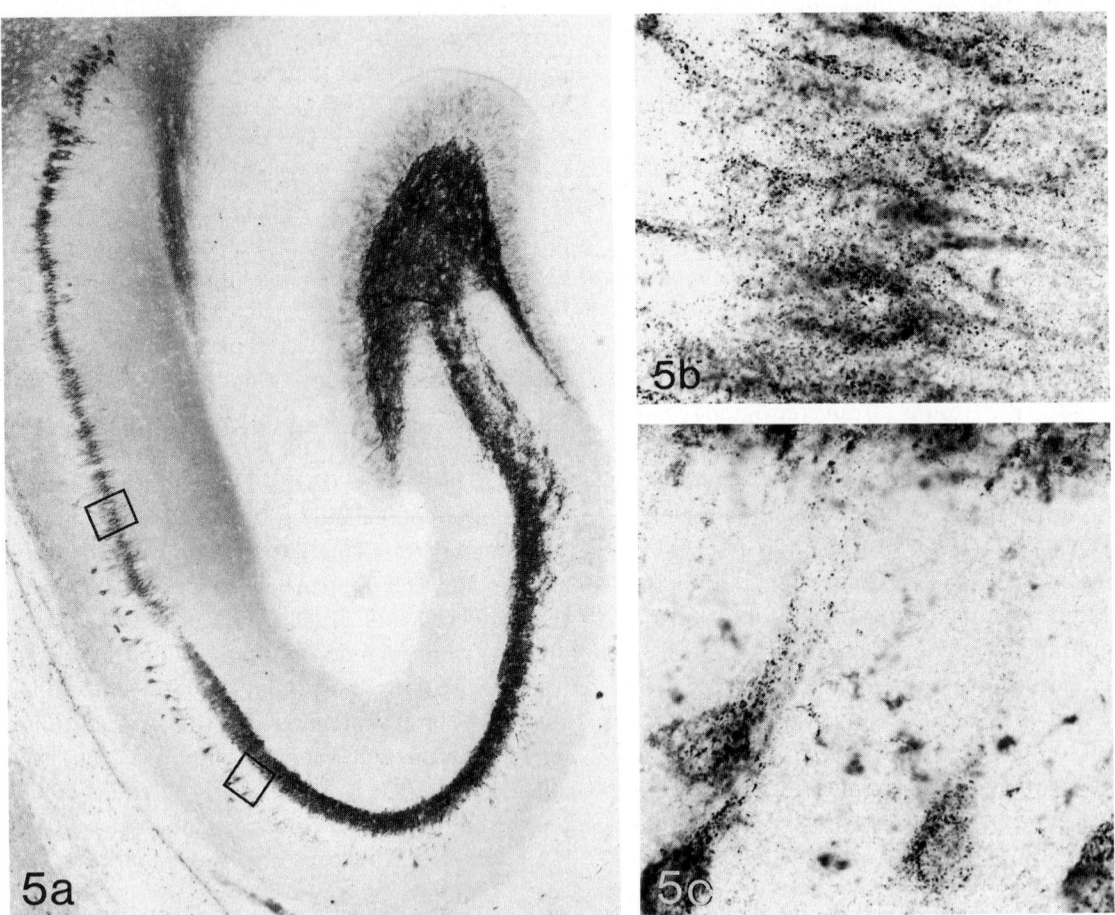

Fig. 5. Retrograde labeling of neurons after prior intravital loading of the zinc-containing boutons by i.p. administration of sodium selenite. The boutons show some residual labeling at this survival delay after the selenium, and neurons have also become labeled. Note the heavy labeling of the most distal CA1 pyramids and the lighter labeling of the main CA3 pyramids. Frames of (b) and (c) in (a). a, ×42; b and c, ×600. Intraventricular colchicine 12 h prior to the selenium administration prevents this labeling of cells (data from Slomianka, L., Frederickson, C.J. and Danscher, G. (1989) Retrograde transport of selenium complexes in neurons used in the identification of cells of origin of zinc-containing axonal boutons, in preparation).

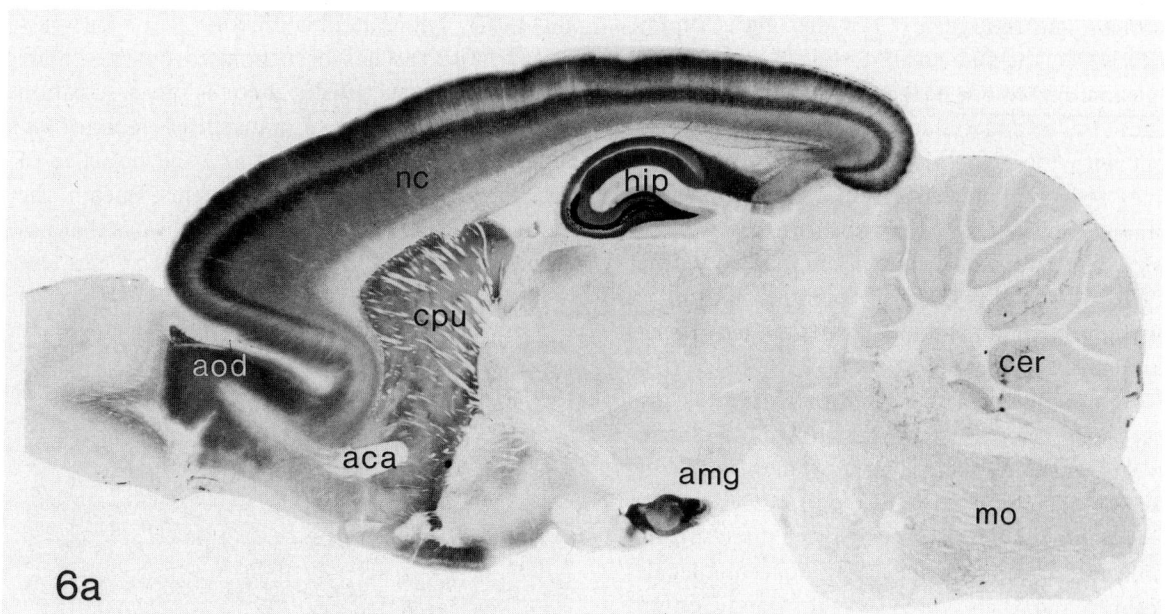

6a

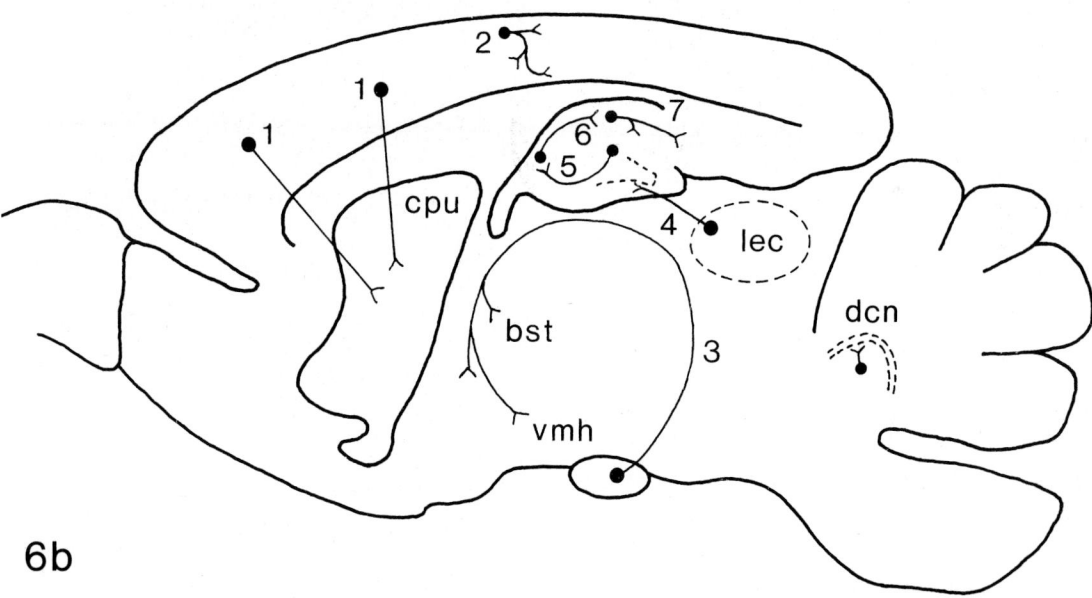

6b

Fig. 6. a: 30-μm sagittal cryostat section from rat treated i.p. with sodium selenite 1 h prior to being sacrificed by transcardial perfusion with saline. The section was autometallographically developed. ×6.3. b: pathways: 1, corticostriatal (Pérez-Clausell et al., 1986; Frederickson et al., 1989); 2, cortico-cortico (Hill and Frederickson, 1988); 3, fimbria/stria terminalis (Howell and Frederickson, 1988; Pérez-Clausell et al., 1989); 4, lateral perforant path (Zimmer, 1973, 1974; Haug, 1976); 5, mossy fiber axons; 6 and 7, Schaffer collaterals, and CA1-to-subiculum (Haug, 1976); granule neuron to dorsal cochlear neurons (Frederickson et al., 1988). Abbreviations: aca, anterior commissure anterior; aod, anterior olfactory nucleus dorsal; amg, amygdala; bst, bed nucleus of stria terminalis; cer, cerebellum; cpu, caudate putamen; dcn, dorsal cochlear nucleus; hip, hippocampus; lec, lateral entorhinal cortex; mo, medulla oblongata; nc, neocortex; vmh, ventromedial hypothalamic nucleus.

theories. The first idea (Crawford and Connor, 1975) is that the zinc-positive vesicles may harbor large amounts of one of the 50-odd zinc metalloenzymes (Vallee and Galdes, 1984). The major problem with these theories is that zinc metalloenzymes (which bind the cation tightly) generally cannot be labeled by zinc histochemistry, whereas vesicle-related zinc is distinguished by the fact that it does react with various zinc staining reagents. A possible role of zinc as an enzyme co-factor is not excluded, however.

The storage co-factor hypothesis suggests that zinc ions serve to stabilize storage of macromolecules in vesicles, perhaps by stabilizing vesicular membranes (Bettger and O'Dell, 1981), pH (Epand et al., 1985), or by some direct ligand-stabilization of aggregates of macromolecules (Colburn and Maas, 1965; Crawford and Connor, 1975). The latter notion gains some support from the study of non-neural secretory cells, many of which selectively sequester histochemically reactive zinc in their secretory granules in a fashion strikingly similar to the storage of zinc in neural vesicles (Frederickson et al., 1987b; Frederickson and Danscher, 1988; Fig. 7). In two such cells, the pancreatic β-cell and the murine salivary granular convoluted tubule (GCT) cell, the role of zinc has been studied in some detail, and the data suggest that the cation coordinates directly with protein molecules (crystalline insulin and 7S-NGF, respectively), preventing their dissociation into active subunits (insulin and β-NGF) (Pattison and Dunn, 1976; Epand et al., 1985). Similar mechanisms have been considered for zinc in other secretory granules (Kerp, 1963).

The major problem with the storage co-factor hypothesis is that no single macromolecule has been identified which has a distribution matching that of the zinc in the CNS. Thus for example, the possibility that zinc might co-localize with one of the ever-growing list of neuropeptides has not been realized. There is some modest association between vesicular zinc and an apparent NGF-like factor, the two of which vary together regionally and temporally in the hippocampus of the rat (Kesslak et

al., 1987), but that link remains to be fully explored. Also, as has been pointed out by others (Storm-Mathisen, 1977), there is an association between the presence of transmitter pools of excitatory amino acids (EAA) and the presence of vesicular zinc in specific fiber systems. Each of the so far identified zinc-containing pathways that has been examined in this respect has been at least ten-

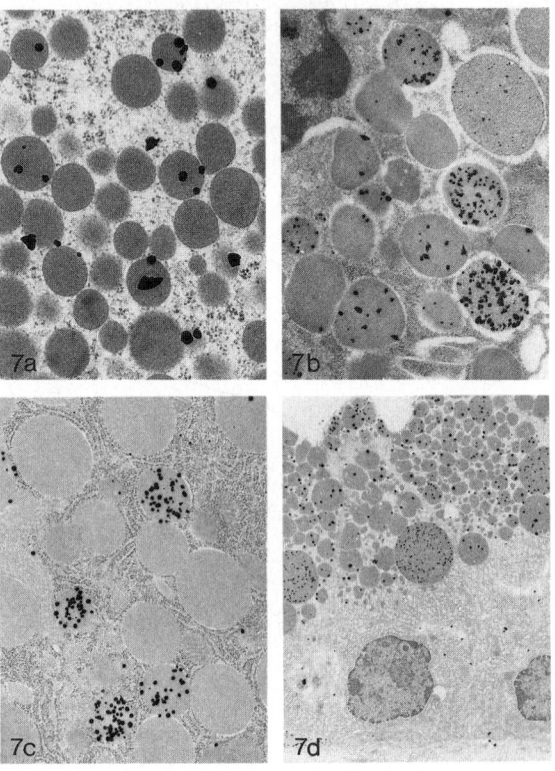

Fig. 7. Silver-amplified zinc in storage granules. Note the similarity in labeling pattern. a: somatotroph cell from adenohypophysis. 3.7 mg selenomethionine/kg body weight; killed 48 h later by transcardial perfusion with buffered glutaraldehyde. × 34,720. b: histamine-heparine granules of the mast cell stained with the Timm/Danscher method. × 12,400. c: acinar excretory cell from rat pancreas. 20 mg selenite i.p. Survival time 1 h and autometallographically developed. The enzymes and proenzymes in the pancreatic juice are exclusively secreted by acinar cells. The significance of this pool of vesicular zinc is not known at present. × 9920. d: silver-enhanced zinc in the secretory granules of granular convoluted tubule cells of murine salivary gland. The demonstrated zinc coexists with 7S-NGF in submandibular glands of adult male mice. × 2480.

tatively identified as an EAA pathway (Cotman, 1987) (Fig. 6). However, the presence of the EAA appears to be a necessary but not a sufficient condition for zinc in the vesicles. EAA systems such as the cerebellar parallel fiber system (Cotman, 1987) do not have histochemically detectable zinc in the boutons (Fig. 3). In other words, zinc-containing neurons are evidently a special subclass of the EAA neurons. Conceivably, the zinc in these neurons could permit storage of especially high concentrations of EAA as a zinc-EAA complex of some type; alternatively, the zinc could be necessary for storage of some co-transmitter or neuromodulator (presently unknown) that might be utilized only by this particular subclass of EAA neurons.

Zinc as a CNS messenger

Whether zinc serves to stabilize the storage of vesicular macromolecules, acts as an enzyme constituent or co-factor, or has some other role in vesicles remains unresolved. Nonetheless, the evidence that the cation is released from the boutons during impulse activity is rather compelling and raises the possibility that zinc might act as an intercellular messenger/neuromodulator substance. Certainly zinc can have profound modulatory effects upon nerve cells. For example, extracellular levels of zinc that could be attained during presynaptic release of zinc (Frederickson et al., 1983; Assaf and Chung, 1984) can modulate the binding affinities of enkephalin (Stengaard-Pedersen et al., 1981), GABA, and glutamate receptors (Ebadi and Hama, 1986), and can alter both membrane fluidity (Bettger and O'Dell, 1981) and the activity of ionic pumps and channels (Ebadi and Hama, 1986) in the membrane (see Frederickson, 1989, for review). Recent evidence indicates that the NMDA receptor is especially sensitive to blockage by Zn^{2+}, whereas the kainic and quisqualate types may be slightly facilitated (Peters et al., 1987; Westbrook and Mayer, 1987). Moreover, because zinc is avidly taken up into cells (e.g. Howell et al., 1984), the released cation could

potentially influence a broad spectrum of processes inside target cells via its effects upon enzymes such as GAD, pyridoxal phosphate, and GDH (Wolf and Schmidt, 1983; Ebadi and Hama, 1986), and indirectly, via suppression of calcium-dependent calmodulin functions (Brewer, 1980). As an inter- and intracellular messenger, zinc has a range of potential actions comparable to that of calcium.

However, concerning the possible role of Zn^{2+} as a transsynaptic messenger, there is one discordant bit of data that suggests some caution. Specifically, when Ca-EDTA (which cannot penetrate into cells or alter zinc staining in boutons (Fredens and Danscher, 1973)) is infused into the extracellular fluids of hippocampal tissue in amounts and concentrations that should effectively block transsynaptic fluxes of Zn^{2+} by chelating the cation in clefts, there are no apparent changes in hippocampal function as assessed electrophysiologically (Danscher et al., 1975) or behaviorally (Frederickson et al., 1986). Because parallel administration of a chelator that can penetrate cells and vesicles, diethyldithiocarbamate (DDC), blocks the zinc-staining (Danscher et al., 1973) and disrupts hippocampal function (Danscher et al., 1975; Frederickson et al., 1986), one is somewhat drawn towards the conclusion that the essential role of the chelatable zinc in boutons may be performed within the boutons, not after release.

Conclusions and implications

Like the amine-containing neurons of the brain, the zinc-containing neurons have been identified by the fact that they can be rendered visible by histochemical procedures which selectively label the contents of their axon boutons. In that context, the zinc-containing neuron stands today approximately where amine-containing neurons stood in the mid 1960s: the boutons can be identified histochemically, activity-dependent neural uptake and release have been established, most of the major projection fields are known, and some of the specific pathways and cells of origin are now being identified and mapped. Whether zinc-containing neurons will prove to be as important in the functional organization of the brain as the amine-containing neurons remains to be seen.

In our view, the anatomical organization of the zinc-containing system is perhaps the best guide to its possible function. Though there are some delicate plexuses in the spinal gray matter (Schrøder, 1979), and the superior colliculus, for example (Danscher, 1984b), what is most striking about the distribution is that the zinc-containing systems are almost entirely associated with limbic or cerebrocortical structures. Within the cerebral cortex, the distinction can be drawn even more finely. The zinc-containing circuitry is apparently part of the intrinsic, intracortical system, arising from small pyramids of laminae II – III and deep VI (according to zinc-selenium retrograde labeling) (Howell and Frederickson, 1989; Slomianka et al., in preparation) and terminating primarily in laminae II – III and V – VI (e.g. Fig. 3). The principal thalamocortical inputs, in contrast, are not zinc-containing (lamina IV), nor apparently are the principal outputs to subcortical targets, inasmuch as the large pyramids of lamina V generally do not label with the zinc-selenium retrograde methods (Howell and Frederickson, 1989; Slomianka et al., in preparation). In Jacobson's (1978) parcellation, then, the Type I neurons of the cortex (large, early developing neurons forming long projection systems) tend not to be zinc-containing.

From the characteristics and locations of the zinc-containing neurons it is tempting to speculate that these neurons are involved in the processes of synaptic lability and plasticity that are especially characteristic of limbic and cortical systems. The EAA synapses in the telencephalon are clearly implicated in processes of functional synaptic change and reorganization, both as pertains to learning and memory (Morris et al., 1986; Cotman, 1987) and the pathological changes underlying epileptogenesis (Ebadi and Hama, 1986). Inasmuch as a substantial component of the EAA neurons in limbic and cerebrocortical circuits are apparently of the zinc-EAA subclass, it is not unreasonable to suppose that the zinc-EAA neurons may be the pivotal agent in processes of synaptic change. Zinc's role in synaptic modification could conceivably be as a transsynaptic messenger working in concert with released EAA to modify postsynaptic cells (Weiss et al., 1989). Alternatively, it could be that the essential role of zinc in these processes is to stabilize the storage of some peptide or protein which itself is the active agent in initiating changes in synaptic potency.

Acknowledgements

Supported in part by an NIMH Fogarty Senior Fellowship and MH 42798 to C.J. Frederickson and Grants from the Danish Medical Research Council to G. Danscher.

References

Aniksztejn, L., Charton, G. and Ben-Ari, Y. (1987) Selective release of endogenous zinc from the hippocampal mossy fibers in situ. *Brain Res.,* 404: 58 – 64.

Assaf, S.Y. and Chung, S.-H. (1984) Release of endogenous Zn^{++} from brain tissue during activity. *Nature (Lond.),* 308: 734 – 736.

Bettger, W. and O'Dell, B. (1981) A critical physiological role of zinc in the structure and function of biomembranes. *Life Sci.,* 28: 1425 – 1438.

Brewer, G.J. (1980) Calmodulin, zinc and calcium in cellular and membrane regulation: an interpretative review. *Am. J. Hematoxicol.,* 8: 231 – 248.

Chafetz, M.D. (1986) Timm's method modified for human tissue and compatible with adjacent section histofluorescence in the rat. *Brain Res. Bull.,* 16: 19 – 24.

Colburn, R.W. and Maas, J.W. (1965) Adenosine triphosphate-metal-norepinephrine ternary complexes and catecholamine binding. *Nature (Lond.),* 50: 37 – 46.

Cotman, C.W. (1987) Anatomical organization of excitatory amino acid receptors and their pathways. *Trends Neurosci.,* 10: 273 – 279.

Crawford, I. (1983) Zinc and the hippocampus. In I. Dreosti and R. Smith (Eds.), *Neurobiology of the Trace Elements,* Clifton, N.J., pp. 163 – 211.

Crawford, I.L. and Connor, J.D. (1975) Zinc and hippocampal function. *J. Orthomol. Psychiatry,* 4: 39 – 52.

Danscher, G. (1981) Histochemical demonstration of heavy metals. A revised version of the sulphide silver method suitable for both light and electronmicroscopy.

Histochemistry, 71: 1–16.

Danscher, G. (1982) Exogenous selenium in the brain. A histochemical technique for light and electron microscopical localization of catalytic selenium bonds. *Histochemistry,* 76: 281–293.

Danscher, G. (1984a) Dynamic changes in the stainability of rat hippocampal mossy fiber boutons after local injection of sodium sulphide, sodium selenite, and sodium diethyldithiocarbamate. In C.J. Frederickson, E.J. Kasarskis and G.A. Howell (Eds.), *The Neurobiology of Zinc. Vol. B,* A.R. Liss, N.Y., pp. 177–191.

Danscher, G. (1984b) Similarities and differences in the localization of metals in rat brains after treatment with sodium sulphide and sodium selenide. In C.J. Frederickson, G.A. Howell and E.J. Kasarskis (Eds.), *The Neurobiology of Zinc. Vol. A,* A.R. Liss, New York, pp. 229–242.

Danscher, G. (1984c) Do the Timm sulphide silver method and the selenium method demonstrate zinc in the brain. In C.J. Frederickson, G.A. Howell and E. Kasarskis (Eds.), *The Neurobiology of Zinc, Part A,* Alan R. Liss, New York, pp. 273–287.

Danscher, G. and Fredens, K. (1972) The effect of oxine and alloxan on the sulfide silver stainability of the rat brain. *Histochemie,* 30: 307–314.

Danscher, G., Haug, F.-M.S. and Fredens, K. (1973) Effect of diethyldithiocarbamate (DEDTC) on sulphide silver stained boutons. Reversible blocking of Timm's sulphide silver stain for ''heavy'' metals in DEDTC treated rats (light microscopy). *Exp. Brain Res.,* 16: 521–532.

Danscher, G., Shipley, M.T. and Andersen, P. (1975) Persistent function of mossy fibre synapses after metal chelation with DEDTC (antabuse). *Brain Res.,* 85: 522–526.

Danscher, G., Howell, G., Pérez-Clausell, J. and Hertel, N. (1985) The dithizone, Timm's sulphide silver and the selenium methods demonstrate a chelatable pool of zinc in CNS. *Histochemistry,* 83: 419–422.

Ebadi, M. and Hama, Y. (1986) Zinc-binding proteins in the brain. In R. Schwarcz and Y. Ben-Ari (Eds.), *Excitatory Amino Acids and Epilepsy,* Plenum, New York, pp. 557–570.

Epand, R.M., Stafford, A.R., Tyers, M. and Nieboer, E. (1985) Mechanism of action of diabetogenic zinc-chelating agents. *Mol. Pharmacol.,* 27: 366–374.

Fleischhauer, K. and Horstmann, E. (1957) Intravitale Dithizonfärbung homologer Felder der Ammonsformation von Säugern. *Z. Zellforsch,* 46: 598–609.

Fredens, K. and Danscher, G. (1973) The effect of intravital chelation with dimercaprol, calcium disodium edetate, 1-10-phenantroline and 2,2′-dipyridyl on the sulfide silver stainability of the rat brain. *Histochemie,* 37: 321–331.

Frederickson, C.J. (1989) Neurobiology of zinc and zinc-containing neurons. *Int. Rev. Neurobiol.,* 31: 145–238.

Frederickson, C.J. and Danscher, G. (1988) Hippocampal zinc, the storage granule pool: localization, physiochemistry, and possible functions. In J.E. Morley, M.B. Sterman and J.H. Walsh (Eds.), *Nutritional Modulation of Brain Function,* Academic Press, San Diego, CA, pp. 289–306.

Frederickson, C.J., Klitenick, M.A., Manton, W.I. and Kirkpatrick, J.B. (1983) Cytoarchitectonic distribution of zinc in the hippocampus of man and the rat. *Brain Res.,* 273: 335–339.

Frederickson, C.J., Kasarskis, E.J., Ringo, D. and Frederickson, R.E. (1987a) A quinoline fluorescence method for visualizing and assaying the histochemically reactive zinc (bouton zinc) in the brain. *J. Neurosci. Methods,* 20: 91–103.

Frederickson, C.J., Pérez-Clausell, J. and Danscher, G. (1987b) Zinc-containing 7S-NGF complex. Evidence from zinc histochemistry for localization in salivary secretory granules. *J. Histochem. Cytochem.,* 35: 579–583.

Frederickson, C.J., Hernandez, M.D., Goik, S.A., Morton, J.D. and McGinty, J.F. (1988a) Loss of zinc staining from hippocampal mossy fibers during kainic acid induced seizures: a histofluorescent study. *Brain Res.,* 446: 383–386.

Frederickson, C.J., Howell, G.A., Haigh, M.D. and Danscher, G. (1988b) Zinc-containing fiber systems in the cochlear nuclei of the rat and mouse. *Hearing Res.,* 36: 203–212.

Frederickson, C.J., Howell, G.A., Christensen M.K. and Montava, P. (1989) Identification of zinc-containing efferents to the neostriatum by retrograde transport of zinc selenide. *Soc. Neurosci. Abstr.,* in press.

Frederickson, R.E., Danscher, G. and Frederickson, C.J. (1986) Reversible chelation of hippocampal zinc causes time-locked disruption of spatial/working memory. *Soc. Neurosci. Abstr.,* 12: 523.

Haug, F.-M.S. (1967) Electron microscopical localization of the zinc in hippocampal mossy fibre synapses by a modified sulfide silver procedure. *Histochemie,* 8: 355–368.

Haug, F.-M.S. (1973) Heavy metals in the brain. A light microscope study of the rat with Timm's sulphide silver method. Methodological considerations and cytological and regional staining patterns. *Adv. Anat. Embryol. Cell Biol.,* 47: 1–71.

Haug, F.-M.S. (1976) Laminar distribution of afferents in the allocortex visualized with Timm's sulphide silver method for ''heavy'' metals. *Exp. Brain Res.,* Suppl. 1: 177.

Haug, F.-M.S. (1984) Sulfide silver stainable (Timm stainable) fiber systems in the brain. In C.J. Frederickson, G.A. Howell and E.J. Kasarskis (Eds.), *The Neurobiology of Zinc. Vol. A,* A.R. Liss, N.Y., pp. 213–228.

Haug, F.-M.S., Blackstad, T.W., Simonsen A.H. and Zimmer, J. (1971) Timm's sulphide silver reaction for zinc during experimental anterograde degeneration of hippocampal mossy fibers. *J. Comp. Neurol.,* 142: 23–32.

Howell, G.A. and Frederickson C.J. (1988) Identification of zinc-containing neurons by retrograde transport of zinc-selenide. *Soc. Neurosci. Abstr.,* 14: 859.

Howell, G.A. and Frederickson C.J. (1989) Retrograde

84

transport method for mapping zinc-containing fiber systems in the brain. *Brain Res.,* in press.

Howell, G.A., Welch, M.G. and Frederickson, C.J. (1984) Stimulation-induced uptake and release of zinc in hippocampal slices. *Nature (Lond.),* 308: 736 – 738.

Hu, K.H. and Friede, R.L. (1968) Topographic determination of zinc in human brain by atomic absorption spectrophotometry. *J. Neurochem.,* 15: 667 – 685.

Jacobson, M. (1978) *Developmental Neurobiology,* Plenum Press, New York.

Kerp, L. (1963) Bedeutung von Zink für die Histaminspeicherung in Mastzellen. *Int. Arch. Allergy,* 22: 112 – 123.

Kesslak, J.P., Frederickson, C.J. and Gage, F.H. (1987) Quantification of hippocampal noradrenalin and zinc changes after selective cell destruction. *Exp. Brain Res.,* 67: 77 – 84.

Lopez-Garcia, C., Soriano, E., Molowny, A., Garcia Vredugo, J.M., Berbel, P. and Regidor, J. (1983) The Timm positive system of axonic terminals of the cerebral cortex of Lacerta. In S. Grisolia, C. Guerri, F. Samson, S. Norton and F. Reinoso-Suarez (Eds.), *Ramón y Cajal's Contribution to the Neurosciences,* Elsevier Science Publishers, B.V., Amsterdam, pp. 137 – 148.

Maske, H. (1955) Über den topochemischen Nachweis von Zink im Ammonshorn verschiedener Säugetiere. *Naturwissenschaften,* 42: 424.

McLardy, T. (1960) Neurosyncytial aspects of the hippocampal mossy fibre system. *Confin. Neurol.,* 20: 1 – 17.

Morris, R.G., Anderson, E., Lynch, G.S. and Baudry, M. (1986) Selective impairment of learning and blockade of long-term potentiation by an *N*-methyl-D-aspartate receptor antagonist, AP5. *Nature (Lond.),* 319: 774 – 776.

Pattison, S.W. and Dunn, M.F. (1976) On the mechanism of divalent metal ion chelator induced activation of the 7S nerve growth factor esteropeptidase. Activation by 2,2′,2-terpyridine and by 8-hydroxyquinoline-5-sulfonic acid. *Biochemistry,* 15: 3691 – 3696.

Pérez-Clausell, J. and Danscher, G. (1985) Intravesicular localization of zinc in rat telencephalic boutons. A histochemical study. *Brain Res.,* 337: 91 – 98.

Pérez-Clausell, J. and Danscher, G. (1986) Release of zinc sulphide accumulations into synaptic clefts after in vivo injection of sodium sulphide. *Brain Res.,* 362: 358 – 361.

Pérez-Clausell, J., Frederickson, C.J., Danscher, G. and Møller-Madsen, B. (1986) Fimbria, stria terminalis, and the cortico-striatal projections contain axons which end in zinc-containing boutons. *Neurosci. Lett.,* 26: S89 (abstract).

Pérez-Clausell, J., Frederickson, C.J. and Danscher, G. (1989) Amygdaloid efferents through the stria terminalis in the rat give origin to zinc-containing boutons. *J. Comp. Neurol.,* 290: 201 – 212.

Peters, S., Koh, J. and Choi, D.W. (1987) Zinc selectively blocks the action of *N*-methyl-D-aspartate on cortical neurons. *Science,* 236: 589 – 593.

Schröder, H.D. (1979) Sulfide silver stainability of a type of bouton in spinal cord motoneuron neuropil: an electron microscopic study with Timm's method for demonstration of heavy metals. *J. Comp. Neurol.,* 186: 439 – 450.

Sloviter, R.S. (1985) A selective loss of hippocampal mossy fiber Timm stain accompanies granule cell seizure activity induced by perforant path stimulation. *Brain Res.,* 330: 150 – 153.

Stengaard-Pedersen, K., Fredens, K. and Larsson, L.I. (1981) Enkephalin and zinc in the hippocampal mossy fiber system. *Brain Res.,* 212: 230 – 233.

Storm-Mathisen, J. (1977) Localization of transmitter candidates in the brain: the hippocampal formation as a model. *Prog. Neurobiol.,* 8: 119 – 181.

Szerdahelyi, P. and Kasa, P. (1984) Histochemistry of zinc and copper. *Int. Rev. Cytol.,* 89: 1 – 33.

Vallee, B.L. and Galdes, A. (1984) The metallobiochemistry of zinc. In A. Meister (Ed.), *Advances in Enzymology and Related Areas of Molecular Biology, Vol. 56,* J. Wiley and Sons, New York, pp. 283 – 430.

Weiss, J.H., Koh, J.-Y., Christine, C.W. and Choi, D.W. (1989) Zinc and LTP. *Nature (Lond.),* 338: 212.

Westbrook, G.L. and Mayer, M.L. (1987) Micromolar concentrations of Zn^{++} antagonize NMDA and GABA responses of hippocampal neurons. *Nature (Lond.),* 328: 640 – 643.

Wolf, G. and Schmidt, W. (1983) Zinc and glutamate dehydrogenase in putative glutamatergic brain structures. *Acta Histochem.,* 72: 15 – 23.

Zimmer, J. (1973) Changes in the Timm sulphide silver staining pattern of the rat hippocampus and fascia dentata following early postnatal deafferentation. *Brain Res.,* 64: 313 – 326.

Zimmer, J. (1974) Proximity as a factor in the regulation of aberrant axonal growth in postnatally deafferented fascia dentata. *Brain Res.,* 72: 143 – 146.

J. Storm-Mathisen, J. Zimmer and O.P. Ottersen (Eds.)
Progress in Brain Research, Vol. 83
© 1990 Elsevier Science Publishers B.V. (Biomedical Division)

CHAPTER 7

Immunocytochemical demonstration of the calcium-binding proteins calbindin-D 28k and parvalbumin in the subiculum, hippocampus and dentate area of the domestic pig

I.E. Holm[1], F.A. Geneser[1], J. Zimmer[1] and K.G. Baimbridge[2]

[1] *Institute of Neurobiology, University Aarhus, DK-8000 Aarhus C, Denmark and* [2] *Department of Physiology, Faculty of Medicine, University of British Columbia, Vancouver, B.C., Canada*

The distribution of the calcium-binding proteins calbindin-D 28k (CaBP) and parvalbumin (PV) in the hippocampal region of the domestic pig was demonstrated by immunocytochemistry. Scattered CaBP-immunoreactive cell bodies were present in the subiculum, stratum oriens, pyramidal cell layer and stratum radiatum of the hippocampal regio superior and inferior, and the outer plexiform layer and outer hilar cell layer of the dentate hilus. Other cell bodies and bundles of stained fibers were present in stratum moleculare of regio superior and inferior, and in the outer third of the molecular layer of the fascia dentata. Terminal-like CaBP-immunoreactivity was seen in the subiculum and around cell bodies in the pyramidal cell layer of regio superior and inferior and the dentate granular cell layer. Scattered PV-immunoreactive cell bodies were present in stratum oriens and the pyramidal cell layer of regio superior and inferior, and in the outer plexiform layer and outer hilar cell layer of the dentate hilus. Terminal-like PV-immunoreactivity surrounded the cell bodies in the pyramidal cell layer of regio superior and inferior and in the dentate granular cell layer. The distribution of CaBP and PV in the pig hippocampus is compared to that of other more commonly used experimental animals. Whereas the distribution of PV-immunoreactivity in the pig hippocampus appears identical to that of the rat hippocampus, the distribution of CaBP-immunoreactivity in the pig hippocampus differs markedly from that of the rat hippocampus, the most prominent feature being a lack of CaBP-immunoreactivity in the granule cells, mossy fibers and pyramidal cells in the pig. The functional implications of calcium-binding proteins in the brain are discussed.

Introduction

Most studies on the hippocampal region have been carried out in rodents, monkeys and non-human primates. For many purposes it would, however be convenient to use larger animals with a closer resemblance to man than rodents, without having to use monkeys and primates. In biomedical research the domestic pig is already widely used due to many similarities in the anatomy and physiology of the different organ systems between pigs and man (Tumbleson, 1986). Although several neuroanatomical studies of the pig have already been carried out (Herre, 1936; Solnitzki, 1938;

Woolsey et al., 1946; Stephan, 1951; Breazile, 1967; Hereć, 1967; Kruska, 1970; Palmieri et al., 1986; Salinas-Zeballos et al., 1986; Freeman et al., 1988; Grandin et al., 1988; Niwa et al., 1988; Pearlmutter et al., 1988), no description of the hippocampal region of the domestic pig has to our knowledge been published previously. As the first step in the description of the pig hippocampal region we have used the Timm staining (Holm and Geneser, 1989, 1990a, b), which besides its histochemical detection of zinc, helps delineate the different areas, subfields and layers.

In the present study, we describe the immunocytochemical localization of two calcium-binding proteins, calbindin-D 28k and parvalbumin, in the pig hippocampal region. The two proteins have previously been demonstrated by immunocytochemistry in the hippocampal region of other species (Jande et al., 1981; Celio and Heizmann, 1981; Baimbridge and Miller, 1982; Rami et al., 1987; Heizmann and Celio, 1987; Kawaguchi et al. 1987; Kosaka et al., 1987; Katsumaru et al., 1988a, b). Calbindin-D 28k and parvalbumin belong to a homologous family of calcium ion binding proteins and both might, in spite of quite different cellular and intracellular distribution, be involved in calcium transport and act as intracellular calcium ion buffers (Heizmann, 1984). The role of calcium ions in the control of neurotransmitter release, neuronal excitability and neural plasticity makes the distribution of the calcium-binding proteins of general interest in neurobiology. The involvement of calcium ions in pathology and cell death, such as neuronal death

associated with NMDA receptor-mediated neurotoxicity (Mayer and Westbrook, 1987; Rothmann and Olney, 1987; Choi, 1988), also adds to the actuality of research in calcium ion homeostasis.

Materials and methods

Four young domestic pigs (two females, two males), weighing 25 – 30 kg, were anesthetized with a combination of midazolam, ketamine and pentobarbital and killed by transcardiac perfusion with 5 liters of 4% paraformaldehyde in 0.15 M Sørensen phosphate buffer (pH 7.3). The brain was then removed from the skull and placed in fixative for an additional 2 hours before a tissue block containing the hippocampus along its entire septotemporal (longitudinal) extent was removed by careful dissection (Figs. 1 and 2). In addition to the hippocampus (proper) the tissue included the dentate area and subiculum. The main block of

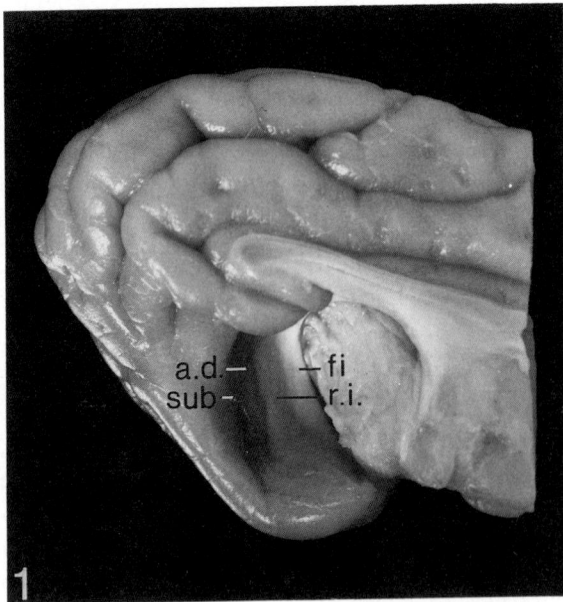 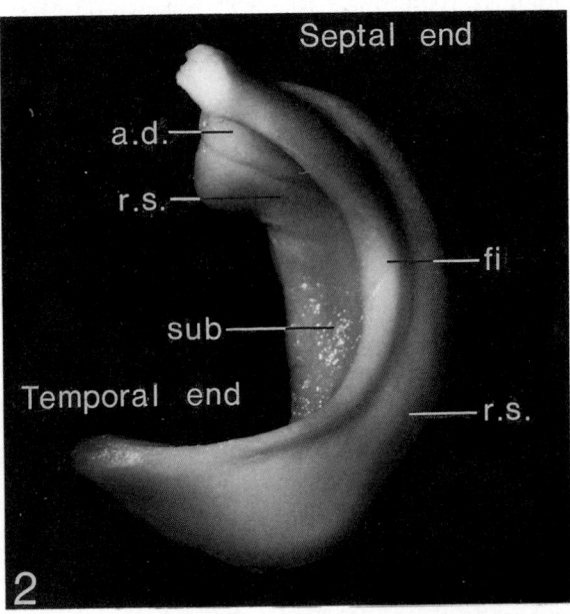

Fig. 1. Medial view of the posterior part of the left cerebral hemisphere of a pig. The thalamus and brainstem were removed to reveal the hippocampus in situ. Abbreviations (some applying to the other figs.): a.d., area dentata; fi, fimbria hippocampi; g, granular cell layer; mf, layer of mossy fibers; m_1, stratum moleculare of regio superior; m, molecular layer of area dentata; o, stratum oriens; ohc, outer hilar cell layer; opl, outer plexiform layer; p, pyramidal cell layer; r, stratum radiatum; r.i., regio inferior; r.s., regio superior; sub, subiculum; ×1.6.

Fig. 2. Anterior view of left hippocampus after dissection. Most of the area dentata and regio inferior is hidden behind the fimbria. ×2.9.

tissue was divided into 4 blocks of equal size along the septotemporal axis, and 50-μm-thick sections were then cut perpendicular to the septotemporal axis of each block on an Oxford Vibratome. The sections were collected in several series in a cryoprotective fluid for deep-freeze storage. The fluid consisted of 30% sucrose, 1% polyvinylpyrrolidone (PVP40, Sigma) and 30% ethyleneglycol in 0.06 M sodium phosphate (Warr et al., 1981).

Immunocytochemistry was performed according to the unlabeled antibody peroxidase-antiperoxidase (PAP) method of Sternberger (1979). After a wash in 0.05 M Tris buffer, pH 7.4, the sections were incubated in 1% swine serum for 30 min at room temperature and then incubated with the primary antibody for 48 h at 4°C.

The calbindin-D 28k (CaBP) antibody (R202) and parvalbumin (PV) antibody (R301) were supplied by one of us (K.G. Baimbridge), and have previously been characterized in other studies (Baimbridge et al., 1982). CaBP was used in 1:1200 dilution, whereas PV was used in 1:500 dilution. After wash in Tris buffer with 1% Triton X-100, the sections were incubated in swine antirabbit immunoglobulin (DAKO, Copenhagen, dilution 1:30) for 30 min at room temperature, washed again, and incubated with a PAP complex (DAKO, Copenhagen, dilution 1:75) for 30 min. The peroxidase was visualized using diaminobenzidine (DAB) as chromogen (50 mg DAB in 100 ml Tris buffer, with 0.033 ml 30% H_2O_2 added just before use). After immunocytochemical staining half of the sections in the different series were counterstained with Toluidine blue. Finally, the sections were dehydrated in alcohol and coverslipped in Dammar resin.

Results

Anatomical terminology

The nomenclature used in the present study for cortical areas and subfields and layers within the hippocampal region of the pig are identical with those used in a previous description based on the Timm staining (Holm and Geneser, 1989, 1990a, b). The latter, in turn, are based on the terms used by Geneser (1986, 1987a,b) in the study of the rabbit hippocampal region. The dentate hilus of the pig will be described accordingly with the following layers: the outer plexiform layer, the outer hilar cell layer, the inner plexiform layer and the inner hilar cell layer. A limiting subzone could not be distinguished with certainty. In Figs. 3a and 4a, the pig dentate area, hippocampus proper and subiculum are shown in Nissl-stained sections at septal and mid-septotemporal levels.

The term terminal-like immunoreactivity designates both diffuse punctate staining and fiber-like staining without direct relation to parent cell bodies. Immunoreactive cell bodies display a Golgi-like impregnation of the perikarya and the proximal parts of the processes.

Calbindin-D 28k (CaBP)

The distribution of CaBP-immunoreactivity in the pig dentate area, hippocampus proper and subiculum is shown at septal and mid-septotemporal levels (Figs. 3b and 4b).

The subiculum

In the subiculum, an area of strong immunoreactivity was seen at all levels, but with an increase in size and staining density towards temporal levels (Figs. 3b and 4b). The area consisted of intensely stained pyramidal-like neurons located in the cell layer, in addition to a diffuse staining of the neuropil (Fig. 5). Stained dendrites extended from the cells in the cell layer into the plexiform layer (Fig. 5) which itself contained scattered immunoreactive stellate cells. Most superficially in the plexiform layer, strongly reactive fibers ran parallel to the pial surface (Fig. 5) continuing from the subiculum into stratum moleculare of the adjacent regio superior hippocampi. This arrangement was most conspicuous at temporal levels.

88

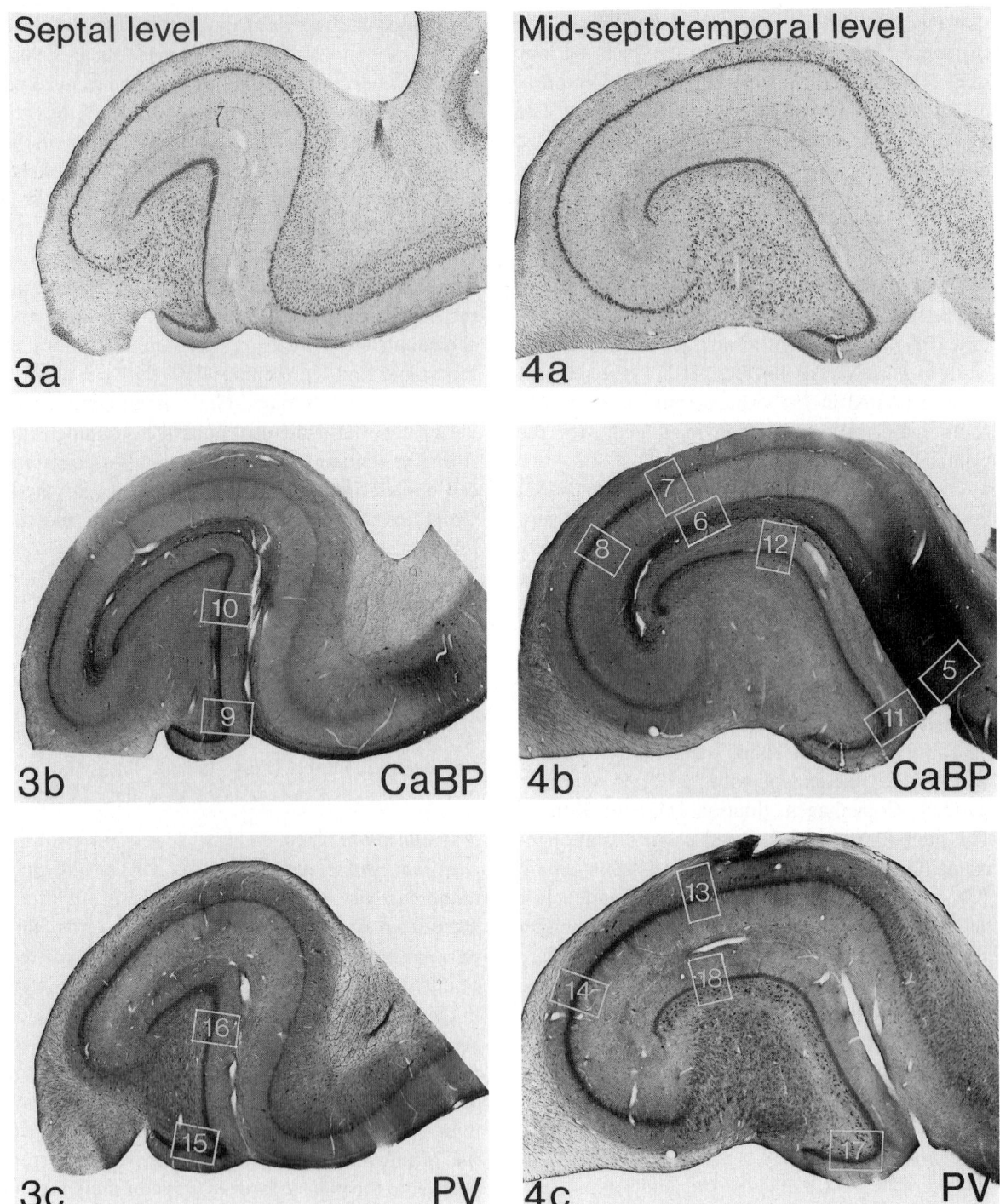

Septal level

Mid-septotemporal level

3a

4a

3b   CaBP

4b   CaBP

3c   PV

4c   PV

Figs. 3 and 4. 50-μm sections from septal (Fig. 3) and mid-septotemporal (Fig. 4) parts of the pig hippocampus, cut perpendicular to the septotemporal axis. The quadrangles mark the positions of Figs. 5–18. a: stained with Toluidine blue. b: CaBP-immunocytochemistry. c: PV-immunocytochemistry. ×12.

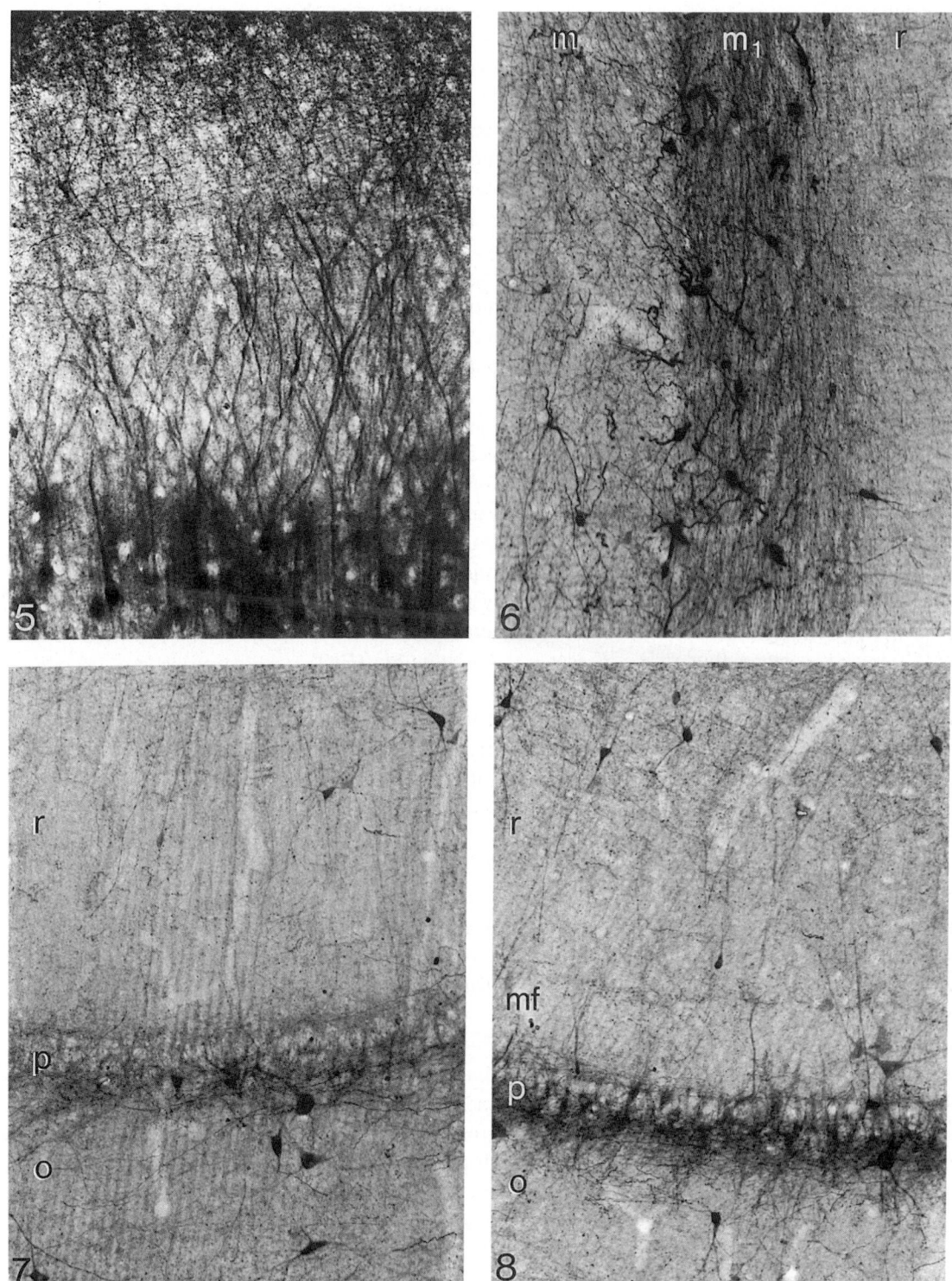

Fig. 5 – 8. CaBP-immunocytochemistry. Fig. 5. Subiculum. ×137. Fig. 6. Stratum moleculare of regio superior. ×137.
Figs. 7 and 8. Stratum radiatum, pyramidal cell layer and stratum oriens of regio superior (Fig. 7) and regio inferior (Fig. 8). ×137.

The hippocampus

Regio superior. Stratum moleculare was densely stained, with an increase in density towards the subiculum, in particular at more temporal levels (Figs. 3b and 4b). Many longitudinally oriented reactive fibers were seen in addition to numerous reactive cell bodies (Fig. 6). In stratum radiatum, a small number of stained bipolar and stellate cells with long, transversely oriented processes were seen (Fig. 7). Long dendrites with a beaded appearance were also present. In the pyramidal cell layer, a weak, scattered terminal-like reactivity was seen as stained punctae around the pyramidal cells (Fig. 7). In addition, a few reactive cell bodies were occasionally encountered. Stratum oriens contained large stellate cells with beaded dendrites (Fig. 7). In the alveus, weakly reactive fibers were seen.

Regio inferior. Stratum moleculare and radiatum presented essentially the same characteristics as in regio superior (Fig. 8). The layer of mossy fibers was almost unreactive, but a thin stripe of scattered terminal-like punctae marked the superficial border of the layer towards stratum radiatum (Fig. 8). Occasionally, reactive cells were encountered in the layer of mossy fibers (Fig. 8). In the pyramidal cell layer, diffuse terminal-like punctae surrounded the pyramidal cells. This staining was somewhat more pronounced than in regio superior and was most prominent immediately basal to the pyramidal cell layer, where reactive cell bodies were seen, too (Fig. 8). Stratum oriens and alveus exhibited the same staining character as in regio superior (Fig. 8).

Area dentata

At all septotemporal levels, the immunoreactivity was stronger in the free medial blade of the dentate area (Figs. 9 and 11) than in the so-called hidden, lateral blade (Figs. 10 and 12). The outer third of the molecular layer contained many intensely stained cells and fibers (Figs. 9–12). In the middle third of the molecular layer, a few reactive stellate cells were encountered (Figs. 9–12), whereas in the inner third of the molecular layer, a punctate terminal-like reactivity and weakly stained fibers were seen, especially at more temporal levels (Figs. 11 and 12). At septal levels, stained processes were seen to radiate from the granular cell layer out in the molecular layer (Figs. 9 and 10). The origin of these processes could not be determined. In the granular cell layer, strong, punctate terminal-like reactivity was seen around the granule cells, especially at septal levels and corresponding to the most superficial cell bodies (Figs. 9–12). In the outer plexiform layer of the hilus, reactive fibers, but also a few stained cell bodies were seen (Figs. 9–12). In the outer hilar cell layer, a plexus consisting of reactive dendrites with a beaded appearance as well as a few reactive cell bodies were found at septal levels (Figs. 9 and 10). This plexus was, however, absent at more temporal levels (Figs. 11 and 12). Corresponding to the inner hilar cell layer, a small number of reactive stellate cells were seen.

Parvalbumin (PV)

The distribution of PV-immunoreactivity in the pig dentate area, hippocampus proper and subiculum is shown at septal and mid-septotemporal levels (Figs. 3c and 4c).

The subiculum

In the subiculum, a few reactive cells were seen in the deep part of the cell layer.

The hippocampus

Regio superior. In stratum moleculare, no immunoreactivity was seen, whereas in stratum radiatum, occasional weakly stained cells were encountered (Fig. 13). The pyramidal cell layer displayed punctate terminal-like reactivity around the pyramidal cells and their apical dendrites. In addition, a few reactive cell bodies were observed (Fig. 13). In stratum oriens, scattered reactive stellate cells and fibers were seen (Fig. 13). In the alveus, faintly stained fibers were present.

Regio inferior. Stratum moleculare, radiatum, oriens and alveus showed the same characteristics as in regio superior (Fig. 14). The layer of mossy fibers was almost unreactive, but occasional reactive cells were present in this layer (Fig. 14). The pyramidal cell layer showed the same characteristics as in regio superior, but seemed more reactive (Fig. 14).

Area dentata

The immunoreactivity was generally strongest in the medial blade of the dentate area at all septotemporal levels (Figs. 15–18). In the molecular layer, stained processes radiating from stellate cells in the granular cell layer and the outer plexiform layer were most prominent at septal levels (Figs. 15 and 16). In the medial blade, the inner third of the molecular layer displayed an additional faint punctate terminal-like reactivity (Figs. 15 and 17). The granular cell layer displayed strong, punctate terminal-like reactivity around the granule cells, especially at septal levels (Figs. 15–18). Corresponding to the outer hilar cell layer and the outer plexiform layer, reactive dendrites with a beaded appearance were seen at septal levels (Figs. 15 and 16), in addition to a few stained stellate cells in the outer hilar cell layer (Figs. 15 and 16). At more temporal levels, the outer hilar cell layer and the outer plexiform layer contained many reactive stellate cells (Figs. 17 and 18), whereas few faintly stained fibers were present in the outer plexiform layer (Fig. 17). A small number of reactive stellate cells were seen in the inner hilar cell layer.

Discussion

In the present study, the immunocytochemical distribution of two calcium ion binding proteins, calbindin-D 28k (CaBP) and parvalbumin (PV) has been described. Whereas the distribution of PV-immunoreactivity in the hippocampal region has only been described in rat (Celio and Heizmann, 1981; Heizmann and Celio, 1987; Kawaguchi et al., 1987; Kosaka et al., 1987; Katsumaru et al., 1988a, b) and man (Berchtold et al.,

1985), the distribution of CaBP-immunoreactivity has been studied in rat (Jande et al., 1981; Baimbridge and Miller, 1982; Miller and Baimbridge, 1983; Rami et al., 1987), guinea pig and hedgehog (Rami et al., 1987). CaBP-immunoreactivity was present in granule cells and the mossy fiber system in all 3 species, whereas stained pyramidal cells were seen in regio superior in the rat and hedgehog, but were absent in the guinea pig. On the outer hand, stained cells were numerous in the subiculum of the guinea pig (Rami et al., 1987). The distribution of CaBP in the pig hippocampus, as described in the present study, differs markedly from that of rat, guinea pig and hedgehog, in that neither granule cells, mossy fibers nor pyramidal cells were stained. On the other hand, the bundle of stained fibers and cell bodies in stratum moleculare and the outer third of the dentate molecular layer described in the pig hippocampus resembles that of the rat (Baimbridge and Miller, 1982; Miller and Baimbridge, 1983), and the staining of cell bodies in the pig subiculum corresponds to that of the guinea pig (Rami et al., 1987). In the pig hippocampus, CaBP-reactive cell bodies were also seen in stratum oriens, the pyramidal cell layer and stratum radiatum of regio superior and inferior as well as in the outer plexiform layer and outer hilar cell layer of the dentate hilus, whereas terminal-like reactivity was present in the pyramidal cell layer of regio superior and inferior and in the granular cell layer. The latter part of the CaBP-staining (reactive cell bodies and terminals) has not been described in other species, but bears a striking resemblance to the distribution of PV-immunoreactivity in the pig both regarding localization of reactivity and morphology of the stained cells. The distribution of PV-immunoreactivity has been thoroughly studied in the rat hippocampus, where PV-reactive cell bodies were concentrated in the pyramidal cell layer and stratum oriens of regio superior and inferior as well as in the granular cell layer, the subgranular zone and hilus of the dentate area, and terminal-like reactivity was observed in the pyramidal cell layer and the granular cell layer

92

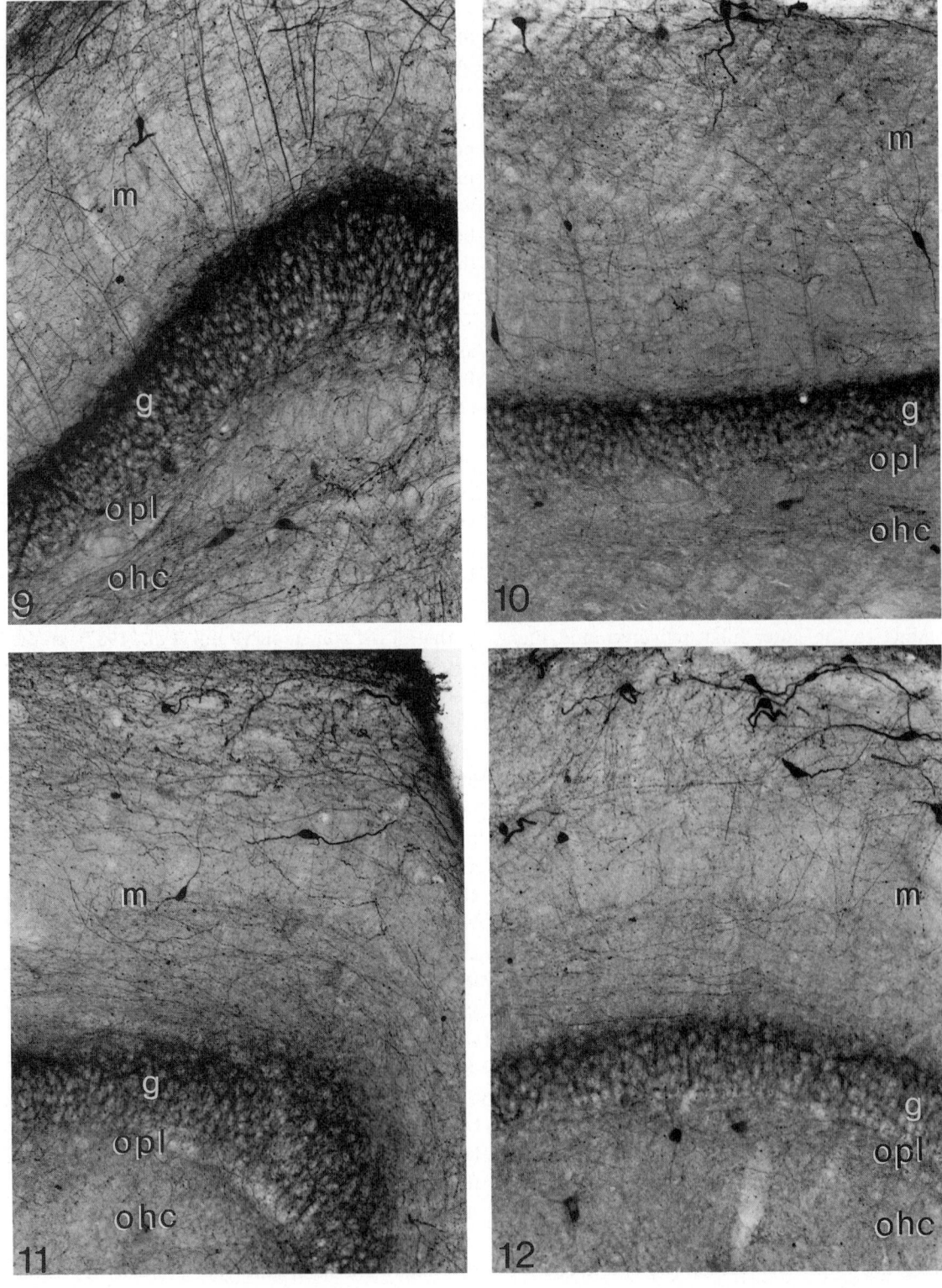

(Celio and Heizmann, 1981; Heizmann and Celio, 1987; Kawaguchi et al., 1987; Kosaka et al., 1987a; Katsumaru et al., 1988a; Kamphuis et al., 1989). The distribution of PV-immunoreactivity in the pig hippocampus as described in the present paper thus appears identical to that of the rat hippocampus.

Although no information on cell morphology in the pig hippocampus is available, it is tempting to assume that some or most of the CaBP- or PV-immunoreactive cell bodies in the pig hippocampus represent non-pyramidal interneurons (basket cells) in that their localization and morphological appearance resemble that of PV-reactive cells in the rat hippocampus, and these have been

classified as interneurons (basket cells and axo-axonic cells (or chandelier cells)) (Celio and Heizmann, 1981; Heizmann and Celio, 1987; Kosaka et al., 1987a; Katsumaru et al., 1988).

The functional significance of CaBP and PV is still not fully understood. At the ultrastructural level the CaBP- and PV-immunoreactivity was found associated with microtubules, postsynaptic densities and intracellular membranes within the perikarya, axons and dendrites of labeled cells (Stichel et al., 1987; Di Figlia et al., 1989), and the proteins are therefore not believed to function as neurotransmitters, neurohormones or neuro-modulators (Pasteels et al., 1986). Whereas CaBP does not seem to be co-localized with any known

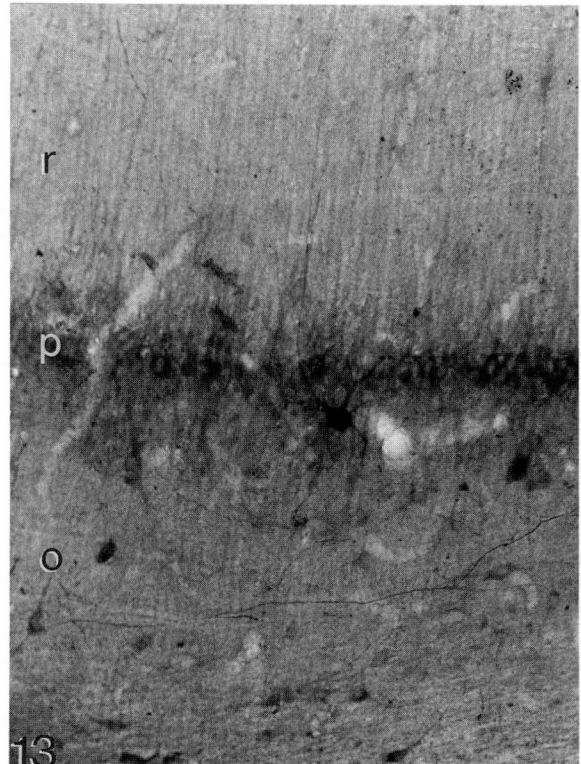 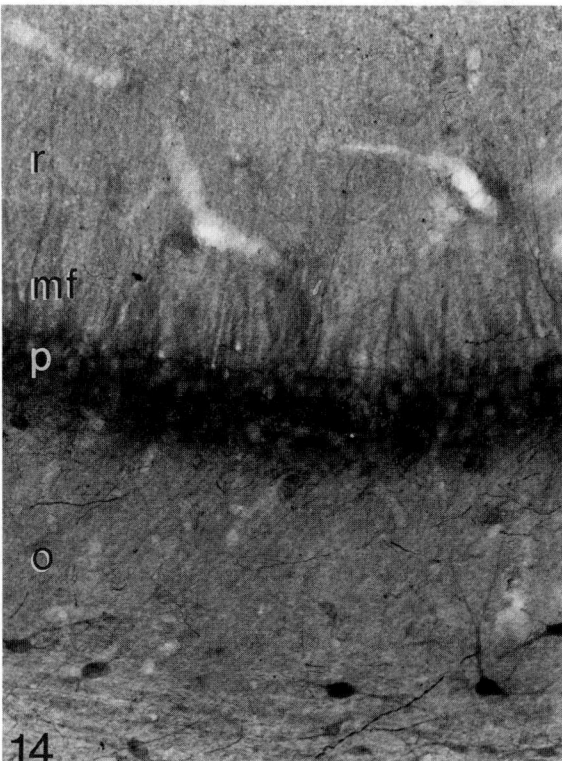

Figs. 13 and 14. Stratum radiatum, pyramidal cell layer and stratum oriens of regio superior (Fig. 13) and regio inferior (Fig. 14). PV-immunocytochemistry. ×145.

Figs. 9–12. Area dentata at septal (Figs. 9 and 10) and mid-septotemporal levels (Figs. 11 and 12). CaBP-immunocytochemistry. Note differences between medial (Figs. 9 and 11) and lateral parts (Figs. 10 and 12). ×145.

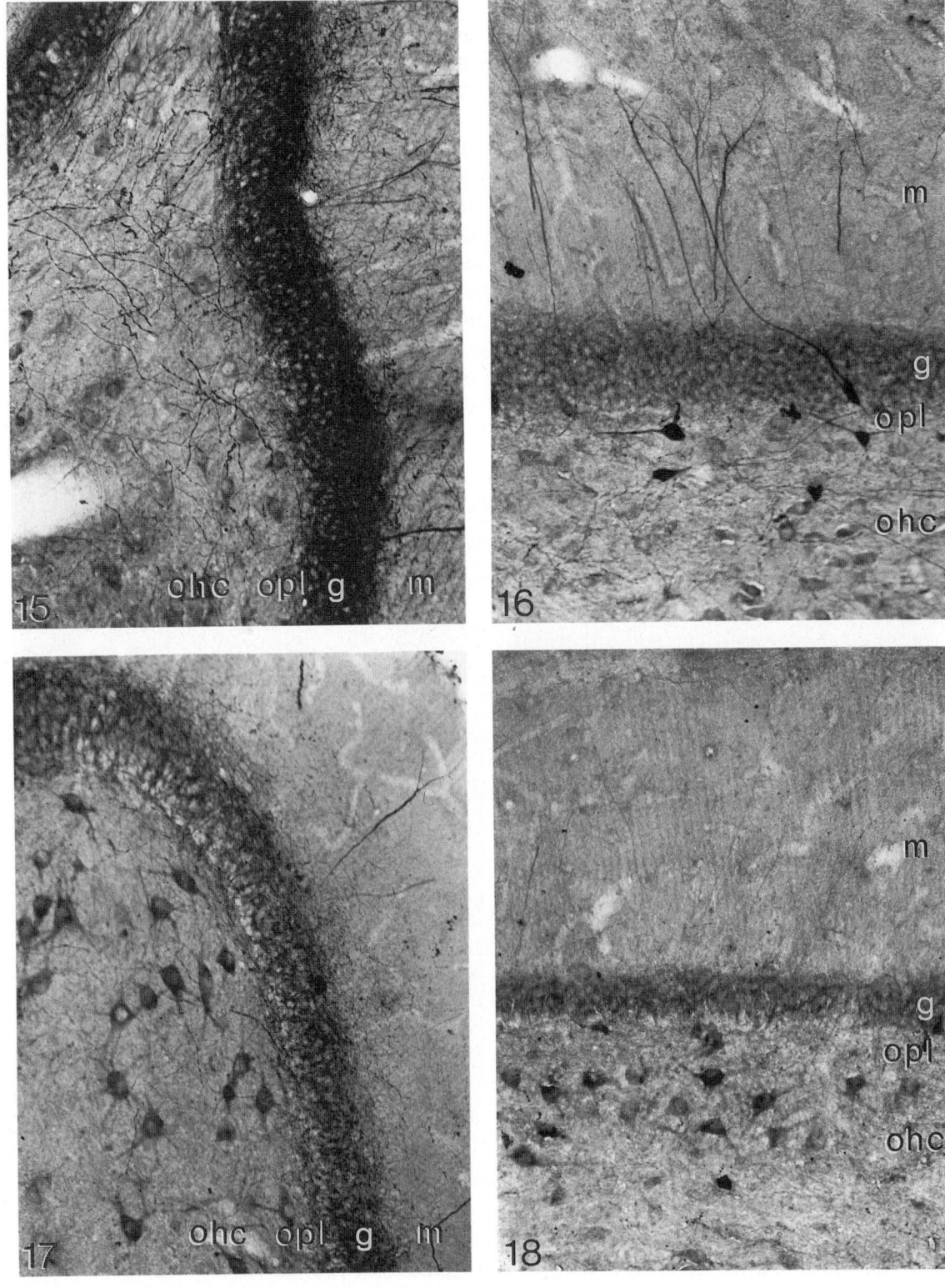

neurotransmitter or neuropeptide, PV has been shown to be present in a subpopulation of GABAergic neurons in both the cerebral cortex (Celio and Heizmann, 1981; Celio, 1986; Stichel et al., 1986; Kosaka et al., 1987b; Heizmann and Celio, 1987; DeFelipe et al., 1989) and hippocampal region (Kosaka et al., 1987a; Kawaguchi et al., 1987; Katsumaru et al., 1988a). In the rat hippocampus, the majority of non-pyramidal neurons contain GABA (Ribak et al., 1978, 1981; Storm-Mathisen et al., 1983), which is the inhibitory transmitter substance in the hippocampus and dentate area (Storm-Mathisen and Ottersen, 1984). Almost all PV-immunoreactive neurons in the rat hippocampus also contain GABA, whereas only 20% of the GABAergic neurons stain for PV. However, the percentage of PV-containing GABAergic neurons depends on the exact localization in the hippocampus (Kosaka et al., 1987a), and it has been shown that PV-containing GABAergic non-pyramidal cells in regio superior differ electrophysiologically from GABAergic non-pyramidal cells with no PV-reactivity in that the former belong to the fast-spiking neurons (Kawaguchi et al., 1987). These observations suggest that PV may act as an intracellular calcium-buffer, suppressing the elevation of the calcium concentration during repetitive firing and blocking the adaptation due to calcium activating potassium conductance in fast spiking cells (Kawaguchi et al., 1987).

Results from kindling experiments also suggest a role for both CaBP and PV in controlling intracellular calcium homeostasis. Following commissural kindling, the concentration of CaBP in the rat hippocampal region was significantly reduced and a localized depletion of CaBP-immunoreactivity was seen in the dentate granule cells and the mossy fiber system (Miller and Baimbridge, 1983). On the other hand, commissural kindling has been shown to cause a decrease in the number of GABAergic cells in the rat hippocampus (Kamphuis et al., 1986, 1987). This reduction was shown to be restricted to GABAergic cells without PV-immunoreactivity, whereas PV-containing GABAergic cells were not reduced in number, suggesting that PV exerts a protective role by buffering a rise in intracellular calcium ion concentration during seizures (Kamphuis et al., 1989).

In Alzheimer-type dementia, a decreased number of cortical neurons containing PV as well as neurons containing CaBP was seen (Arai et al., 1987; Ichimiya et al., 1988), and it is possible that both proteins by buffering calcium ions, reduce neuronal vulnerability to excitotoxic effects of excitatory amino acids which are possibly involved in the pathogenesis of Alzheimer-type dementia (Mayer and Westbrook, 1987).

In the present study, the distribution of the calcium-binding proteins CaBP and PV was described in the hippocampal region of normal pigs. In view of the extensive use of pigs in biomedical research it is our hope that the present description may serve as a useful basis for future experimental studies of calcium ion involvement in various pathological states.

Acknowledgements

The present study was supported by the Danish MRC, Grant No. 12-8818.

References

Arai, H., Emson, P.C., Mountjoy, C.Q., Carasso, L.H. and Heizmann, C.W. (1987) Loss of parvalbumin-immunoreactive neurones from cortex in Alzheimer-type dementia. *Brain Res.*, 418: 164 – 169.

Baimbridge, K.G. and Miller, J.J. (1982) Immunohistochemical localization of calcium-binding protein in the cerebellum, hippocampal formation and olfactory bulb of the rat. *Brain Res.*, 245: 223 – 229.

Baimbridge, K.G., Miller, J.J. and Parkes, C.O. (1982)

Figs. 15 – 18. Area dentata at septal (Figs. 15 and 16) and mid-septotemporal levels (Figs. 17 and 18). PV-immunocytochemistry. Note differences between medial (Figs. 15 and 17) and lateral parts (Figs. 16 and 18). × 145.

Calcium-binding protein distribution in the rat brain. *Brain Res.*, 239: 519 – 525.

Berchtold, M.W., Celio, M.R. and Heizmann, C.W. (1985) Parvalbumin in human brain. *J. Neurochem.*, 45: 235 – 239.

Breazile, J.E. (1967) The cytoarchitecture of the brain stem of the domestic pig. *J. Comp. Neurol.*, 129: 169 – 188.

Celio, M.R. (1986) Parvalbumin in most γ-aminobutyric acid-containing neurons of the rat cerebral cortex. *Science*, 231: 995 – 997.

Celio, M.R. and Heizmann, C.W. (1981) Calcium-binding protein parvalbumin as a neuronal marker. *Nature*, 293: 300 – 302.

Choi, D.W. (1988) Calcium-mediated neurotoxicity: relationship to specific channel types and role in ischemic damage. *Trends Neurosci.*, 11: 465 – 469.

DeFelipe, J., Hendry, S.H.C. and Jones, E.G. (1989) Visualization of chandelier cell axons by parvalbumin immunoreactivity in monkey cerebral cortex. *Proc. Natl. Acad. Sci. U.S.A.*, 86: 2093 – 2097.

DiFiglia, M., Christakos, S. and Aronin, N. (1989) Ultrastructural localization of immunoreactive calbindin-D$_{28k}$ in the rat and monkey basal ganglia, including subcellular distribution with colloidal gold labeling. *J. Comp. Neurol.*, 279: 653 – 665.

Freeman, T.B., Wojak, J.C., Brandeis, L., Michel, J.P., Pearson, J. and Flamm, E.S. (1988) Cross-species intracerebral grafting of embryonic swine dopaminergic neurons. *Prog. Brain Res.*, 78: 473 – 477.

Geneser, F.A. (1986) Distribution of acetylcholinesterase in the hippocampal region of the rabbit: I. Entorhinal area, parasubiculum, and presubiculum. *J. Comp. Neurol.*, 254: 352 – 368.

Geneser, F.A. (1987a) Distribution of acetylcholinesterase in the hippocampal region of the rabbit: II. Subiculum and hippocampus. *J. Comp. Neurol.*, 262: 90 – 104.

Geneser, F.A. (1987b) Distribution of acetylcholinesterase in the hippocampal region of the rabbit. III. The dentate area. *J. Comp. Neurol.*, 262: 594 – 606.

Grandin, T., Demotte, O.D., Greenough, W.T. and Curtis, S.E. (1988) Perfusion method for preparing pig brain cortex for Golgi-Cox impregnation. *Stain Technol.*, 63: 177 – 181.

Heizmann, C.W. (1984) Parvalbumin, an intracellular calcium-binding protein; distribution, properties and possible roles in mammalian cells. *Experientia*, 40: 910 – 921.

Heizmann, C.W. and Celio, M.R. (1987) Immunolocalization of parvalbumin. *Methods Enzymol.*, 139: 552 – 570.

Hereć, S. (1967) Structure of the olfactory tubercle and nucleus of the diagonal tract of Broca in the pig. *Folia Morph.*, 26: 452 – 458.

Herre, W. (1936) Untersuchungen an Hirnen von Wild- und Hausschweinen. *Verh. Dtsch. Zool. Ges.*, pp. 200 – 211.

Holm, I.E. and Geneser, F.A. (1989) Histochemical demonstration of zinc in the hippocampal region of the domestic pig: I. Entorhinal area, parasubiculum, and presubiculum. *J.*

Comp. Neurol.*, 287: 145 – 163.

Holm, I.E. and Geneser. F.A. (1990a) Histochemical demonstration of zinc in the hippocampal region of the domestic pig: II. Subiculum and hippocampus. *J. Comp. Neurol.*, submitted.

Holm, I.E. and Geneser, F.A. (1990b) Histochemical demonstration of zinc in the hippocampal region of the domestic pig: III. The dentate area. *J. Comp. Neurol.*, submitted.

Ichimiya, Y., Emson, P.C., Mountjoy, C.Q., Lawson, D.E.M. and Heizmann, C.W. (1988) Loss of calbindin-28k immunoreactive neurones from the cortex in Alzheimer-type dementia. *Brain Res.*, 475: 156 – 159.

Jande, S.S., Maler, L. and Lawson, D.E.M. (1981) Immunohistochemical mapping of vitamin D-dependent calcium-binding protein in brain. *Nature (Lond.)*, 294: 765 – 767.

Kamphuis, W., Wadman, W.J., Buijs, R.M. and Lopes da Silva, F.H. (1986) Decrease in number of hippocampal gamma-aminobutyric acid (GABA) immunoreactive cells in the rat kindling model of epilepsy. *Exp. Brain Res.*, 64: 491 – 495.

Kamphuis, W., Wadman, W.J., Buijs, R.M. and Lopes da Silva, F.H. (1987) The development of changes in hippocampal gamma-aminobutyric acid (GABA) in the rat kindling model of epilepsy: a light microscopic study with GABA-antibodies. *Neuroscience*, 23: 433 – 446.

Kamphuis, W., Huisman, E., Wadman, W.J., Heizmann, C.W. and Lopes da Silva, F.H. (1989) Kindling induced changes in parvalbumin immunoreactivity in rat hippocampus and its relation to long-term decrease in GABA-immunoreactivity. *Brain Res.*, 479: 23 – 34.

Katsumaru, H., Kosaka, T., Heizmann, C.W. and Hama, K. (1988a) Immunocytochemical study of GABAergic neurons containing the calcium-binding protein parvalbumin in the rat hippocampus. *Exp. Brain Res.*, 72: 347 – 362.

Katsumaru, H., Kosaka, T., Heizmann, C.W. and Hama, K. (1988b) Gap junctions on GABAergic neurons containing the calcium-binding protein parvalbumin in the rat hippocampus (CA1 region). *Exp. Brain Res.*, 72: 363 – 370.

Kawaguchi, Y., Katsumaru, H., Kosaka, T., Heizmann, C.W. and Hama, K. (1987) Fast spiking cells in rat hippocampus (CA$_1$ region) contain the calcium-binding protein parvalbumin. *Brain Res.*, 416: 369 – 374.

Kosaka, T., Heizmann, C.W., Tateishi, K., Hamaoka, Y. and Hama, K. (1987a) An aspect of the organizational principle of the γ-aminobutyric acidergic system in the cerebral cortex. *Brain Res.*, 409: 403 – 408.

Kosaka, T., Katsumaru, H., Hama, K., Wu, J.-Y. and Heizmann, C.W. (1987b) GABAergic neurons containing the Ca^{2+}-binding protein parvalbumin in the rat hippocampus and dentate gyrus. *Brain Res.*, 419: 119 – 130.

Kruska, D. (1970) Vergleichende cytoarchitektonische Untersuchungen an Gehirnen von Wild- und Hausschweinen. *Z.*

Anat. Entwickl. -Gesch., 131: 291 – 324.

Mayer, M.L. and Westbrook, G.L. (1987) The physiology of excitatory amino acids in the vertebrate central nervous system. *Prog. Neurobiol.,* 28: 197 – 276.

Miller, J.J. and Baimbridge, K.G. (1983) Biochemical and immunohistochemical correlates of kindling-induced epilepsy: role of calcium binding protein. *Brain Res.,* 278: 322 – 326.

Niwa, M., Shigematsu, K., Kurihara, M., Kataoka, Y., Maeda, T., Nakao, K., Imura, H., Matsuo, H., Tsuchiyama, H. and Ozaki, M. (1988) Receptor autoradiographic evidence of specific brain natriuretic peptide binding sites in the porcine subfornical organ. *Neurosci. Lett.,* 95: 113 – 118.

Palmieri, G., Farina, V., Panu, R., Asole, A., Sanna, L., de Riu, P.L., and Gabbi, C. (1987) Course and termination of the pyramidal tract in the pig. *Arch. Anat. Microsc.,* 75: 167 – 176.

Pasteels, J.L., Pochet, R., Surardt, L., Hubeau, C., Chirnoaga, M., Parmentier, M. and Lawson, D.E.M. (1986) Ultrastructural localization of brain "vitamin D-dependent" calcium binding proteins. *Brain Res.,* 384: 294 – 303.

Pearlmutter, A.F., Szkrybalo, M., Kim, Y. and Harik, S.I. (1988) Arginine vasopressin receptors in pig cerebral microvessels, cerebral cortex and hippocampus. *Neurosci. Lett.,* 87: 121 – 126.

Rami, A., Bréhier, A., Thomasset, M. and Rabié, A. (1987) The comparative immunocytochemical distribution of 28 kDa cholecalcin (CaBP) in the hippocampus of rat, guinea pig and hedgehog. *Brain Res.,* 422: 149 – 153.

Ribak, C.E., Vaughn, J.E. and Saito, K. (1978) Immunocytochemical localization of glutamic acid decarboxylase in neuronal somata following colchicine inhibition of axonal transport. *Brain Res.,* 140: 315 – 332.

Ribak, C.E., Vaughn, J.E. and Barber, R.P. (1981) Immunocytochemical localization of GABA-ergic neurones at the electron microscopic level. *Histochem. J.,* 13: 555 – 582.

Rothman, S.M. and Olney, J.W. (1987) Excitotoxicity and the NMDA receptor. *Trends Neurosci.,* 10: 299 – 302.

Salinas-Zeballos, M.-E., Zeballos, G.A. and Gootman, P.M. (1986) A stereotaxic atlas of the developing swine (*Sus scrofa*) forebrain. In M.E. Tumbleson (Ed.), *Swine in Biomedical Research, Vol. 2,* Plenum Press, New York, pp. 887 – 906.

Solnitzky, O. (1938) The thalamic nuclei of *Sus scrofa. J. Comp. Neurol.,* 69: 121 – 169.

Stephan, H. (1951) Vergleichende Untersuchungen über den Feinbau des Hirnes von Wild- und Haustieren. (Nach Studien am Schwein und Schaf.) *Zool. Jb., Abt. Anat. Ontog.,* 71: 487 – 586.

Sternberger, L.A. (1979) Immunocytochemistry. Wiley, New York.

Stichel, C.C., Kägi, U. and Heizmann, C.W. (1986) Parvalbumin in cat brain: isolation, characterization, and localization. *J. Neurochem.,* 47: 46 – 53.

Stichel, C.C., Singer, W., Heizmann, C.W. and Norman, A.W. (1987) Immunohistochemical localization of calcium-binding proteins, parvalbumin and calbindin-D 28k, in the adult and developing visual cortex of cats: a light and electron microscopic study. *J. Comp. Neurol.,* 262: 563 – 577.

Storm-Mathisen, J., Leknes, A.K., Bore, A.T., Vaaland, J.L., Edminson, P., Haug, F.-M.S. and Ottersen, O.P. (1983) First visualization of glutamate and GABA in neurones by immunocytochemistry. *Nature (Lond.),* 301: 517 – 520.

Storm-Mathisen, J. and Ottersen, O.P. (1984) Neurotransmitters in the hippocampal foramation. In F. Reinoso-Suárez and C. Ajmone-Marsan (Eds.), *Cortical Integration,* Raven Press, New York, pp. 105 – 130.

Tumbleson, M.E. (Ed.) (1986) *Swine in Biomedical Research, Vol. 1 – 3,* Plenum Press, New York.

Warr, W.B., de Olmos, J.S. and Heimer, L. (1981) Horseradish peroxidase. The basic procedure. In L. Heimer and M.J. Robards (Eds.), *Neuroanatomical Tract – Tracing Methods,* Plenum Press, New York, pp. 207 – 262.

Woolsey, C.N. and Fairman, D. (1946) Contralateral, ipsilateral, and bilateral representation of cutaneous receptors in somatic areas I and II of the cerebral cortex of pig, sheep, and other mammals. *Surgery,* 19: 684 – 702.

J. Storm-Mathisen, J. Zimmer and O.P. Ottersen (Eds.)
Progress in Brain Research, Vol. 83
© 1990 Elsevier Science Publishers B.V. (Biomedical Division)

CHAPTER 8

A quantitative electron microscopic immunocytochemical study of the distribution and synaptic handling of glutamate in rat hippocampus

Ole P. Ottersen[1], Jon Storm-Mathisen[1], Clive Bramham[2], Reidun Torp[1], Jon Laake[1] and Vidar Gundersen[1]

[1] *Anatomical Institute, University of Oslo, Karl Johans gate 47, N-0162 Oslo 1, Norway and* [2] *Department of Physiology, University of Bergen, N-5000 Bergen, Norway*

One of the major problems in glutamate immunocytochemistry has been the difficulty involved in separating immunocytochemical labelling due to metabolic glutamate from the labelling caused by transmitter glutamate. Another problem appears to be the accessibility of antigenic sites in conventional light microscopic preparations. In the present report, we have applied the primary glutamate antiserum onto ultrathin tissue sections, followed by the use of a colloidal gold detection system. The use of this postembedding immunogold procedure allows equal access of antibodies to all cellular compartments exposed at the section surface, allows quantitative assessment of the immunoreactivity, and affords a high resolution compatible with studies at the organelle level. When applied to slice preparations the immunogold procedure can be used to identify releasable pools of glutamate. These methodological advances have greatly increased the usefulness of glutamate immunocytochemistry as a tool to study putative glutamatergic terminals in the CNS.

Introduction

Glutamate serves many important roles in the brain: it is assumed to be the predominant mediator of fast excitation in CNS synapses, but it is also indirectly engaged in inhibitory neurotransmission as substrate for the GABA synthesizing enzyme, glutamic acid decarboxylase. Further, as in other tissues, glutamate is involved in several biochemical pathways in the "intermediary metabolism" and is a building block of proteins. Consonant with its multiple functions, glutamate is ubiquitously present in brain tissue and shows rather modest concentration differences among different brain regions (Balcom et al., 1976), and different hippocampal laminae (Berger et al., 1977).

It follows from the above considerations that a demonstration of glutamate in a cellular compartment is not easily interpreted in a functional context. A particularly important question is how to differentiate between transmitter and nontransmitter ("metabolic") glutamate. Biochemical data suggest that the size of the metabolic pool of glutamate is by no means insignificant: indeed, some calculations indicate that it may exceed the size of the transmitter pool (Fonnum, 1984). The routes of glutamate synthesis are probably not qualitatively different in the two pools. As a consequence, the development of an immunocytochemical technique for the localization of glutamate (Storm-Mathisen et al., 1983; Ottersen and Storm-Mathisen, 1984) initially did not provide a breakthrough in the identification of glutamatergic terminals. This was not due to problems with serum specificity (the sera were shown to react with fixed glutamate in a highly selective manner) but rather reflected the interference of "metabolic" glutamate as well as the limitations inherent in standard immunocytochemical procedures (e.g. antigen masking, incomplete and uneven penetration of the tissue by the immunoreagents).

A recent advance in the field of glutamate immunocytochemistry is the adaptation of the postembedding immunogold procedure (Somogyi et al., 1986; Ottersen, 1987; De Biasi and Rustioni, 1988; Ehinger et al., 1988; Liu et al., 1989). With this procedure, ultrathin sections of plastic-embedded tissue specimens are first incubated in the primary antiserum, and then in a colloidal gold-labelled secondary antibody or protein with high affinity for the primary antibodies. The use of this approach alleviates problems related to antigen masking and uneven tissue permeability since only antigenic sites at the surface of the section will be accessible to the immunoreagents. Moreover, the gold particles are easily detected and counted, permitting a semiquantitative assessment of the immunolabelling (Somogyi et al., 1986; Ottersen, 1987). Indeed, with the use of model systems it is possible to go one step further, namely to translate gold particle densities into absolute concentrations of fixed glutamate (Ottersen, 1989a, b). The gold particles signal the position of the antigens with an accuracy of about $20 - 30$ nm (depending on the gold particle size) and thus provide a resolution unattainable with the standard peroxidase-antiperoxidase technique.

In the present paper we have used the postembedding immunogold procedure as a tool to investigate whether the transmitter and metabolic pools of glutamate can be distinguished on the basis of differences in their distribution, concentration, or response to experimental manipulation. Hippocampus is a favourable model for such studies: not only does it contain some of the best documented glutamatergic pathways in the mammalian brain (Cotman et al., 1987; Ottersen and Storm-Mathisen, 1989), but the terminals of the different pathways are usually easily identified due to their segregated distribution and ultrastructural characteristics. Parts of the results on perfusion-fixed material have been published previously (Ottersen and Bramham, 1988; Ottersen, 1989a).

Methods

Adult male Wistar rats ($n = 9$) were fixed by transcardial perfusion with a mixture of 2.5% glutaraldehyde and 1% paraformaldehyde in 0.1 M sodium phosphate buffer, pH 7.4 (20°C, 50 ml/min for 10 min), following a brief wash ($10 - 15$ s) with buffer containing 2% dextran (4°C). Realizing the considerable risk for amino acid redistribution due to hypoxia (Benveniste et al., 1984) or other perturbations of systemic parameters, the necessary surgical procedures were completed as quickly as possible so that fixation (judged by neck stiffness) was achieved within $60 - 90$ s after thoracotomy. The brains were postfixed for $3 - 24$ h in the same fixative as above. For in vitro studies, rats ($n = 6$) were perfused with ice-cold buffer after which the hippocampus was rapidly dissected out and cut on a Vibratome at 400 μm. The slices thus obtained were preincubated in artificial cerebrospinal fluid (ACSF)[a] for 40 min $-$ 1 h and subsequently transferred to fresh ACSF containing "physiological" (5 mM) or "high" (40 or 55 mM) K^+ concentrations ($3 - 30$ min). Adjacent slices were simultaneously processed in media composed exactly as above except that the concentration of Ca^{2+} had been reduced from 2.4 mM to 0.1 mM, and that of Mg^{2+} increased from 1.3 mM to 10 mM. The media (pH 7.4, 33°C) were continuously gassed with 95% O_2/5% CO_2. All incubations were performed in 40 ml of fluid circulating past the tissue slices which were suspended on a nylon net. The slices were fixed by immersion (1 h) in a fixative identical to that used for perfusion (see above).

---

[a] The composition of the ACSF was as follows: 74 mM NaCl, 3.8 mM KCl, 26 mM $NaHCO_3$, 1.2 mM KH_2PO_4, 1.3 mM $MgSO_4$, 50 mM Tris/HCl, 10 mM glucose, and 2.4 mM $CaCl_2$. When 40 or 55 mM K^+ was added, the concentration of Tris/HCl was decreased correspondingly (to maintain a constant Na^+ concentration).

Tissue specimens from the perfusion-fixed and immersion-fixed hippocampi were osmicated, dehydrated and embedded in an epoxy resin (Durcupan ACM, Fluka) as previously described (Ottersen, 1987, 1988). Ultrathin sections were treated sequentially with $HIO_4/NaIO_4$ (to alleviate the masking effect of osmium), the primary antiserum (glutamate antiserum 13 or 03; Storm-Mathisen et al., 1983; Ottersen and Storm-Mathisen, 1984, 1985), and a secondary antibody coupled to colloidal gold particles (GAR G15; Janssen). The procedure has been described in full detail in previous reports (Ottersen, 1987, 1989a, b). Throughout the immunocytochemical processing, the tissue sections were accompanied by test sections (for assessing the specificity of the immunocytochemical reaction; Ottersen, 1987) and graded sections (for defining the relationship between the gold particle density and the concentration of fixed glutamate; Ottersen, 1989b). The test sections contained glutaraldehyde-brain protein conjugates of the 6 most abundant amino acids in the brain, whereas the graded sections comprised conjugates made at a series of different glutamate concentrations. All conjugates were prepared so as to mimic the amino acid conjugates that are formed in the brain during fixation.

The test sections were used to establish the optimum incubation parameters. The best results were obtained when the antisera (which had previously been purified in solid phase; Ottersen and Storm-Mathisen, 1984) were preadsorbed in liquid phase with glutaraldehyde fixation complexes (Ottersen et al., 1986) of glutamate and aspartate (100 µM of each with respect to the amino acid). The optimum serum dilution was 1 : 300 to

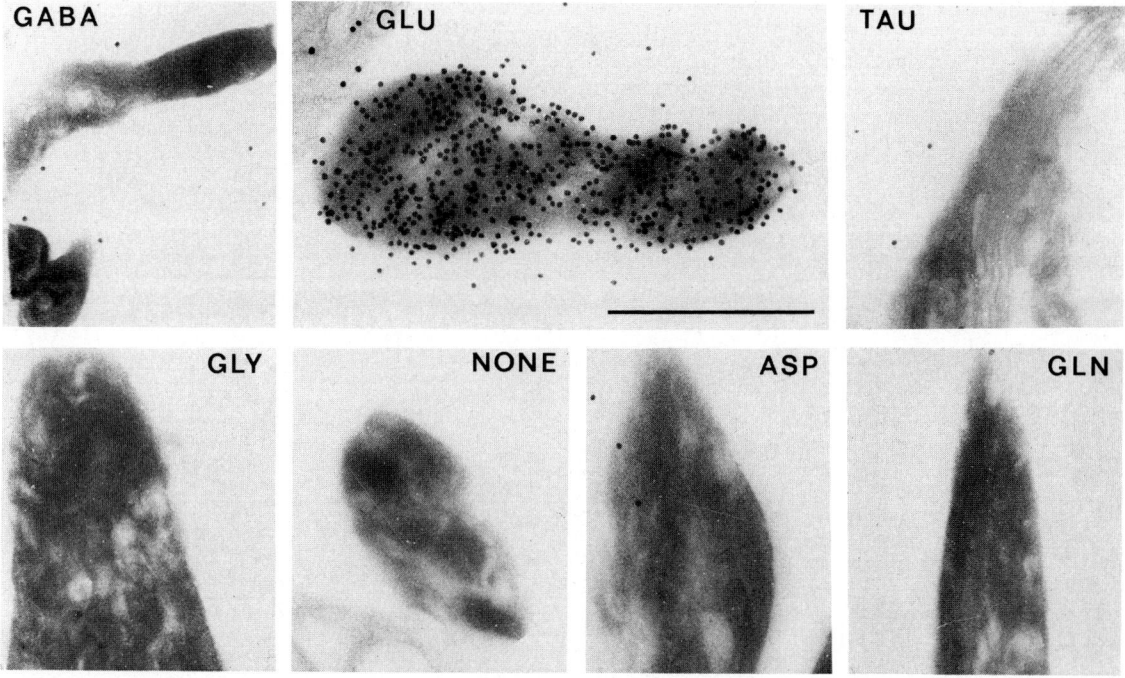

Fig. 1. Electron micrographs of test conjugates incubated together with tissue sections. The test conjugates were prepared by reacting an amino acid with the fixative (glutaraldehyde) used for animal perfusion in the presence of a brain protein extract. The conjugates thus formed were freeze-dried, embedded, and arranged in a sandwich as previously described (Ottersen, 1987). In ultrathin sections through this sandwich, the conjugates appear as discrete clumps, the gold particle covering of which can readily be assessed in the electron microscope. Note highly selective labelling of the glutamate conjugates. (From Ottersen and Bramham (1988). *Frontiers in Excitatory Amino Acid Research*, pp. 93–100. Reprinted with permission.) Bar: 0.5 µm.

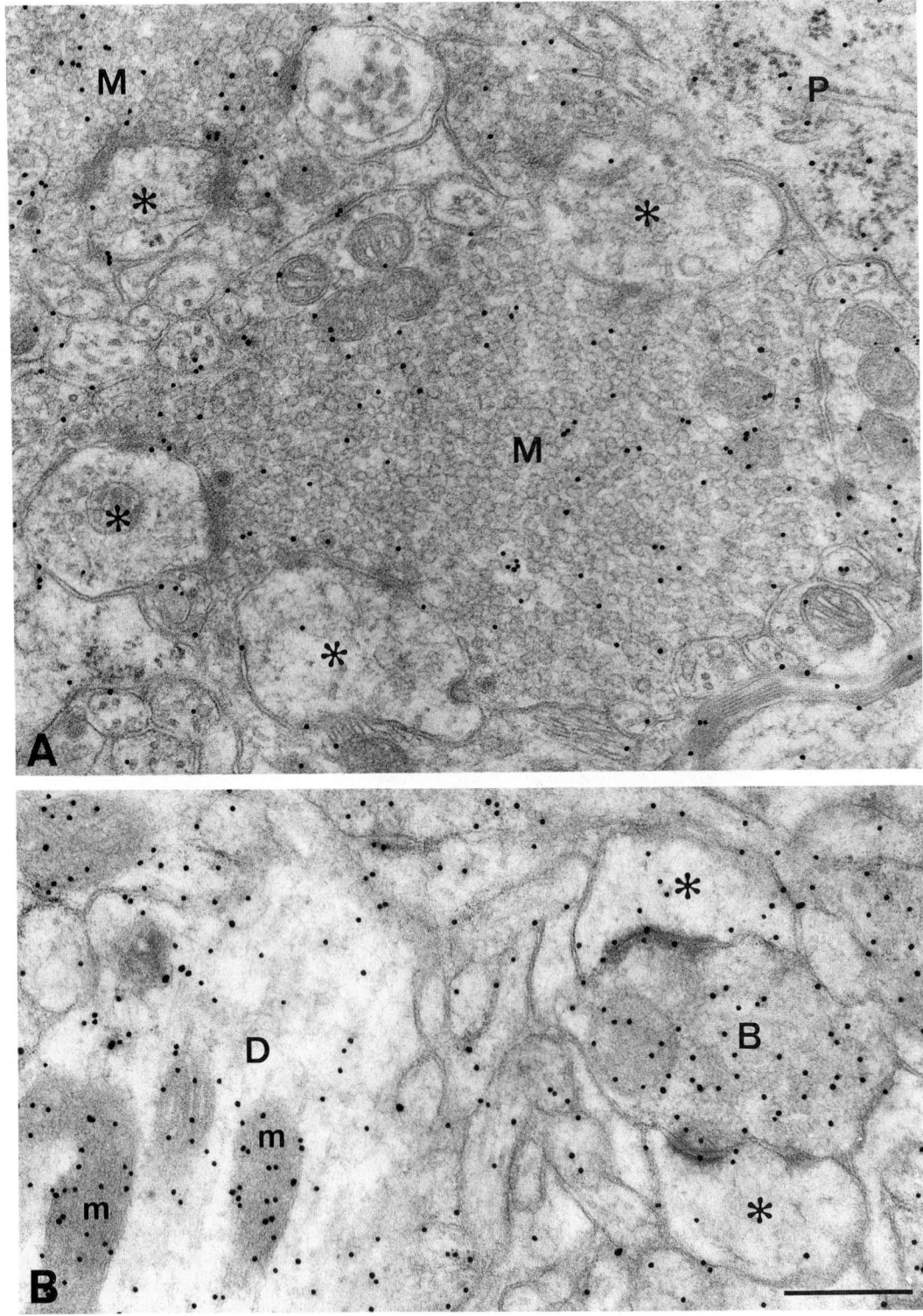

1 : 1500. One percent human serum albumin was added to the serum to decrease background labelling. Under these conditions, the glutamate antiserum produced a highly selective labelling of the glutamate conjugates (Fig. 1).

Quantitative analyses. A computer program (MORFOREL) has been designed to aid in the calculation of particle densities (Blackstad et al., 1989). The program is based on the use of a digitizer for recording the areas of cell profiles in electron micrographs. Particle numbers are fed into the computer after manual counting. The program permits basic statistical calculations, and provides a facility for export of data into commercial statistical packages.

Results

Perfusion-fixed material

Gold particles indicative of glutamate-like immunoreactivity are found in varying concentrations in all tissue profiles (Fig. 2). Supporting the impression gained by visual inspection of the electron micrographs, the quantitative analysis shows that the gold particle density is particularly high over certain populations of nerve terminals (Table I). The terminals that are enriched in glutamate-like immunoreactivity correspond to those of known excitatory pathways in the hippocampus (i.e., the perforant path, the commissural/Schaffer collateral fibre system, the hilar associational/commissural fibre system, and the mossy fibres). However, the gold particle density was not identical across these classes of excitatory fibre terminals: e.g., the terminals establishing asymmetric synapses in stratum radiatum of CA1 (commissural/Schaffer collateral terminals) displayed a

higher concentration of gold particles than did the mossy fibre terminals. This was true for all but one animal, in which these two types of terminals displayed the same labelling intensity. Terminals of asymmetric junctions in the outer zone of the dentate molecular layer showed gold particle densities equal to or exceeding those of the commissural/Schaffer collateral terminals. The lowest gold particle densities were found in boutons establishing symmetric contacts on dendritic stems or cell somata, and in glial processes (Table I). Intermediate labelling intensities occurred in cell bodies, dendrites, and dendritic spines of the granule and pyramidal cells. These findings imply that, in the case of the commissural/Schaffer collateral and mossy fibre system, the nerve terminals contain a higher level of glutamate-like immunoreactivity than their respective parent cell bodies (Table I).

Although the absolute concentrations of gold particles varied from animal to animal (as a consequence of inadvertent fluctuations in the incubation parameters), in all animals the tissue profiles could be divided into 3 broad groups which differed with regard to their relative gold particle concentrations: a strongly labelled group of profiles, comprising the terminals of the major excitatory fibre pathways in the hippocampus, an intermediately labelled group of profiles comprising the dendrosomatic parts of the pyramidal and granule cells, and a weakly labelled group of profiles, comprising terminals forming symmetric contacts and glial cell processes. It should be emphasized that even the last group of profiles contains a significantly higher concentration of gold particles than background (i.e. over empty resin), suggesting that even these profiles contain noteworthy concentrations of glutamate.

Fig. 2. Electron micrographs from the stratum lucidum (A) and CA1 stratum radiatum (B) from perfusion-fixed rat hippocampus. Gold particles indicate glutamate-like immunoreactivity. Note enrichment of gold particles over mossy fibre terminals (M) and over terminals establishing asymmetric junctions in stratum radiatum (B). There is also an accumulation of gold particles over mitochondria (m). Asterisks, postsynaptic spines; D, dendrite; P, pyramidal cell body. The section represented here was subjected to a computer-assisted analysis of the immunolabelling pattern (Table I). Bar: 0.5 μm.

TABLE I

Quantitative assessment of glutamate-like immunoreactivity in different cell profiles of perfusion-fixed rat hippocampus

Group No.	Profile	Mean gold particle density ± S.E.M. (n)	Statistical comparison Group No.														
			1	2	3	4	5	6	7	8	9	10	11	12	13	14	15
1	glial processes CA3	18.1 ± 2.0 (21)															
2	symm. bout. CA1	23.8 ± 3.8 (10)															
3	spines CA1	28.9 ± 2.7 (35)															
4	pyramidal dendr. CA1	31.6 ± 3.0 (14)															
5	spines CA3	39.6 ± 2.2 (33)	*														
6	pyramidal somata CA1	43.5 ± 2.1 (9)	*														
7	spines Mo	45.7 ± 3.6 (28)	*	*	*												
8	pyramidal dendr. CA3	46.3 ± 2.0 (17)	*	*	*												
9	granule somata	50.2 ± 2.6 (7)	*														
10	pyramidal somata CA3	56.5 ± 2.8 (10)	*	*	*	*											
11	mossy fibre term.	86.1 ± 2.4 (22)	*	*	*	*	*	*	*	*	*	*					
12	asymm. term. Mm	88.4 ± 5.4 (20)	*	*	*	*	*	*	*	*	*	*					
13	asymm. term. Mi	92.2 ± 4.8 (18)	*	*	*	*	*	*	*	*	*	*					
14	asymm. term. CA1 rad.	97.5 ± 6.9 (25)	*	*	*	*	*	*	*	*	*	*					
15	asymm. term. Mo	125.9 ± 7.3 (17)	*	*	*	*	*	*	*	*	*	*	*	*	*	*	

Data were obtained from an ultrathin section (shown in Fig. 2) incubated with glutamate antiserum 13 diluted 1 : 500. Values represent number of gold particles/μm^2 ± S.E.M. corrected for particle density over empty resin (2.3 particles/μm^2). The number of measured profiles is shown in parentheses (n). Mi, Mm and Mo, inner, middle and outer zones of the dentate molecular layer. Asterisks denote pairs of groups significantly different at the 0.05 level (multiple range test, Student – Newman – Keuls procedure, SPSS/PC$^+$). Based on data also presented in Blackstad et al. (1989). Similar results were obtained in 20 experiments from a total of 9 animals.

Immersion-fixed material

Compared with perfusion-fixed material, hippocampal slices that were fixed by immersion showed a much greater contrast in labelling intensity between different tissue compartments (Figs. 3, 4). When sections from perfusion-fixed and immersion-fixed material were incubated in the same drops of immunoreagents to allow direct comparison, it became clear that this increased contrast was due partly to an enhanced accumulation of gold particles over presumed excitatory terminals, partly to a decrease in the gold particle covering of the remaining tissue elements. Thus, in vitro incubation of hippocampal slices seems to favour a nerve terminal pattern of labelling, a conclusion that was previously arrived at on the basis of light microscopic preparations (Storm-Mathisen et al., 1983, 1986a, b; Storm-Mathisen and Ottersen, 1988). Why the in vitro conditions induce these changes in the labelling pattern is not known. However, a plausible explanation is that the preparation of the slices and the subsequent incubation lead to a non-selective efflux of glutamate from all cell compartments. Glutamate will only remain in high concentrations at sites where the rate of synthesis is sufficient to keep pace with the efflux. The apparent increase in intraterminal glutamate in the in vitro experiments could be explained if the activity of the phosphate-activated glutaminase is less tightly coupled to the glutamate concentration (Kvamme et al., 1988) in

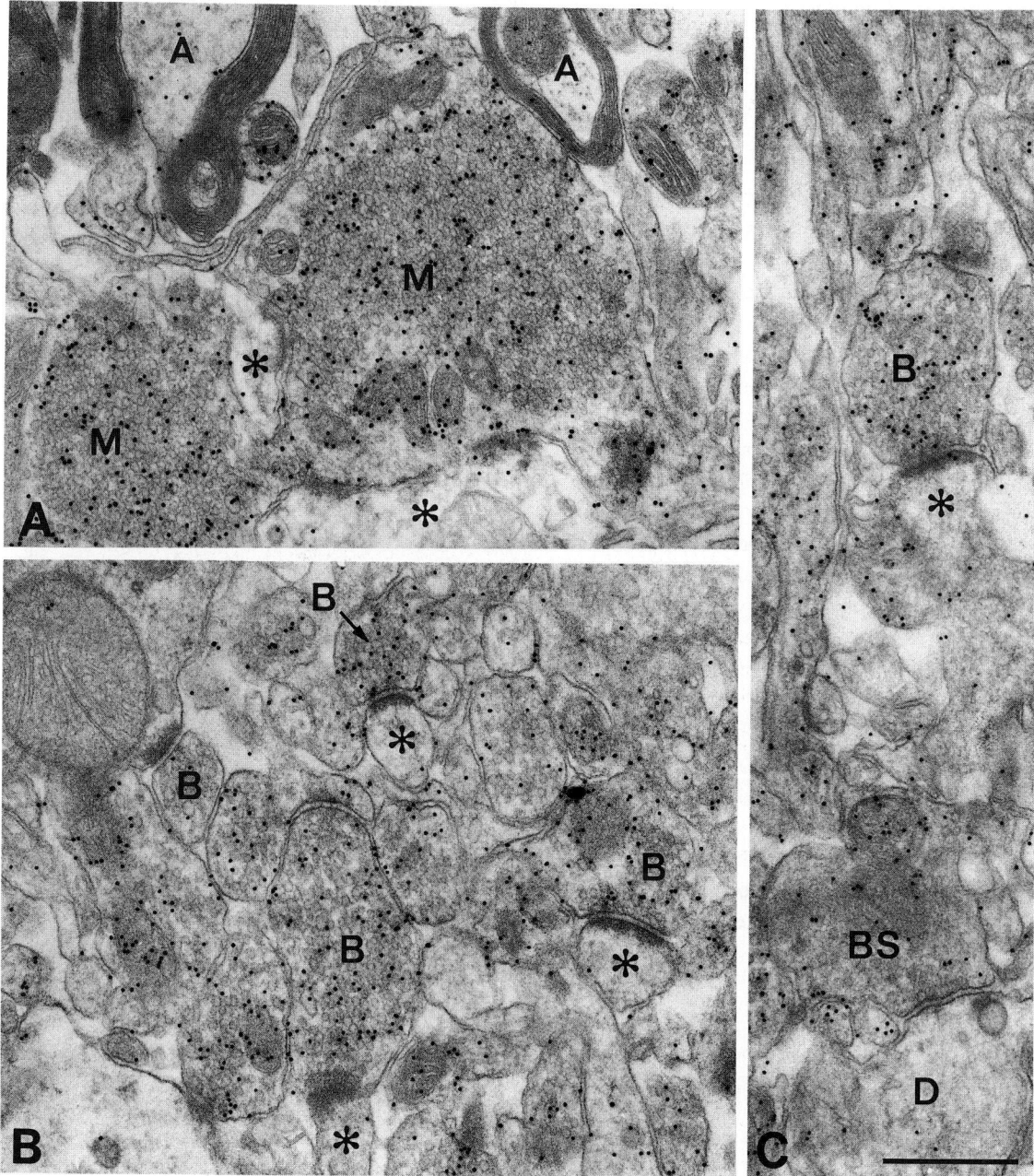

Fig. 3. Electron micrographs from the stratum lucidum (A) and CA1 stratum radiatum (B,C) of immersion-fixed rat hippocampus. The mossy fibre terminals (M) are from the hilus-near portion of the stratum lucidum. Note that in this material the mossy fibre terminals and terminals establishing asymmetric junctions in the stratum radiatum (B) display a higher density of gold particles (relative to the rest of the tissue) than do corresponding terminals in perfusion-fixed material (Fig. 2). BS, poorly labelled terminal engaged in symmetric contact with a dendritic stem (D); A, myelinated axons; asterisks, postsynaptic elements of asymmetric synapses. Bar: 0.6 μm.

vitro than in vivo. A high glutamate turnover may be characteristic of the transmitter pool of glutamate (Engelsen and Fonnum, 1983). Thus, it is tempting to speculate that the nerve terminals that show a high density of gold particles after in vitro incubation (and a slightly lower density of gold particles after perfusion fixation) are identical to those that release glutamate as neurotransmitter.[b]

Whether this is indeed the case can be explored by testing whether the terminals can be depleted of immunoreactivity under conditions known to induce synaptic release. Exposing the slices to 55 mM K^+ for 20–30 min led to a significant drop in the level of immunoreactivity in all categories of presumed excitatory nerve terminals. This drop was particularly pronounced for the mossy fibre terminals (Figs. 5, 6). (It should be emphasized that sections from the depolarized slices were processed for immunocytochemistry together with, and thus under exactly the same conditions as, sections from slices that had been maintained under physiological K^+ concentrations.) In the presence of low Ca^{2+} and high Mg^{2+}, the effect of high K^+ was nearly abolished (Fig. 6), suggesting that the observed changes were caused by a Ca^{2+}-dependent process.

The effect of stimulation with high K^+ was confined to the presynaptic element of the asymmetric synapses: the postsynaptic spines did not show

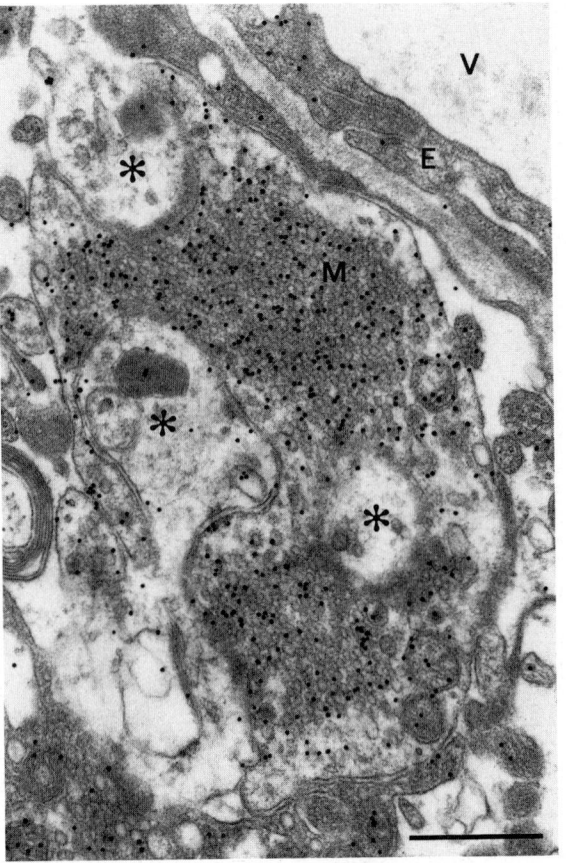

Fig. 4. Electron micrograph of mossy fibre terminal (M) from immersion-fixed rat hippocampus. Note that the gold particles are enriched over the vesicle-containing parts of the terminal (see Table II). Asterisks, postsynaptic spines; V, vessel lumen; E, endothelial cell. Bar: 0.36 μm.

[b] The mossy fibres (sampled from the hilus-near part of CA3, i.e. "CA3c") showed a non-uniform labelling after in vitro incubation. Whereas most of the mossy fibres appear intensely labelled, a minority contains a low concentration of gold particles. Whether this finding reflects a true heterogeneity among the mossy fibres, or whether it is due to technical factors (the very large mossy fibre terminals may be particularly vulnerable to mechanical damage during the preparation of the slices) remains to be resolved. The preparation and incubation procedure used here (Vibratome slicing, mechanical support, medium and temperature close to physiological conditions) preserve the glutamate immunoreactivity of the mossy fibres better than a previously used procedure (Fig. 2B of Cotman et al., 1987).

significant changes in gold particle densities in response to K^+ stimulation (Fig. 6). Glial cell processes differed from all other tissue elements in displaying an *increased* labelling intensity following depolarization with high K^+ (Fig. 6).

Exposure of the slices to 40 mM K^+ for 20–30 min led to a redistribution of glutamate-like immunoreactivity that was similar to, but less pronounced than that caused by 55 mM K^+. No detectable redistribution was noted when the time of exposure to high K^+ (40 or 55 mM) was reduced to 3 min.

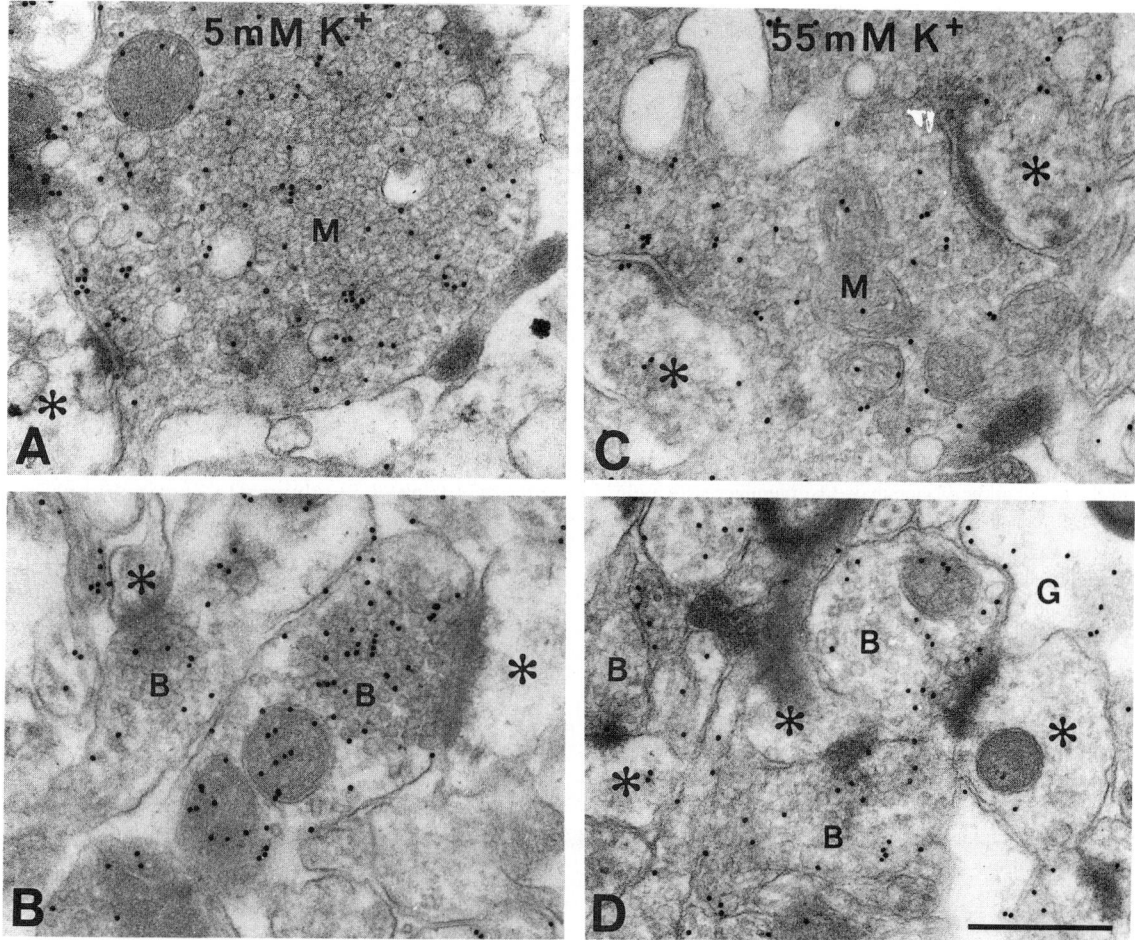

Fig. 5. Electron micrographs of mossy fibres (M; A,C) and terminals enganged in asymmetric junctions in CA1 stratum radiatum (B; B,D) from hippocampal slice incubated in vitro in the presence of 5 mM K$^+$ (A,B), or 55 mM K$^+$ (C,D). Depolarization with high K$^+$ leads to a decreased level of glutamate-like immunoreactivity in the two types of terminals illustrated (see Fig. 6 for a quantitative analysis). Asterisks, postsynaptic spines; G, glial process. Bar: 0.42 μm.

Subcellular distribution of glutamate-like immunoreactivity

Gold particles indicating glutamate-like immunoreactivity were more concentrated over clusters of vesicles than over areas of axoplasm devoid of vesicles and other organelles. This was particularly clear in immersion-fixed material (Fig. 4). A distinct accumulation of gold particles was also found over mitochondria (Figs. 2B, 3, Table II). However, the net particle density over vesicles, calculated assuming the lowest possible contribu-

tion of cytosol to the observed value, was higher than that over mitochondria (Table II). Nuclei were labelled at the same intensity as the surrounding cytoplasm.

Discussion

There are good reasons to believe that the glutamate immunolabelling pattern observed in immunogold preparations of perfusion-fixed tissue closely reflects the in vivo distribution of free glutamate. We know from model experiments with

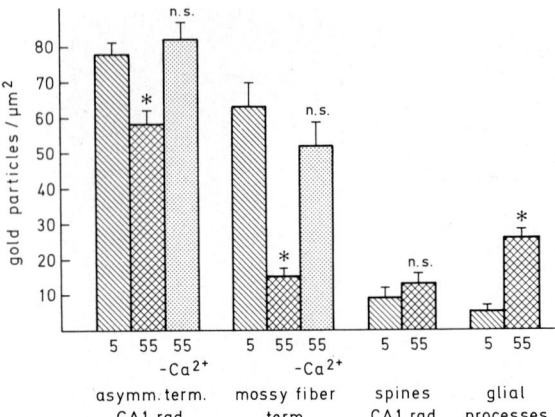

Fig. 6. Diagram showing the effect of depolarization with high K$^+$ on the distribution of glutamate-like immunoreactivity in different cell compartments in the hippocampus. Glutamate-like immunoreactivity is expressed as gold particles per μm^2. Values below columns indicate the mM concentration of K$^+$ in the incubation medium. Stippled columns represent values obtained from slices that were exposed to 55 mM K$^+$ under "Ca^{2+}-free conditions" (0.1 mM Ca^{2+}/10 mM Mg^{2+}). Asterisks indicate values significantly different ($P < 0.001$; Student's t-test) from first value in each group. n.s., not significantly different from first value in the group. Note that the depolarization is followed by a reduced level of immunoreactivity in the two categories of nerve terminals, by an increased level of immunoreactivity in glial processes, and by no statistically significant change in the level of immunoreactivity in postsynaptic spines.

radiolabelled taurine as a tracer that a major proportion (up to 90%) of the free amino acid pool in the brain is retained when the brain is perfusion-fixed according to the procedure presently used, i.e., with rapid surgery and relatively high concentrations of glutaraldehyde (S. Madsen and O.P. Ottersen, unpublished). A series of control experiments have been performed which indicate that no gross redistribution of glutamate occurs during the perfusion procedure (Storm-Mathisen and Ottersen, 1986). It should be remembered, however, that it is impossible to fix brain tissue quickly enough to completely rule out minor changes in the localization of glutamate, particularly at the subcellular level.

With this caveat in mind, the present results indicate that the terminals of the main excitatory

pathways in the hippocampus are enriched in glutamate, compared to terminals of symmetric, presumed inhibitory synapses and glial elements. The intermediate labelling intensity that is found over cell bodies and dendrites of granule and pyramidal cells may reflect predominantly a metabolic pool of glutamate, since it is not reduced by prolonged depolarization (Fig. 6) and since light microscopic studies have shown that levels of labelling comparable to those of hippocampal pyramidal cell bodies may be found also in cell bodies and dendrites of presumed non-glutamatergic neurons (Ottersen and Storm-Mathisen, 1984). The categories of nerve terminals that are enriched in glutamate-like immunoreactivity after perfusion fixation show an even greater accumulation of gold particles when fixed by immersion after incubation in vitro. As mentioned above, this may reflect a high rate of glutamate

TABLE II

Quantitative assessment of the subcellular distribution of glutamate-like immunoreactivity in mossy fibre terminals from a rat hippocampal slice

Subcellular compartment	Mean gold particle density ± S.E.M.
Mitochondria	128.9 ± 7.0
Clusters of synaptic vesicles	97.2 ± 5.8*
Cytosol	44.2 ± 6.0**
Whole terminal	64.0 ± 7.7[†]
Synaptic vesicles (calculated net)	150

Data were obtained from 14 mossy fibre terminals of a hippocampal slice incubated in vitro under "physiological" K$^+$ concentration (5 mM). Antiserum 03 diluted 1 : 500. Values represent number of gold particles/μm^2 ± S.E.M. corrected for particle density over empty resin (2.0 particles/μm^2). The value for clusters of synaptic vesicles reflects the labelling over vesicles as well as over the intervening cytosol. The net density in synaptic vesicles was calculated assuming that the intervening cytosol has the same particle density as the surrounding cytosol and that its volume equals the volume of vesicles, i.e. that the vesicles are densely packed and of equal size.
Asterisks denote value significantly different from the previous (*) or the two previous (**) values (*, $P < 0.01$; **, $P < 0.001$; Student's t-test, two tails). Dagger denotes statistically significant difference from two first values ($P < 0.002$).

synthesis in these terminals. Our finding that the same types of terminals show a Ca^{2+}-dependent loss of immunoreactivity upon stimulation with high K^+ supports previous light microscopic observations (Storm-Mathisen et al., 1986a, b; Gundersen et al., 1990), and suggests that the glutamate they contain belongs to or may enter a transmitter pool. This would be consistent with our observation that glutamate-like immunoreactivity tends to be concentrated over clusters of synaptic vesicles relative to the surrounding cytosol.

We propose therefore that putative glutamatergic terminals in the CNS may be identified in immunocytochemical preparations by virtue of their following characteristic features: (1) a high level of glutamate-like immunoreactivity compared to other tissue elements; (2) an enrichment of immunoreactivity over clusters of synaptic vesicles relative to surrounding cytosol; (3) a Ca^{2+}-dependent loss of glutamate-like immunoreactivity during depolarizing conditions. Each of these points will be considered in more detail below.

Level of glutamate-like immunoreactivity vs level of glutamate

One of the most important questions regards the relationship between gold particle densities and glutamate concentrations. For example, what does the difference in labelling intensity between putative excitatory and putative inhibitory terminals in the hippocampus correspond to in terms of concentration of fixed glutamate? In an attempt to resolve this issue we prepared a series of different glutamate-glutaraldehyde-brain protein conjugates, each containing a different concentration of fixed glutamate. These model conjugates were embedded in Durcupan in such a way that they could be retrieved in ultrathin sections ("graded sections") and incubated together with the tissue sections (Ottersen, 1989a, b). With this model system it was possible to show that the relationship between gold particle densities and ab-

solute concentration of fixed glutamate was close to linear, at least in the upper part of the biologically relevant range of glutamate concentrations. This was confirmed in the graded sections that were incubated together with the hippocampal sections used for the present study. Thus, in this material, an n-fold difference in gold particle density roughly corresponds to an n-fold difference in the concentration of fixed glutamate.

Subcellular distribution of glutamate-like immunoreactivity

Our finding of an enrichment of glutamate-like immunoreactivity over synaptic vesicles is in accord with the large amount of data that favour an exocytotic release of transmitter glutamate (Nicholls, 1989). Our finding would also be consistent with the demonstration by Naito and Ueda (1985) that cortical synaptic vesicles, isolated by means of synapsin I antibodies, show an ATP-dependent uptake of L-glutamate. With one recent exception (Riveros et al., 1986), biochemical studies have failed to demonstrate an enrichment of glutamate in synaptic vesicle preparations, but this may easily be explained by a loss of glutamate during the preparation procedures.

Although glutamate-like immunoreactivity is clearly enriched over clusters of synaptic vesicles, the resolution of the procedure used does not at present allow this observation to be confirmed at the level of individual vesicles. Thus, the maximum distance between the centre of a gold particle and the corresponding epitope is 20 – 25 nm, similar to or exceeding the radius of the synaptic vesicles.

Our finding of a high concentration of gold particles over mitochondria probably reflects the mitochondrial localization of phosphate-activated glutaminase, which is one of the key enzymes in glutamate synthesis (Kvamme et al., 1988; also see Palaiologos et al., 1988, 1989). The mitochondria were even more strongly labelled than synaptic vesicle clusters (Table II). However, the vesicles in these clusters are "diluted" by the intervening cytosol, leading to an underestimation of the vesicular contents of antigen. A conservative correction for this, i.e. assuming that the intervening cytosol has the theoretically least possible volume, suggests that the intravesicular glutamate concentration is indeed higher than the intramitochondrial concentration (Table II). A further factor reducing the observed labelling of synaptic vesicles is that, due to their small size, some of them will not be cut open on the section surface and hence their contents will not be accessible to the antibodies.

When interpreting the subcellular distribution of glutamate-like immunoreactivity, one must take into account the fact that a small proportion of the free glutamate in the brain will inevitably be lost during the fixation procedure or subsequent handling of the tissue (see above). Artifactual contrasts in immunolabelling intensity could thus arise if the loss of free amino acids occurs to different extents in the different cellular compartments. As discussed previously (Ottersen et al., 1986), the exact proportion of the free glutamate that is fixed in a given subcellular compartment may depend on the availability of lysine residues, which are favoured sites for reaction with glutaraldehyde, and on the presence of compounds that interfere with fixation (for example, excess amounts of amino acids other than glutamate). Furthermore, we cannot exclude the possibility that the subcellular immunolabelling pattern is also influenced by some redistribution of glutamate during the perfusion procedure.

However, the finding that taurine-like immunoreactivity is much more uniformly distributed between vesicles and cytosol (unpublished observations in the cerebellar cortex) suggests that these factors do not invalidate the results on glutamate.

Depolarization-induced redistribution of glutamate-like immunoreactivity

The present approach to the study of glutamate release (Storm-Mathisen et al., 1986a, b; V. Gundersen, O.P. Ottersen and J. Storm-Mathisen, in preparation) differs considerably from biochemical approaches. Notably, release is evidenced by reduction of intracellular glutamate, instead of by an increased efflux. Further, in the hippocampal slices used here the close spatial relationship between glial and neuronal elements is retained, which is in contrast to the situation in synaptosome preparations. These differences have important consequences for the design and interpretation of our release experiments. First, the depolarization stimulus must be so strong that the release it induces exceeds the capacity for glutamate replenishment. This capacity is likely to be much greater in slices than in synaptosome preparations. Thus, instead of being diluted in the medium (as in synaptosome preparations), in slices the glutamate is released into a confined extracellular space from which the glutamate can be taken up by the presynaptic and glial uptake mechanisms. Further, the presence of functioning astrocytes permits the operation of the glutamate-glutamine shuttle, which is considered an important mechanism for the renewal of the transmitter pool of glutamate (Bradford et al., 1978; Hamberger et al., 1979). Reflecting the high capacity for glutamate replenishment, it was necessary to increase the K^+ concentrations to 40 mM or above to produce a demonstrable decrease in the nerve terminal level of glutamate-like immunoreactivity. Further, the depolarization stimulus had to be of a sufficiently long duration; no changes were observed after depolarization with 55 mM K^+ for 3 min or less. This is in apparent contrast to the observations by Nicholls (1989) who found that the Ca^{2+}-dependent glutamate release in synaptosomes was depleted after $3-5$ min of stimulation. The availability in slices of precursors from glia is a possible explanation of the discrepancy.

Our results showed that the K^+-induced depletion of glutamate-like immunoreactivity could be abolished in the absence of Ca^{2+}. This finding must not be taken to indicate that the *release* is entirely Ca^{2+}-dependent. On the contrary, a considerable proportion of the release is probably independent of Ca^{2+} as demonstrated in synaptosome preparations (Nicholls, 1989). A likely interpretation of our findings is as follows: in the presence of Ca^{2+}, depolarization by K^+ induces a release that consists of a Ca^{2+}-dependent as well as a Ca^{2+}-independent component. The sum of these components exceeds the capacity for glutamate replenishment, and thus leads to a gradual depletion of the glutamate contents in the nerve terminals. In the absence of Ca^{2+}, the K^+-induced release consists of the Ca^{2+}-independent component only. This component is not large enough to exceed the capacity of glutamate replenishment, and will therefore not lead to detectable changes in the nerve terminal contents of glutamate-like immunoreactivity.

Electron microscopic vs light microscopic immunocytochemistry

Although the procedures outlined in the present paper should prove to be potent tools for the identification of putative glutamatergic terminals, they are relatively time-consuming. An important question is whether it will prove possible to obtain the same type of information at the light microscopic level. As stated in the Introduction, the pattern of glutamate-like immunoreactivity obtained in routine light microscopic preparations of perfusion-fixed brains is commonly very difficult to interpret. Nerve terminal staining is often weak compared to cell body staining, suggesting that the nerve terminal pool of glutamate is relatively inaccessible to the immunoreagents under these conditions. However, the magnitude of this problem appears to vary among regions. Thus, at the light microscopic level, glutamate-enriched nerve terminals are quite conspicuous in the vestibular nuclei (Walberg et al., 1990) and in the lateral cervical nucleus (Broman et al., 1990), but difficult to distinguish in, e.g., the hippocampal formation. Recent studies by Streit and colleagues (Liu et al., 1989) indicate that this problem may be partly method-dependent. They showed that even nerve terminals in the perfusion-fixed hippocampus may show up as intensely labelled in light microscopic

preparations. However, for unidentified reasons, the results varied between individual rats. These authors used a monoclonal glutamate antibody in combination with a silver enhancement procedure. Why the LM preparations of the latter group differ from ours is presently unclear, but the differences are more likely to be related to differences in the tissue preparation procedure than to differences between the antisera or immunocytochemical procedures used.

Glial labelling

We have presently confirmed previous light microscopic observations (Storm-Mathisen et al., 1986a, b; Gundersen et al., 1990) that high K^+ stimulation not only leads to a depletion of glutamate-like immunoreactivity from nerve terminals, but also to an increase in this immunoreactivity in astroglial cells. The observations indicate that part of the released glutamate is being taken up into glia. Biochemical data suggest that the uptake of glutamate into glia is the first step in a shuttle of glutamate carbon between neurons and glia, acting to replenish the releasable stores of glutamate (van den Berg et al., 1975; Quastel, 1978; Schousboe and Hertz, 1983). The subsequent steps in this shuttle involve a transformation of glutamate to glutamine in the glial cells, and then transfer of the glutamine to the neurons where it acts as the main precursor of transmitter glutamate. Our findings indicate that glutamate immunocytochemistry may be used not only as a tool to study release, but also as a means to investigate glutamate uptake and metabolism in the different tissue compartments. Such phenomena have long been important objects of biochemical analyses, but can now be studied in a quantitative manner in preparations with a reasonable structural integrity.

Conclusion

Glutamate immunocytochemistry has now matured to a stage at which it can be used to identify putative glutamatergic terminals in the CNS. It follows from the above considerations that a combined analysis of perfusion-fixed and immersion-fixed material should ideally be carried out before drawing conclusions about transmitter identity: the perfusion-fixed material is valuable for revealing the in vivo distribution of free glutamate, whereas the immersion-fixed material offers the possibility of studying glutamate release. We have shown in the hippocampus as well as in the cerebellum (Ottersen, 1989a, b; Ottersen and Laake, 1990) that the terminals that are enriched in glutamate-like immunoreactivity in perfusion-fixed material are of the same morphological types as those that sustain glutamate release, as judged from immersion-fixed slices. The question thus arises whether an analysis of perfusion-fixed material is sufficient to identify putative glutamatergic synapses. In other words, are all terminals that are enriched in glutamate-like immunoreactivity glutamatergic? It would still seem premature to answer this question. There is certainly good evidence from the hippocampus and cerebellum that putative glutamatergic terminals contain a several-fold higher concentration of glutamate-like immunoreactivity than putative GABAergic terminals, but does this difference also apply to terminals using other transmitters, such as acetylcholine or monoamines (cf. Bradford et al., 1989)? Pending an answer to the latter question, it seems prudent, whenever possible, to base one's conclusions on both perfusion-fixed material and slice experiments.

Acknowledgements

The expert technical assistance of A.T. Bore (preparation of antisera), J. Knutsen and B. Riber (immunocytochemistry) is gratefully acknowledged. We also wish to thank C. Ingebrigtsen and G. Lothe for photographical assistance, T. Eliassen for typing and editing the manuscript, T.W. Blackstad for developing the computer program, and P. Somogyi for invaluable advice on the immunogold technique. Supported by the Norwegian Council for Science and the Humanities, and the Norwegian Council on Cardiovascular Disease.

References

Balcom, G.J., Lenox, R.H. and Meyerhoff, J.L. (1976) Regional glutamate levels in rat brain determined after microwave fixation. *J. Neurochem.,* 26: 423 – 425.

Benveniste, H., Drejer, J., Schousboe, A. and Diemer, N.H. (1984) Elevation of the extracellular concentrations of glutamate and aspartate in rat hippocampus during transient cerebral ischemia monitored by intracerebral microdialysis. *J. Neurochem.,* 43: 1369 – 1374.

Berger, S.J., Carter, J.G. and Lowry, O.H. (1977) The distribution of glycine, GABA, glutamate and aspartate in rabbit spinal cord, cerebellum and hippocampus. *J. Neurochem.,* 28: 149 – 158.

Blackstad, T.W., Karagülle, T. and Ottersen, O.P. (1989) MORFOREL, a computer program for two-dimensional analysis of micrographs of biological specimens, with emphasis on immunogold preparations, *Comp. Biol. Med.,* in press.

Bradford, H.F., Ward, H.K. and Thomas, A.J. (1978) Glutamine – a major substrate for nerve endings. *J. Neurochem.,* 30: 1453 – 1459.

Bradford, H.F., Docherty, M., Wu, J.-Y., Cash, C.D., Ehret, M., Maitre, M. and Joh, T.H. (1989) The immunolysis, isolation, and properties of subpopulations of mammalian brain synaptosomes. *Neurochem. Res.,* 14: 301 – 310.

Broman, J., Westman, J. and Ottersen, O.P. (1990) Ascending afferents to the lateral cervical nucleus are enriched in glutamate-like immunoreactivity: a combined anterograde transport-immunogold study in the cat. *Brain Res.,* in press.

Cotman, C.W., Monaghan, D.T., Ottersen, O.P. and Storm-Mathisen, J. (1987) Anatomical organization of excitatory amino acid receptors and their pathways. *Trends Neurosci.,* 10: 273 – 280.

De Biasi, S. and Rustioni, A. (1988) Glutamate and substance P coexist in primary afferent terminals in the superficial laminae of spinal cord. *Proc. Natl. Acad. Sci. U.S.A.,* 85: 7820 – 7824.

Ehinger, B., Ottersen, O.P., Storm-Mathisen, J. and Dowling, J.E. (1988) Bipolar cells in the turtle retina are strongly immunoreactive for glutamate. *Proc. Natl. Acad. Sci. U.S.A.,* 85: 8321 – 8325.

Engelsen, B. and Fonnum, F. (1983) Effects of hypoglycemia on the transmitter pool and the metabolic pool of glutamate in rat brain. *Neurosci. Lett.,* 42: 317 – 322.

Fonnum, F. (1984) Glutamate: a neurotransmitter in mammalian brain. *J. Neurochem.,* 42: 1 – 11.

Hamberger, A.C., Chiang, G.H., Nylén, E.S., Scheff, S.W. and Cotman, C.W. (1979) Glutamate as a CNS transmitter. I. Evaluation of glucose and glutamine as precursors for the synthesis of preferentially released glutamate. *Brain Res.,* 168: 513 – 530.

Kvamme, E., Svenneby, G. and Torgner, I. Aa. (1988) Glutaminases. In E. Kvamme (Ed.), *Glutamine and Glutamate in Mammals, Vol. I.,* CRC Press, Inc., Boca Raton, FL, pp. 53 – 67.

Liu, C.-j., Grandes, P., Matute, C., Cuénod, M. and Streit, P. (1989) Glutamate-like immunoreactivity revealed in rat olfactory bulb, hippocampus and cerebellum by monoclonal antibody and sensitive staining method. *Histochemistry,* 90: 427 – 445.

Naito, S. and Ueda, T. (1985) Characterization of glutamate uptake into synaptic vesicles. *J. Neurochem.,* 44: 99 – 109.

Nicholls, D.G. (1989) Release of glutamate, aspartate and γ-aminobutyric acid from isolated nerve terminals. *J. Neurochem.,* 52: 331 – 341.

Ottersen, O.P. (1987) Postembedding light- and electron microscopic immunocytochemistry of amino acids: description of a new model system allowing identical conditions for specificity testing and tissue processing. *Exp. Brain Res.,* 69: 167 – 174.

Ottersen, O.P. (1988) Quantitative assessment of taurine-like immunoreactivity in different cell types and processes in rat cerebellum: an electronmicroscopic study based on a postembedding immunogold labelling procedure. *Anat. Embryol.,* 178: 407 – 421.

Ottersen, O.P. (1989a) Quantitative electron microscopic immunocytochemistry of amino acids. *Anat. Embryol.,* 180: 1 – 15.

Ottersen, O.P. (1989b) Postembedding immunogold labelling of fixed glutamate: an electron microscopic analysis of the relationship between gold particle density and antigen concentration. *J. Chem. Neuroanat.,* 2: 57 – 66.

Ottersen, O.P. and Bramham, C.R. (1988) Quantitative electron microscopic immunocytochemistry of excitatory amino acids. In E.A. Cavalheiro, J. Lehmann and L. Turski (Eds.), *Frontiers in Excitatory Amino Acid Research,* Alan R. Liss, New York, pp. 93 – 100.

Ottersen, O.P. and Laake, J.H. (1989) Light and electron microscopic immunocytochemistry of putative neurotransmitter amino acids in the cerebellum with a note on the distribution of glutamine. In R. Llinás and C. Sotelo (Eds.), *Neurobiology of the Cerebellar Systems: A Centenary of Ramón y Cajal's Description of the Cerebellar Circuits,* in press.

Ottersen, O.P. and Storm-Mathisen, J. (1984) Glutamate- and GABA-containing neurons in the mouse and rat brain, as demonstrated with a new immunocytochemical technique. *J. Comp. Neurol.,* 229: 374 – 392.

Ottersen, O.P. and Storm-Mathisen, J. (1985) Different neuronal localization of aspartate-like and glutamate-like immunoreactivities in the hippocampus of rat, guinea pig, and Senegalese baboon *(Papio papio),* with a note on the distribution of GABA. *Neuroscience,* 16: 589 – 606.

Ottersen, O.P. and Storm-Mathisen, J. (1989) Excitatory and inhibitory amino acids in the hippocampus. In V. Chan-Palay and C. Köhler (Eds.), *The Hippocampus: New Vistas,* Alan R. Liss, New York, pp. 97 – 117.

Ottersen, O.P., Storm-Mathisen, J., Madsen, S., Skumlien, S. and Strømhaug, J. (1986) Evaluation of the immunocytochemical method for amino acids. *Med. Biol.,* 64: 147 – 158.

Palaiologos, G., Hertz, L. and Schousboe, A. (1988) Evidence that aspartate aminotransferase activity and ketodicarboxylate carrier function are essential for biosynthesis of transmitter glutamate. *J. Neurochem.,* 51: 317 – 320.

Palaiologos, G., Hertz, L. and Schousboe, A. (1989) Role of aspartate aminotransferase and mitochondrial dicarboxylate transport for release of endogenously and exogenously supplied neurotransmitter in glutamatergic neurons. *Neurochem. Res.,* 14: 359 – 366.

Quastel, J.H. (1978) Cerebral glutamate – glutamine interrelations in vivo and in vitro. In E. Schoffeniels, G. Franck, L. Hertz, and D.B. Tower (Eds.), *Dynamic Properties of Glia Cells,* Pergamon Press, Oxford, pp. 153 – 162.

Riveros, N., Fiedler, J., Lagos, N., Muñoz, C. and Orrego, F. (1986) Glutamate in rat brain cortex synaptic vesicles: influence of the vesicle isolation procedure. *Brain Res.,* 386: 405 – 408.

Schousboe, A. and Hertz, L. (1983) Regulation of glutamatergic and GABAergic neuronal activity by astroglial cells. In N.N. Osborne (Ed.), *Dale's Principle and Communication Between Neurones,* Pergamon Press, Oxford, pp. 113 – 141.

Somogyi, P., Halasy, K., Somogyi, J., Storm-Mathisen, J. and Ottersen, O.P. (1986) Quantification of immunogold labelling reveals enrichment of glutamate in mossy and parallel fibre terminals in cat cerebellum. *Neuroscience,* 19: 1045 – 1050.

Storm-Mathisen, J. and Ottersen, O.P. (1986) Antibodies against amino acid transmitters. In P. Panula, H. Päivärinta and S. Soinila (Eds.), *Neurochemistry: Modern Methods and Applications,* Alan R. Liss, New York, pp. 107 – 136.

Storm-Mathisen, J. and Ottersen, O.P. (1988) Localization of excitatory amino acid transmitters. In D. Lodge (Ed.), *Excitatory Amino Acids in Health and Disease,* John Wiley, Chichester, pp. 107 – 141.

Storm-Mathisen, J., Leknes, A.K., Bore, A.T., Vaaland, J.L., Edminson, P., Haug, F.-M. and Ottersen, O.P. (1983) First visualization of glutamate and GABA in neurones by immunocytochemistry. *Nature (Lond.),* 301: 517 – 520.

Storm-Mathisen, J., Ottersen, O.P. and Fu-long, T. (1986a) Antibodies for the localization of excitatory amino acids. In P.J. Roberts, J. Storm-Mathisen and H.F. Bradford (Eds.), *Excitatory Amino Acids,* Macmillan, London, pp. 101 – 116.

Storm-Mathisen, J., Ottersen, O.P., Fu-long, T., Gundersen, V., Laake, J.H. and Nordbø, G. (1986b) Metabolism and transport of amino acids studied by immunocytochemistry.

114

Med. Biol., 64: 127 – 132.

Van den Bergh, C.J., Matheson, D.F., Ronda, G., Reijnierse, G.L.A., Blokhuis, G.G.D., Kroon, M.C., Clarke, D.D. and Garfinkel, D. (1975) A model of glutamate metabolism in brain: a biochemical analysis of a heterogeneous structure. In S. Berl, D.D. Clarke and D. Schneider (Eds.), *Metabolic Compartmentation and Neurotransmission. Relation to*

Brain Structure and Function, Plenum Press, New York, pp. 515 – 543.

Walberg, F., Ottersen, O.P. and Rinvik, E. (1990) GABA, glycine, aspartate, glutamate and taurine in the vestibular nuclei. An immunocytochemical investigation in the cat. *Exp. Brain Res.,* in press.

J. Storm-Mathisen, J. Zimmer and O.P. Ottersen (Eds.)
Progress in Brain Research, Vol. 83
© 1990 Elsevier Science Publishers B.V. (Biomedical Division)

CHAPTER 9

Regulation of glutamate and aspartate release from the Schaffer collaterals and other projections of CA3 hippocampal pyramidal cells

J. Victor Nadler, David Martin, Gonzalo A. Bustos*, Stephan P. Burke and Mark A. Bowe

Departments of Pharmacology and Neurobiology, Duke University Medical Center, Durham, NC 27710, U.S.A.

Excitatory synaptic transmission in the CNS can be modulated by endogenous substances and metabolic states that alter release of the transmitter, usually glutamate and/or aspartate. To explore this issue, we have studied the release of endogenous glutamate and aspartate from synaptic terminals of the CA3-derived Schaffer collateral, commissural and ipsilateral associational fibers in slices of hippocampal area CA1. These terminals release glutamate and aspartate in about a 5 : 1 ratio. The release process is modulated by adenosine, by the transmitters themselves and by nerve terminal metabolism. Adenosine inhibits the release of both amino acids by acting upon an A1 receptor. The transmitters, once released, can regulate their further release by acting upon both an NMDA and a non-NMDA (quisqualate/kainate) receptor. Activation of the NMDA receptor enhances the release of both glutamate and aspartate, whereas activation of the non-NMDA receptor depresses the release of aspartate only. Superfusion of CA1 slices with a glucose-deficient medium increases the release of both amino acids and reduces the glutamate/aspartate ratio. These results have implications for the regulation of excitatory synaptic transmission in the CA1 area and for the mechanism of hypoglycemic damage to CA1 pyramidal cells.

Introduction

The demonstration that excitatory pathways of the mammalian CNS release glutamate and/or aspartate (Roberts, 1974; Nadler et al., 1976; Collins, 1979; Reubi and Cuénod, 1979) was a major advance in the identification of these amino acids as neurotransmitters. There is now general agreement that glutamate or a closely related compound serves as the transmitter utilized by the vast majority of these pathways (Fonnum, 1984; Ottersen and Storm-Mathisen, 1986). This discovery has permitted the detailed exploration of excitatory synaptic mechanisms. Important advances have been made in our understanding of postsynaptic receptor mechanisms at excitatory CNS synapses and in the way these mechanisms impact on higher brain function. However, much less is known about presynaptic mechanisms, in particular about the regulation of excitatory amino acid release. In principle, the complex functions mediated by excitatory amino acid pathways could be modulated by influences that act upon the transmitter release process as readily as by influences on postsynaptic receptor function. The results summarized in this chapter suggest that glutamate/aspartate release is subject to regulation by neuroactive compounds normally present extracellularly at the synapse and by nerve terminal metabolism.

---

* Permanent address: Laboratory of Biochemical Pharmacology, Faculty of Biological Sciences, Catholic University of Chile, P.O. Box 114-D, Santiago, Chile.

Methodological considerations

The preparation used to study the release process must be carefully considered. Glutamate/aspartate release should preferably be studied with a preparation in which the excitants are released from only one source. One should not assume that transmitter release from all excitatory amino acid pathways will be regulated in the same manner. This consideration rules out the use of synaptosomal preparations for many studies, unless it has been shown that the structures in the preparation which release glutamate and/or aspartate were derived predominantly from a single population of nerve endings. Similarly, slice preparations of neocortex or whole hippocampal formation do not meet our criterion. A problem with many studies of modulatory substances is that the cellular locus of action has not been specifiable, that is, whether the test compound acted upon the synaptic terminal itself, on the cell bodies or dendrites of the presynaptic neuron or on another cell in the proximity of the synaptic terminal. This ambiguity derives, in part, from the use of preparations that include all parts of the excitatory amino acid-releasing neuron. Dissociated neuronal preparations, explant cultures and most brain slice preparations suffer from this limitation. Indeed a major virtue of synaptosomal preparations for release studies is that the nerve endings have been separated from the remainder of their parent neurons, although the utility of most such preparations is limited by their heterogeneity. A third consideration is the metabolic intactness of the tissue. Electrophysiological studies of brain slices have indicated approaches to slice preparation, incubation and superfusion that maximize tissue viability (Dingledine, 1984). Our results suggest that the metabolic state of the preparation can dramatically influence both the quantity of glutamate and aspartate released and the ability to detect certain types of modulation. One must also carefully consider the choice of stimulus. Ideally, the stimulus should be as close to physiological as possible, that is, transmitter release should be evoked entirely by action potentials generated in the presynaptic fibers of interest. A few such studies have been reported (Collins, 1979; Corradetti et al., 1983). In our hands, however, it has been exceedingly difficult to evoke a readily measurable release of glutamate and/or aspartate from a single pathway by orthodromic electrical stimulation. This difficulty undoubtedly arises, at least in part, from the presence of robust acidic amino acid uptake systems at the synapse and from the fact that in slices a large proportion of the nerve endings is severed from the parent axons. Alternative approaches include the use of electrical field stimulation, elevated K^+ and veratrum alkaloids. Potential drawbacks of these stimuli include their lack of specificity for the pathway of interest, their essentially non-physiological nature and the possibility that some forms of modulation will not be detected because the modulator alters glutamate/aspartate release by changing the amplitude of the presynaptic action potential, the duration of the action potential or the ability of the action potential to invade the synaptic terminal. Furthermore, these stimuli can potentially evoke glutamate/aspartate efflux from both transmitter and non-transmitter stores. In other words, the efflux may not be entirely Ca^{2+}-dependent. Although these considerations do not invalidate the use of non-specific stimuli to study glutamate/aspartate release, one must always be aware of the limitations their mechanisms of action impose on the conclusions that can be drawn from these studies. Finally, we believe it essential to study the release of endogenous amino acid transmitters. Preloading the tissue with [^{3}H]glutamate or D-[^{3}H]aspartate simplifies the quantitation of amino acid efflux, but a number of reports have demonstrated that the release of preloaded amino acid is not equivalent to the release of endogenous transmitter (Nadler et al., 1977; Fagg and Lane, 1979; Levi et al., 1982; Ferkany and Coyle, 1983; Virgili et al., 1986). This is especially obvious in studies of modulation.

Based upon these considerations, we developed a method of studying glutamate/aspartate release that (1) quantitated the release of endogenous excitatory amino acid evoked predominantly from just one CNS pathway, (2) eliminated the cell bodies and dendrites of the presynaptic neuron (although not of the postsynaptic neuron) from the preparation, (3) preserved tissue viability as best as possible and (4) assured that nearly all the release of glutamate and aspartate was Ca^{2+}-dependent.

The Schaffer collateral-commissural-ipsilateral associational (SCCIA) projection

The SCCIA projection was one of the first CNS pathways shown to release glutamate and aspartate (Nadler et al., 1976) and subsequent investigations strongly supported the view that one or both amino acids serve a transmitter role at SCCIA synapses (Storm-Mathisen, 1977; Storm-Mathisen and Iversen, 1979; Collingridge et al., 1983; Ottersen and Storm-Mathisen, 1985; Ganong et al., 1986). SCCIA fibers originate from the pyramidal cells of hippocampal area CA3 and terminate upon the dendrites of pyramidal cells in the CA1 area (Gottlieb and Cowan, 1973; Swanson et al., 1978). One branch of the CA3 pyramidal cell axon, the Schaffer collateral (sc, Fig. 1), innervates stratum radiatum of the ipsilateral CA1 area. A second axonal branch (a, Fig. 1) follows a similar trajectory to the Schaffer collateral, but remains in stratum oriens. This branch lacks a specific name upon which all neuroanatomists agree. We refer to this portion of the SCCIA projection as the "ipsilateral associational pathway" or the "ipsilateral stratum oriens pathway". A third axonal branch projects to the contralateral hippocampal formation. This "commissural" fiber (c, Fig. 1) divides several times within the contralateral CA3 area. One branch co-mingles with the Schaffer collaterals and another with the ipsilateral associational pathway. Because the Schaffer collateral, commissural and ipsilateral associational fibers originate from the same neuronal population and, at least in many instances, from the same neurons (Laurberg and Sørensen, 1981), it seems reasonable to treat them as a single pathway for purposes of transmitter release studies. A major advantage of the SCCIA projection for such studies is that the SCCIA terminal field in area CA1 can be separated by dissection (Fig. 1) from both the cell bodies and dendrites of the CA3 pyramidal cells and from any other significant projection that is known or suspected to release excitatory amino acids.

Methods and their rationale (Burke and Nadler, 1988)

Transverse slices of the rostral hippocampal formation were prepared from female Sprague–Dawley rats. The CA1 area (excluding stratum lacunosum-moleculare) was isolated while viewing each slice individually through a dissecting microscope (Fig. 1). Dissection along the border of stratum radiatum and stratum lacunosum-moleculare was facilitated by the distinctly whiter appearance of stratum lacunosum-moleculare, due presumably to the presence of heavily myelinated axons in that layer. Removing stratum lacunosum-moleculare from the CA1 slice eliminated the temporo-ammonic pathway, which is likely to release excitatory amino acids (Ottersen and

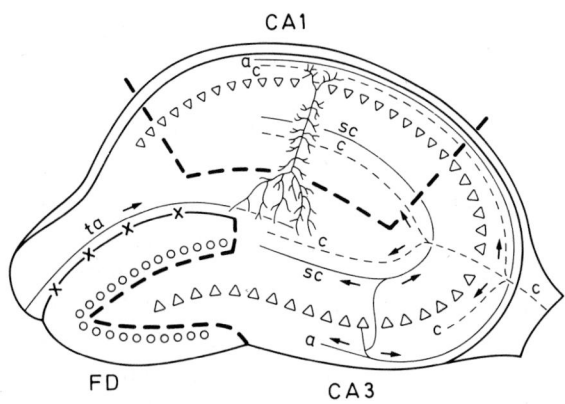

Fig. 1. Preparation of CA1 and fascia dentata (FD) slices from a slice of the whole hippocampal formation. Hippocampal regions were dissected along the heavily dashed lines and the fascia dentata was separated from CA1-subiculum by cutting along the hippocampal fissure (x). △, hippocampal pyramidal cells; ○, dentate granule cells. Pathways: a, ipsilateral associational fibers; c, commissural fibers; sc, Schaffer collaterals; ta, temporo-ammonic fibers. Small arrows indicate the direction of orthodromic impulse flow.

Storm-Mathisen, 1986).

These microdissected CA1 slices were transferred to small chambers and superfused dropwise from above with artificial CSF (Elliott, 1969). The flow rate was $0.8-1.0$ ml/min and the temperature within the chambers was maintained at 32°C. The chambers were surrounded by an atmosphere of water-saturated 95% O_2/5% CO_2. The outflow from the bottom of the chamber was maintained slightly faster than the inflow, so that the tissue would be covered most of the time by only a thin layer of medium. CA1 slices were superfused in this fashion in order to reproduce as closely as possible conditions found to be optimal for the preservation of pyramidal cell viability in vitro. Indeed we confirmed that normal-appearing Schaffer collateral-commissural field potentials can be recorded from these slices.

Potential modulatory substances were tested routinely by the conventional twin-pulse method. That is, transmitter release was provoked by increasing the K^+ concentration of the superfusion medium for a 1-min period, beginning 60 and 100 min after the start of superfusion. Test compounds were present in the superfusion medium only for the 5 min immediately before and during the second exposure to elevated K^+ (45 min in the case of phencyclidine (PCP)). Basal samples (B1 and B2) were collected during the 1 min preceding the K^+ pulses and total release samples (T1 and T2) were collected during the pulses. Superfusate samples were assayed for primary amino acids by high-pressure liquid chromatography (HPLC) after derivatization with o-phthalaldehyde (Lindroth and Mopper, 1979). For the minislices in each chamber, an S2/S1 ratio was calculated for release of each transmitter amino acid as follows: $(T2 - B2)/(T1 - B1) = S2/S1$. This ratio provided a consistent measure of release against which the effects of modulators could be tested, eliminating between-chamber differences in the size or orientation of minislices. Most studies utilized 50 mM K^+ to evoke transmitter amino acid release, because this stimulus released a substantial, but submaximal, quantity of each transmitter amino acid.

This protocol was developed with the objectives of maximizing the quantity of glutamate and aspartate released, minimizing K^+-evoked, Ca^{2+}-independent amino acid efflux and minimizing basal efflux. Delaying the first exposure to elevated K^+ for 60 min and the second exposure for an additional 40 min maximized transmitter amino acid release, presumably because these long delays permitted the restoration of ionic and metabolic homeostasis before each K^+ stimulus was applied. Under the present experimental conditions, the release of both glutamate and aspartate was better than 90% Ca^{2+}-dependent when a K^+ concentration of less than 60 mM (or veratridine concentration of 25 μM or less) was used. For this reason, there was no need to correct for effects of the depolarizing agent that do not depend on extracellular Ca^{2+}. Our use of a 1-min stimulation period at least partially accounts for this high degree of Ca^{2+}-dependence (Nicholls and Sihra, 1986). Basal efflux of transmitter amino acids was not measurable in these experiments. Minimal glutamate and aspartate was detected in the B1 and B2 samples and the quantities present in these samples were found to have originated predominantly from contamination of the medium. This finding suggested that the CA1 slices maintained a robust uptake mechanism for glutamate/aspartate, another indication of healthy tissue. Indeed 50 μM DL-threo-β-hydroxyaspartate, a selective inhibitor of glutamate/aspartate uptake, doubled the overflow of glutamate. Finally, it should be noted that elevated K^+ or veratridine released only a small quantity of non-transmitter amino acids from the tissue under our experimental conditions. Those detected were serine, glycine, glutamine, taurine and alanine. Efflux of these amino acids was unaffected by removing Ca^{2+} from the superfusion medium.

Relative proportions of glutamate and aspartate released

K^+ concentrations of 20 to 70 mM ($23.5-73.5$ mM final concentrations) and veratridine concentrations of 10 or 25 μM released $4-7$ times as much glutamate as aspartate from CA1 slices (Burke and Nadler, 1988). Similar results were obtained with electrical field stimulation of whole hippocampal slices (Szerb and O'Regan, 1987; Szerb, 1988). A relatively high ratio of glutamate to aspartate released appears to characterize healthy tissue, because metabolically stressed slices exhibit much lower ratios. For example, preincubating CA1 slices for much less than 60 min not only reduces the K^+-evoked release of both glutamate and aspartate, but also greatly reduces the glutamate/aspartate ratio. Some of the early studies on amino acid release from area CA1 had reported glutamate/aspartate ratios close to unity (Nadler et al., 1976; Spencer et al., 1981; Corradetti et al., 1983). It seems likely that, in these studies, tissue metabolism was poorly preserved.

Origin of glutamate and aspartate release

To determine the extent to which the K^+-evoked

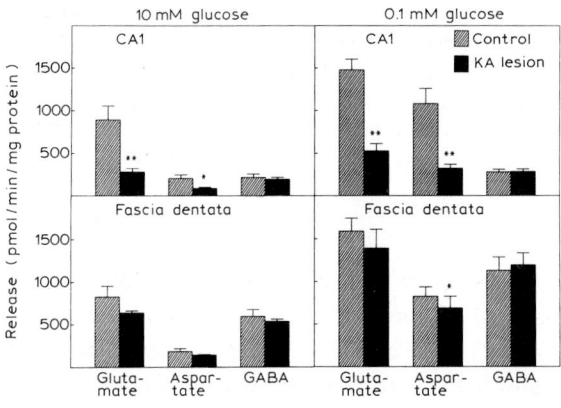

Fig. 2. K^+-evoked transmitter amino acid release after bilateral destruction of CA3 hippocampal pyramidal cells with i.c.v. KA. Microdissected slices of area CA1 and the fascia dentata (Fig. 1) were prepared 6 days after the lesion. Each tissue sample was exposed to 50 mM K^+ for 1 min in the presence of the indicated glucose concentration. (Under the present conditions the evoked release of glutamate, aspartate and GABA are greater than 90% Ca^{2+}-dependent, at 10 mM as well as at 0.1 mM glucose.) Values are means ± S.E.M. for 6 animals in each group. Lesion and control groups differed at * $P < 0.05$; **$P < 0.01$ (two-tailed Student's t-test). Adapted from Burke and Nadler (1988, 1989).

release of glutamate and aspartate originated from the SCCIA projection, the CA3 pyramidal cells were destroyed with intracerebroventricular kainic acid (i.c.v. KA; Nadler et al., 1980). When CA1 slices from these animals were studied, the KA lesion was found to reduce the K^+-evoked release of both amino acids by about $60-65\%$ (Fig. 2). This figure was only slightly less than the estimated percentage of CA3 pyramidal cells destroyed. The lesion appeared to be selective for CA3 pyramidal cells, because i.c.v. KA did not significantly reduce GABA release from CA1 slices and little affected the release of excitatory amino acids from slices of the fascia dentata, which does not receive a projection from CA3 pyramidal cells. Therefore, in conjunction with the demonstrated Ca^{2+}-dependence of the release process, our results suggested that the release of both glutamate and aspartate originated from a transmitter store within the SCCIA projection.

Modulation by adenosine

Adenosine is released from many compartments in the brain as a consequence of ATP hydrolysis and exerts a depressant effect on neuronal activity (Dunwiddie, 1985). Adenosine can block synaptic transmission at SCCIA synapses (Dunwiddie and Hoffer, 1980; Siggins and Schubert, 1981). Evidence from studies of other systems suggests that it acts, at least in part, by inhibiting glutamate/aspartate release (Dolphin and Archer, 1983; Scholfield and Steel, 1988). It has been assumed that adenosine also reduces SCCIA synaptic transmission by inhibiting transmitter release, but a previous attempt to test this hypothesis produced rather ambiguous results (Corradetti et al., 1984). Furthermore, adenosine can hyperpolarize CA1 pyramidal cells directly (Haas and Greene, 1984) and thus might block synaptic transmission through a postsynaptic action. Our studies provided firm evidence that adenosine does indeed inhibit transmitter release at SCCIA synapses and yielded insight into the mechanism by which adenosine acts (Burke and Nadler, 1988).

Adenosine inhibited the release of both glutamate and aspartate to a comparable extent and in a concentration-dependent manner (Fig. 3, Table I). Depressant effects were consistently obtained with concentrations as low as 1 μM and the estimated EC_{50} was about 0.7 μM. A maximal reduction of about 60% was obtained with concentrations of 30 – 100 μM.

Similar results were obtained with a series of adenosine receptor agonists. Concentration – response curves were essentially parallel and the relative potencies suggested the activation of a presynaptic A1 receptor. Furthermore, the depressant action of adenosine on glutamate/aspartate release could be completely reversed with the adenosine receptor antagonist 8-phenyltheophylline (Table I). Adenosine also inhibits transmission at SCCIA synapses by activating an A1 receptor and this action can be reversed with specific antagonists (Reddington et al., 1982; Dunwiddie and Fredholm, 1984, 1989). Some evidence suggested that adenosine can also enhance release by activating an A2 receptor.

8-Phenyltheophylline by itself increased gluta-

TABLE I

Effects of adenosine-related compounds and baclofen on evoked glutamate and aspartate release

Treatment	Release (S2/S1)	
	Glutamate	Aspartate
10 mM Glucose		
Control (28)	0.97 ± 0.03	0.83 ± 0.05
3 μM Adenosine (9)	0.53 ± 0.07**	0.51 ± 0.07**
3 μM Adenosine + 1 μM 8-Phenyltheophylline (4)	1.10 ± 0.11	0.97 ± 0.09
10 μM 8-Phenyltheophylline (9)	1.77 ± 0.07**	1.42 ± 0.08**
25 μM Dipyridamole (6)	0.61 ± 0.03**	0.48 ± 0.03**
100 μM Baclofen (4)	0.95 ± 0.07	0.89 ± 0.08
0.1 mM Glucose		
Control (7)	0.87 ± 0.04	1.05 ± 0.03
100 μM Adenosine (4)	0.93 ± 0.02	0.98 ± 0.05
10 μM 8-Phenyltheophylline (3)	2.22 ± 0.08**	2.56 ± 0.09**
50 μM Baclofen (4)	0.92 ± 0.04	1.07 ± 0.04

Values are ratios of release evoked by 50 mM K$^+$ in the presence (S2) and absence (S1) of the compounds indicated, expressed as means ± S.E.M. for the number of experiments in parentheses. When negative results were obtained with 100 μM adenosine or 50 – 100 μM baclofen, the experiments were repeated with lower concentrations of the compound. These experiments also yielded negative results. Experimental slices differed from controls at **$P < 0.01$ (Dunnett test).

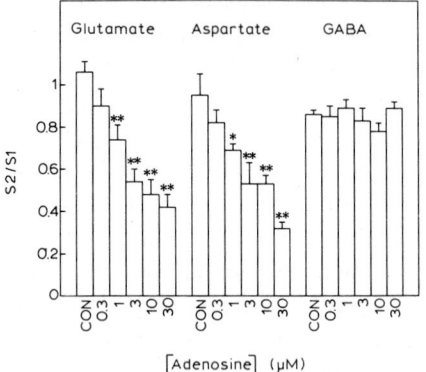

Fig. 3. Effects of adenosine on transmitter amino acid release evoked by 50 mM K$^+$. Values are ratios of K$^+$-evoked release with (S2) and without (S1) adenosine. They are expressed as means ± S.E.M. for 5 experiments. Experimental slices differed from controls at *$P < 0.05$; **$P < 0.01$ (Dunnett test). (From Burke and Nadler (1988). *J. Neurochem.*, 51: 1541 – 1551. Reprinted with permission.)

mate/aspartate release, whereas dipyridamole, an inhibitor of adenosine uptake, reduced the release (Table I). These results suggested that endogenous adenosine was released from CA1 slices in a concentration sufficient to inhibit glutamate/aspartate release. Thus the maximal inhibition produced by endogenous adenosine and exogenous adenosine together approached 80%. Nevertheless, concentrations of adenosine that abolish SCCIA synaptic transmission, as determined by recording field potentials in hippocampal slice preparations (Reddington et al., 1982; Dunwiddie et al., 1984), never abolished glutamate or aspartate release. We have discussed possible explanations for this discrepancy (Burke and Nadler, 1988). Two of these possibilities appear especially attractive: that adenosine is more effective against release evoked by an action potential than by 50 mM K$^+$ and that the residual 20% of the release is insufficient to evoke a postsynaptic response that can be detected in extracellular recordings.

A significant finding was that adenosine and other A1 receptor agonists reduce glutamate/aspartate release evoked by elevated K$^+$, but not release evoked by veratridine. One difference between depolarization of nerve endings with K$^+$ and veratridine is that Ca^{2+} entry proceeds largely through different mechanisms. Elevated K$^+$ favors Ca^{2+} entry through voltage-sensitive Ca^{2+} channels, whereas veratridine, at concentrations of 25 μM or less, mainly activates Ca^{2+} influx through voltage-sensitive Na$^+$ channels (Adam-Vizi and Ligeti, 1986). Ca^{2+} that enters the terminal by either route gains access to the transmitter release sites, but only release that is evoked in the normal way, by Ca^{2+} influx through its own voltage-sensitive channels, appears subject to modulation by adenosine. Adenosine can reduce the stimulus-evoked influx of Ca^{2+} into SCCIA terminals (Schubert et al., 1986). This action might involve a direct or indirect coupling between the A1 receptor and Ca^{2+} channel. Some studies suggest that adenosine inhibits transmitter release by activating K$^+$ channels, thus shortening the duration of the presynaptic action potential and reducing Ca^{2+} influx (Michaelis et al., 1988; Scholfield and Steel, 1988). Other studies, however, suggest that adenosine more importantly modulates a step beyond the passage of Ca^{2+} through its voltage-sensitive channels (Dunwiddie, 1984; Silinsky et al., 1987).

Modulation by excitatory amino acids

A number of transmitters, once released, can regulate their further release by activating autoreceptors located on the synaptic terminal (Bartfai et al., 1988). With respect to the release of excitatory amino acids, however, little attention has been paid to the possible existence of a feed-back regulation. McBean and Roberts (1981) reported that activation of a "glutamate-preferring" receptor reduced the K$^+$-evoked release of preloaded D-[^{3}H]aspartate from rat hippocampal prisms. However, these investigators made no attempt to identify the source of amino acid release in their preparation and the receptor involved in the modulation appeared to be distinct from any of the physiologically characterized excitatory amino acid receptors. Our results suggest that autoreceptor activation modulates glutamate/aspartate release from SCCIA terminals in area CA1 and that the receptors involved closely resemble those types that have been identified on hippocampal pyramidal cells.

NMDA (100 μM) did not affect the release of glutamate or aspartate evoked by 50 mM K$^+$, even in the absence of Mg^{2+}. When the K$^+$ stimulus was reduced to 30 mM, however, NMDA selectively and substantially enhanced the release of aspartate (Fig. 4). Conversely, the NMDA

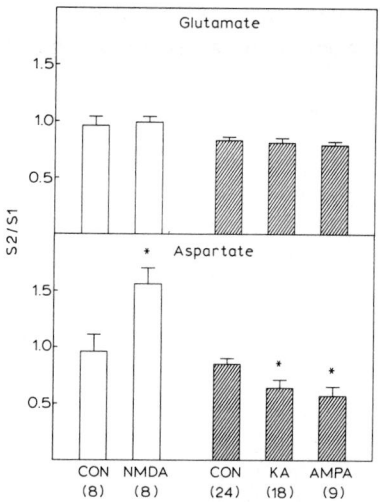

Fig. 4. Effects of prototypic agonists of excitatory amino acid receptors on the release of glutamate and aspartate. Open bars, nominally Mg^{2+}-free medium; striped bars, 1.2 mM Mg^{2+}. Effects of KA and AMPA were tested with 50 mM K$^+$ and effects of NMDA with 30 mM K$^+$. Values are ratios of K$^+$-evoked release with (S2) and without (S1) the excitant. They are expressed as means ± S.E.M. for the number of experiments indicated in parentheses. Experimental slices differed from controls at *$P < 0.05$ (Dunnett test).

receptor antagonists 3-((±)-2-carboxypiperazin-4-yl)-propyl-1-phosphonic acid (CPP; 20 μM) and PCP (20 μM) reduced the 50 mM K^+-evoked release of both glutamate and aspartate (Fig. 5). Effects of NMDA receptor antagonists were usually easier to demonstrate in the absence of Mg^{2+}. While this study was in progress, other groups reported that the NMDA receptor antagonists 2-amino-5-phosphonovalerate (AP5 or APV) and 2-amino-7-phosphonoheptanoate (AP7 or APH) inhibited the release of excitatory amino acids from whole hippocampal slices (Chapman and Bowker, 1987; Crowder et al., 1987; Connick and Stone, 1988).

These findings suggest the presence of NMDA autoreceptors on SCCIA terminals. Feedback activation of these receptors by both glutamate and aspartate (Olverman et al., 1984; Mayer and Westbrook, 1987) enhances the further release of these amino acids, possibly by increasing Ca^{2+} influx into the terminal (Arvin et al., 1987). NMDA receptor activation discriminates between glutamate release and aspartate release. Even the small quantities of excitatory amino acids released by 30

mM K^+ maximally enhance glutamate release, whereas exogenous NMDA can further increase the release of aspartate. Thus conditions that favor activation of the NMDA receptor could shift the balance of glutamate/aspartate release in favor of aspartate.

(RS)-α-amino-hydroxy-5-methyl-4-isoxazole-propionate (AMPA; 20 μM) and KA (10 – 800 μM) selectively depressed the K^+-evoked release of aspartate (Fig. 4). Conversely, the quisqualate/kainate receptor antagonist 6-cyano-2,3-dihydroxy-7-nitroquinoxaline-2,3-dione (CNQX; 20 μM) selectively enhanced aspartate release (Fig. 5). These results suggest the presence of quisqualate and/or kainate receptors on aspartate-releasing SCCIA terminals. Because aspartate has little affinity for either the quisqualate or the kainate receptor (London and Coyle, 1979; Honoré et al., 1982; Mayer and Westbrook, 1987), the endogenous ligand for these autoreceptors is presumably glutamate. Thus glutamate, once released, appears to inhibit the further release of aspartate by acting upon a non-NMDA excitatory amino acid receptor.

Our results suggest that the feedback activation of NMDA receptors, on the one hand, and non-NMDA receptors, on the other, have quite different effects on glutamate/aspartate release from SCCIA terminals. Both receptor interactions mainly influence aspartate release. However, their effects are in opposite directions. This finding contrasts with the depolarizing effect on hippocampal pyramidal cells of activating either receptor type. Thus the autoreceptor modulation of glutamate/aspartate release appears to be rather complex. Activation of these receptors can potentially increase transmitter release, reduce transmitter release or alter the proportion of glutamate release to aspartate release, depending on whether and to what extent NMDA receptor activation or non-NMDA receptor activation predominates.

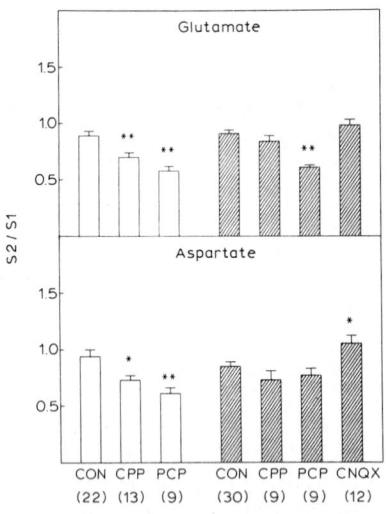

Fig. 5. Effects of excitatory amino acid antagonists on the release of glutamate and aspartate evoked by 50 mM K^+. Open bars, nominally Mg^{2+}-free medium; striped bars, 1.2 mM Mg^{2+}. Values are ratios of K^+-evoked release with (S2) and without (S1) the antagonist. They are expressed as means ± S.E.M. for the number of experiments stated in parentheses. Experimental slices differed from controls at *$P < 0.05$; **$P < 0.01$ (Dunnett test).

Failure to confirm modulation by GABA agonists

GABA has been reported to modulate glutamate/aspartate release by interacting with either

GABA$_A$ or GABA$_B$ receptors. Activation of cerebellar GABA$_A$ receptors enhances the K$^+$-evoked release of glutamate (Levi and Gallo, 1981). In contrast, the prototypic GABA$_B$ receptor agonist baclofen has been shown to inhibit glutamate/aspartate release in several different preparations (Potashner, 1979; Collins et al., 1982; Kato et al., 1982). Baclofen can block synaptic transmission at SCCIA synapses and indirect evidence suggests that it, like adenosine, acts mainly by suppressing transmitter release (Ault and Nadler, 1982; Inoue et al., 1985b). However, baclofen also resembles adenosine in its ability to hyperpolarize CA1 pyramidal cells (Inoue et al., 1985a; Newberry and Nicoll, 1985). Therefore a postsynaptic mechanism of action cannot be ruled out. Numerous GABA terminals are intermixed with SCCIA terminals in the dendritic layers of area CA1 (Gamrani et al., 1986). Any GABA that overflows from these inhibitory synapses could potentially modulate glutamate/aspartate release. To explore this possibility, we tested the actions of agonists and antagonists for the two GABA receptors in our release system (Burke and Nadler, 1988).

To our surprise, baclofen, at concentrations ranging from 3 to 100 μM, did not alter the K$^+$-evoked or veratridine-induced release of glutamate or aspartate (Table I). One possible explanation of this result appeared to be that an inhibitory action of baclofen was masked by endogenous adenosine. A1 and GABA$_B$ receptors may regulate the same limited pool of adenylate cyclase in synaptic membranes (Wojcik et al., 1985). We reasoned therefore that the activation of A1 receptors by adenosine may have been so great as to preclude any additional effect of baclofen. This possibility was excluded, however, by the inability of 8-phenyltheophylline to unmask an inhibitory action of baclofen. A second likely possibility seemed to be that 50 mM K$^+$ released enough endogenous GABA from the minislices to occupy all the GABA$_B$ receptors, thus eliminating any action of added baclofen. We first tested this hypothesis by exposing the tissue to pulses of 35, instead of 50, mM K$^+$. The lesser evoked GABA release might

have been expected to leave more presynaptic GABA$_B$ receptors available for occupancy by baclofen. However, baclofen still did not alter the release of either glutamate or aspartate. Secondly, we tested the GABA$_B$ receptor antagonist phaclofen. If the GABA$_B$ receptors were normally saturated with GABA, we expected phaclofen to enhance glutamate/aspartate release by competing with GABA for these receptors. Phaclofen, however, was without effect. This result was interpreted to suggest either that baclofen does not inhibit transmission at SCCIA synapses by reducing transmitter release or that it does so in a way that cannot be detected when a chemical depolarizing agent is employed. One mechanism compatible with the latter possibility is a reduction in the amplitude or duration of the presynaptic action potential. Such a change would depress transmitter release by reducing the stimulus-evoked Ca^{2+} influx, but it might only be readily detected if release were evoked by discrete electrical stimulation.

After these studies had been completed, Dutar and Nicoll (1988) reported that phaclofen does not reverse the baclofen-induced depression of SCCIA synaptic transmission, even though phaclofen does block the baclofen-induced hyperpolarization of the pyramidal cells. In light of this finding, we must reconsider the possibility that baclofen failed to inhibit glutamate/aspartate release because the presynaptic GABA$_B$ receptors were fully occupied by GABA. A definitive test of this idea awaits the development of a GABA$_B$ receptor antagonist that is effective upon the phaclofen-resistant receptor subtype.

Neither the GABA$_A$ receptor agonist muscimol (10 μM) nor the GABA$_A$ receptor antagonist bicuculline methiodide (100 μM) significantly affected the K$^+$-evoked release of glutamate or aspartate. Thus glutamate/aspartate release from SCCIA terminals appears not to be modulated by the activation of GABA$_A$ receptors.

Effects of glucose deficiency

CA1 pyramidal cells are among the most vulnerable neurons in the brain to hypoglycemia-induced cell death (Brierley and Graham, 1984). Both insulin-induced hypoglycemia in vivo (Sandberg et al., 1986) and superfusion of brain slices with a glucose-deficient medium (Fonnum et al., 1986; Szerb and O'Regan, 1987; Szerb, 1988) enhance the evoked overflow of glutamate and aspartate. It has been proposed that it is the excessive extracellular concentration of neuroexcitants which initiates the sequence of events culminating in neuronal cell death (Simon et al., 1986; Westerberg and Wieloch, 1987). Thus overflow of glutamate and/or aspartate from the SCCIA projection could at least partially explain the death of CA1 pyramidal cells after hypoglycemia. To address this issue, we tested the effects of hypoglycemic conditions on glutamate/aspartate release from the SCCIA projection in vitro (Burke and Nadler, 1989).

CA1 slices were superfused with control medium (10 mM glucose) for 60 min before exposure to medium that contained 0.1 or 1 mM glucose. Elevated K^+ was applied 30 and 60 min later. The switch to 0.1 mM glucose increased the K^+-evoked release of both glutamate and aspartate

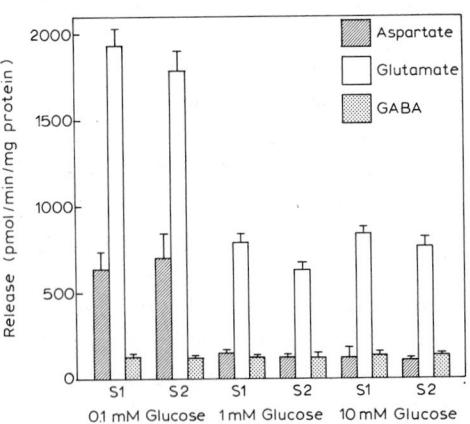

Fig. 6. Effects of varying the glucose concentration on transmitter amino acid release evoked by 50 mM K^+. CA1 slices were exposed to two 1-min pulses of 50 mM K^+ 30 (S1) and 60 (S2) min after changing the glucose concentration of the superfusion medium from 10 mM as indicated. Values are means ± S.E.M. for 6 experiments. From Burke and Nadler (1989).

(Fig. 6). Glucose-deficient medium enhanced the release of aspartate more than that of glutamate. Hence the glutamate/aspartate ratio dropped from about 5 to between 1.5 and 3 in response to the first K^+ pulse (Figs. 2, 6), and the ratio dropped even farther when the minislices were exposed to a second K^+ pulse. In general, glucose-deficient medium altered glutamate/aspartate release from the SCCIA projection in vitro much as insulin-induced hypoglycemia alters the extracellular concentration of these amino acids in vivo. Lowering the glucose concentration to 1 mM was insufficient to produce these changes. Under our conditions, glucose-deficient medium did not affect the K^+-evoked release of GABA.

Further studies revealed that the K^+-evoked release of glutamate and aspartate obtained in glucose-deficient medium was better than 90% Ca^{2+}-dependent and was markedly reduced by the prior destruction of CA3 pyramidal cells with i.c.v. KA (Fig. 2). Therefore the additional release, like the release in control medium, originated largely from a transmitter store within the SCCIA projection. In addition, glucose-deficient medium abolished the depressant effect of adenosine on glutamate/aspartate release and increased the effect of 8-phenyltheophylline (Table I). This result reflects the presence of a saturating extracellular adenosine concentration (Butcher et al., 1987).

The increased ratio of aspartate release to glutamate release probably reflected corresponding changes in the tissue content of these amino acids. Lowering the glucose concentration of the superfusion medium to 0.1 mM for 30 min reduced the glutamate content of CA1 slices by an average of 32% and increased the aspartate content by an average of 73%. Assuming that these changes apply specifically to the transmitter stores within SCCIA terminals, they are large enough to account for the entire shift in the glutamate/aspartate release ratio. Other investigators who used different slice preparations reached a similar conclusion (Fonnum et al., 1986; Szerb and O'Regan, 1987).

As to the enhanced release of both glutamate and aspartate in glucose-deficient medium, other investigators suggested that reduced energy-dependent amino acid uptake accounts for this effect (Kauppinen et al., 1988; Szerb and O'Regan, 1988). Although a reduction in glial and/or neuronal uptake of glutamate/aspartate may partially explain the increased overflow we obtained, for several reasons the enhancement of overflow expected from this factor alone appears inadequate to explain the full effect of glucose-deficient medium. For one thing, glucose-deficient medium failed to increase the overflow of GABA in our study, even though GABA uptake is probably as dependent on the cellular energy supply as glutamate/aspartate uptake. For another, even essentially complete suppression of glutamate/aspartate uptake with threo-β-hydroxyaspartate only doubled the release of glutamate. Yet the reduction in glutamate/aspartate uptake due to glucose deprivation was probably far less than complete, because uptake was still adequate to prevent the overflow of glutamate and aspartate under basal conditions and because 0.1 mM glucose has been shown to support normal levels of ATP and phosphocreatine in hippocampal slices (Bachelard et al., 1984). Thus one must also consider the possible effects of hypoglycemia on the release process itself. We have suggested that the enhanced release of glutamate and aspartate results in part from a rise in intraterminal Ca^{2+} concentration (Burke and Nadler, 1989).

Despite its facilitatory effect on excitatory transmitter release, a 40-min superfusion with glucose-deficient medium abolished transmission at Schaffer collateral-commissural synapses in area CA1. This effect did not signify hypoglycemic damage to the pyramidal cells, because it could be reversed by paired-pulse potentiation, frequency potentiation or restoring the glucose concentration of the medium to 10 mM. Glucose-deficient medium most readily reduces the ability of the EPSP to evoke cell firing (Bachelard et al., 1984; Fan et al., 1988), but lowering the glucose concentration to 0.1 mM also abolished the EPSP. Two explanations for the latter observation seem especially worthy of consideration. The use of intense artificial stimuli, such as elevated K^+, in in vitro studies could have masked an impairment of the release process that is effective when transmitter release is evoked by physiological low-frequency stimulus pulses. In addition, the substitution of aspartate for glutamate might impair synaptic transmission, as explained in the following section.

The increased release of potentially neurotoxic excitants from the SCCIA projection during hypoglycemia could, in itself, destroy CA1 pyramidal cells. The much enhanced release of aspartate may be particularly relevant here, because aspartate is about 3 times as potent a hippocampal excitotoxin as glutamate (Nadler et al., 1981).

Simultaneous release of glutamate and aspartate: implications for excitatory synaptic transmission

The simultaneous release of glutamate and aspartate is by no means unique to SCCIA terminals. Indeed, with a few notable exceptions, nearly every study on CNS preparations has demonstrated the release of both excitants (Ottersen and Storm-Mathisen, 1986). The question arises whether glutamate and aspartate are released from the same terminals or from different subsets of terminals within the same population. Available evidence, including the close correspondence between the ratio of glutamate to aspartate released and the ratio of these amino acids in the tissue, appears to favor release of both amino acids from the same terminals (Fonnum et al., 1986; Szerb, 1988). It is difficult to propose a vesicular model for the co-release of both amino acids, however. Both glutamate release and aspartate release require extracellular Ca^{2+} and thus presumably proceed through an exocytotic mechanism. Yet synaptic vesicles that accumulate and sequester glutamate cannot take up aspartate (Naito and Ueda, 1983). No aspartate-accumulating population of synaptic vesicles has yet been identified. The idea that excitatory amino acid terminals release both amino acids implies the presence in these terminals of either synaptic vesicles that take up glutamate and aspartate indiscriminately or two separate populations of synaptic vesicles, each selective for one excitatory amino acid. Therefore it is important to investigate whether glutamate/aspartate-accumulating and/or aspartate-accumulating synaptic vesicles exist. If the synaptic vesicles of excitatory amino acid terminals are found to accumulate only glutamate, then one would have to consider the possibility that aspartate and glutamate are released by fundamentally different mechanisms.

Our finding that prototypic excitatory amino acids alter the release of aspartate, but not of glutamate, also relates to the localization of these release processes. Evidence from other transmitter systems consistently indicates that modulators similarly affect the release of all co-localized transmitters (Bartfai et al., 1988). The action of amino acid excitants would violate this rule, if glutamate and aspartate were released from the same terminals. We conclude that the two excitatory amino acids must be released either from separate terminal populations or from separately-regulated stores within the same terminals.

The issue of co-release or separate release of glutamate and aspartate has important implications for the physiological operation of excitatory amino acid synapses. During low-frequency stimulation of SCCIA fibers, synaptic transmission normally involves activation of only the postsynaptic quisqualate receptor (Collingridge et al., 1983; Ganong et al., 1986). Quisqualate receptor activation probably depends on the release of glutamate only, because aspartate interacts only very weakly with this receptor. Aspartate can activate postsynaptic NMDA receptors, which also exist at these synapses, but these receptors are largely non-functional at low stimulus frequencies under physiological conditions. Thus, if aspartate alone is released at a subpopulation of SCCIA synapses, those synapses would presumably be silent during low-frequency stimulation. They would be expected to contribute to the postsynaptic response only under conditions that permit the activation of NMDA receptors, in particular dur-

ing high-frequency stimulation (Herron et al., 1986; Collingridge et al., 1988b) and when synaptic inhibition is reduced (Dinglediine et al., 1986; Collingridge et al., 1988a). Glutamate can activate both the quisqualate and the NMDA receptor. Therefore, if glutamate and aspartate are released from the same terminals, the precise effect on synaptic transmission of modulators or of pathological states that alter release would depend on whether the release of glutamate, aspartate or both was altered, as well as on whether conditions existed that favored the activation of normally dormant NMDA receptors.

Receptor-mediated modulation of glutamate/aspartate release: a model and some caveats

Our results favor the view that some of the receptors present postsynaptically at SCCIA synapses are also expressed on the synaptic terminal membrane and serve to modulate glutamate/aspartate release (Fig. 7). Specifically, endogenous adenosine depresses the release of both amino acids by activating an A1 receptor. The transmitters themselves modulate their release by interacting with at least two different receptors: an NMDA receptor, whose activation enhances glutamate/aspartate release, and a non-NMDA receptor, whose activation selectively depresses aspartate release. However, activation of the same receptor type can have different effects on transmitter release and postsynaptic membrane potential. This point is illustrated by the depressant effect of quisqualate/kainate receptor agonists on the release of aspartate, compared with their excitatory action on CA1 pyramidal cells. Even when pre- and postsynaptic actions are in the same direction, receptor activation may produce its ultimate effect through different coupling mechanisms. For example, adenosine could potentially inhibit glutamate/aspartate release by activating K^+ conductance, inactivating Ca^{2+} conductance or reducing cAMP content. Rather little is known about the mechanisms by which the activation of presynaptic receptors modulates the release process and the SCCIA projection appears well suited to a detailed study of these mechanisms. It would be particularly interesting to know whether excitatory amino acid receptor mechanisms differ on the two sides of the synapse.

Although the model portrayed in Fig. 7 is consistent with the available data, some details remain uncertain. First, the model postulates that glutamate and aspartate are released in about a 5:1 ratio from the same SCCIA terminals. As discussed above, the evidence for co-release of these amino acids from the same terminals is not conclusive and indeed the preferential effect of most excitatory amino acid receptor ligands on aspartate release could be viewed as evidence against co-release. An alternative model would place the QUIS/KA receptor exclusively on a separate aspartate-releasing terminal. Second, neither our results nor the results of other groups prove that receptors which modulate transmitter release are actually located on the synaptic terminal. Our dissection of the CA1 area rules out the possibility that modulators acted on the cell bodies or dendrites of the CA3 pyramidal cells or through a polysynaptic circuit. Nevertheless, they still could have acted indirectly, such as by releasing the actual modulatory substance from the CA1 pyramidal cells or from astrocytes. Lesion studies suggest that SCCIA terminals do indeed possess adenosine A1 receptors (Deckert and Jørgensen, 1988), but no comparable information about excitatory amino acid receptors is presently available. Third, we cannot be certain at this point whether one, two or several non-NMDA receptors mediate the inhibition of aspartate release. Resolution of this issue awaits a more complete pharmacological characterization of this phenomenon, including the use of more selective excitants and antagonists. Finally, it is possible that modulatory actions identified with K^+ depolarization in vitro do not significantly affect synaptic transmission in vivo. There is good reason to believe that endogenous adenosine does inhibit glutamate/aspartate release and synaptic transmission in vivo. However, there is as yet no electrophysiological action of excitatory amino acids or their antagonists in area CA1 that can be attributed to the modulation of transmitter release. Conversely, as discussed earlier, modulatory effects that alter synaptic transmission in vivo may escape detection when in vitro preparations are depolarized with elevated K^+. Correlative studies of transmitter release and synaptic physiology are essential to resolve this issue. The SCCIA projection is especially suitable for these studies, because both processes can be investigated with similar slice preparations.

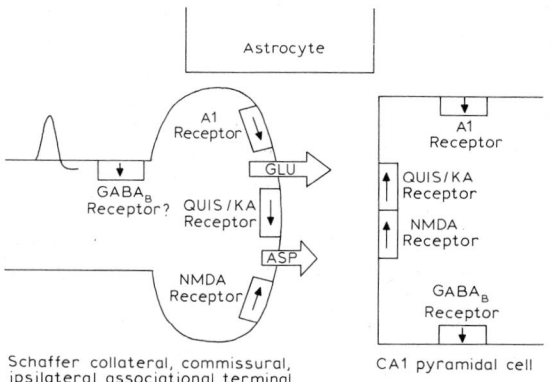

Fig. 7. Tentative localization of the adenosine A1 receptor, GABA$_B$ receptor, NMDA receptor and non-NMDA (QUIS/KA) excitatory amino acid receptor at a Schaffer collateral-commissural-ipsilateral associational (SCCIA) synapse. Open arrows of different sizes signify that SCCIA terminals release more glutamate than aspartate. Upward solid arrows denote either enhancement of transmitter release or postsynaptic depolarization. Downward solid arrows denote either inhibition of transmitter release or postsynaptic hyperpolarization.

Acknowledgements

We thank Ms. Sherrilynn Bray, Ms. Regina Thomas and Mr. Michael Thompson for their expert technical assistance. We also acknowledge the generous support of our research provided by NIH Grant NS 16064 and by a grant from the Burroughs Wellcome Fund.

References

Adam-Vizi, V. and Ligeti, E. (1986) Calcium uptake of rat brain synaptosomes as a function of membrane potential under different depolarizing conditions. *J. Physiol. (Lond.)*, 372: 363 – 377.

Arvin, B., Roberts, P.J. and McMaster, O.G. (1987) *N*-Methyl-D-aspartate increases rat brain synaptosomal free calcium. *Biochem. Soc. Trans.*, 15: 501.

Ault, B. and Nadler, J.V. (1982) Baclofen selectively inhibits transmission at synapses made by axons of CA3 pyramidal cells in the hippocampal slice. *J. Pharmacol. Exp. Ther.*, 223: 291 – 297.

Bachelard, H.S., Cox, D.W.G. and Drower, J. (1984) Sensitivity of guinea-pig hippocampal granule cell field potentials to hexoses in vitro: an effect on cell excitability? *J. Physiol. (Lond.)*, 352: 91 – 102.

Bartfai, T., Iverfeldt, K., Fisone, G. and Serfözö, P. (1988) Regulation of the release of coexisting neurotransmitters. *Annu. Rev. Pharmacol. Toxicol.*, 28: 285 – 310.

Brierley, J.B. and Graham, D.I. (1984) Hypoxia and vascular disorders of the central nervous system. In J.H. Adams, J.A.N. Corsellis and L.W. Duchen (Eds.), *Greenfield's Neuropathology*, Wiley, New York, pp. 125 – 207.

Burke, S.P. and Nadler, J.V. (1988) Regulation of glutamate and aspartate release from slices of the hippocampal CA1 area: effects of adenosine and baclofen. *J. Neurochem.*, 51: 1541 – 1551.

Burke, S.P. and Nadler, J.V. (1989) Effects of glucose deficiency on glutamate/aspartate release and excitatory synaptic responses in the hippocampal CA1 area in vitro. *Brain Res.*, 500: 333 – 342.

Butcher, S.P., Sandberg, M., Hagberg, H. and Hamberger, A. (1987) Cellular origins of amino acids released into the extracellular fluid of the rat striatum during severe insulin-induced hypoglycemia. *J. Neurochem.*, 48: 722 – 728.

Chapman, A.G. and Bowker, H.M. (1987) Inhibition of hippocampal ³H-D-aspartate release by 2-APB, 2-APV, and 2-APH. In T.P. Hicks, D. Lodge and H. McLennan (Eds.), *Excitatory Amino Acid Transmission, Neurology and Neurobiology, Vol. 24*, Liss, New York, pp. 165 – 168.

Collingridge, G.L., Kehl, S.J. and McLennan, H. (1983) Excitatory amino acids in synaptic transmission in the Schaffer collateral-commissural pathway of the rat hippocampus. *J. Physiol. (Lond.)*, 334: 33 – 46.

Collingridge, G.L., Herron, C.E. and Lester, R.A.J. (1988a) Synaptic activation of *N*-methyl-D-aspartate receptors in the Schaffer collateral-commissural pathway of rat hippocampus. *J. Physiol. (Lond.)*, 399: 283 – 300.

Collingridge, G.L., Herron, C.E. and Lester, R.A.J. (1988b) Frequency-dependent *N*-methyl-D-aspartate receptor-mediated synaptic transmission in rat hippocampus. *J. Physiol. (Lond.)*, 399: 301 – 312.

Collins, G.G.S. (1979) Evidence of a neurotransmitter role for aspartate and γ-aminobutyric acid in the rat olfactory cortex. *J. Physiol. (Lond.)*, 291: 51 – 60.

Collins, G.G.S., Anson, J. and Kelly, E.P. (1982) Baclofen: effects on evoked field potentials and amino acid neurotransmitter release in the rat olfactory cortex slice. *Brain Res.*, 238: 371 – 383.

Connick, J.H. and Stone, T.W. (1988) Excitatory amino acid antagonists and endogenous aspartate and glutamate release from rat hippocampal slices. *Br. J. Pharmacol.*, 93: 863 – 867.

Corradetti, R., Moneti, G., Moroni, F., Pepeu, G. and Wieraszko, A. (1983) Electrical stimulation of the stratum radiatum increases the release and neosynthesis of aspartate, glutamate, and γ-aminobutyric acid in rat hippocampal slices. *J. Neurochem.*, 41: 1518 – 1525.

Corradetti, R., Lo Conte, G., Moroni, F., Passani, M.B. and Pepeu, G. (1984) Adenosine decreases aspartate and glutamate release from rat hippocampal slices. *Eur. J. Pharmacol.*, 104: 19 – 26.

Crowder, J.M., Croucher, M.J., Bradford, H.F. and Collins, J.F. (1987) Excitatory amino acid receptors and depolarization-induced Ca^{2+} influx into hippocampal slices. *J. Neurochem.*, 48: 1917 – 1924.

Deckert, J. and Jørgensen, M.B. (1988) Evidence for pre- and postsynaptic localization of adenosine A1 receptors in the CA1 region of rat hippocampus: a quantitative autoradiographic study. *Brain Res.*, 446: 161 – 164.

Dingledine, R. (1984) *Brain Slices*, Plenum, New York, pp. 381 – 437.

Dingledine, R., Hynes, M.A. and King, G.L. (1986) Involvement of *N*-methyl-D-aspartate receptors in epileptiform burst firing in the rat hippocampal slice. *J. Physiol. (Lond.)*, 380: 175 – 189.

Dolphin, A.C. and Archer, E.R. (1983) An adenosine agonist inhibits and a cyclic AMP analogue enhances the release of glutamate but not GABA from slices of rat dentate gyrus. *Neurosci. Lett.*, 39: 49 – 54.

Dunwiddie, T.V. (1984) Interactions between the effects of adenosine and calcium on synaptic responses in rat hippocampus *in vitro*. *J. Physiol. (Lond.)*, 350: 545 – 559.

Dunwiddie, T.V. (1985) The physiological role of adenosine in the central nervous system. *Int. Rev. Neurobiol.*, 27: 63 – 139.

Dunwiddie, T.V., Basile, A.S. and Palmer, M.R. (1984) Electrophysiological responses to adenosine analogs in rat hippocampus and cerebellum: evidence for mediation by adenosine receptors of the A_1 subtype. *Life Sci.*, 34: 37 – 47.

Dunwiddie, T.V. and Fredholm, B.B. (1984) Adenosine receptors mediating inhibitory electrophysiological responses in rat hippocampus are different from receptors mediating cyclic AMP accumulation. *Naunyn-Schmiedebergs Arch. Pharmacol.*, 326: 294 – 301.

Dunwiddie, T.V. and Fredholm, B.B. (1989) Adenosine A_1

receptors inhibit adenylate cyclase activity and neurotransmitter release and hyperpolarize pyramidal neurons in rat hippocampus. *J. Pharmacol. Exp. Ther.*, 249: 31–37.

Dutar, P. and Nicoll, R.A. (1988) Pre- and postsynaptic GABA$_B$ receptors in the hippocampus have different pharmacological properties. *Neuron*, 1: 585–591.

Elliott, K.A.C. (1969) The use of brain slices. In A. Lajtha, (Ed.), *Handbook of Neurochemistry, Vol. 2*, Plenum, New York, pp. 103–114.

Fagg, G.E. and Lane, J.D. (1979) The uptake and release of putative amino acid neurotransmitters. *Neuroscience*, 4: 1015–1036.

Fan, P., O'Regan, P.A. and Szerb, J.C. (1988) Effect of low glucose concentration on synaptic transmission in the rat hippocampal slice. *Brain Res. Bull.*, 21: 741–747.

Ferkany, J.W. and Coyle, J.T. (1983) Evoked release of aspartate and glutamate: disparities between prelabeling and direct measurement. *Brain Res.*, 278: 279–282.

Fonnum, F. (1984) Glutamate: a neurotransmitter in mammalian brain. *J. Neurochem.*, 42: 1–11.

Fonnum, F., Paulsen, R.H., Fosse, V.M. and Engelsen, B. (1986) Synthesis and release of amino acid transmitters. In R. Schwarcz and Y. Ben-Ari (Eds.). *Excitatory Amino Acids and Epilepsy, Advances in Experimental Medicine and Biology, Vol. 203*, Plenum, New York, pp. 285–293.

Gamrani, H., Onteniente, B., Seguela, P., Geffard, M. and Calas, A. (1986) Gamma-aminobutyric acid-immunoreactivity in the rat hippocampus. A light and electron microscopic study with anti-GABA antibodies. *Brain Res.*, 364: 30–38.

Ganong, A.H., Jones, A.W., Watkins, J.C. and Cotman, C.W. (1986) Parallel antagonism of synaptic transmission and kainate/quisqualate responses in the hippocampus by piperazine-2,3-dicarboxylic acid analogs. *J. Neurosci.*, 6: 930–937.

Gottlieb, D.I. and Cowan, W.M. (1973) Autoradiographic studies of the commissural and ipsilateral association connections of the hippocampus and dentate of the rat. *J. Comp. Neurol.*, 149: 393–422.

Haas, H.L. and Greene, R.W. (1984) Adenosine enhances afterhyperpolarization and accommodation in hippocampal pyramidal cells. *Pflügers Arch.*, 402: 244–247.

Herron, C.E., Lester, R.A.J., Coan, E.J. and Collingridge, G.L. (1986) Frequency-dependent involvement of NMDA receptors in the hippocampus: a novel synaptic mechanism. *Nature (Lond.)*, 322: 265–268.

Honoré, T., Lauridsen, J. and Krogsgaard-Larsen, P. (1982) The binding of [^{3}H]AMPA, a structural analogue of glutamic acid, to rat brain membranes. *J. Neurochem.*, 38: 173–178.

Inoue, M., Matsuo, T. and Ogata, N. (1985a) Baclofen activates voltage-dependent and 4-aminopyridine sensitive K$^+$ conductance in guinea-pig hippocampal pyramidal cells maintained *in vitro*. *Br. J. Pharmacol.*, 84: 833–841.

Inoue, M., Matsuo, T. and Ogata, N. (1985b) Characterization

of pre- and postsynaptic actions of (−) baclofen in the guinea-pig hippocampus *in vitro*. *Br. J. Pharmacol.*, 84: 843–851.

Kato, K., Goto, M. and Fukuda, H. (1982) Baclofen: inhibition of the release of L-[^{3}H]glutamate and L-[^{3}H]aspartate from rat whole brain synaptosomes. *Gen. Pharmacol.*, 13: 445–447.

Kauppinen, R.A., Enkvist, K., Holopainen, I. and Åkerman, K.E.O. (1988) Glucose deprivation depolarizes plasma membrane of cultured astrocytes and collapses transmembrane potassium and glutamate gradients. *Neuroscience*, 26: 283–289.

Laurberg, S. and Sørensen, K.E. (1981) Associational and commissural collaterals of neurons in the hippocampal formation (hilus fasciae dentatae and subfield CA3). *Brain Res.*, 212: 287–300.

Levi, G. and Gallo, V. (1981) Glutamate as a putative transmitter in the cerebellum: stimulation by GABA of glutamic acid release from specific pools. *J. Neurochem.*, 37: 22–31.

Levi, G., Gordon, R.D., Gallo, V., Wilkin, G.P. and Balazs, R. (1982) Putative acidic amino acid transmitters in the cerebellum. I. Depolarization-induced release. *Brain Res.*, 239: 425–445.

Lindroth, P. and Mopper, K. (1979) High performance liquid chromatographic determination of subpicomole amounts of amino acids by precolumn fluorescence derivatization with σ-phthaldialdehyde. *Anal. Chem.*, 51: 1667–1674.

London, E.D. and Coyle, J.T. (1979) Specific binding of [^{3}H]kainic acid to receptor sites in rat brain. *Mol. Pharmacol.*, 15: 492–505.

Mayer, M.L. and Westbrook, G.L. (1987) The physiology of excitatory amino acids in the vertebrate central nervous system. *Prog. Neurobiol.*, 28: 197–276.

McBean, G.J. and Roberts, P.J. (1981) Glutamate-preferring receptors regulate the release of D-[^{3}H]aspartate from rat hippocampal slices. *Nature (Lond.)*, 291: 593–594.

Michaelis, M.L., Johe, K.K., Moghadam, B. and Adams, R.N. (1988) Studies on the ionic mechanism for the neuromodulatory actions of adenosine in the brain. *Brain Res.*, 473: 249–260.

Nadler, J.V., Vaca, K.W., White, W.F., Lynch, G.S. and Cotman, C.W. (1976) Aspartate and glutamate as possible transmitters of excitatory hippocampal afferents. *Nature (Lond.)*, 260: 538–540.

Nadler, J.V., White, W.F., Vaca, K.W. and Cotman, C.W. (1977) Calcium-dependent γ-aminobutyrate release by interneurons of rat hippocampal regions: lesion-induced plasticity. *Brain Res.*, 131: 241–258.

Nadler, J.V., Perry, B.W., Gentry, C. and Cotman, C.W. (1980) Loss and reacquisition of hippocampal synapses after selective destruction of CA3–CA4 afferents with kainic acid. *Brain Res.*, 191: 387–403.

Nadler, J.V., Evenson, D.A. and Cuthbertson, G.J. (1981) Comparative toxicity of kainic acid and other excitatory amino acids toward rat hippocampal neurons. *Neuroscience*, 6: 2505 – 2517.

Naito, S. and Ueda, T. (1983) ATP-dependent uptake of glutamate into protein I-associated synaptic vesicles. *J. Biol. Chem.*, 258: 696 – 699.

Newberry, N.R. and Nicoll, R.A. (1985) Comparison of the action of baclofen with γ-aminobutyric acid on rat hippocampal pyramidal cells *in vitro. J. Physiol. (Lond.)*, 360: 161 – 185.

Nicholls, D.G. and Sihra, T.S. (1986) Synaptosomes possess an exocytotic pool of glutamate. *Nature (Lond.)*, 321: 772 – 773.

Olverman, H.J., Jones, A.W. and Watkins, J.C. (1984) Glutamate has higher affinity than other amino acids for [^{3}H]-D-AP5 binding sites in rat brain membranes. *Nature (Lond.)*, 307: 460 – 462.

Ottersen, O.P. and Storm-Mathisen, J. (1985) Different neuronal localization of aspartate-like and glutamate-like immunoreactivities in the hippocampus of rat, guinea pig, and Senegalese baboon *(Papio papio)*, with a note on the distribution of γ-aminobutyrate. *Neuroscience*, 16: 589 – 606.

Ottersen, O.P. and Storm-Mathisen, J. (1986) Excitatory amino acid pathways in the brain. In R. Schwarcz and Y. Ben-Ari (Eds.), *Excitatory Amino Acids and Epilepsy, Advances in Experimental Medicine and Biology, Vol. 203*, Plenum, New York, pp. 263 – 284.

Potashner, S.J. (1979) Baclofen: effects on amino acid release and metabolism in slices of guinea pig cerebral cortex. *J. Neurochem.*, 32: 103 – 109.

Reddington, M., Lee, K.S. and Schubert, P. (1982) An A$_1$-adenosine receptor, characterized by [^{3}H]cyclohexyladenosine binding, mediates the depression of evoked potentials in a rat hippocampal slice preparation. *Neurosci. Lett.*, 28: 275 – 279.

Reubi, J.C. and Cuénod, M. (1979) Glutamate release in vitro from corticostriatal terminals. *Brain Res.*, 176: 185 – 188.

Roberts, P.J. (1974) The release of amino acids with proposed neurotransmitter function from the cuneate and gracile nuclei of the rat *in vivo. Brain Res.*, 67: 419 – 428.

Sandberg, M., Butcher, S.P. and Hagberg, H. (1986) Extracellular overflow of neuroactive amino acids during severe insulin-induced hypoglycemia: in vivo dialysis of the rat hippocampus. *J. Neurochem.*, 47: 178 – 184.

Scholfield, C.N. and Steel, L. (1988) Presynaptic K-channel blockade counteracts the depressant effect of adenosine in olfactory cortex. *Neuroscience*, 24: 81 – 91.

Schubert, P., Heinemann, U. and Kolb, R. (1986) Differential effect of adenosine on pre- and postsynaptic calcium fluxes. *Brain Res.*, 376: 382 – 386.

Siggins, G.R. and Schubert, P. (1981) Adenosine depression of hippocampal neurons in vitro: an intracellular study of dose-dependent actions on synaptic and membrane potentials. *Neurosci. Lett.*, 23: 55 – 60.

Silinsky, E.M., Hirsh, J.K. and Vogel, S.M. (1987) Intracellular calcium mediating the actions of adenosine at neuromuscular junctions. In E. Gerlach and B.F. Becker (Eds.), *Topics and Perspectives in Adenosine Research*, Springer-Verlag, Berlin, pp. 537 – 548.

Simon, R.P., Schmidley, J.W., Meldrum, B.S., Swan, J.H. and Chapman, A.G. (1986) Excitotoxic mechanisms in hypoglycaemic hippocampal injury. *Neuropathol. Appl. Neurobiol.*, 12: 567 – 576.

Spencer, H.J., Tominez, G. and Halpern, B. (1981) Mass spectrographic analysis of stimulated release of endogenous amino acids from rat hippocampal slices. *Brain Res.*, 212: 194 – 197.

Storm-Mathisen, J. (1977) Glutamic acid and excitatory nerve endings: reduction of glutamic acid uptake after axotomy. *Brain Res.*, 120: 379 – 386.

Storm-Mathisen, J. and Iversen, L.L. (1979) Uptake of [^{3}H]glutamic acid in excitatory nerve endings: light and electron-microscopic observations in the hippocampal formation of the rat. *Neuroscience*, 4: 1237 – 1253.

Swanson, L.W., Wyss, J.M. and Cowan, W.M. (1978) An autoradiographic study of the organization of intrahippocampal association pathways in the rat. *J. Comp. Neurol.*, 172: 49 – 84.

Szerb, J.C. (1988) Changes in the relative amounts of aspartate and glutamate released and retained in hippocampal slices during stimulation. *J. Neurochem.*, 50: 219 – 224.

Szerb, J.C. and O'Regan, P.A. (1987) Reversible shifts in the Ca^{2+}-dependent release of aspartate and glutamate from hippocampal slices with changing glucose concentrations. *Synapse*, 1: 265 – 272.

Szerb, J.C. and O'Regan, P.A. (1988) Increase in the stimulation-induced overflow of excitatory amino acids from hippocampal slices: interaction between low glucose concentration and fluoroacetate. *Neurosci. Lett.*, 86: 207 – 212.

Vergili, M., Poli, A., Contestabile, A., Migani, P. and Barnabei, O. (1986) Synaptosomal release of newly-synthesized or recently accumulated amino acids. Differential effects of kainic acid on naturally occurring excitatory amino acids and on [D-^{3}H]aspartate. *Neurochem. Int.*, 9: 29 – 33.

Westerberg, E. and Wieloch, T. (1987) Excitatory amino acids and hypoglycemic brain damage. In T.P. Hicks, D. Lodge and H. McLennan, (Eds.), *Excitatory Amino Acid Transmission, Neurology and Neurobiology, Vol. 24*, Liss, New York, pp. 225 – 232.

Wojcik, W.J., Cavalla, D. and Neff, N.H. (1985) Colocalized adenosine A1 and γ-amino-butyric acid B (GABA$_B$) receptors of cerebellum may share a common adenylate cyclase catalytic unit. *Mol. Pharmacol.*, 232: 62 – 66.

J. Storm-Mathisen, J. Zimmer and O.P. Ottersen (Eds.)
Progress in Brain Research, Vol. 83
© 1990 Elsevier Science Publishers B.V. (Biomedical Division)

CHAPTER 10

Dendritic excitation by glutamate in CA1 hippocampal cells

Øivind Hvalby

Institute of Neurophysiology,
University of Oslo, Karl Johans gate 47, N-0162 Oslo 1, Norway

In order to reveal properties and effects of glutamate excitation, CA1 pyramidal cells in rat hippocampal slices were impaled and responses to iontophoresis of glutamate onto sensitive spots in the dendrites were analyzed. The glutamate-elicited response consisted of a steady depolarization; its amplitude was dose-dependent. The cellular response to repeated applications of glutamate showed a striking degree of stability. Both dendritic and somatic depolarization, induced by glutamate and current, respectively, elicited similar discharge patterns. The sensitivity to glutamate was highly localized, corresponding to the dendritic tree of a given cell. Short, repeated glutamate pulses did not interfere with an orthodromic test response, whereas longer glutamate ejections often depressed the EPSP. Combined temporal and spatial pairing of glutamate and orthodromic activation was followed by a lasting increase in synaptic efficiency, similar to LTP.

Introduction

The hippocampus serves as a particularly attractive model system for electrophysiological studies of neuronal excitability. This is due to its stratified structure, with the cell bodies gathered in a single layer, the parallel arrangement of dendrites and the relatively precise organization of the afferents making synapses on the dendrites (Ramón y Cajal, 1911; Lorente de Nó, 1936; Blackstad, 1956). The transverse lamellar organization (Andersen et al., 1971) permits the use of hippocampal slices with preserved circuitry (Skrede and Westgaard, 1971) where stable, long-lasting, and high-quality intracellular recordings can be performed (Schwartzkroin, 1975).

L-Glutamate has been shown to fulfil several of the criteria for a neurotransmitter in the synapses between the Schaffer collateral/commissural fibres and the CA1 pyramidal cells (Nadler et al., 1976; Storm-Mathisen et al., 1983; Storm-Mathisen and Ottersen, 1984). The CA1 pyramidal cells respond to glutamate with a powerful excitation in extracellular (Biscoe and Straughan, 1966) and intracellular studies (Schwartzkroin and Andersen, 1975). Glutamate acts as an agonist on both the N-methyl-D-aspartate (NMDA) type and the quisqualate/kainate (non-NMDA) types of receptors (Watkins and Evans, 1981). This dual receptor system is densely distributed in stratum radiatum (Monaghan et al., 1983). The receptors serving single volley transmission across these synapses are of the non-NMDA receptor type (Collingridge et al., 1983). During high-frequency stimulation, however, both requirements for NMDA channel opening are provided: the signal is delivered by synaptic transmission per se and the synaptic current creates a sustained depolarization of sufficient magnitude to relieve the voltage-dependent Mg^{2+} block of the channel (Nowak et al., 1984; Mayer et al., 1984). In accordance with the properties of the NMDA receptor/channel complex a synaptic component sensitive to the NMDA receptor blocker 2-amino-5-phosponovale-

132

rate (APV) is unmasked during high-frequency activation (Wigström and Gustafsson, 1984; Herron et al., 1986). Since the excitatory synapses are located on the dendrites in these cells (Andersen et al., 1966), local, dendritic application of glutamate is expected to mimic the effects of a synaptic bombardment.

Because hippocampal excitatory pathways show a marked degree of plasticity we decided to analyze the properties and the effects of the responses elicited by iontophoretically applied L-glutamate. The study is based on intracellular recordings from 118 CA1 pyramidal cells in rat hippocampal slices. The methods used for slice preparation, fluid composition, stimulation and recording have been described previously (Storm and Hvalby, 1985; Hvalby et al., 1987).

Properties and discharge patterns of the glutamate induced responses

In addition to require an appropriate position of the iontophoretic electrode, the response to dendritically applied glutamate depended upon the size and duration of the ejection current. With increasing amount of current, the cellular depolarization occurred with shorter latency and greater rate of rise. The amplitude of the induced depolarization increased and the latency to cell discharge decreased (Fig. 1A,B). Above a certain amount of iontophoretic current, however, no further decrease in the spike latency or increase in the amplitude of the induced depolarization were observed (Fig. 2A), in accordance with earlier reports (Hablitz and Langmoen, 1982). The duration of the depolarization after the cessation of the glutamate ejection also changed in a dose-dependent manner (Fig. 1A,B). The speed of repolarization was nearly constant, however, irrespective of the amount of ejected glutamate (Fig. 1A,B). In response to a glutamate pulse some cells showed a double rising phase before reaching a plateau level of depolarization. A two-step repolarization phase was seen after the end of the glutamate pulse (Fig. 1C).

Repeated ejections of glutamate elicited responses with a remarkable degree of stability. When short glutamate pulses (duration < 100 ms, repetition rate 0.2 or 0.5 Hz for 3 – 5 min) were delivered, the latency to the initial spike and the level of depolarization were both unchanged from one response to the next in 42 cells (Fig. 2B). The regularity of the responses was also maintained when the rate of delivery was increased (Fig. 2C). Only at the fastest repetition rates, however, was there an increased duration of the depolarizing plateau, similar to that seen in the dose-response experiments.

The dose- and frequency-dependent increase in duration of the induced depolarizations may possibly be caused by a dose-dependent saturation of the glutamate uptake system. In addition, transient local changes in ion composition and effects due to the diffusion of glutamate may contribute to the observed phenomenon.

In twenty cells, once a hot spot was found, the subthreshold response to repeated application of

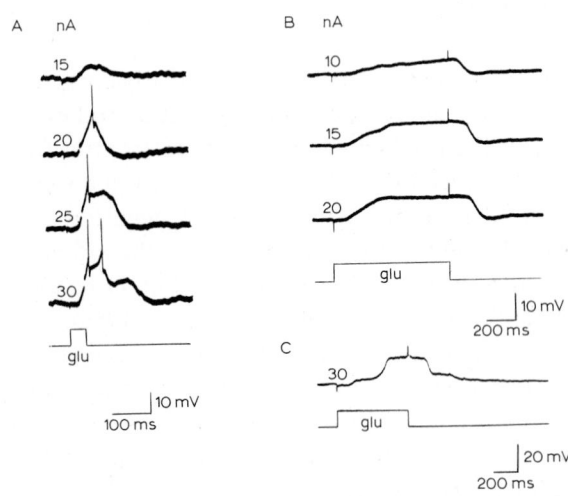

Fig. 1. A: cellular responses to glutamate ejected by rectangular pulses (40 ms duration) of increasing current in the apical dendritic region. The intensity of the stimulus current is indicated to the left of each trace. The ejection pulse is indicated at the bottom. The spikes have been retouched and are truncated. B: as A, but taken from another CA1 cell (glutamate pulses of 800 ms duration). C: an example from another cell which showed a biphasic response induced by a 600 ms long glutamate pulse.

longer glutamate pulses (0.3 – 1.5 s duration, 0.2 – 0.5 Hz repetition rate and a total of 30 – 120 ejections) remained stable throughout the series (Fig. 5A). In some cells, however, there was a tendency towards an improved response with repeated glutamate applications (Fig. 5C), a feature which may bear resemblance to the agonist-induced enhancement seen in layer V of the sensorimotor cortex (Flatman et al., 1986).

As previously described (Storm and Hvalby, 1985), iontophoretic application of glutamate to sensitive spots in the dendritic territory of a CA1 pyramidal cell elicited at low intensities an initial depolarization leading up to a slow repetitive firing

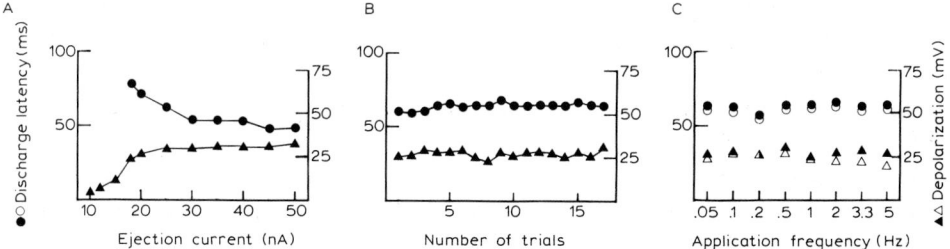

Fig. 2. A: graphic representation of the dose-dependent action of glutamate. The latency to the initial spike (filled circles) was measured from the onset of the glutamate ejection pulse (40 ms pulse duration). The amplitude of the induced depolarization (filled triangles) was measured at a fixed time after the onset. Both are plotted as a function of the stimulus current (nA). B: stability of the glutamate response. As A, but in response to a constant ejection current of 20 nA with a repetition rate of 0.2 Hz. The latency to the spike and the depolarization amplitude are plotted as a function of repeated responses. C: frequency dependence of the glutamate response. Two pulses of glutamate (40 ms duration, 18 nA stimulus current) were given with increasing frequency. Open symbols show the parameters in response to the first, filled symbols the parameters in response to the second glutamate application, respectively.

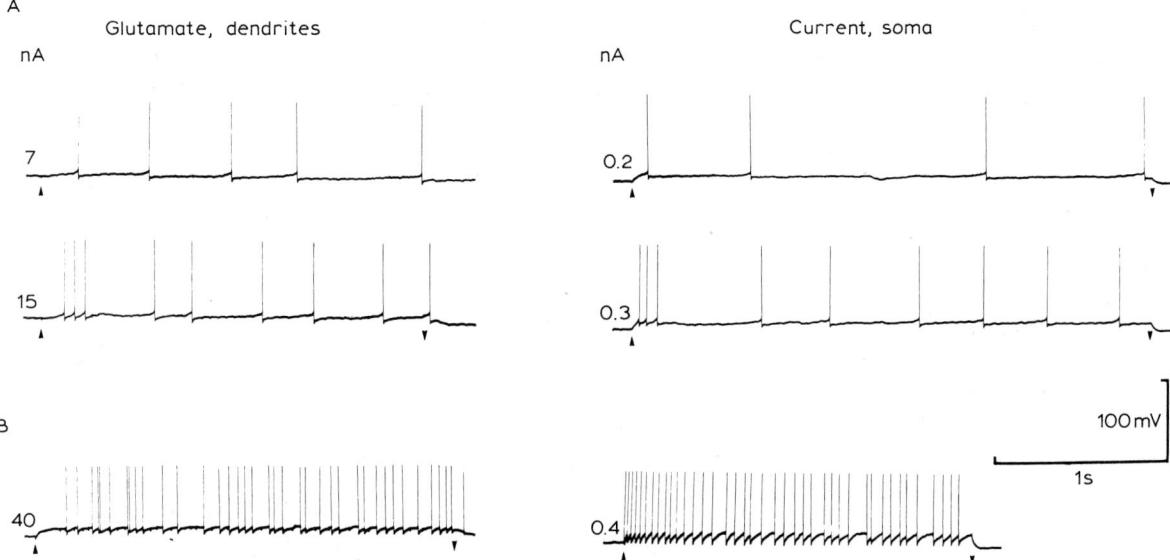

Fig. 3. A: responses from a CA1 pyramidal cell to depolarization, induced either by application of glutamate delivered iontophoretically at a sensitive spot in the apical dendrites (left panel) or by pulses of depolarizing current injected into the soma (right panel). The intensity of the stimulus current is indicated (nA). Arrowheads mark the onset and the end of each stimulus. The spikes have been retouched (Modified from Fig. 1, Storm and Hvalby, 1985). B: as A, but responses from another pyramidal cell.

with slow prepotentials and fast and slow after-hyperpolarizations (Fig. 3A). At moderate intensities the pattern of discharge was characterized by an initial burst of action potentials followed by a pause and thereafter a relatively regular discharge. In some cells, which did not show a burst – pause pattern, a gradual adaptation developed instead of a complete pause between the initial and the tail discharge (Fig. 3B). When high doses of glutamate were applied the responses were characterized by an initial firing followed by a plateau of depolarization with spike inactivation (Schwartzkroin and Andersen, 1975).

At low and moderately strong stimulus intensities CA1 pyramidal cells respond in a strikingly similar manner to depolarization, whether imposed by current injection at the soma or in the dendrites by glutamate (Fig. 3A,B; Storm and Hvalby, 1985). The glutamate induced depolarization shows a slower onset which complicates a comparison between the two stimuli, although the difference most probably can be ascribed to the time needed for diffusion of glutamate. With comparable stimuli the slow afterhyperpolarization (sAHP) was more pronounced after glutamate than after current stimulation. In both cases a Ca^{2+} dependent potassium current underlies the sAHP (Nicoll and Alger, 1981), but an electrogenic sodium pump may additionally contribute to the post-glutamate hyperpolarization (Segal, 1981).

Localization of glutamate-sensitive spots

The responsive area of a CA1 pyramidal cell to iontophoretically applied glutamate corresponds to a volume shaped as a double cone, where the tips meet each other at the level of the stratum pyramidale (Fig. 4A). Within this volume, roughly equivalent to the dendritic tree of the cell, a number of sensitive, highly localized, spots can be

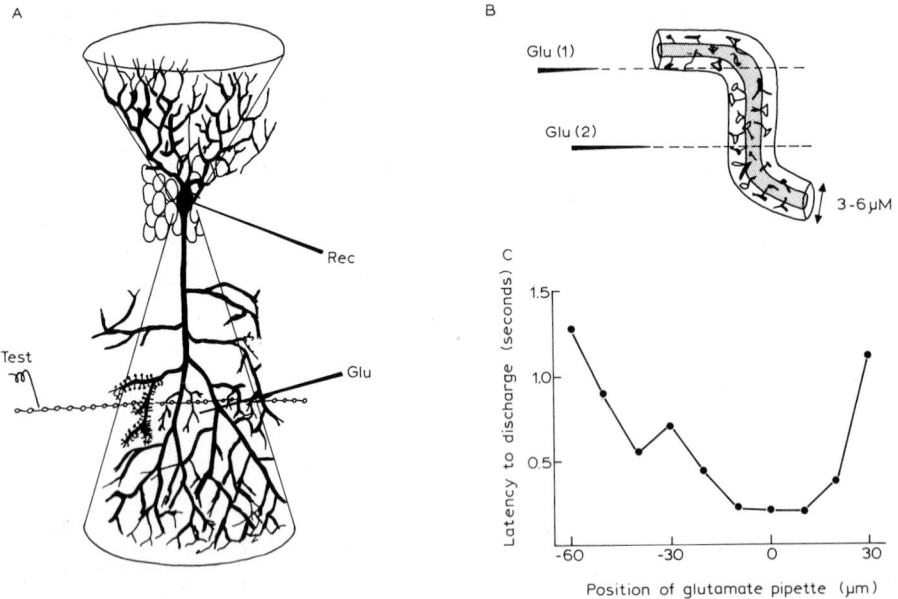

Fig. 4. A: dendritic territory of a CA1 pyramidal cell. Responses of a CA1 pyramidal cell to iontophoretically applied L-glutamate (1.0 M, pH 8.0, Glu) and to orthodromic activation of the afferent fibres in stratum radiatum (Test) were recorded intracellularly (Rec). B: possible explanation for the different sizes of the glutamate-sensitive areas. Schematic drawing of a dendritic branch and two different glutamate pipette tracks (Glu 1 and Glu 2). C: localization of the sensitivity to glutamate. The glutamate pipette was lowered vertically through the slice in the apical dendritic region, 300 μm from the soma. For every 10 μm, a pulse of glutamate (30 nA) was ejected. The latency to discharge has been plotted against the distance from the point of minimum latency.

found (Dudar, 1974; Schwartzkroin and Andersen, 1975; Hablitz and Langmoen, 1982). At a given distance from the soma a vertical movement of the glutamate pipette through the slice typically discloses from 0 to 3 separate areas, each with a maximal sensitivity along a stretch of $10-20$ μm (Fig. 4C). The relative variation in size between the areas might be explained by the trajectory of the glutamate pipette: in some tracks it might run perpendicular to the dendritic branches, in others it might run parallel to them (Fig. 4B).

The glutamate-induced depolarization is not caused by simple diffusion of the compound to the soma, because the hot spots can be found at any distance from 20 to 400 μm from the soma. Intermediate positions may give considerably weaker responses than more distal sensitive spots (Schwartzkroin and Andersen, 1975; Storm and Hvalby, 1985). Furthermore, the spread of glutamate in cortex and the caudate nucleus was reported to be $2-3$ orders of magnitude slower (Herz et al., 1969) than the observed response latency in the CA1 region. This can be as fast as 6 ms with an appropriately placed electrode in stratum radiatum (Hvalby, Bliss and Andersen, unpublished observations). In addition, with glutamate electrodes situated in the apical and basal dendrites, respectively, the distance precluding any direct effect, the summation resulted from depolarization of the soma membrane itself (Schwartzkroin and Andersen, 1975). Taken together, the most probable explanation is that each sensitive region represents a dendritic branch with its attached spines and glutaminergic receptor regions.

Glutamate ejections and orthodromic activation

When low-frequency orthodromic stimulation of the afferent fibres and iontophoretic application of short glutamate pulses (duration < 400 ms, subthreshold depolarization) were given alternately to the same dendritic region (Fig. 4A), the responses to orthodromic activation remained unchanged (Fig. 5B). When the duration and intensity of the ejection current was increased, however, there was a transient or often a long-lasting (in some cells up to 30 min) depression of the orthodromically evoked EPSPs (Fig. 5D), in accordance with earlier extracellular reports (Collingridge et al., 1983).

The induced depression could conceivably be due to desensitization of one or more of the glutamate receptor subtypes as earlier reported in hippocampal slices (Fagni et al., 1983; Mohan and Sastry, 1985). A desensitization mechanism lasting for seconds in our experiments appears unlikely because the responses to the repeated glutamate pulses did not show any significant changes, neither in the start or discharge latency nor of the depolarization (Figs. 2B, 5A,C). However, possible presynaptic effects of glutamate may well be present since the existence of glutamatergic, presynaptic receptors has been proposed (McBean and Roberts, 1981; Collins et al., 1983; Errington et al., 1987).

The long-lasting improvement of synaptic transmission following high-frequency trains of afferent impulses which occurs in hippocampal excitatory pathways (long-term potentiation – LTP), is expressed as an increased amplitude of the EPSP and an improved probability of action potential generation with shorter spike latency (Bliss and Lømo, 1973). During the induction of LTP in hippocampal synapses, a slow depolarization of dendritic origin seemed to be important for subsequent LTP-development (Andersen et al., 1984; Wigström and Gustafsson, 1984).

In order to mimic the high-frequency synaptic bombardment of a restricted part of the dendritic tree we combined temporal and spatial coupling between subthreshold depolarizations caused by glutamate ejections and low-frequency orthodromic activation. The lasting enhancement of the orthodromically evoked response expressed itself as an increased probability of firing and a shorter spike latency (Hvalby et al., 1986; 1987). Albeit the EPSPs were significantly increased in most cells, they were depressed in a few cells, similar to the observed depression when long glutamate pulses were applied alone. The effect of the conjunction was furthermore input-specific because the transmission across control synapses in stratum oriens was unchanged (Fig. 6) and no changes in soma excitability were observed. Coupling with comparable strong current-induced soma depolarization did not elicit any change in synaptic transmission.

Conjunction with considerably stronger soma depolarizing currents (3 – 8 nA), however, induces an enhancement of synaptic transmission expressed as an increased EPSP (Kelso et al., 1986; Sastry et al., 1986; Wigström et al., 1986). Taken together, these results suggest that the conjunction effect is generated at, or close to the dendritic

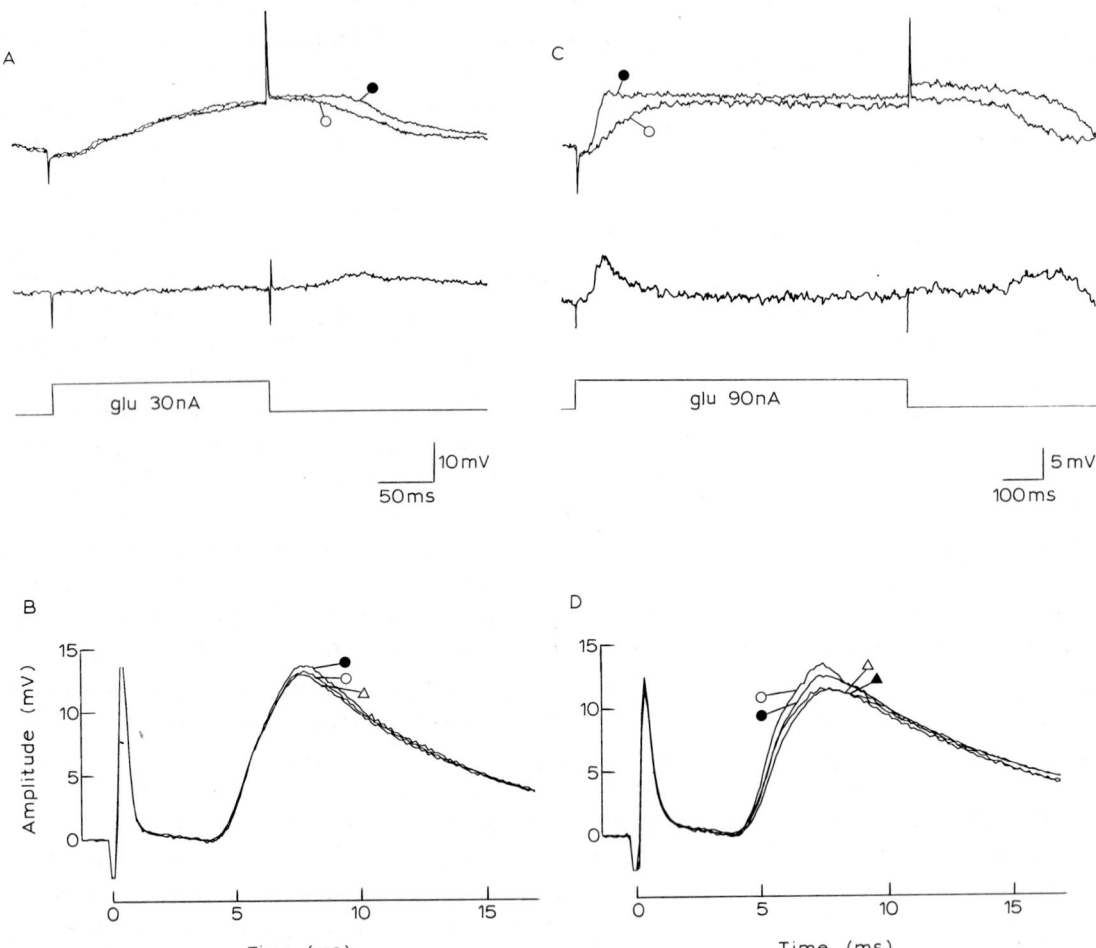

Fig. 5. Dose-dependent interference between responses to glutamate application and orthodromic activation. A: average records of the responses to the 10 first (open circle) and the 10 last (filled circle) applications of glutamate in a series of 60 (30 nA, 200 ms, repetition rate 0.25 Hz), alternating with orthodromic activation (0.25 Hz) of the radiatum fibres activating the same dendritic territory of the cell. The lower panel shows the difference in response between the two averages. B: average records of the EPSPs based on 20 trials before (open circle), during (open triangle) and 5 min after (filled circle) the 60 glutamate ejections described in A. C: as A, but from another cell to which stronger and longer glutamate pulses were applied (90 nA, 830 ms). D: average records of the EPSPs based on 20 trials before (open circle), during (open triangle), immediately after (filled triangle), and 5 min after (filled circle) the stimulation paradigm described in A. Note the improved response to glutamate applications (C, lower panel) contrasting the depressed orthodromic response (D).

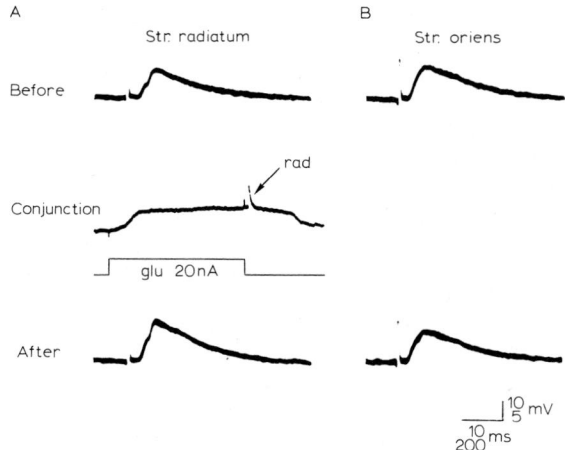

A   Str. radiatum   B   Str. oriens

Before

rad

Conjunction

glu 20nA

After

10
5 mV
10
200 ms

Fig. 6. Cellular responses before and after conjunction. A: two superimposed responses to orthodromic stimulation of radiatum fibres before (upper panel) and 25 min after (lower panel) conjunction. The coupling (middle panel) consisted of 30 glutamate pulses delivered in str. radiatum (20 nA, 650 ms duration, 0.2 Hz) simultaneously with the same number of orthodromic synaptic responses (rad). B: a separate, orthodromic activation in str. oriens served as a control and was delivered alternately. Two superimposed responses following stimulation of str. oriens before and 25 min after the conjunction in str. radiatum are shown. The little notch on the upstroke of the EPSP is a field effect of the population spike, generated by the synchronous discharge of surrounding cells.

synapses. Furthermore, simultaneous pre- and postsynaptic activation is necessary since neither is sufficient by itself.

The NMDA receptor/channel complex plays a pivotal role during the induction of LTP functioning as a postsynaptic Ca^{2+} injector (Collingridge and Bliss, 1987). Both requirements for activation of NMDA gated channels – agonist and depolarization – are met when pulses of glutamate are ejected. The lack of an enhanced synaptic transmission following glutamate application alone in our experiments, therefore, seems to be a paradox. Kauer et al. (1988a), have, however, observed a decremental potentiation following glutamate ejection similar to the one following NMDA application (Collingridge et al., 1983; Kauer et al., 1988a).

Recently, it has been shown that although

NMDA channel activation is a necessary requirement for the induction of LTP, the long-lasting improved transmission is expressed as a non-NMDA mediated response (Kauer et al., 1988b; Muller et al., 1988; Davies et al., 1989).

Glutamate may well have effects in addition to the induced depolarization. Whereas single ion channel electrophysiology strongly supports a direct linkage between excitatory amino acids and ion channels (Cull-Candy and Usowicz, 1987; Jahr and Stevens, 1987), the reported coupling between excitatory amino acids and second messenger systems may have a multitude of effects on neuronal function (Smart, 1989). In hippocampus, activation of receptors of the quisqualate type by some excitatory amino acid agonists enhances the hydrolysis of membrane inositol phospholipids (Nicoletti et al., 1986), whereas others apparently inhibit the activation of the phosphatidylinositol second messenger system (Baudry et al., 1986). The glutamate-induced increase in intracellular Ca^{2+}, as visualized in acutely dissociated hippocampal neurones (Connor et al., 1988), may alone have crucial effects on a diversity of processes. The correlation between activation of the NMDA receptor and the encoding of a presumed transcription regulatory factor important for changes in gene expression (Cole et al., 1989) makes it likely that glutamate has profound effects on a variety of neuronal functions, among them excitability and plasticity.

Acknowledgements

I thank Dr. Per Andersen, Dr. Johan Storm, Dr. Jean-Claude Lacaille and Dr. G.-Y. Hu for the collaboration during many of the experiments. This work was supported by the Norwegian Research Council for Science and the Humanities.

References

Andersen, P., Avoli, M. and Hvalby, Ø. (1984) Evidence for both pre- and postsynaptic mechanisms during long-term potentiation in hippocampal slices. *Exp. Brain Res.*, Suppl. 9: 315–324.

138

Andersen, P., Blackstad, T.W. and Lømo, T. (1966) Location and identification of excitatory synapses on hippocampal pyramidal cells. *Exp. Brain Res.*, 1: 236–248.

Andersen, P., Bliss, T.V.P. and Skrede, K.K. (1971) Lamellar organization of hippocampal excitatory pathways. *Exp. Brain Res.*, 13: 222–238.

Baudry, M., Evans, J. and Lynch, G. (1986) Excitatory amino acids inhibit stimulation of phosphatidylinositol metabolism by aminergic agonists in hippocampus. *Nature (Lond.)*, 319: 329–331.

Biscoe, T.J. and Straughan, D.W. (1966) Micro-electrophoretic studies of neurones in the cat hippocampus. *J. Physiol. (Lond.)*, 183: 341–359.

Blackstad, T.W. (1956) Commissural connections of the hippocampal region in the rat, with special reference to their mode of termination. *J. Comp. Neurol.*, 105: 417–537.

Bliss, T.V.P. and Lømo, T. (1973) Long-lasting potentiation of synaptic transmission in the dentate area of the anaesthetized rabbit following stimulation of the perforant path. *J. Physiol. (Lond.)*, 232: 331–356.

Cole, A.J., Saffen, D.W., Baraban, J.M. and Worley, P.F. (1989) Rapid increase of an immediate early gene messenger RNA in hippocampal neurons by synaptic NMDA receptor activation. *Nature (Lond.)*, 340: 474–476.

Collingridge, G.L. and Bliss, T.V.P. (1987) NMDA receptors – their role in long-term potentiation. *Trends Neurosci.*, 10: 288–293.

Collingridge, G.L., Kehl, S.J. and McLennan, H. (1983) Excitatory amino acids in synaptic transmission in the Schaffer collateral-commissural pathway of the rat hippocampus. *J. Physiol. (Lond.)*, 334: 33–46.

Collins, G.G.S., Anson, J. and Surtees, L. (1983) Presynaptic kainate and N-methyl-D-aspartate receptors regulate excitatory amino acid release in the olfactory cortex. *Brain Res.*, 265: 157–159.

Connor, J.A., Wadman, W.J., Hockberger, P.E. and Wong, R.K.S. (1988) Sustained dendritic gradients of Ca^{2+} induced by excitatory amino acids in CA1 hippocampal neurons. *Science*, 240: 649–653.

Cull-Candy, S.G. and Usowicz, M.M. (1987) Multiple-conductance channels activated by excitatory amino acids in cerebellar neurons. *Nature (Lond.)*, 325: 525–528.

Davies, S.N., Lester, R.A.J., Reymann, K.G. and Collingridge, G.L. (1989) Temporally distinct pre- and post-synaptic mechanisms maintain long-term potentiation. *Nature (Lond.)*, 338: 500–503.

Dudar, J.D. (1974) *In vitro* excitation of hippocampal pyramidal cell dendrites by glutamic acid. *Neuropharmacology*, 13: 1083–1089.

Errington, M.L., Lynch, M.A. and Bliss, T.V.P. (1987) Long-term potentiation in the dentate gyrus: induction and increased glutamate release are blocked by D(−) aminophosphonovalerate. *Neuroscience*, 20: 279–284.

Fagni, L., Baudry, M. and Lynch, G. (1983) Classification and properties of acidic amino acid receptors in hippocampus. I. Electrophysiological studies of an apparent desensitization and interactions with drugs which block transmission. *J. Neurosci.*, 3: 1538–1546.

Flatman, J.A., Schwindt, P.C. and Crill, W.E. (1986) The induction and modification of voltage-sensitive response in cat neocortical neurons by N-methyl-D-aspartate. *Brain Res.*, 363: 62–77.

Hablitz, J.J. and Langmoen, I.A. (1982) Excitation of hippocampal pyramidal cells by glutamate in the guinea-pig and rat. *J. Physiol. (Lond.)*, 325: 317–331.

Herron, C.E., Lester, R.A.J., Coan, E.J. and Collingridge, G.L. (1986) Frequency-dependent involvement of NMDA receptors in the hippocampus: a novel synaptic mechanism. *Nature (Lond.)*, 322: 265–268.

Herz, A., Zieglgänsberger, W. and Färber, G. (1969) Microelectrophoretic studies concerning the spread of glutamic acid and GABA in brain tissue. *Exp. Brain Res.*, 9: 221–235.

Hvalby, Ø, Andersen, P., Lacaille, J.-C. and Hu, G.-Y. (1986) Post-synaptic depolarization, a necessary condition for the development of LTP? *Adv. Biosci.*, 59: 61–66.

Hvalby, Ø., Lacaille, J.-C., Hu, G.-Y. and Andersen, P. (1987) Postsynaptic long-term potentiation follows coupling of dendritic glutamate application and synaptic activation. *Experientia*, 43: 599–601.

Jahr, C.E. and Stevens, C.F. (1987) Glutamate activates multiple single channel conductances in hippocampal neurones. *Nature (Lond.)*, 325: 522–525.

Kauer, J.A., Malenka, R.C. and Nicoll, R.A. (1988a) NMDA application potentiates synaptic transmission in the hippocampus. *Nature (Lond.)*, 334: 250–252.

Kauer, J.A., Malenka, R.C. and Nicoll, R.A. (1988b) A persistent postsynaptic modification mediates long-term potentiation in the hippocampus. *Neuron*, 1: 911–917.

Kelso, S.R., Ganong, A.H. and Brown, T.H. (1986) Hebbian synapses in hippocampus. *Proc. Natl. Acad. Sci. U.S.A.*, 83: 5326–5330.

Lorente de Nó, R. (1934) Studies on the structure of the cerebral cortex. II. Continuation of the study of the Ammonic system. *J. Psychol. Neurol.*, 46: 113–177.

Mayer, M.L., Westbrook, G.L. and Guthrie, P.B. (1984) Voltage-dependent block by Mg^{2+} of NMDA responses in spinal cord neurones. *Nature (Lond.)*, 309: 261–263.

McBean, G.J. and Roberts, P.J. (1981) Glutamate-preferring receptors regulate the release of D-[³H]aspartate from rat hippocampal slices. *Nature (Lond.)*, 291: 593–594.

Mohan, P.M. and Sastry, B.R. (1985) Calcium and unit response decrement to locally applied glutamate on rat hippocampal CA1 neurones. *Eur. J. Pharmacol.*, 114: 335–341.

Monaghan, D.T., Holets, V.R., Toy, D.W. and Cotman, C.W. (1983) Anatomical distributions of four pharmacologically distinct ³H-L-glutamate binding sites. *Nature (Lond.)*, 306:

176 – 179.

Muller, D., Joly, M. and Lynch, G. (1988) Contribution of quisqualate and NMDA receptors to the induction and expression of LTP. *Science*, 242: 1694 – 1697.

Nadler, J.V., Vaca, K.W., White, W.F., Lynch, G.S. and Cotman, C.W. (1976) Aspartate and glutamate as possible transmitters of excitatory hippocampal afferents. *Nature (Lond.)*, 260: 538 – 540.

Nicoletti, F., Meek, J.L., Iadarola, M.J., Chuang, D.M., Roth, B.L. and Costa, E. (1986) Coupling of inositol phospholipid metabolism with excitatory amino acid recognition sites in rat hippocampus. *J. Neurochem.*, 46: 40 – 46.

Nicoll, R.A. and Alger, B.E. (1981) Synaptic excitation may activate a calcium dependent potassium conductance in hippocampal pyramidal cells. *Science*, 212: 957 – 959.

Nowak, L., Bregestovski, P., Ascher, P., Herbet, A. and Prochiantz, A. (1984) Magnesium gates glutamate-activated channels in mouse central neurones. *Nature (Lond.)*, 307: 462 – 465.

Ramón y Cajal, S. (1911) *Histologie du Système Nerveux de l'Homme et des Vertébrés*. A. Maloine, Paris, 993 pp.

Sastry, B.R., Goh, J.W. and Auyeung, A. (1986) Associative induction of posttetanic and long-term potentiation in CA1 neurons of rat hippocampus. *Science*, 232: 988 – 990.

Schwartzkroin, P.A. (1975) Characteristics of CA1 neurons recorded intracellularly in the hippocampus *in vitro* preparation. *Brain Res.*, 85: 423 – 436.

Schwartzkroin, P.A. and Andersen, P. (1975) Glutamic acid sensitivity of dendrites in hippocampal slices *in vitro*. In G.W. Kreutzberg (Ed.), *Physiology and Pathology of Dendrites, Advances in Neurology, Vol. 12*, Raven Press, New York, pp. 45 – 51.

Segal, M. (1981) The actions of glutamic acid on neurons in the rat hippocampal slice. In G. Di Chiara and G.L. Gessa (Eds.), *Glutamate as a Neurotransmitter*, Raven Press, New York, pp. 217 – 225.

Skrede, K.K. and Westgaard, R.H. (1971) The transverse hippocampal slice: a well-defined cortical structure maintained *in vitro*. *Brain Res.*, 35: 589 – 593.

Smart, T.G. (1989) Excitatory amino acids: the involvement of second messengers in the signal transduction process. *Cell. Mol. Neurobiol.*, 9: 193 – 206.

Storm, J. and Hvalby, Ø. (1985) Repetitive firing of CA1 hippocampal pyramidal cells elicited by dendritic glutamate: slow prepotentials and burst – pause pattern. *Exp. Brain Res.*, 60: 10 – 18.

Storm-Mathisen, J., Leknes, A.K., Bore, A.T., Vaaland, J.L., Edminson, P., Haug, F.-M.S. and Ottersen, O.P. (1983) First visualization of glutamate and GABA in neurones by immunocytochemistry. *Nature (Lond.)*, 301: 517 – 520.

Storm-Mathisen, J. and Ottersen, O.P. (1984) Neurotransmitters in the hippocampal formation. In F. Reinoso-Suárez and C. Ajmone-Marsan (Eds.), *Cortical Integration*, Raven Press, New York, pp. 105 – 130.

Watkins, J.C. and Evans, R.H. (1981) Excitatory amino acid transmitters. *Annu. Rev. Pharmacol. Toxicol.*, 21: 165 – 206.

Wigström, H. and Gustafsson, B. (1984) A possible correlate of the postsynaptic condition for long-lasting potentiation in the guinea pig hippocampus in vitro. *Neurosci. Lett.*, 44: 327 – 332.

Wigström, H., Gustafsson, B., Huang, Y.-Y. and Abraham, W.C. (1986) Hippocampal long-term potentiation is induced by pairing single afferent volleys with intracellularly injected depolarizing current pulses. *Acta Physiol. Scand.*, 126: 317 – 319.

J. Storm-Mathisen, J. Zimmer and O.P. Ottersen (Eds.)
Progress in Brain Research, Vol 83
© 1990 Elsevier Science Publishers B.V. (Biomedical Division)

CHAPTER 11

Membrane currents in hippocampal neurons

David A. Brown[1], Beat H. Gähwiler[2], William H. Griffith[3] and James V. Halliwell[4]

[1] *Department of Pharmacology, University College London, Gower Street, London WC1E 6BT, U.K.,* [2] *Brain Research Institute, University of Zürich, August Forel Strasse 1, CH-8029 Zürich, Switzerland,* [3] *Department of Medical Pharmacology, Texas A. & M. University, College Station, TX 77077, U.S.A. and* [4] *Department of Physiology, Royal Free Hospital School of Medicine, University of London, London NW3 2PF, U.K.*

This chapter reviews properties and functions of endogenous ionic currents in hippocampal neurones. Currents considered are: Na currents $I_{Na(fast)}$ and $I_{Na(slow)}$; Ca currents; K currents – delayed rectifier $I_{K(DR)}$, transient $I_{K(A)}$, 'delay' current $I_{K(D)}$ and M current $I_{K(M)}$; inward rectifiers I_Q, $I_{K(IR)}$ and $I_{Cl(V)}$; Ca-activated currents $I_{K(Ca)}$ (I_C and I_{AHP}), $I_{Cl(Ca)}$ and $I_{cation(Ca)}$; Na-activated currents; and anoxia-induced currents.

Introduction

This chapter provides a short review of membrane ionic currents in hippocampal pyramidal neurones as deduced from voltage-clamp data, plus an indication of their likely role in membrane voltage responses. The specific role of K currents is discussed in more detail in the chapter by Storm (this volume). A summary of the principal currents is given in Table I. Before discussing these individually, some general points about the origin of the data in Table I need mentioning.

Preparations

The data in Table I are culled from observations on a variety of preparations using several different voltage-clamp techniques. Early attempts at recording ionic currents were performed on fresh slices of hippocampus, using a single-electrode voltage-clamp method (e.g. Johnston et al., 1980; Halliwell and Adams, 1982; Brown and Griffith, 1983a, b). This has the advantage of reproducing the "normal" state as closely as possible, but is limited by the slow speed of the single microelec-

trode clamp method and by the difficulties of achieving an adequate space-clamp with a point somatic current source (see below). Alternative approaches have used a variety of tissue-cultured preparations, combined with single microelectrode, twin microelectrode or patch-clamp techniques. Although providing better conditions for electrophysiology, where these preparations preserve the dendritic tree, they suffer from the same problems of dendritic clamp control as those encountered with fresh slices (see below) and may have the further disadvantage of remoteness from the normal in situ state. Patch-clamp techniques allow better clamp control, but at the cost of disturbing the intracellular milieu. (It would be very nice indeed to see a really careful comparison of the electrophysiological characteristics of hippocampal cells impaled with a microelectrode and dialysed with a patch-clamp electrode, but this has not yet been done.) Two recent refinements have been the use of freshly dissociated adult cells (see below) and the application of patch-clamp methods to the "cleaned slice" preparation, using either cultured slices (Llano et al., 1988) or fresh slices (Edwards et al., 1989).

TABLE I

Some membrane currents recorded from hippocampal neurones (see text for details and references)

Current	Code	Ion	V_{thr}	Inactivation	Blocked by	Transmitter action	Function
1. Voltage-gated (depolarization)							
Na currents							
Fast	$I_{Na(fast)}$	Na	−60	Fast	TTX		Spike (rising phase)
Slow	$I_{Na(slow)}$	Na	−65	Slow	TTX		Prepotential (soma)
Ca currents							
High-threshold Sustained	$I_{Ca(L)}$	Ca	−50	Slow	Cd, wCTX DHP	Noradrenaline +	Ca-spike
Low-threshold Transient	$I_{Ca(T)}$	Ca	−60	Fast	Ni, Cd DHP		Prepotential
High-threshold Transient	$I_{Ca(N)}$	Ca	?	Medium	DHP	Noradrenaline + Adenosine −	Ca-spike (?)
K currents							
Delayed rectifier	$I_{K(DR)}$	K	−40	Slow	TEA (10 mM)		?
Transient	$I_{K(A)}$	K	−60	Fast	4-AP (> 0.1 mM) DTX	Acetylcholine −	Spike repolarization
Delay current	$I_{K(D)}$	K	−75	Slow	4-AP (< 0.1 mM)		Delayed firing
M current	$I_{K(M)}$	K	−65	None	Ba	Acetylcholine − 5-HT − Somatostatin +	Spike train accommodation
2. Voltage-gated (hyperpolarization)							
Slow inward rectifier	I_Q	Na + K	−80	None	Cs		Membrane stabilization
Fast inward rectifier	$I_{K(IR)}$	K	−60	Slow	Cs, Ba		?
Time-dependent Cl currents	$I_{Cl(V)}$	Cl	−20	None	Cd Phorbol esters		Dendritic resting conductance
		Cl	−60	None	Cd		?

3. Ca-gated currents

	Symbol	Ion		Blocker	Modulator	Function
Fast K current	I_C	K	−40	TEA (1 mM)		Spike repolarization, Early AHP
Slow K current	I_{AHP}	K	None	Ba	Acetylcholine −, Noradrenaline −, 5-HT −, Histamine −	Spike train accommodation, Late AHP
Cl current	$I_{Cl(Ca)}$	Cl				
Cation current		Na + K (?)	None	None	Acetylcholine +	Spike after depolarization (?)

4. Other currents

	Symbol	Ion		Blocker	Modulator	Function
Leak current	$I_{K(L)}$	K	None	None	Acetylcholine −	Resting membrane potential
Chloride		Cl				(Channels only recorded)
Anoxic current	$I_{K(ATP)}$	K			Cromakalin +, Galanin +, Sulphonylureas −	Anoxic hyperpolarization

Clamp fidelity

Although hippocampal pyramidal cells are relatively compact electronically, with a steady-state length constant of about unity (Johnston, 1979; Brown et al., 1981; Turner and Schwartzkroin, 1981; Johnston and Brown, 1983), their dendritic tree is extensive, so considerable voltage attenuation will occur in the dendrites following a somatic voltage perturbation. This will be particularly severe for high-frequency signals (> 50 Hz: Johnston and Brown, 1983), for which the effective length constant will fall appreciably below that predicted from steady-state analysis. Also, hippocampal cell dendrites are electrically excitable, so they possess voltage-gated ion currents (Wong and Prince, 1979; Wong et al., 1979; Traub and Llinás, 1979; Benardo et al., 1982; Turner and Schwartzkroin, 1983). These currents will not be adequately clamped using a somatic point-clamp: this not only limits study of dendritic currents, but their presence can also seriously compromise the study of the somatic currents. This can be obviated by removing the dendrites – e.g., using freshly dissociated cells in which dendritic arborizations are reduced in extent or retracted into the soma (Kay and Wong, 1987). However, this has its own limitations, and it is clear that some of the more interesting currents are not well preserved by this method.

Voltage-gated currents

Na currents

Two Na currents have been reported in hippocampal neurones: a fast current $I_{Na(fast)}$ and a slowly inactivating current $I_{Na(slow)}$.

$I_{Na(fast)}$

The fast Na current, as recorded from dissociated adult guinea-pig hippocampal neurones at 22°C (Sah et al., 1988a), behaves as an orthodox Hodgkin–Huxley current with an activation threshold of – 60 mV and a time-to-peak of about 0.9 ms at 0 mV. Activation could be described by a Boltzmann expression with a half-activation voltage (V_o) of – 39 mV and a slope factor (k) of 6.6 mV/e-fold voltage change, giving an effective gating particle valency of about 4. Current decay at 0 mV was bi-exponential in most cells, with a half-decay time of about 2 ms. In 15/120 cells a much more rapid (< 1 ms) decay was observed. Inactivation fitted a Boltzmann expression with a half-inactivation at – 75 mV and slope factor 7.7 mV. Inactivation was complete throughout the activation range, with no overlap between activation and inactivation curves, implying negligible steady-state Na conductance. Assuming a single channel conductance of 18 pS, the maximal Na-conductance of about 1.2 nS corresponded to a channel density of 5 – 10 channels/μm^2. The charge transfer was calculated to yield a maximum rate of rise of a Na spike of 600 – 1200 V/s at 22°C, which corresponded with that measured under these conditions. The Q_{10} for the current amplitude between 20 and 27°C was 1.5, giving an appropriately faster rate of rise at 37°C. Kaneda et al. (1988) have recorded a similar amplitude (5 nA) fast Na current from dissociated rat hippocampal neurons, with a similar activation range. The permeability sequence for this current was comparable to that previously reported in squid axons, frog nodes of Ranvier and rat ventricular muscle (Li > Na > hydrazine > formamidine > guanidine > methylguanidine > monomethylamine).

The Na currents reported in these experiments were principally somatic in origin, and account for the fast, TTX-sensitive somatic action potentials. Intracellular recordings from isolated dendrites (Benardo et al., 1982) revealed similar fast spikes to those usually recorded from the soma. Two forms were described, with similar rise-times but somewhat different decay rates, giving mean durations 1.21 and 2.85 ms at 37°C. Both were blocked by intracellular QX-312, implying that both were Na-spikes. Direct evidence for the presence of dendritic Na currents, of comparable time-course and current density to those in the soma, has recently been obtained by Hugenard et al. (1989) in freshly-dissociated neocortical neurones. Equivalent experiments have not been completed on hippocampal cells. However, in their recordings from dissociated guinea-pig hippocampal cells, Sah et al. (1988) noted the presence of delayed "breakthrough" inward currents in cells with long (> 50 μm) processes, due to activation of (presumably lower threshold) Na currents in dendritic or axonal processes.

$I_{Na(slow)}$

When depolarizing currents are injected into hippocampal cell somata, the cells fire repetitive Na spikes. These appear to be triggered by depolarizing prepotentials (Lanthorn et al., 1984). These are blocked by TTX, and hence arise from the activation of subthreshold Na currents (MacVicar, 1985). This process also confers a degree of TTX-sensitive "inward rectification" on the steady voltage deflexions produced by such current injections (Hotson et al., 1979; MacVicar, 1985). An appropriate slowly inactivating Na current has been recorded from CA1 neurones in rat hippocampal slices using the single microelectrode clamp technique (French and Gage, 1985). This had an activation threshold of about 5 to 10 mV positive to rest potential, and was sustained during a 400 ms depolarizing command. It persisted in 50 μM Ca with added Cd (1 mM) or Mn (5 mM), and hence was not a Ca-current; instead it was blocked in low (18 mM) Na or by TTX.

This slow Na current may be confined to the soma, since the equivalent anomalous rectification in isolated dendrites was not blocked by intracellular injection of the local anaesthetic QX 314, but was instead depressed by Mn (Benardo et al., 1982) whereas that in the soma was blocked by QX 314. Hence, in dendrites it appears to be replaced by a slow inward Ca current. Interestingly, isolated dendrites did not fire repetitive Na spikes (unlike intact dendrites or somata). This might be explained if the dendritic prepotential Ca current arrested firing by activating a Ca-dependent K current (see below), which a Na-

prepotential may not do. A slow Na current would therefore be a more effective "pacemaker" current.

Ca currents

Hippocampal neurones appear to possess 3 types of Ca-current − a high-threshold, sustained current, a low-threshold transient current and a high-threshold, inactivating current (see below). These may correspond to the L, T and N currents recorded in sensory neurones (Fox et al., 1987a, b). At the single channel level channels with 3 conductances (7 − 8 pS, 13 − 15 pS and 25 − 27 pS) have been recorded from acutely dissociated guinea-pig neurones with cell-attached patch pipettes containing 110 mM Ba (Gray and Johnston, 1986). The former were clustered at the beginning of the voltage step, so may accord with the transient (T) current (Gray and Johnston, 1986). The 13 − 15 pS channel may underlie the N current and the 25 − 27 pS channel the L current (Gray and Johnston, 1987; cf. Fox et al., 1987b).

High-threshold sustained (L) current

Early experiments from cells in intact or tissue-cultured slices using the single-microelectrode voltage-clamp method, in which K currents were reduced by filling the pipette with Cs solution and/or by adding external tetraethylammonium (TEA) or tetrabutylammonium (TBA), revealed a slowly-activating sustained inward current which was enhaned by Ba and blocked in Ca-free solution or by adding Co or Cd (Johnston et al., 1980; Brown and Griffith, 1983a; Brown et al., 1984; Docherty and Brown, 1986; Gähwiler and Brown, 1987a). With Ba as the principle charge-carrier, this current showed little inactivation over several hundred ms, and indeed appeared capable of contributing a persistent inward component to the steady membrane current between − 50 and − 10 mV such that the membrane potential oscillated between these two potentials (Johnston et al., 1980; Brown and Griffith, 1983a). The current was blocked by verapamil (100 μM: Brown and Griffith, 1983a) and by dihydropyridine Ca-antagonists such as nimodipine (50 nM – 10 μM), nifedipine (1 μM) or PY 108 – 068 (1 μM) and was enhanced by the dihydropyridine "Ca-agonist" BAY K8644 (1 – 10 μM) (Brown et al., 1984; Docherty and Brown, 1986; Segal and Barker, 1986; Gähwiler and Brown, 1987a), in accordance with observations on L currents in sensory neurones (Fox et al., 1987a). This current has subsequently been studied in more detail in freshly dissociated (Kay and Wong, 1987) or tissue-cultured (Yaari, et al., 1987; Meyers and Barker, 1989) cells by whole-cell patch-clamp method. In the dissociated cells, the current was sustained over 200 ms using Ca as charge carrier, with internal Ca buffered to < 100 nM and with leupeptin and ATP in the patch pipette. Activation could be described by a Boltzmann equation with a threshold of about – 50 mV, half-activation at – 20 mV, a slope factor of 10 mV and a cooperativity factor of 2 (Kay and Wong, 1987).

Transient (T) current

Initial experiments suggested that neither the Ca-dependent potentials recorded from hippocampal neurones (see below) nor the clamp currents themselves could be adequately explained by a single Ca current (Brown and Griffith, 1983a). Halliwell (1983) showed the presence of an additional, low-threshold transient current in guinea-pig CA1 neurones which could be activated in depolarizing to about – 60 mV from potentials down to – 100 mV, and which was totally inactivated at – 50 mV. (In the experiments of Johnston et al. (1980) and Brown and Griffith (1983a), the usual holding potential was – 40 mV.) This current has been characterized in more detail by Yaari et al. (1987) in cultured rat embryonic neurones using the whole-cell clamp method. With 10 mM Ca as charge-carrier, the current was activated above – 50 mV (about 30 mV negative to the sustained current) and inactivated in 50 ms or so. Unlike the sustained current, it was reduced on substituting Ba for Ca. In agreement with Halliwell (1983), both transient and sustained cur-

rents were suppressed by 100 μM Cd. Both currents were also blocked by 100 μM verapamil, but the T current was much more sensitive to phenytoin (see below). Takahashi et al. (1989) have recently recorded a low-threshold T-type current from dissociated rat CA1 neurones at various stages of development (2 weeks, 8 weeks and 44 weeks old) by the suction-pipette method. With 10 mM Ca as charge carrier and holding potential – 100 mV the current threshold was – 60 mV and current peak around – 30 mV. Inactivation was mono-exponential with a time-constant of 25 – 30 ms. Current amplitude and kinetics were unchanged throughout development. The current was blocked by Ni^{2+} ions (IC_{50} 0.2 – 0.4 mM), as reported for T currents in sensory neurones (Fox et al., 1987a). However, it was also blocked by quite low concentrations of the dihydropyridine nicardipine (IC_{50} 1 – 2 μM). This accords with previous tests on dihydropyridines in slice preparations (Docherty and Brown, 1986; Gähwiler and Brown, 1987a), suggesting that these compounds may not differentiate as strongly between L and T currents in hippocampal cells as in peripheral neurones (cf. Fox et al., 1987a).

High-threshold inactivating (N) current

Madison et al. (1987a) report an early component to the envelope current seen on depolarizing from – 90 to + 10 mV which decays over 100 ms or so and which is absent on holding at – 30 mV. This may correspond to the N current seen in other neurones (see Fox et al., 1987a). Interestingly, Kay and Wong (1987) failed to detect a second component to the Ca current in freshly dissociated neurones, and concluded that both activation and deactivation kinetics could be accommodated by a single Ca-channel type.

Effect of transmitters

Both high-threshold currents are modifiable by neurotransmitters. Gray and Johnston (1987) report that high-threshold currents in acutely dissociated guinea-pig neurones are augmented by noradrenaline and isoprenaline, and that this is replicated by cyclic AMP so may be due to activation of adenylate cyclase. Involvement of a soluble cytoplasmic messenger is indicated by the fact that single-channel activity in cell-attached patches was augmented by extra-patch application of isoprenaline. The opening probability of both large (19 pS) and intermediate (14.5 pS) channels was increased, suggested a possible effect on both N- and L-type channels. Madison et al. (1987a) report that adenosine inhibits an N-type current in cultured rat CA3 neurones. In contrast, Halliwell and Scholfield (1984) could detect no effect of adenosine on either the sustained high-threshold or transient low-threshold current in intact guinea-pig hippocampal neurones. Gähwiler and Brown (1987b) and Toselli and Lux (1989) show a reduction of the composite high-threshold Ca current by muscarinic acetylcholine-receptor stimulation: to what extent this reflects an effect in N- or L-type currents is unclear but the former might be the more likely.

Contribution of Ca currents to voltage responses

Three "Ca-dependent" voltage responses of hippocampal neurones have been reported – slow Ca-spikes (Schwartzkroin and Slawsky, 1977; Wong and Prince, 1978; Peacock and Walker, 1983); burst potentials (Wong and Prince, 1978 and 1981; Schwartzkroin, 1980; Hablitz and Johnston, 1981); and a subthreshold prepotential conferring a Ca-dependent component of inward rectification (Hotson et al., 1979; Benardo et al., 1982). From their original description, Johnston et al. (1980) suggested that the sustained high-threshold current might be responsible for hippocampal burst-behaviour, particularly after Ba application. Traub (1982) successfully modelled both burst and slow Ca-spikes in the basis of a single Ca current which showed partial, Ca-dependent inactivation. However, Brown and Griffith (1983a) pointed out that the threshold for the slow Ca current is substantially positive to that for inducing burst-firing and suggested the burst potential and Ca spike could more easily be accommodated by assuming at least two Ca currents. The

above data suggest that the prepotential and the initial phase of burst-potential might be triggered by the T current, and that the higher threshold currents might be responsible for the sustained phase of the burst potential and the Ca spikes. The apparently selective effect of phenytoin in the T current (Yaari et al., 1987) should help in clarifying its role in low-threshold events. A role for the high-threshold sustained current in generating the Ca spike is suggested by the ability of BAY K8644 to lengthen the spike (Gähwiler and Brown, 1987a). This effect is reversed by Ca-antagonist dihydropyridines. On the other hand, dihydropyridine Ca antagonists have little effect on the duration or amplitude of the normal Ca spike in the absence of BAY K8644 pretreatment (Gähwiler and Brown, 1987a). This may reflect the voltage-sensitivity of the drug's action or it may imply an additional, and major, role for the inactivating N current in spike generation. Further careful analysis of the effects of adenosine (see above) may assist in clarifying the contributions of the two high-threshold currents to the Ca spike.

Somatic/dendritic location of Ca channels

Intradendritic recording has established that dendrites may be the primary site of Ca-dependent bursts and Ca spikes, particularly in CA1 neurones (Wong and Prince, 1979; Wong et al., 1979; Benardo et al., 1982). Indeed, the dendritic Ca spike is appreciably larger than the somatic Ca spike (though this could reflect differences in other membrane currents). On the other hand, the Ca-dependent subthreshold depolarization appears to be restricted to the soma. In keeping with these observations, Yaari et al. (1987) have noted that, in cultured rat embryonic neurones, the low-threshold transient current (which probably underlies the subthreshold depolarizations: see above) was present within a few hours of plating, before the appearance of processes, and hence is indubitably present in the soma. In contrast, the appearance of the high-threshold current was more gradual and associated with the acquisition of neurites. However, this does not mean that channels carrying the high-threshold current were *restricted* to processes, and indeed two lines of evidence suggest that they are also present on the soma. Firstly, the high-threshold sustained current can be recorded from freshly dissociated adult cells, in which the contribution of dendritic currents is reduced (Kay and Wong, 1987). Secondly, Jones et al. (1989) have shown that fluorescent or biotinylated derivatives of ω-conotoxin, which bind to neuronal N and L channels, tagged both soma and processes of cultured hippocampal neurones. These cells showed multiple clusters of tagged sites, which became organized into single clusters around sites of synaptic contact when the cells became cross-innervated. Photobleaching tests indicated that a high proportion of these putative Ca channels (50 – 70% of somatic channels and 85% of dendritic channels) were essentially "fixed" in location, with a lateral mobility 30 times less than that of the pool of more mobile channels. This provides direct evidence for a concentration of high-threshold Ca channels in "hot spots", frequently associated with synaptic contacts.

K currents

At least 5 voltage-gated K currents have been recorded from hippocampal neurones – a delayed rectifier current $I_{K(DR)}$; a transient current or A current $I_{K(A)}$; a "delay" current akin to a slowly inactivating A current $I_{K(D)}$; a subthreshold, non-inactivating current or "M current" $I_{K(M)}$; and an inwardly rectifying K current $I_{K(IR)}$ activated by hyperpolarization. The function of these (and other) K currents is considered in more detail elsewhere in this volume; hence only a brief account is given here.

Delayed rectifier current $I_{K(DR)}$

A current corresponding broadly to the classical delayed rectifier current has been recorded under a variety of conditions on depolarizing hippocampal neurones above – 40 mV (Segal and Barker, 1984; Numann et al., 1987; Sah et al., 1988b). This can

be distinguished from the large Ca-activated current (see below) by its resistance to Ca-channel block (though it can be directly blocked by some Ca-channel blockers such as Co and Cd in mM concentrations: Sah et al., 1988) and from the A and D currents by its greater sensitivity to TEA (IC_{50} about 10 mM: Segal and Barker, 1984) and insensitivity to 4-aminopyridine (4-AP). The most striking feature of the hippocampal delayed rectifier current is its slow activation, with a time-to-peak of some 50 – 200 ms at 0 mV. This is not due to recording limitations, since single channels recorded in cell-attached patch pipettes also show a slow increase in opening following a depolarizing step command (time constant about 100 ms near threshold: Rogawski, 1986). Hence $I_{K(DR)}$ seems ill-suited to accomplish its traditional function of accelerating spike repolarization in hippocampal cells, a point confirmed by Storm (1987a).

Transient (A) current $I_{K(A)}$

This is a prominent current which can be recorded from hippocampal neurones in situ (Gustafsson et al., 1982; Zbicz and Weight, 1985) or in culture (Segal et al., 1984; Segal and Barker, 1984) and in acutely dissociated neurones (Numann et al., 1987; Alger and Doerner, 1988; but see Sah et al., 1988). It activates much more rapidly than $I_{K(DR)}$, within 5 – 10 ms, but also inactivates rapidly (time constant 20 – 30 ms) and completely (or nearly so) throughout its activation range (from – 60 mV upwards). Some authors (Gustafsson et al., 1982; Zbicz and Weight, 1986) have noted (or show) a slower component to the inactivation, which may represent another current (see below). The A current itself does not appear to be Ca-activated but a faster, Ca-sensitive component has been noted by Zbicz and Weight (1986) and Doerner and Alger (1988). The current is insensitive to TEA but is readily blocked by 4-AP at > 100 μM and also by dendrotoxin (DTX) between 50 and 300 nM (Halliwell et al., 1986). Inhibition has also been reported by noradrenaline (Sah et al., 1985) and acetylcholine (Nakajima et al., 1986). Its activation is sufficiently rapid to allow a role in spike repolarization, and Storm (1987) has obtained some evidence for such a role using 4-AP though interpretation of this is confounded somewhat by the presence of another 4-AP sensitive current (see below). As in invertebrates (Connor and Stevens, 1971), $I_{K(A)}$ may also contribute to the maintenance of repetitive firing (Segal et al., 1984; Storm, 1987a).

Slowly-inactivating "delay" current $I_{K(D)}$

Like the A current, $I_{K(D)}$ shows rapid activation and complete inactivation throughout its activation range. However it differs from the A current in that: (a) $I_{K(D)}$ shows much slower, multi-component inactivation over several seconds; (b) activation and inactivation curves for $I_{K(D)}$ are $15-20$ mV negative to those for $I_{K(A)}$, with an activation threshold of about -75 mV; and (c) $I_{K(D)}$ is more sensitive to 4-AP, being completely blocked at $30-40$ μM (Storm, 1988). In many respects it resembles the current recorded by Stansfeld et al. (1986) from certain sensory neurones and labelled I_{DTX} on the basis of its very high sensitivity to dendrotoxin (DTX). The effect of DTX in the hippocampal current is unknown, but the hippocampus contains a high density of DTX binding sites (Halliwell et al., 1986) and reconstitution of brain DTX-binding protein in lipid vesicles yields K channels with similar conductance properties (20 pS in symmetrical high K) to the DTX-sensitive channels in sensory neurones (Rehm et al., 1989; cf. Stansfeld and Feltz, 1988). With hindsight, evidence for a slowly inactivating component of the A current, with high sensitivity to 4-AP (presumably representing $I_{K(D)}$) may be gleaned from earlier experiments (e.g. Gustafsson et al., 1982; Zbicz and Weight, 1986; see also Fig. 1). One effect of $I_{K(D)}$ on the electrical behaviour of hippocampal cells is to introduce a long delay in the firing induced by just-threshold depolarizations from rest potential: firing is inhibited by the rapid activation of $I_{K(D)}$ and can only commence when $I_{K(D)}$ inactivates (Storm, 1988). Slow inactivation of $I_{K(D)}$ also leads to a form of "recruitment" with repetitive depolarizations. Storm (1987) has

also shown that 4-AP can retard the initial phase of spike repolarization in hippocampal neurones: the relative contribution of $I_{K(A)}$ and $I_{K(D)}$ to this component of spike repolarization remains to be determined. It is also worth noting that 4-AP can induce an inward shift in the resting membrane current within a range of $I_{K(D)}$ activation (see Fig. 1), suggesting that a small "window" of incompletely inactivated $I_{K(D)}$ or $I_{K(A)}$ might contribute a minor component of outward current to the resting membrane potential.

M-current $I_{K(M)}$

This is a non-inactivating, subthreshold, voltage-gated K current originally identified in sympathetic neurones (Brown and Adams, 1980). Its presence in hippocampal cells was first reported by Halliwell and Adams (1982) in CA1 cells in slices of guinea pig hippocampus and has since been confirmed in these cells and in guinea pig CA3 neurones (Brown and Griffith, 1983b) and in both freshly dissected (Madison et al., 1987b) and tissue-cultured (Gähwiler and Brown, 1985a) rat

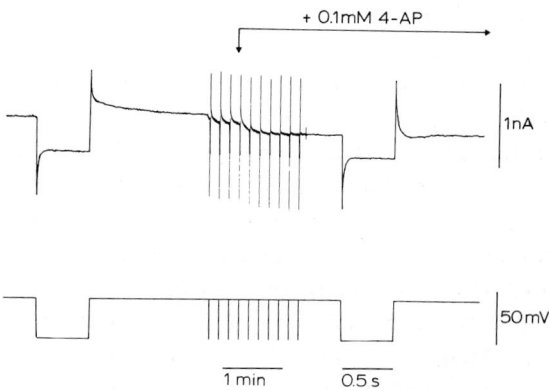

Fig. 1. Suppression of a slowly-decaying component of outward current ($I_{K(D)}$? See Storm, 1988) by 4-aminopyridine (4-AP) in a CA3 neurone in a tissue-cultured rat hippocampal slice preparation. The cell was impaled with a KCl-filled microelectrode, voltage-clamped at about 50 mV and commanded to -90 mV for 500 ms at 10-s intervals. Note that an outward current was activated on repolarizing to -50 mV which decayed over several seconds and that this was suppressed by bath-application of 100 μM 4-AP. (B.H. Gähwiler and D.A. Brown, unpublished; see Gähwiler and Brown, 1985 (and references cited therein) for technical details.)

hippocampal slices. It has not so far been reported in dissociated cells. The current is activated from about -70 mV upwards. Thus, although it does not inactivate, it probably does not contribute significantly to the steady membrane current at normal resting potentials of -70 mV or more. However, it does form a component of the outward rectification seen in these cells when they are depolarized, and, although small in amplitude, can constitute an appreciable fraction of the membrane conductance between -70 and -40 mV. The current is slow to activate (τ about 90 ms at -45 mV at 30°C: Halliwell and Adams, 1982) so, even though appreciably faster at higher temperatures, it is too slow to affect the configuration of the action potential. However, it does appear to generate a component of postspike hyperpolarization (Storm, 1989) and also contributes to the accommodation seen during trains of action potentials (Madison and Nicoll, 1984), in conjunction with the slow Ca-activated K current (see below). $I_{K(M)}$, like several other K currents, is inhibited by Ba and by muscarinic acetylcholine-receptor agonists (Halliwell and Adams, 1982; Gähwiler and Brown, 1985a; Madison et al., 1987b). However, it is less sensitive to acetylcholine than the slow Ca-activated K current or than a voltage-insensitive leak current (Madison et al., 1987b; Benson et al., 1988). Hence, although inhibition of $I_{K(M)}$ can contribute a voltage-dependent component to the slow synaptic current produced by stimulating cholinergic septal inputs (Gähwiler and Brown, 1985a), this may normally be manifest only after rather intense stimulation (Madison et al., 1987b). The mechanism whereby acetylcholine inhibits $I_{K(M)}$ is not yet clear, but may involve the generation and action of inositol 1,4,5-trisphosphate (Dutar and Nicoll, 1988). $I_{K(M)}$ can also be reduced by 5-HT (Colino and Halliwell, 1987) and may be increased by somatostatin (Moore et al., 1988; Watson and Pittman, 1988).

Currents activated by hyperpolarization

Q-current I_Q

This is a mixed cation (Na + K) current activated when hippocampal cells are hyperpolarized to -80 mV or more (Adams and Halliwell, 1982; Halliwell and Adams, 1982; see Fig. 2). Activation is relatively slow (τ about 100 ms at 30°C at -82 mV) but accelerates with increasing hyperpolarization ($\tau = 37$ ms at -130 mV: Halliwell and Adams, 1982). I_Q is unaffected by Ba ions but is completely blocked by 1 mM external Cs. It therefore resembles the current termed I_h/I_f in cardiac cells (Yanagihara and Irisawa, 1980; Brown and DiFrancesco, 1980). It is also reduced by tetrahydroaminoacridine (Brown et al., 1988). I_Q does not appear to contribute to the normal resting potential of hippocampal cells but its activation serves to resist hyperpolarizing deviations from the resting potential, inducing a characteristic rebound depolarization during a hyperpolarizing current pulse (Fig. 2c), and hence stabilizing the membrane potential. Deactivation of the current also contributes to the rebound depolarization and excitation following a hyperpolarizing pulse (Fig. 2c). Unlike cortical cells, where I_Q is activated at rest potentials (Spain et al., 1987), it does not contribute to normal spike after-hyperpolarization but may do so when spikes are initiated from membrane potentials negative to the normal resting potential (Storm, 1989). I_Q can also be recorded from cells in tissue-cultured slices (B.H. Gähwiler and D.A. Brown, unpublished) and from dissociated cells in culture (Segal and Barker, 1984).

Inwardly-rectifying K current $I_{K(IR)}$

In addition to the time-dependent cation current I_Q, a rapidly activating (< 10 ms) K current similar to the "fast inward rectifier" (I_{fir}) in cortical neurones (Constanti and Galvan, 1983) can be recorded from some hippocampal neurones

(Owen, 1987). $I_{K(IR)}$ can also be detected in the presence of I_Q if the latter is blocked by THA (but not by Cs since $I_{K(IR)}$ is blocked by Cs) (J.V. Halliwell, personal communication). Blockade of

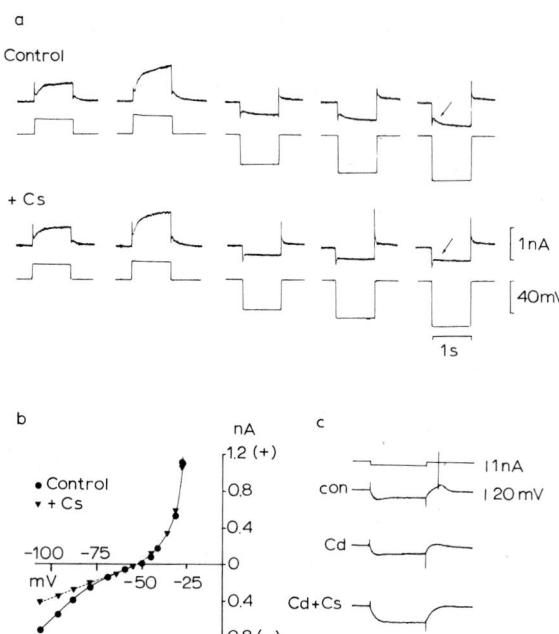

a
Control

+ Cs

b

nA
1.2 (+)

0.8

0.4

0

0.4

0.8 (-)

• Control
▼ + Cs

-100 -75

mV   -50   -25

c

con

Cd

Cd+Cs

I1nA
I20mV

0.5 s

Fig. 2. Some properties of the Q-current (I_Q) recorded from CA1 neurones in guinea-pig hippocampal slices in vitro. a: membrane currents (upper trace) recorded in response to 1-s voltage steps (lower trace) from about -50 mV before and after adding 1 mM CsCl to the perfusion fluid. The Q-current is seen as a slow inward current (arrowed) during the hyperpolarizing steps in normal solution and is blocked by Cs (see Halliwell and Adams, 1982). b: current – voltage curves constructed from the records in (a) by measuring currents at the end of the voltage steps, measured before (●) and after (▼) adding Cs. Note the inward rectification at potentials negative to -80 mV and its block by Cs. c: voltage trajectories induced by hyperpolarizing current injection before and after adding 1 mM Cd and then with 1 mM additional Cs. Note that activation of I_Q by hyperpolarization produces a repolarizing sag in the voltage trajectory during the current injection and a rebound depolarization after the current is removed, both of which are blocked by Cs. Under normal conditions this rebound depolarization activates a Ca current (leading to a spike); the Ca current is blocked by Cd. (Records (a) and (b): W.H. Griffith and D.A. Brown, unpublished; record (c): J.V. Halliwell, unpublished. See Brown and Griffith, 1983a and Halliwell and Adams, 1982, respectively, for technical details.)

$I_{K(IR)}$ by Ba may account for the reduction of the "instantaneous" component of current during a hyperpolarizing voltage step described by Halliwell and Adams (1982). $I_{K(IR)}$ appears to be partly activated at rest potential (-60 mV) but inactivates at potentials negative to -100 mV (Owen, 1987).

A variety of neurotransmitters, including GABA (via $GABA_B$ receptors), 5-hydroxytryptamine and adenosine can induce an inward-rectifying K current in hippocampal neurones (Gähwiler and Brown, 1985b; Newberry and Nicoll, 1985; Colino and Halliwell, 1987; Andrade and Nicoll, 1987). These effects are probably mediated through a common, pertussis-toxin sensitive GTP-binding protein (Andrade et al., 1986; Zgombik et al., 1989). Application of the α-subunit of the GTP-binding protein G_0 to the inside of isolated patches of hippocampal cell membranes induces the opening of several K channels, some of which show marked inward rectification (VanDongen et al., 1988). However, it is not yet known whether these channels are active in the absence of neurotransmitters or their GTP-binding protein, or to what extent they might contribute to the cell's normal rectification.

Chloride current $I_{Cl(V)}$

Madison et al. (1986) have described a slow Cl current in pyramidal cells in rat hippocampal slices which was activated by hyperpolarizing steps between -20 and -100 mV. The reversal potential for the current was $+9.5$ mV in cells impaled with Cl^--filled microelectrodes and -71 mV in cells impaled with electrodes filled with $MeSO_4$ anion. Although the current persisted in a Ca-free medium (and hence was not "Ca-dependent"), it was blocked by Cd ions, like a similar current previously detected in sympathetic neurones (Selyanko, 1984). $I_{Cl(V)}$ was also strikingly suppressed by phorbol dibutyrate. Madison et al. (1986) suggested that $I_{Cl(V)}$ was restricted to pyramidal cell processes since it could only be detected with a somatic microelectrode when K currents were suppressed (e.g. by injecting Cs ions and/or adding TEA, Cs or carbachol to the

152

bathing medium). If so, since the current is quite large and strongly activated at rest potential, it must exert a strong influence in the resting dendritic conductance and space constant, effectively isolating them from the soma. By suppressing $I_{Cl(V)}$, phorbol esters, or other procedures activating protein kinase C, might then facilitate dendritic/somatic coupling.

We (Gähwiler and Brown, unpublished; see Fig. 3) have observed a rather similar current in CA3 neurones in rat hippocampal slices in culture with the difference that it is only activated at potentials negative to -60 mV and hence contributes minimally to resting membrane current. In this it more closely resembles the Cl current seen in rat sympathetic neurones (Selyanko, 1984); like the latter, and like the current described by Madison et al. (1986), it was reduced by Cd ions (Fig. 3).

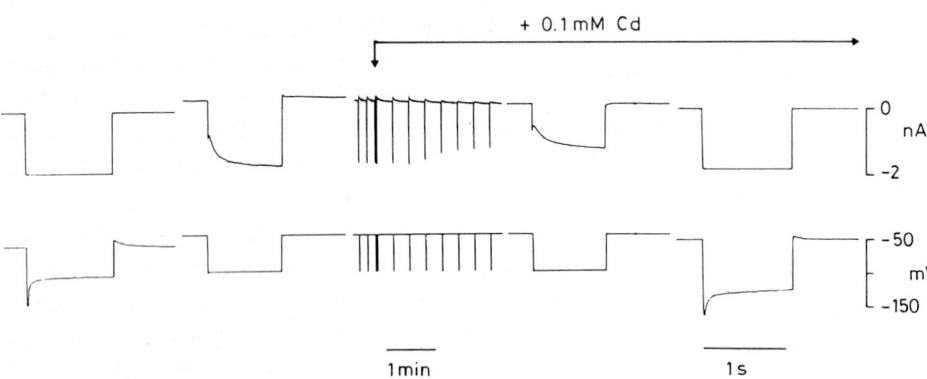

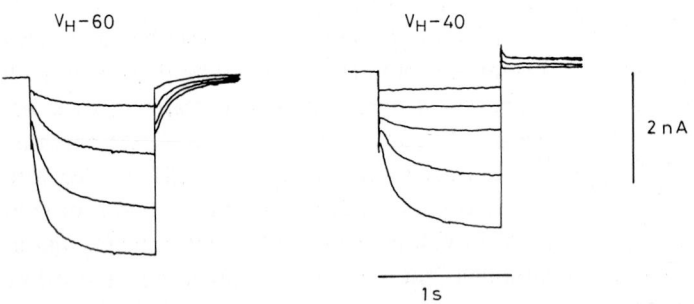

Fig. 3. Hyperpolarization-activated Cl current in a CA3 neurone in a cultured hippocampal slice. The cell was impaled with a KCl-filled electrode. Upper records show current (upper trace) and voltage (lower trace) before and after adding 100 μM CdCl$_2$ to the perfusion medium. Hyperpolarizing current injection at the initial resting potential (-45 mV) revealed strong time-dependent rectification in the voltage trajectory (first record). Under voltage clamp (at -40 mV), a hyperpolarizing voltage step induces a slow inward current accompanied by a large increase in membrane conductance. This inward current is reduced by Cd and the rectification of the voltage response correspondingly diminishes (last panel). The records below show families of slow inward currents induced by 10 mV incremental hyperpolarizing steps from holding potentials of -60 and -40 mV, recorded before adding Cd. Note that the threshold for activating the slow current is about -60 mV and that the reversal potential of the tail currents lies between the two holding potentials (corresponding to E_{Cl} in this KCl-impaled cell as judged from the reversal potential for the Cl current induced by GABA, see Gähwiler and Brown, 1985b). (B.H. Gähwiler and D.A. Brown, unpublished; see Gähwiler and Brown, 1985, for technical details.)

Ca-activated currents

Hippocampal cells possess several currents gated by intracellular Ca, including two K currents, a Cl current and (probably) a cation current. These may be activated by the rise in intracellular Ca produced by Ca entry through voltage-gated Ca channels (as during an action potential, see above) or through ligand-gated channels such as those (presumed NMDA-type) activated by glutamate (Nicoll and Alger, 1981; Kudo and Ogura, 1986), or possibly by the release of intracellular Ca resulting from activation of muscarinic receptors (Kudo et al., 1988) or of the "metabotropic" glutamate receptor (Furuya et al., 1989).

Ca-activated K currents $I_{K(Ca)}$

Two quite distinct Ca-activated K currents have been identified in hippocampal neurones: a large, time- and voltage-dependent current termed I_C (Brown and Griffith, 1983b) by analogy to comparable currents in molluscan neurones (Thompson, 1977) and frog sympathetic neurones (Adams et al., 1982); and a smaller, voltage-independent form dubbed I_{AHP} (Lancaster and Adams, 1986) because it underlies the slow Ca-dependent after-hyperpolarization (AHP) previously reported in hippocampal pyramidal cells (Hotson and Prince, 1980; Alger and Nicoll, 1980; Gustafsson and Wigström, 1981; Schwartzkroin and Stafstrom, 1980).

I_C

This is a large current which is activated rapidly (probably within 1 – 2 ms) when a Ca charge flows through voltage-gated Ca channels following their activation by a depolarizing voltage-clamp pulse or during an action potential (Brown and Griffith, 1983b; Lancaster and Adams, 1986; Storm, 1987a; Lancaster and Nicoll, 1987). When the cell is repolarized, the current then deactivates within 50 – 150 ms, depending on the voltage (Brown and Griffith, 1983b). The current is blocked by concentrations of TEA (1 – 10 mM) below those needed to block the delayed rectifier current. It is probably carried by the high-conductance (150 – 270 pS) "BK" channels which have been detected in membrane patches from cultured rat hippocampal neurones (Brett and Lancaster, 1985; Brett et al., 1986; Franciolini, 1988; Ikemoto et al., 1989). These channels require a relatively high concentration of Ca for their activation (threshold $> 1 \ \mu M$; $P_{0.5}$ at 4 μM at $- 15$ mV: Franciolini, 1988) and also show strong voltage-sensitivity (slope factor 14 mV: Franciolini, 1988). When Ca-concentration jumps are applied to isolated patches, some delay occurs before channel opening, dependent upon the applied concentration of Ca and the recording voltage (Brett et al., 1986; Ikemoto et al., 1989). Thus, even at $+ 40$ mV, delay times were 100, 87, 29 and 13 ms at 3.2, 12.6, 11 and 1000 μM Ca respectively (Ikemoto et al., 1989). Unless some factor normally favouring a more rapid opening was lost in the isolation procedure, this implies that the channels responsible for I_C must be close to those mediating Ca entry in order for them to see a sufficiently high concentration of Ca and open within the 1 – 2 ms necessary for their activation during an action potential (see below). A close relationship to the Ca channels has also been proposed from the fact that spike-activated I_C is not prevented by intracellular EGTA injection, only by injection of the "fast" buffer BAPTA, in spite of the fact that EGTA can readily inhibit I_{AHP} which is more sensitive to Ca (Storm, 1987b; Lancaster and Nicoll, 1987).

Tests with TEA and charybdotoxin, and with intracellular BAPTA injections, suggests that I_C is strongly activated during a single pyramidal cell action potential and that its activation contributes to spike repolarization and generates the early phase of the spike after-hyperpolarization (Lancaster and Nicoll, 1987; Storm, 1987a, b). This initial after-hyperpolarization has an influence on the initial firing frequency during a spike train, but dissipates too rapidly (because of the fast, voltage-dependent deactivation of I_C) to affect later events.

I$_{AHP}$

In comparison to I_C, I_{AHP} is smaller in amplitude, rises more slowly following Ca entry, and declines more slowly (time constant $1-1.6$ s) on repolarization (Lancaster and Adams, 1986). Moreover, the decay rate is insensitive to voltage over the range -50 to -90 mV (Lancaster and Adams, 1986) and instead seems to be determined primarily by the rate of decline of intracellular Ca (Knöpfel et al., 1989 and unpublished observations). It is clearly activated by much lower Ca concentrations than those required to activate. I_C, such that an AHP current can be recorded in cells in slice cultures when the intracellular Ca measured with Fura-2 rises from 30 to 60 nM (Knöpfel et al., 1989). The delay in the rise of I_{AHP} suggests that the channels might be relatively remote from the source of Ca entry. In addition to its higher sensitivity to Ca and lack of voltage sensitivity, I_{AHP} further differs from I_C in being insensitive to TEA or charybdotoxin (Lancaster and Adams, 1986; Storm, 1987a; Lancaster and Nicoll, 1987). These properties suggest that I_{AHP} might be mediated by low-conductance "SK" channels (see Blatz and Magleby, 1986) (except that the hippocampal I_{AHP} is not blocked by apamin, unlike that in muscle and in some peripheral neurones). Appropriate channels of about 14 pS conductance have been detected in hippocampal membrane patches (Lancaster et al., 1987).

A further important feature of I_{AHP} is that it can be inhibited by a variety of neurotransmitters, including acetylcholine (Cole and Nicoll, 1983; Madison et al., 1987), noradrenaline (Madison and Nicoll, 1982; Haas and Konnerth, 1983; Lancaster and Adams, 1986), histamine (Haas and Konnerth, 1983) and 5-hydroxytryptamine (Andrade et al., 1987; Colino and Halliwell, 1987). These substances depress I_{AHP} by inhibiting the K current itself rather than by blocking the Ca transient (Knöpfel et al., 1989).

I_{AHP} generates the long after-hyperpolarization following hippocampal action potentials (Lancaster and Adams, 1986; Lancaster and Nicoll, 1987). Its most important role, however, lies in its

contribution to the decline in firing frequency, and eventual cessation of firing, during spike trains induced by prolonged depolarization ("spike frequency accommodation": Madison and Nicoll, 1984). Thus, accommodation is strongly reduced when Ca entry is blocked or internal Ca buffered with EGTA or BAPTA, or when I_{AHP} is selectively inhibited with noradrenaline (Madison and Nicoll, 1982 and 1984; Cole and Nicoll, 1983). A possible role for physiological buffering of intracellular Ca as a mechanism for controlling the amount of adaptation is indicated by the observation of Kawaguchi et al. (1987) that fast-firing interneurones contain high levels of the Ca-binding protein parvalbumin. However, it should be noted that I_{AHP} is not only the determinant of accommodation: its effect is reinforced by other K currents such as the M current (see above: Madison and Nicoll, 1984), so that hippocampal cells can still show substantial accommodation when I_{AHP} is suppressed (Jones and Heinemann, 1988). In spite of the apparent sensitivity of I_{AHP} to intracellular Ca, there is no evidence that it contributes to the resting membrane current in the absence of a spike- or transmitter-induced Ca transient. Resting concentrations of Ca have been estimated at $20-30$ nM in CA3 neurones in tissue-cultured rat hippocampal slices impaled with Fura-2/K-acetate microelectrodes (Knöpfel et al., 1989 and unpublished observations) – presumably too low to activate I_{AHP}.

Ca-activated Cl currents $I_{Cl(Ca)}$

Voltage-insensitive, Ca-activated Cl channels of 20 pS conductance, activated by > 0.5 μM Ca, have been noted in hippocampal cell membrane patches (Owen et al., 1988). These probably contribute to the long Ca-dependent "tail currents" previously noted in some voltage-clamp studies following Cl-loading coupled with suppression of Ca-activated K currents (e.g. Brown and Griffith, 1983b). In sensory and spinal neurones such Ca-activated Cl currents can generate depolarizing after-potentials (Owen et al., 1984; Meyer, 1985); whether this current contributes to after-potentials in hippocampal cells is not yet clear.

Ca-activated cation currents

Following suppression of I_{AHP} with muscarinic agonists, the normal after-hyperpolarization is replaced with an after-depolarization (Benardo and Prince, 1982; Gähwiler, 1984). Recent experiments with parallel Fura-2 recording show that the corresponding inward current coincides with the peak of the Ca transient (Knopfel et al., 1989). Since E_{Cl} is about -60 mV or so in K acetate impaled cells, this cannot be due to the Ca-activated Cl current, but might instead represent a Ca-activated cation current. There is some evidence for a similar current in cortical neurones in the presence of muscarine (Schwindt et al., 1988).

Other membrane currents

"Leak" currents

These refer to the passive currents which remain around rest potential when voltage- and Ca-gated currents are suppressed. Under normal circumstances, the hippocampal pyramidal cell membrane potential is "squeezed" into a region of high membrane resistance between -60 and -80 mV by the inwardly rectifying Q current on the one hand and the outwardly rectifying M current on the other (see Fig. 5a in Brown, 1988). When these currents are suppressed the residual current – voltage curve negative to -50 mV is linear with a slope conductance of under 10 nS in microelectrode-impaled cells (Brown and Griffith, 1983b and unpublished observations: see Fig. 2).

One component of this residual conductance is a voltage-insensitive K conductance which can be reduced by muscarinic agonists (Madison et al., 1987b; Benson et al., 1988). This effect is probably mediated by a pertussis-toxin insensitive GTP-binding protein (Brown et al., 1988).

Several types of Cl channel have also been described in cultured hippocampal cell membranes which might carry a component of this leak current (Franciolini and Nonner, 1987; Franciolini and Petris, 1988; Owen et al., 1988). If so, then these would be expected to stabilize the membrane potential around -60 to -70 mV unless the cells were Cl-loaded with Cl-containing electrodes.

Na-activated currents

Tetanic stimulation of CA3 neurones produces a prolonged ($50-200$ s) after-hyperpolarization (Gustaffson and Wigström, 1983). In part, this is probably due to electrogenic Na extrusion stimulated by the Na load, since it was reduced and slowed by Na pump inhibition. However, a residual potential persisted in the presence of ouabain which reversed with membrane hyperpolarization. It was suggested that this might result from a Na-activated K current (Gustafsson and Wigström, 1983). Constanti and Sim (1987) and Schwindt et al. (1989) have presented evidence for a prolonged Na-activated K current in voltage-clamped cortical neurones, capable of affecting cell excitability. There is no clear evidence that the electrogenic Na pump contributes to the resting potential (McCarren and Alger, 1987); the significance of the posttetanic Na-activated currents to hippocampal cell behaviour has not been studied extensively.

Anoxic current: ATP-gated K channels?

Short periods of anoxia induce a hyperpolarization of rat hippocampal CA1 neurones, resulting from an increased K conductance (Hansen et al., 1982). One possible mechanism for this is an anoxic-induced release of Ca and consequent activation of Ca-dependent K channels (Krnjević, 1975), but the hyperpolarization is only partly suppressed (if at all) by injecting a Ca chelator (Krnjević and Leblond, 1987; Fujiwara et al., 1987). An alternative mechanism might be a reduction of ATP and consequent activation of ATP-blocked K channels (cf. Ashcroft, 1988), since Mourre et al. (1989) have reported that the hyperpolarization is

156

inhibited by sulphonylurea compounds, which block ATP-regulated K channels. Such channels have been detected in cortical and cerebellar cell membranes (Ashford et al., 1988). Further evidence for their presence in hippocampal cell membranes (albeit in low density) might be adduced from the hyperpolarizing action of cromakalim (Alzheimer et al., 1988), which activates ATP-regulated channels in smooth muscle (Standen et al., 1989), and from the occasional (but small) hyperpolarizing effect of galanin (Dutar et al., 1989), which activates ATP-blocked channels in pancreatic β-cells (de Weille et al., 1988). However, these channels do not seem to play a prominent role in controlling the membrane potential under normal conditions since no reduction in resting potential or conductance occurs in the absence of anoxia on applying sulphonylurea-blocking drugs (Krnjević and Leblond, 1988; Mourre et al., 1989).

References

Adams, P.R., Constanti, A., Brown, D.A. and Clark, R.B. (1982) Intracellular Ca^{2+} activates a fast voltage sensitive K^+ current in vertebrate sympathetic neurones. *Nature (Lond.)*, 296: 746 – 749.

Adams, P.R. and Halliwell, J.V. (1982) A hyperpolarization-induced inward current in hippocampal pyramidal cells. *J. Physiol. (Lond.)* 324: 62 – 63P.

Alger, B.E. and Doerner, D. (1988) Whole-cell voltage-clamp study of two distinct components of "A-current" in hippocampal neurons. *Soc. Neurosci. Abstr.*, 14: 947.

Alger, B.E. and Nicoll, R.A. (1980) Epileptiform burst afterhyperpolarization: calcium-dependent potassium potential in hippocampal CA1 pyramidal cells. *Science*, 210: 1122 – 1124.

Alzheimer, C. (1988) Cromakalim (BRL 34915) activates a Ba^{2+} and Cs^+ sensitive K^+-conductance in hippocampal CA3 pyramidal cells in vitro. *Pflüg. Arch.*, 412: R17.

Andrade, R., Malenka, R.C. and Nicoll, R.A. (1986). A G-protein couples serotonin and $GABA_B$ receptors to the same channels in hippocampus. *Science*, 234: 1261 – 1265.

Andrade, R. and Nicoll, R.A. (1987) Pharmacologically distinct actions of serotonin on single pyramidal neurones of the rat hippocampus recorded in vitro. *J. Physiol. (Lond.)*, 394: 99 – 124.

Ashcroft, F.M. (1988) Adenosine 5-triphosphate sensitive potassium channels. *Ann. Rev. Neurosci.*, 11: 97 – 118.

Ashford, M.L.J., Sturgess, N.C., Trout, N.J., Gardner, N.J. and Hales, C.N. (1988) Adenosine-5-triphosphate-sensitive ion channels in neonatal rat cultured central neurones. *Pflüg. Arch.*, 412: 297 – 304.

Benardo, L.S., Masukawa, L.M. and Prince, D.A. (1982) Electrophysiology of isolated hippocampal cell dendrites. *J. Neurosci.*, 2: 1614 – 1622.

Benardo, L.S. and Prince, D.A. (1982) Cholinergic excitation of mammalian hippocampal pyramidal cells. *Brain Res.*, 249: 315 – 331.

Benson, D.M., Blitzer, R.D. and Landau, E.M. (1988) An analysis of the depolarization produced in guinea-pig hippocampus by cholinergic receptor stimulation. *J. Physiol. (Lond.)*, 404: 479 – 496.

Blatz, A.L. and Magleby, K.L. (1987) Calcium-activated potassium channels. *Trends Neurosci.*, 10: 463 – 467.

Brett, R.S., Dilger, J.P., Adams, P.R. and Lancaster, B. (1986) A method for the rapid exchange of solutions bathing excised membrane patches. *Biophys. J.*, 50: 987 – 992.

Brett, R.S. and Lancaster, B (1985) Activation of potassium channels by rapid application of calcium to inside-out patches of cultured hippocampal neurons. *Soc. Neurosci. Abstr.*, 10: 241.

Brown, D.A. (1988) M-currents. In T. Narahashi (Ed.), *Ion Channels. Vol. 1*, Plenum, New York, pp. 55 – 94.

Brown, D.A. and Adams, P.R. (1980) Muscarinic suppression of a novel voltage-sensitive K^+ current in a vertebrate neurone. *Nature (Lond.)*, 242: 673 – 676.

Brown, D.A., Constanti, A., Docherty, R.J., Galvan, M., Gähwiler, B. and Halliwell, J.V. (1984) Pharmacology of calcium currents in mammalian central neurones. *Iuphar Proc. 9th Int. Pharmacol. Congr.*, 2: 343 – 348.

Brown, D.A. and Griffith, W.H. (1983a) Persistent slow inward calcium current in voltage-clamped hippocampal neurones of the guinea-pig. *J. Physiol. (Lond.)*, 337: 303 – 320.

Brown, D.A. and Griffith, W.H. (1983b) Calcium-activated outward current in voltage-clamped hippocampal neurons of the guinea-pig. *J. Physiol. (Lond.)*, 337: 287 – 301.

Brown, D.A., Grove, E.A. and Halliwell, J.V. (1988) Tetrahydroaminoacridine (THA) blocks the Q-currents in hippocampal CA1 neurones. *Neurosci. Lett.*, Suppl. 32: S8.

Brown, H. and DiFrancesco, D. (1980) Voltage-clamp investigation of membrane currents underlying pacemaker activity in rabbit sino-atrial node. *J. Physiol. (Lond.)*, 308: 331 – 351.

Brown, L.D., Nakajima, S. and Nakajima, Y. (1988) Acetylcholine modulates resting K-current through a pertussis-toxin-resistant G-protein in hippocampal neurones. *Soc. Neurosci. Abstr.*, 14: 1328.

Brown, T.H., Fricke, R.A. and Perkel, D.H. (1981) Passive electrical constants in three classes of hippocampal neurons. *J. Neurophysiol.*, 46: 812 – 827.

Cole, A.E. and Nicoll, R.A. (1983) Acetylcholine mediates a slow synaptic potential in hippocampal pyramidal cells.

Science, 221: 1299–1301.

Colino, A. and Halliwell, J.V. (1987) Differential modulation of three separate K-conductances in hippocampal CA1 neurones by serotonin. *Nature (Lond.)*, 327: 73–77.

Connor, J.A. and Stevens, C.F. (1971) Voltage clamp studies of a transient outward membrane current in gastropod neural somata. *J. Physiol. (Lond.)*, 213: 21–30.

Constanti, A. and Galvan, M. (1983) Fast inward-rectifying current accounts for anomalous rectification in olfactory cortex neurones. *J. Physiol. (Lond.)*, 335: 153–178.

Constanti, A. and Sim, J.A. (1987) Calcium-dependent potassium conductance in guinea-pig olfactory cortex in vitro. *J. Physiol. (Lond.)*, 387: 173–194.

DeWeille, J., Schmid-Antomarchi, H., Fosset, M. and Lazdunski, M. (1988) ATP-sensitive K^+ channels that are blocked by hypoglycemia-inducing sulfonylureas in insulin-secreting cells are activated by galanin, a hyperglycemia-inducing hormone. *Proc. Natl. Acad. Sci. U.S.A.*, 85: 1312–1316.

Docherty, R.J. and Brown, D.A. (1986) Interaction of 1,4-dihydropyridines with somatic Ca currents in hippocampal CA1 neurones of the guinea-pig in vitro. *Neurosci. Lett.*, 70: 110–115.

Dutar, P. and Nicoll, R.A. (1988) Classification of muscarinic responses in hippocampus in terms of receptor subtypes and second-messenger systems: electrophysiological studies in vitro. *J. Neurosci.*, 8: 4214–4224.

Dutar, P., Lamour, Y. and Nicoll, R.A. (1989) Galanin blocks the slow cholinergic EPSP in CA1 pyramidal cells from ventral hippocampus. *Eur. J. Pharmacol.*, 164: 355–360.

Edwards, F.A., Konnerth, A., Sakmann, B. and Takahashi, T. (1989) *Pflüg. Arch.*, 414: 600–612.

Fox, A.P., Nowycky, M.C. and Tsien, R.W. (1987a) Kinetic and pharmacological properties distinguishing three types of calcium currents in chick sensory neurones. *J. Physiol. (Lond.)*, 394: 149–172.

Fox, A.P., Nowycky, M.C. and Tsien, R.W. (1987b) Single channel recordings of three types of calcium channels in chick sensory neurones. *J. Physiol. (Lond.)*, 394: 173–200.

ffrench-Mullen, J.M.H., Rogawski, M.A. and Barker, J.L. (1988) Phencyclidine at low concentration selectively blocks the sustained but not the transient voltage-dependent potassium current in cultured hippocampal neurons. *Neurosci. Lett.*, 88: 325–330.

Franciolini, F. (1988) Calcium and voltage dependence of single Ca^{2+}-activated K^+ channels from cultured hippocampal neurones of rat. *Biochim. Biophys. Acta*, 943: 419–427.

Franciolini, F. and Nonner, W. (1987) Anion and cation permeability of a chloride channel in rat hippocampal neurones. *J. Gen. Physiol.*, 90: 453–478.

Franciolini, F. and Petris, A. (1988) Single chloride channels in cultured rat neurones. *Arch. Biochem. Biophys.*, 261: 97–102.

French, C.R. and Gale, P.W. (1985) A threshold sodium current in pyramidal cells in rat hippocampus. *Neurosci. Lett.*, 56: 289–293.

Fujiwara, N., Higashi, H., Shimoji, K. and Yoshimura, M. (1987) Effects of hypoxia on rat hippocampal neurones in vitro. *J. Physiol. (Lond.)*, 384: 131–151.

Furuya, S., Ohmori, H., Shigemoto, T. and Sugiyama, H. (1989) Intracellular calcium mobilization by a glutamate receptor in rat cultured hippocampal cells. *J. Physiol. (Lond.)*, 414: 539–548.

Gähwiler, B.H. (1984) Facilitation by acetylcholine of tetrodotoxin resistant spikes in rat hippocampal pyramidal cells. *Neuroscience*, 11: 381–388.

Gähwiler, B.H. and Brown, D.A. (1985a) Functional innervation of cultured hippocampal neurones by cholinergic afferents from co-cultured septal explants. *Nature (Lond.)*, 313: 577–579.

Gähwiler, B.H. and Brown, D.A. (1985b) $GABA_B$-receptor-activated K^+ current in voltage-clamped CA3 pyramidal cells in hippocampal cultures. *Proc. Natl. Acad. Sci. U.S.A.*, 82: 1558–1562.

Gähwiler, B.H. and Brown, D.A. (1987a) Effects of dihydropyridines on calcium currents in CA3 pyramidal cells in slice cultures of rat hippocampus. *Neuroscience*, 20: 731–738.

Gähwiler, B.H. and Brown, D.A. (1987b) Muscarine affects calcium-currents in rat hippocampal pyramidal cells in vitro. *Neurosci. Lett.*, 76; 301–306.

Gray, R.A. and Johnston, D. (1986) Multiple types of calcium channels in acutely exposed neurones from the adult guinea-pig hippocampus. *J. Gen. Physiol.*, 88: 25a.

Gray, R. and Johnston, D. (1987) Noradrenaline and β-adrenoceptor agonists increase activity of voltage-dependent calcium channels in hippocampal neurones. *Nature (Lond.)*, 327: 620–622.

Gustafsson, H., Galvan, M., Grafe, P. and Wigström, H. (1982) A transient outward current in a mammalian central neurone blocked by 4-aminopyridine. *Nature (Lond.)*, 299: 252–254.

Gustafsson, B. and Wigström, H. (1981) Evidence for two types of after-hyperpolarization in CA1 pyramidal cells in the hippocampus. *Brain Res.*, 206: 462–468.

Gustafsson, B. and Wigström, H. (1983) Hyperpolarization following long-lasting tetanic activation of hippocampal pyramidal cells. *Brain Res.*, 275: 159–163.

Haas, H.L. and Konnerth, A. (1983) Histamine and noradrenaline decrease calcium-activated potassium conductance in hippocampal pyramidal cells. *Nature (Lond.)*, 302: 432–434.

Hablitz, J.J. and Johnston, D. (1981) Endogenous nature of spontaneous bursting in hippocampal pyramidal neurones. *Cell. Mol. Neurobiol.*, 1: 325–334.

Halliwell, J.V. (1983) Calcium-loading reveals two distinct Ca-currents in voltage-clamped guinea-pig hippocampal neurones in vitro. *J. Physiol. (Lond.)*, 341: 10P.

Halliwell, J.V. and Adams, P.R. (1982) Voltage-clamp analysis

158

of muscarinic excitation in hippocampal neurones. *Brain Res.*, 250: 71 – 92.

Halliwell, J.V., Othman, I.B., Pelchen-Matthews, A. and Dolly, J.O. (1986) Central action of dendrotoxin: selective reduction of a transient K conductance in hippocampus and binding to localized acceptors. *Proc. Natl. Acad. Sci. U.S.A.*, 83: 493 – 497.

Halliwell, J.V. and Scholfield, C.N. (1984) Somatically recorded Ca-currents in guinea-pig hippocampal and olfactory cortex neurones are resistant to adenosine action. *Neurosci. Lett.*, 50: 13 – 18.

Hansen, A.J., Hounsgaard, J. and Jahnsen, H. (1982) Anoxia increases potassium conductance in hippocampal nerve cells. *Acta. Physiol. Scand.*, 115: 301 – 310.

Hotson, J.R. and Prince, D.A. (1980) A calcium-activated hyperpolarization follows repetitive firing in hippocampal neurons. *J. Neurophysiol.*, 43: 409 – 419.

Hotson, J.R., Prince, D.A. and Schwartzkroin, P.A. (1979) Anomalous inward rectification in hippocampal neurones. *J. Neurophysiol.*, 42: 889 – 895.

Huguenard, J.R., Hamill, O.P. and Prince, D.A. (1989) Sodium channels in dendrites of rat cortical pyramidal neurons. *Proc. Natl. Acad. Sci., U.S.A.*, 86: 2473 – 2477.

Ikemoto, Y., Ono, K., Yoshida, A. and Akaike, N. (1989) Delayed activation of large-conductance Ca^{2+}-activated K channels in hippocampal neurones of the rat. *Biophys. J.*, 56: 207 – 212.

Johnston, D. (1981) Passive cable properties of hippocampal Ca3 pyramidal neurones. *Cell. Mol. Neurobiol.*, 1: 41 – 55.

Johnston, D. and Brown, T.H. (1983) Interpretation of voltage-clamp measurements in hippocampal neurons. *J. Neurophysiol.*, 50: 464 – 486.

Johnston, D., Hablitz, J.J. and Wilson, W.A. (1980) Voltage-clamp discloses slow inward current in hippocampal burst-firing neurons. *Nature (Lond.)*, 286: 391 – 393.

Jones, O.T., Kunze, D.L. and Angelides, K.J. (1989) Localization and mobility of ω-conotoxin-sensitive Ca^{2+} channels in hippocampal CA1 neurones. *Science*, 244: 1189 – 1193.

Jones, R.S.G. and Heinemann, U. (1988) Verapamil blocks the after-hyperpolarization but not the spike frequency accommodation of rat CA1 pyramidal cells in vitro. *Brain Res.*, 462: 367 – 371.

Kaneda, M., Oomura, Y., Ishibashi, O. and Akaike, N. (1988) Permeability to various cations of the voltage-dependent sodium channel of isolated rat hippocampal neurons. *Neurosci. Lett.*, 88: 253 – 256.

Kawaguchi, Y., Katsumaru, A., Kosaka, T., Heizmann, C.W. and Hamma, K. (1987) Fast spiking cells in rat hippocampus (CA1 region) contain the calcium-binding protein parvalbumin. *Brain Res.*, 416: 369 – 374.

Kay, A.R. and Wong, R.K.S. (1987) Calcium current activation kinetics in isolated pyramidal neurones of the CA1 of the mature guinea-pig hippocampus. *J. Physiol. (Lond.)*, 392: 603 – 616.

Knöpfel, T., Brown, D.A., Vranesic, I. and Gähwiler, B.H. (1989) Depression of Ca^{2+} activated potassium conductance by muscarine and isoproterenol without alteration of depolarization-induced transient rise in cytosolic free Ca^{2+} in hippocampal CA3 pyramidal cells. *Eur. J. Neurosci.*, Suppl. 2: 92.

Krnjević (1975) Coupling of neuronal metabolism and electrical activity. In D.H. Ingvar and N.A. Lassen (Ed.), *Brain Work*, Munksgaard, Copenhagen, pp. 65 – 78.

Krnjević, K. and Leblond, J. (1987) Mechanism of hyperpolarizing response of hippocampal cells to anoxia in isolated slices of rat hippocampus. *J. Physiol. (Lond.)*, 382: 79P.

Krnjević, K. and Leblond, J. (1988) Are there hippocampal ATP-sensitive K channels that are activated by anoxia? *Pflüg. Arch.*, 211: R145.

Kudo, Y. and Ogura, A. (1986) Glutamate-induced increase in intracellular Ca^{2+} concentration in isolated hippocampal neurons. *Br. J. Pharmacol.*, 89: 191 – 198.

Kudo, Y., Ogura, A. and Iljima, T. (1988) Stimulation of muscarinic receptor in hippocampal neuron induces characteristic increase in cytosolic free Ca^{2+} concentration. *Neurosci. Lett.*, 85: 345 – 350.

Lancaster, B. and Adams, P.R. (1986) Calcium-dependent current generating the afterhyperpolarization of hippocampal neurons. *J. Neurophysiol.*, 55: 1268 – 1282.

Lancaster, B. and Nicoll, R.A. (1987) Properties of two calcium-activated hyperpolarizations in rat hippocampal neurones. *J. Physiol. (Lond.)*, 389: 187 – 203.

Lancaster, B., Perkel, D.J. and Nicoll, R.A. (1987) Small conductance Ca^{2+}-activated K^+ channels in hippocampal neurons. *Neurosci. Abstr.*, 13: 176.

Lanthorn, T., Storm, J. and Andersen, P. (1984) Current-to-frequency transduction in Ca1 hippocampal pyramidal cells: slow potentials dominate the primary range firing. *Exp. Brain. Res.*, 53: 431 – 443.

Llano, I., Marty, A., Johnson, J.W., Ascher, P. and Gähwiler, B.H. (1988) Patch-clamp recording of amino acid-activated responses in "organotypic" slice cultures. *Proc. Natl. Acad. Sci. U.S.A.*, 85: 3221 – 3225.

Macvicar, B.A. (1985) Depolarizing prepotentials are Na^+ dependent in CA1 pyramidal neurons. *Brain Res.*, 333: 378 – 381.

Madison, D., Fox, A.P. and Tsien, R.W. (1987a) Adenosine reduces an inactivating component of calcium current in hippocampal CA3 neurons. *Biophys. J.*, 51: 30a.

Madison, D.V., Lancaster, B. and Nicoll, R.A. (1987b) Voltage-clamp analysis of cholinergic action in the hippocampus. *J. Neurosci.*, 7: 733 – 741.

Madison, D.V., Malenka, R.C. and Nicoll, R.A. (1986) Phorbol esters block a voltage-sensitive chloride current in hippocampal pyramidal cells. *Nature (Lond.)*, 321: 695 – 697.

Madison, D.V. and Nicoll, R.A. (1982) Noradrenaline blocks accommodation of pyramidal cell discharge in the hippocampus. *Nature (Lond.)*, 299: 636 – 638.

Madison, D.V. and Nicoll, R.A. (1964) Control of the repetitive discharge of rat CA1 pyramidal neurons in vitro. *J. Physiol. (Lond.)*, 354: 319–331.

Mayer, M.L. (1985) A calcium-activated chloride current generates the after-depolarization of rat sensory neurons in culture. *J. Physiol. (Lond.)*, 364: 217–239.

McCarren, M. and Alger, B.E. (1987) Sodium-potassium pump inhibitors increase neuronal excitability in the rat hippocampal slice: role of Ca^{2+}-dependent conductance. *J. Neurophysiol.*, 57: 496–509.

Meyers, D.E.R. and Barker, J.L. (1989) Whole-cell patch-clamp analysis of voltage-dependent calcium conductances in cultured embryonic rat hippocampal neurons. *J. Neurophysiol.*, 61: 467–477.

Moore, S.D., Madamba, S.G., Joels, M. and Siggins, G.R. (1988) Somatostatin augments the M-current in hippocampal neurones. *Science*, 239: 278–280.

Mourre, C., Ben-Ari, Y., Benardi, H., Fosset, M. and Lazdunski, M. (1989) Antidiabetic sulfonylureas: localization of binding sites in the brain and effect on the hyperpolarization induced by anoxia in hippocampal slices. *Brain Res.*, 486: 159–164.

Nakajima, Y., Nakajima, S., Leonard, R.J. and Yamagichi, K. (1986) Acetylcholine raises excitability by inhibiting the fast transient potassium current in cultured rat sympathetic neurons. *Proc. Natl. Acad. Sci. U.S.A.*, 83: 3022–3026.

Newberry, N. and Nicoll, R.A. (1985) Comparison of the action of baclofen with gamma-aminobutyric acid on rat hippocampal pyramidal cells in vitro. *J. Physiol. (Lond.)*, 348: 239–254.

Nicoll, R.A. and Alger, B.E. (1981) Synaptic excitation may activate a calcium-dependent potassium conductance in hippocampal pyramidal cells. *Science*, 212: 957–959.

Numann, R.E., Wadman, W.J. and Wong, R.K.S. (1987) Outward currents of single hippocampal cells obtained from the adult guinea-pig. *J. Physiol. (Lond.)*, 393: 334–353.

Owen, D.G. (1987) Three types of inward rectifier currents in cultured hippocampal neurones. *Neurosci. Lett.*, Suppl 29: 518.

Owen, D.G., Harrison, N.L. and Barker, J.L. (1988) Three types of chloride channels in cultured rat hippocampal neurons. *Soc. Neurosci. Abstr.*, 14: 1203.

Owen, D.G., Segal, M. and Barker, J.L. (1984) A Ca-dependent Cl^- conductance in cultured mouse spinal neurons. *Nature (Lond.)*, 311: 567–570.

Peacock, J.H. and Walker, C.R. (1983) Development of calcium action potentials in mouse hippocampal cell cultures. *Dev. Brain Res.*, 8: 39–52.

Rehm, H., Pelzer, S., Cochet, C., Chambard, E., Tempel, B.L., Trautwein, W., Pelzer, D. and Lazdunski, M. (1989) The dendrotoxin binding brain membrane protein displays a K^+ channel activity which is stimulated both by cAMP-dependent and endogenous phosphorylations. *Biochemistry*, 28: 6455–6460.

Rogawski, M.A. (1986) Single voltage-dependent potassium channels in cultured rat hippocampal neurones. *J. Neurophysiol.*, 56: 481–493.

Sah, P., French, C.R. and Gage, P.W. (1985) Effects of noradrenaline on some potassium currents in CA1 neurones in rat hippocampal slices. *Neurosci. Lett.*, 60: 295–300.

Sah, P., Gibb, A.J. and Gage, P.W. (1988a) The sodium current underlying action potentials in guinea-pig hippocampal CA1 neurons. *J. Gen. Physiol.*, 91: 373–398.

Sah, P., Gibb, A.J. and Gage, P.W. (1988b) Potassium current activated by depolarization of dissociated neurons from adult guinea-pig hippocampus. *J. Gen. Physiol.*, 92: 263–278.

Schwartzkroin, P.A. (1980) Ionic and synaptic determinants of burst generation. In J.S. Lockard and A.A.Ward Jr. (Eds.), *Epilepsy: a Window to Brain Mechanisms*, Raven Press, New York, pp. 83–95.

Schwartzkroin, P.A. and Slawsky, M. (1977) Probable calcium spikes in hippocampal neurones. *Brain Res.*, 135: 157–161.

Schwartzkroin, P.A. and Stafstrom, C.E. (1980) Effects of EGTA on the calcium-activated after-hyperpolarization in hippocampal CA3 pyramidal cells. *Science*, 210: 1125–1126.

Schwindt, P.C., Spain, W.J. and Crill, W.E. (1989) Long-lasting reduction of excitability by a sodium-dependent potassium current in cat neocortical neurons. *J. Neurophysiol.*, 61: 233–244.

Schwindt, P.C., Spain, W.J., Foehring, R.C., Chubb, M.C. and Crill, W.E. (1988) Slow conductances in neurons from cat sensorimotor cortex *in vitro* and their role in slow excitability changes. *J. Neurophysiol.*, 59: 450–467.

Segal, M. and Barker, J.L. (1984) Rat hippocampal neurons in culture: potassium conductances. *J. Neurophysiol.*, 51: 1409–1433.

Segal, M. and Barker, J.L. (1986) Rat hippocampal neurons in culture: Ca^{2+} and Ca^{2+}-dependent K^+ conductances. *J. Neurophysiol.*, 55: 752–766.

Segal, M., Rogawski, M.A. and Barker, J.L. (1984) A transient potassium conductance regulates the excitability of cultured hippocampal and spinal neurons. *J. Neurosci.*, 4: 604–609.

Selyanko, A.A. (1984) Cd^{2+} suppresses a time-dependent Cl^- current in rat sympathetic neurone. *J. Physiol. (Lond.)*, 350: 49P.

Spain, W.J., Schwindt, P.C. and Crill, W.E. (1987) Anomalous rectification in neurons from cat sensorimotor cortex in vitro. *J. Neurophysiol.*, 57: 1555–1576.

Stansfeld, C.E. and Feltz, A. (1988) Dendrotoxin-sensitive K^+ channels in dorsal rat ganglion cells. *Neurosci. Lett.*, 93: 49–55.

Stansfeld, C.E., Marsh, S.J., Halliwell, J.V. and Brown, D.A. (1986) 4-aminopyridine and dendrotoxin induced repetitive firing in rat visceral sensory neurones by blocking a slowly-inactivating outward current. *Neurosci. Lett.*, 64: 299–304.

Standen, N.B., Guayle, J.M., Davies, N.W., Brayden, J.E., Huang, Y. and Nelson, M.T. (1989) Hyperpolarizing

160

vasodilators activate ATP-sensitive K^+ channels in arterial smooth muscle. *Science*, 245: 177 – 180.

Storm, J.F. (1987a) Action potential repolarization and a fast after-hyperpolarization in rat hippocampal pyramidal cells. *J. Physiol. (Lond.)*, 385: 733 – 759.

Storm, J.F. (1987b) Intracellular injection of a Ca^{2+} chelator inhibits spike repolarization in hippocampal neurons. *Brain Res.*, 435: 387 – 392.

Storm, J.F. (1988) A slowly inactivating K^+ current mediates integration in hippocampal neurones. *Nature (Lond.)*, 336: 379 – 381.

Storm, J.F. (1989) An after-hyperpolarization of medium duration in rat hippocampal pyramidal cells. *J. Physiol. (Lond.)*, 409: 171 – 190.

Takahashi, K., Tateishi, N., Kaneda, M. and Akaike, N. (1989) Comparison of low-threshold Ca^{2+} currents in the hippocampal CA1 neurons among the newborn, adult and aged rats. *Neurosci. Lett.*, 103: 29 – 33.

Thompson, S.H. (1977) Three pharmacologically distinct potassium channels in molluscan neurones. *J. Physiol. (Lond.)*, 265: 465 – 488.

Toselli, M. and Lux, H.D. (1989) GTP-binding proteins mediate acetylcholine inhibition of voltage-dependent calcium channels in hippocampal neurons. *Pflüg. Arch.*, 413: 319 – 321.

Traub, R.D. (1982) Simulation of intrinsic bursting in CA3 hippocampal neurons. *Neuroscience*, 7: 1233 – 1242.

Traub, R.D. and Llinas, R. (1979) Hippocampal pyramidal cells: significance of dendritic ionic conductances for neuronal function and epileptogenesis. *J. Neurophysiol.*, 42: 476 – 496.

Turner, D.A. and Schwartzkroin, P.A. (1980) Steady-state electronic analysis of intracellularly stained hippocampal neurons. *J. Neurophysiol.*, 44: 184 – 199.

Turner, D.A. and Schwartzkroin, P.A. (1983) Electrical

characteristics of dendrites and dendritic spines in intracellularly stained CA3 and dentate hippocampal neurons. *J. Neurosci.*, 3: 2381 – 2394.

Vandongen, A.M.J., Codina, J., Olate, J., Mattera, R., Joh, O.R., Birnbaumer, L. and Brown, A.M. (1988) Newly identified brain potassium channels gated by the guanine nucleotidine binding protein G_0. *Science*, 242: 1433 – 1437.

Watson, T.W.J. and Pittman, Q.J. (1988) Pharmacological evidence that somatostatin activates the M-current in hippocampal pyramidal neurons. *Neurosci. Lett.*, 91: 172 – 176.

Wong, R.K.S. and Prince, D.A. (1978) Participation of calcium spikes during intrinsic burst firing in hippocampal neurons. *Brain Res.*, 159: 385 – 390.

Wong, R.K.S. and Prince, D.A. (1979) Dendritic mechanisms underlying penicillin-induced epileptiform activity. *Science*, 204: 1228 – 1232.

Wong, R.K.S., Prince, D.A. and Basbaum, A.I. (1979) Intradendritic recordings from hippocampal neurones. *Proc. Natl. Acad. Sci. U.S.A.*, 76: 986 – 990.

Yaari, Y., Hamon, B. and Lux, H.D. (1987) Development of two types of calcium channels in cultured mammalian hippocampal neurons. *Science*, 235: 80 – 82.

Yanagihara, K. and Irisawa, H. (1980) Inward current activated during hyperpolarization in the isolated rabbit sino atrial node cell. *Pflüg. Arch.*, 385: 11 – 19.

Zbicz, K.L. and Weight, F.F. (1985) Transient voltage and calcium-dependent outward currents in hippocampal CA3 pyramidal cells. *J. Neurophysiol.*, 53: 1038 – 1058.

Zgombik, J.M., Beck, S.G., Mahle, C.D., Craddock-Royal, B. and Maayani, S. (1989) Pertussis-toxin-sensitive guanine nucleotide-binding protein(s) couple adenosine A_1 and 5-hydroxy-tryptamine 1_A receptors to the same effector systems in rat hippocampus: biochemical and electrophysiological studies. *Mol. Pharmacol.*, 35: 484 – 494.

J. Storm-Mathisen, J. Zimmer and O.P. Ottersen (Eds.)
Progress in Brain Research, Vol. 83
© 1990 Elsevier Science Publishers B.V. (Biomedical Division)

CHAPTER 12

Potassium currents in hippocampal pyramidal cells

Johan F. Storm

Institute of Neurophysiology, Karl Johans gate 47, N – 0162 Oslo 1, Norway

The hippocampal pyramidal cells provide an example of how multiple potassium (K) currents co-exist and function in central mammalian neurones. The data come from CA1 and CA3 neurones in hippocampal slices, cell cultures and acutely dissociated cells from rats and guinea-pigs. Six voltage- or calcium(Ca)-dependent K currents have so far been described in CA1 pyramidal cells in slices. Four of them (I_A, I_D, I_K, I_M) are activated by depolarization alone; the two others (I_C, I_{AHP}) are activated by voltage-dependent influx of Ca ions (I_C may be both Ca- and voltage-gated). In addition, a transient Ca-dependent K current (I_{CT}) has been described in certain preparations, but it is not yet clear whether it is distinct from I_C and I_A. (1) I_A activates fast (within 10 ms) and inactivates rapidly (time constant typically $15 - 50$ ms) at potentials positive to -60 mV; it probably contributes to early spike-repolarization, it can delay the first spike for about 0.1 s, and may regulate repetitive firing. (2) I_D activates within about 20 ms but inactivates slowly (seconds) below the spike threshold (-90 to -60 mV), causing a long delay ($0.5 - 5$ s) in the onset of firing. Due to its slow recovery from inactivation (seconds), separate depolarizing inputs can be "integrated". I_D probably also participates in spike repolarization. (3) I_K activates slowly (time constant, τ, $20 - 60$ ms) in response to depolarizations positive to -40 mV and inactivates (τ about 5s) at -80 to -40 mV; it probably participates in spike repolarization. (4) I_M activates slowly (τ about 50 ms) positive to -60 mV and does not inactivate; it tends to attenuate excitatory inputs, it reduces the firing rate during maintained depolarization (adaptation) and contributes to the medium after-hyperpolarization (mAHP); I_M is suppressed by acetylcholine (via muscarinic receptors), but may be enhanced by somatostatin. (5) I_C is activated by influx of Ca ions during the action potential and is thought to cause the final spike repolarization and the fast AHP (although I_{CT} may be involved). Like I_M, it also contributes to the medium AHP and early adaptation. It differs from I_{AHP} by being sensitive to tetraethylammonium (TEA, 1 mM), but insensitive to noradrenaline and muscarine. Large-conductance (BK; about 200 pS) Ca-activated K channels, which may mediate I_C, have been recorded. (6) I_{AHP} is slowly activated by Ca-influx during action potentials, causing spike-frequency adaptation and the slow AHP. Thus, I_{AHP} exerts a strong negative feedback control of discharge activity. It is suppressed by noradrenaline via cyclic AMP, muscarinic agonists, serotonin, histamine, corticotropin-releasing factor and phorbol esters (activators of protein kinase C), and it is enhanced by adenosine. In addition to the above K currents, there are resting K currents, and receptor-operated K currents which contribute to the effects of acetylcholine, noradrenaline, serotonin, GABA, adenosine. In conclusion, a variety of different voltage-dependent K currents co-exist in these cells, apparently contributing specifically to various aspects of the cell's electrical properties, such as the resting potential ($I_{K,rest}$), spike repolarization (I_A, I_D, I_K, I_C, I_{CT} ?), spike-frequency adaptation and after-hyperpolarizations (I_{AHP}, I_M, I_C), delayed excitation, slow repetitive firing and temporal integration (I_A, I_D); – and in mediating the effects of transmitter substances such as acetylcholine (I_{AHP}, I_M, I_A), noradrenaline, histamine, serotonin, adenosine, corticotropin-releasing factor (I_{AHP}) and somatostatin (I_M). These multiple roles may help to explain why the cells are equipped with so many channel types.

Introduction

The basic mechanism for the electrical activity of nerve cells was first described for the squid giant axon about 4 decades ago (Hodgkin and Huxley, 1952). This preparation showed just two "active" ionic currents (or conductances): a fast inward sodium current which produces the upstroke of the action potential, and a delayed outward potassium (K) current which causes spike repolarization. Subsequent studies of other neurones have revealed a multitude of different ion currents, each presumably corresponding to a distinct type of ion channel. In accordance with their more complex functions, neuronal cell bodies and dendrites are usually equipped with a larger set of membrane currents than are axons. The K currents constitute a particularly large and varied group; some cells have more than 5 different kinds (Hille, 1984; Adams and Galvan, 1986; Rudy, 1988). What are the functions of these different K channels? Why are there so many kinds?

To answer questions like these a fairly detailed analysis is required, both for separating and characterizing the different currents, and for determining their function. A complete description of all the major currents was first attempted in some invertebrate and peripheral vertebrate axons and somata. However, in recent years, there has been progress also for some vertebrate central neurones, and hippocampal pyramidal cells have become one of the best studied cell types. Although our present knowledge of K currents in hippocampal pyramidal cells is far from complete, the following description may serve to illustrate how multiple K currents co-exist and play different functional roles in a class of mammalian brain cells.

Preparations and methods

Membrane currents can be studied with voltage clamp or current clamp techniques. In voltage clamp, the ionic currents are measured while the voltage, which determines the activity of most channels, is varied in a simple and controlled manner. Thus, the properties of the channels can be studied when their behaviour is at its simplest. In current clamp the situation is far more complex because the membrane potential is allowed to vary spontaneously along with the membrane currents, while only the current injected into the cell is controlled (clamped). Still, current clamp data can give valuable information, particularly about the functions of the currents.

Spinal motoneurones were the first vertebrate central neurones to be studied systematically with voltage clamp technique, as they were large enough to sustain dual impalement (Barrett and Crill, 1972; Barrett and Barrett, 1976; Schwindt and

Crill, 1977; Barrett et al., 1980). However, the advent of the in vitro brain slice (Yamamoto and McIlwain, 1966), the single-electrode voltage clamp (Wilson and Goldner, 1975), and patch-clamp techniques (Hamill et al., 1981) made it easier to study smaller cells, including those of the hippocampus. Hippocampal cells have been extensively studied, partly because they survive well in slices and the localization of the cell bodies in a dense visible layer make them convenient targets for micro-electrodes.

The conventional hippocampal slice has been supplemented by 5 other preparations: (1) cultures of hippocampal cells dissociated from embryonic or newborn animals (Peacock, 1979; Dreyfus et al., 1979; Segal, 1983; Segal and Barker, 1984); (2) organotypic cultures of slices from young animals (Gähwiler, 1981); (3) acutely exposed cells in enzyme-digested slices from adult animals (Gray and Johnston, 1985); (4) acutely dissociated cells, isolated from young or adult animals by enzyme digestion (Kay and Wong, 1986); and (5) mechanically cleaned cells in thin slices (Edwards et al., 1988 and 1989).

The main advantages of these preparations over the traditional slice are that individual cells can be visualized and patch-clamped, and that test solutions can be applied and washed off quickly. On the other hand, it is possible that cells grown in culture may develop properties which differ from those of the intact tissue. The organotypic cell cultures, however, combine some of the advantages of traditional slices and cultures. The "thin slice" technique has so far mainly been used for analysis of synaptic currents (Edwards et al., 1988, 1989) but it should also be useful for studying intrinsic membrane currents. In acutely dissociated cells, the recording conditions are excellent, but some of their membrane currents may have been lost or changed during the dissociation procedure.

In voltage-clamp experiments, two problems must be solved: (1) how to control the voltage near the tip of the electrode (point clamp), and (2) how to control the voltage in remote parts of the cell (space clamp). The speed and accuracy of the point clamp is determined primarily by the kind of clamp employed and by the electrode properties (see e.g. Jones, 1989). The lower the resistance and capacitance of the electrodes, the faster and better the clamp. The space clamp, on the other hand, depends mainly on the properties of the cell itself; even with a perfect point clamp at the soma, the voltage control in remote processes will be limited. Due to the extensive dendrites of hippocampal neurones, space clamp is a major consideration when interpreting voltage clamp data from these cells (Johnston and Brown, 1983). The space clamp limitations not only hampers the measurements of dendritic currents; currents arising in unclamped processes may also contaminate the somatic currents. Still, useful data can be obtained. One reason is that hippocampal pyramidal cells are electrically fairly compact, partly due to a high specific membrane resistivity. Thus, the passive electrotonic length of a hippocampal pyramidal cell is only about 0.9 (Johnston, 1979; Brown et al., 1981; Turner and Schwartzkroin, 1980, 1984), and the predicted steady state attenuation of a voltage step applied at the soma is only 33% at the tip of the dendrites (Johnston, 1979). For voltage transients, the attenuation will be far greater, and the situation is still worse when the opening of ion channels reduces the space constant. However, the space clamp can be improved by changing the geomery of the cell (e.g. removing processes), its membrane properties, or the distribution of active currents. One great advantage with the acutely dissociated cells is that they have lost most of their processes and are electrically compact (Numann et al., 1987).

Like the different preparations, the various recording techniques are in many ways complementary. (1) The discontinuous single electrode voltage clamp (DSEVC) allowed the first voltage clamp recordings in the hippocampus to be done, with a single microelectrode in slices (Johnston et al., 1980; Halliwell and Adams, 1982). This method has provided much of the data considered below. It is suited for cells situated deep in the tissue, which have so far been inaccessible for pat-

ching, and when minimal disturbance of the intracellular milieu is desired (see below). However, the discontinuous mode limits the speed of the clamp and adds noise to the recordings (Finkel and Redman, 1984). The switching frequency is limited by the time constant of the electrode, since the voltage drop which arises across the electrode tip during each current injection has to decay before the voltage can be measured. Thus, only current transients which are very slow with respect to the electrode time constant can be accurately measured. The DSEVC has also been combined with a low-impedance patch electrode to allow large and fast currents to be recorded (Sah et al., 1989). (2) Two-electrode voltage clamp with microelectrodes has been used in cell culture by Segal and Barker (1984). This method can handle larger and faster currents than the microelectrode-DSEVC, but can only be used when the cell is visible, and the insertion of two electrodes cause extra damage to the cell. (3) Continous whole-cell voltage clamp with a patch pipette has been used in cultured (Nakajima et al., 1986) or acutely dissociated cells (Numann et al., 1987). This technique gives excellent low-noise recording conditions, and the rapid exchange of small molecules between the cell interior and the pipette allows the composition of the intracellular fluid to be controlled. However, this can also be a problem, since some channels may be altered by the changed intracellular milieu. (4) Single-channel recordings have been obtained in cell-attached or isolated patches from the soma and dendrites of cultured, acutely exposed or dissociated cells (e.g. Gray and Johnston, 1985; Brett and Lancaster, 1985; Kay and Wong, 1986; Rogawski, 1986; Masukawa and Hansen, 1987; Llano et al., 1988; VanDongen et al., 1988). This method provides invaluable details about individual channels, but cannot replace studying currents of the cell as a whole.

Overview of hippocampal K currents

Fig. 1 gives an overview of some relatively well-defined voltage- and calcium (Ca)-dependent membrane currents in hippocampal pyramidal cells, and also includes a few of the more controversial currents. It should be noted that no "macroscopic" (i.e. whole cell) hippocampal current has yet been shown to be due to a single channel type, and some of the currents discussed below may well be mediated by "families" of related channels. Conversely, identical channels may conceivably mediate seemingly different macroscopic currents.

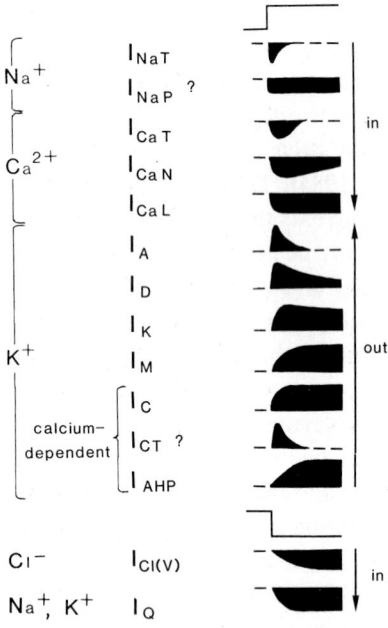

Fig. 1. Schematic overview over 13 of the voltage- and Ca-dependent ionic currents which have been postulated to exist in hippocampal pyramidal cells: transient Na current (I_{NaT}), persistent Na current (I_{NaP}), transient low-threshold Ca current (I_{CaT}), transient high-threshold Ca current (I_{CaN}), persistent high-threshold Ca current (I_{CaL}), fast transient K current (I_A), delay current (I_D), delayed rectifier current (I_K), M-current (I_M), fast Ca-dependent K current (I_C), transient Ca-dependent K current (I_{CT}), slow Ca-dependent K current (I_{AHP}), voltage-dependent chloride current ($I_{Cl(V)}$), and slow inward rectifier current (I_Q). The silhouettes illustrate qualitative features of the time course of each current following a voltage step (indicated above). Most of the currents are activated by depolarization, whereas $I_{Cl(V)}$ and I_Q are activated by hyperpolarization. $I_{Cl(V)}$ is inward, assuming that the activating step goes negative to E_{Cl-}. I_{NaP} and I_{CT} are marked with "?" because it has not been clearly shown that they are distinct from other currents.

Six voltage-dependent K currents have so far been described in CA1 pyramidal cells in hippocampal slices. Four of them seem to be purely voltage-gated (I_A, I_D, I_K, I_M), whereas two are activated by influx of Ca ions through voltage-gated Ca channels (I_C, I_{AHP}).

Three other Ca-dependent K currents have also been described: a transient one (here called "I_{CT}") in CA3 and CA1 cells (Zbicz and Weight, 1985; Storm, 1987c; Alger and Doerner, 1988), and two others ($I_{K1(Ca)}$, $I_{K2(Ca)}$) in acutely dissociated CA1 cells (Numann et al., 1987). However, it is not yet clear whether these currents are distinct from I_A, I_C and I_{AHP} (see below).

In addition to the voltage- and Ca-gated K currents, hippocampal pyradimal cells also have "leak" (i.e. largely voltage- and time-independent) and "resting" K currents, and receptor-operated K currents, which seem to underlie the resting potential and several responses to transmitter-substances.

For each of the voltage- and Ca-gated K currents, 8 topics will be considered: (1) in which hippocampal preparations and cells has the current been studied, (2) its relationship to other currents, (3) voltage- and time-dependence, (4) Ca-dependence, (5) sensitivity to ion channel blockers and other pharmacological manipulations, (6) functional role, (7) modulation by neurotransmitters, and (8) single channel data.

Voltage-gated calcium-independent K currents

I_A, the fast transient K current (synonym: $I_{K(A)}$)

(1) I_A was first reported in CA3 cells in slices from adult guinea-pigs by Gustafsson et al. (1982) and by Zbicz and Weight (1985). In these studies, the time course of inactivation could not be described by a single exponential. At least part of the current inactivated slowly (over hundreds of milliseconds), and could be blocked by low concentrations (0.1 – 0.5 mM of 4-aminopyridine (4-AP). In contrast, only an A current, which is less sensitive to fast-inactivating (mono-exponential) 4-AP, was found in cultured hippocampal pyramidal cells

from newborn rats (Segal and Barker, 1984; Segal et al., 1984; Alger and Doerner, 1988; Doerner et al., 1988) and in acutely dissociated pyramidal cells from adult guinea pigs (Numann et al., 1987; Alger and Doerner, 1988; Doerner et al., 1988). This suggests that there are at least two transient K currents (it is even possible that there are more than two kinds). Recently, two such currents (I_A and I_D) were found to co-exist in CA1 pyramidal cells (Storm, 1988a). Before this distinction was made, the term I_A usually included all 4-AP-sensitive Ca-independent transient K currents in hippocampal cells (e.g. Gustafsson et al., 1982; Storm, 1984; 1986a; see p. 735 in Storm, 1987a). Here, I will concentrate on the typical fast A-current; the slower current, I_D, will be discussed below.

(2 – 3) The fast hippocampal I_A resembles the A-currents in many other neurones (Connor and Stevens, 1971; Hille, 1984; Rogawsky, 1985; Rudy, 1988). It is activated by depolarization beyond about – 60 mV, and it inactivates between – 60 and – 40 mV (i.e. the inactivation starts at – 60 mV and is complete at – 40 mV). Both the activation (peaks within 10 ms at 30°C) and inactivation are quite fast (time constant typically 15 – 50 ms). I_A also recovers quickly from inactivation (time constant 10 – 50 ms; Storm, 1988a), in contrast to I_D.

(4) I_A persists in Ca-free medium and in the presence of Ca-channel blockers like cadmium (Cd), cobalt (Co) or manganese (Mn), so it is not Ca-dependent. Still, divalent cations tend to shift the activation and inactivation curves to more depolarized levels (Gustafsson et al., 1982; Numann et al., 1987; Storm, 1988a), probably due to surface-charge effects.

(5) I_A is blocked by 1 – 5 mM 4-amino-pyridine (4-AP) (Segal et al., 1984; Segal and Barker, 1984; Nakajima et al., 1986; Numann et al., 1987; Storm, 1988a). The 4-AP-block of I_A is voltage and time-dependent, being slowly relieved by depolarization (Numann et al., 1987; Storm, unpublished observations). In contrast, tetraethylammonium (TEA, 3 – 30 mM; Gustafsson et al., 1982; Segal and Barker, 1984) has little effect on

I_A. Dendrotoxin (DTX, 50 – 300 nM) from mamba snake venom (Harvey and Karlsson, 1980, 1982) inhibits I_A in CA1 pyramidal cells (Dolly et al., 1984; Halliwell et al., 1986), and this may contribute to the neurotoxicity of this peptide. However, recent evidence suggests that I_D may be partly responsible for the effects of DTX (see below).

(6) A classical role of I_A in invertebrates is to delay the onset of discharge in response to a depolarizing stimulus, and to permit slow repetitive firing. Thus, Connor and Stevens (1971) found that I_A recovers from inactivation during the after-hyperpolarization (AHP) after each spike, and turns on as the cell again depolarizes towards the spike threshold, thus delaying further depolarization until I_A has inactivated. Thereby, I_A prolongs each AHP, and slows down the firing rate.

I_A has been reported to play a similar role in some vertebrate neurones (Aghajanian, 1985), but it remains to be tested whether I_A is functionally important during repetitive firing in hippocampal pyramidal cells and most other cells where I_A exists. This cannot be tested simply by blocking I_A (e.g. with 4-AP), because the ensuing spike broadening (Storm, 1987a, 1988c) will cause secondary changes in a number of other voltage- and Ca-dependent currents, which also influence the firing rate. Still, it seems clear that the hippocampal I_A can delay the onset of firing for up to 100 ms or so (Gustafsson et al., 1982; Segal et al., 1984; Storm, 1984, 1988a).

I_A also seems to be involved in repolarization of the action potential, since the spike is broadened when I_A is blocked by 4-AP (Storm, 1987a, 1988c). This effect is not only due to blockade of I_D, because a further broadening is seen when 1 mM 4-AP (which blocks I_A) is applied after I_D has already been blocked by 40 μM 4-AP (Storm, unpublished observations). I_A and I_D seem to be particularly important for the early phase of repolarization, before I_C is fully turned on (Storm, 1987a, 1988c). I_A is also involved in spike repolarization in invertebrate nerve and muscle cells (e.g. Shimahara, 1983; Salkoff and Wyman, 1983) and mammalian sympathetic ganglia (Beluzzi et al., 1985; Beluzzi and Sacchi, 1988).

(7) I_A is subject to modulation by neurotransmitters both in invertebrate (Strong, 1984) and vertebrate (Aghajanian, 1985) neurones. In cultured hippocampal pyramidal cells, I_A can be reduced by muscarinic agonist (Nakajima et al., 1986). The effect resembled that of 4-AP in that both the activation and inactivation were shifted in the depolarizing direction, and both 4-AP (2.5 mM) and acetylcholine (0.1 μM) increased the amplitude and duration of the spike. However, muscarinic agonists do not seem to have these effects in slices from adult rats (Lancaster and Nicoll, 1987: 2 μM carbachol; Storm, unpublished: 1–100 μM carbachol). Phorbol esters, which activate protein kinase C and inhibit certain K currents (see below) do not seem to affect I_A (Doerner et al., 1988).

(8) VanDongen et al. (1988) reported single transient K channels in excised patches from the soma of cultured CA1 pyramidal cells. The conductance was 15 pS, the mean open time was 5 ms, and there were 1.5 openings per burst. The channels were insensitive to the G_o protein which is thought to couple K channels to $GABA_B$, serotonin and adenosine receptors.

I_D, the delay current (synonym: $I_{K(D)}$)

(1) I_D is found in CA1 pyramidal cells in rat hippocampal slices, where it co-exists with the faster I_A (Storm, 1988a, b). It differs from I_A in at least 3 respects: (a) I_D has slow kinetics, particularly inactivation and recovery from inactivation, (b) it has more negative thresholds for activation and inactivation, and (c) it is more sensitive to 4-AP. The transient K current of CA3 cells may also contain an I_D-like component, judged from the slow time course and sensitivity to 4-AP (Gustafsson et al., 1982; Zbicz and Weight, 1985). However, I_D has not been reported in cultured neurones from embryonic rats (Segal and Barker, 1984; Segal et al., 1984). Nor has it been reported from acutely dissociated cells from adult guinea pig hippocampus (Numann et al. 1987), although a similar current has been observed in some acutely dissociated rat hippocampal cells (Hernandes-Cruz and Storm, unpublished).

The term "I_D" has also been used to designate a *depolarizing* (inward) after-current in *Aplysia* neurones (Adams and Benson, 1985), and recently also the muscarine-induced *depolarizing* cation current in bullfrog sympathetic neurones (Tsuji and Kuba, 1988). When necessary to avoid confusion, the term $I_{K(D)}$ may be used.

(2) I_D resembles the slowly inactivating, highly

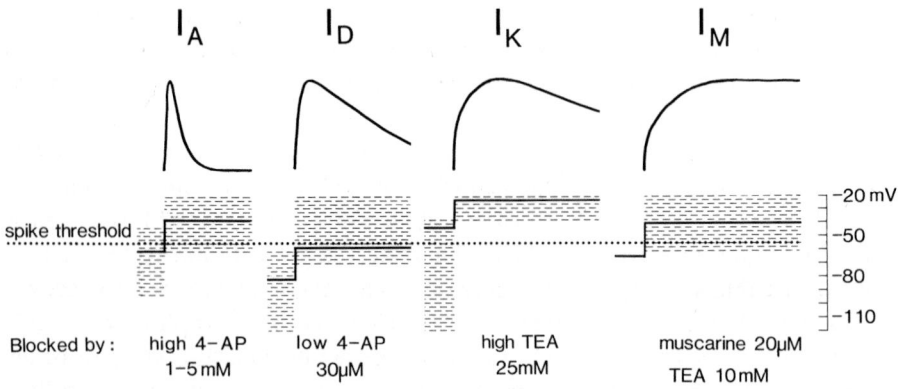

Fig. 2. Schematic representation of the four voltage-gated, Ca-independent currents, I_A, I_D, I_K and I_M, indicating roughly the time-course (drawings of idealized currents), the approximate voltage ranges of inactivation and activation (shaded areas), typical voltage steps used to activate the currents (solid lines), and effective blocking agents and their concentrations. Note that I_A, I_K, and I_M start to activate below the spike threshold (dotted line), whereas I_K can only be activated during action potentials. (Adapted from Storm, 1988.)

4-AP-sensitive K current found in some visceral sensory neurones (Stansfield et al., 1986, 1987). The latter current is also highly sensitive to dendrotoxin, and has been dubbed I_{DTX} (Stansfeld and Feltz, 1988). I_{DTX} resembles I_D in being quite resistant to TEA, barium (Ba) and caesium (Cs). However, I_{DTX} inactivates incompletely, and its main effect was to inhibit repetitive firing; it has not been shown to cause discharge delays. A DTX-sensitive K current found in dorsal root ganglion cells (I_K^s) shows even less inactivation (Penner et al., 1986). One of the fast-activating K currents in frog myelinated axons (I_{Kfl}; Schwartz and Vogel, 1971; Dubois, 1981, 1983) resembles I_D in being highly sensitive to 4-AP and DTX, but differs from I_D by being far more sensitive to TEA (and capsaicin) and in its kinetics of inactivation and recovery. All of these currents may belong to a subgroup of "delayed rectifier" K currents (Rudy, 1988), although it has also been suggested that some of them are more related to the A currents. Current clamp evidence suggests that currents similar to I_D may also exist in other vertebrate central neurones, e.g. in the inferior olive (Yarom and Llinas, 1987), neocortical pyramidal cells (Spain et al., 1988) and cerebellar Purkinje cells (Hounsgaard and Midtgaard, 1988, 1989).

(3) I_D is activated by depolarizations beyond -70 mV, within about 20 ms, and inactivates over several seconds. The exact time course of the activation is not known, but the current obtained by subtraction of records before and after 30 μM 4-AP, peaks in about 20 ms at 30°C. Inactivation starts at about -120 mV and is complete at -60 mV. The inactivation time course can usually not be fitted by a single exponential. The recovery from inactivation is extremely slow (time constant about 5 s at -90 mV), and this accounts for its ability to "integrate" depolarizing inputs over seconds (Storm, 1988a and below).

(4 – 5) I_D persist after blockade of Ca channels by cadmium (Cd, 200 – 600 μM), so it is not dependent on Ca influx. It is highly sensitive to 4-AP, being blocked by about 30 μM. The ability of micromolar concentrations of 4-AP to facilitate synaptic transmission and cause seizures in the hippocampus and other cortical regions (Buckle and Haas, 1982; Galvan et al., 1982; Rutecki et al., 1987), may be due to blockade of I_D or a related K current in the synaptic terminals, since higher concentrations of 4-AP are required to inhibit I_A and other known cortical K currents. In contrast to 4-AP, other K channel blockers have little effect on I_D. Thus, it resists TEA (25 mM), Ba (1 mM), Cs (1 mM), and capsaicin (20 μM, which inhibits I_{Kf} in frog axons; Dubois, 1983). Preliminary data suggest that dendrotoxin (DTX) and Toxin 1 from mamba snake venom block I_D at nanomolar concentrations (unpublished). Thus, I_D channels may contribute to the binding and convulsive effects of these and related toxins (Othman et al., 1982; Rehm and Betz, 1982, 1984; Dolly et al., 1984; Halliwell et al., 1986).

(6) I_D can cause a several seconds long delay in the onset of firing in response to long-lasting depolarizing stimuli. This is because I_D activates rapidly upon depolarization and tends to keep the cell from depolarizing further; only as I_D slowly inactivates will the cell reach threshold and fire with a delay. This is similar to the classical function of I_A (Connor and Stevens, 1971), but I_D can cause far longer delays, up to about 15 seconds. In Aplysia ink motoneurones, a similar slowly inactivating K current plays a behavioural role in delaying the inking reflex (Carew and Kandel, 1977; Byrne, 1980).

I_D is largely inactivated when the resting potential is positive to -65 mV, and its effect can be masked by I_M and I_Q which cause an initial overshoot in response to a depolarizing current pulse. Therefore, I_D seems to be effective only in cells with a highly negative resting potential.

Because I_D takes up to about 20 s to recover from inactivation it enables the cell to "integrate" separate depolarizing inputs over several seconds. Thus, the response of the cell does not only reflect the immediate synaptic input; it will also take into account what happened in the preceding seconds (Storm, 1988a). In cerebellar Purkinje cells, a current resembling I_D has been suggested to participate in dendritic processing (Hounsgaard and Midtgaard, 1988, 1989).

The rapid activation of I_D suggest that it may also participate in spike repolarization. This is supported by the finding that $30-100$ μM 4-AP broadens the action potential (Storm, 1987a, 1988c and unpublished). Micromolar concentrations of 4-AP also facilitate transmitter release, both in the periphery (Thesleff, 1980) and in the brain (Buckle and Haas, 1982; Galvan et al., 1982; Rutecki et al., 1987), presumably by broadening the presynaptic action potential and thus increasing the influx of calcium (Haas et al., 1983). If I_D or a similar current exists in the presynaptic terminals of cortical neurones, it could contribute to the synaptic facilitation caused by 4-AP, DTX and mast-cell degranulating peptide (Othman et al., 1982; Docherty et al., 1983; Cherubini et al., 1987; Bidard et al., 1987; Stansfeld et al., 1987; Rehm and Lazdunski, 1988; Schmidt et al., 1988).

In some hippocampal pyramidal cells, low concentrations of 4-AP or DTX cause a small depolarization of the resting potential, accompanied by an increase in input resistance, and similar effects can be seen under voltage clamp when the holding potential is near -70 mV (Storm, unpublished). This may reflect a steady I_D (or I_A) "window" current, due to the overlap of the activation and inactivation curves (Storm,

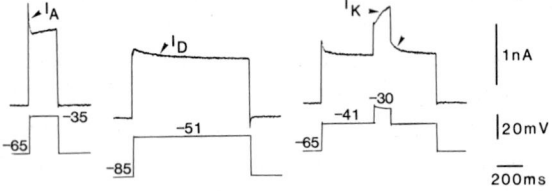

Fig. 3. Example of how 3 of the voltage-gated currents, I_A, I_D and I_K can be separated by using different voltage-clamp commands. I_A is activated by a step from a holding potential of -65 mV (where I_D is largely inactivated) to -35 mV. I_D is activated by stepping from -85 mV to -51 mV. I_K is brought out by first inactivating I_A with a step to -41 mV, and then stepping to -30 mV to activate I_K. In this cell, I_{Na} was blocked by 1 μM TTX, I_{Ca}, I_C and I_{AHP} were blocked by 200 μM Cd, I_M was blocked (and I_K slightly reduced) by 5 mM TEA and I_Q and $I_{Cl(V)}$ were blocked by 2 mM Cs and 0.5 mM 9-anthracene carboxylate, respectively. (Unpublished experiment.)

1988a). Thus, I_D may slightly contribute to the resting potential.

(7 – 8) No evidence for modulation of I_D has been reported, and single channel data for the hippocampal I_D have not been presented so far. The DTX-sensitive channels of sensory neurones have conductances ranging from 17 to 23 pS in symmetrical KCl (Stansfeld and Feltz, 1988).

I_K, the "delayed rectifier" potassium current (synonym: $I_{K(DR)}$)

(1) I_K has been recorded in dissociated cell cultures from fetal rats (Segal and Barker, 1984), in acutely dissociated hippocampal pyramidal cells from adult guinea pigs (Numann et al., 1988) and in CA1 cells in slices from adult rats (Madison et al., 1987; Storm, 1988a, b).

(2) The term "delayed rectifier" has generally been applied to several different kinds of K currents (Hille, 1984; Rudy, 1988). The hippocampal I_K seems to belong to the high-threshold, slow, TEA-sensitive group of "delayed rectifier" currents (Rudy, 1988).

(3) I_K is activated by depolarization beyond -40 mV. Thus, unlike I_A, I_D and I_M, it activates only during action potentials, not at subthreshold levels. The activation is rather slow ($\tau = 20-80$ ms in slices at 30°C: Storm, unpublished; τ, about 180 ms in cultured cells at 23°C: Segal and Barker, 1984; time to peak, 180 ms in acutely dissociated cells: Numann et al., 1987). This slowness is probably not an artefact due to poor space clamp, because a similar time course is seen both in acutely dissociated cells which have lost most of their dendrites (Numann et al., 1987) and in single channel recordings (Rogawsky, 1986; see however Maukawa et al., 1987).

The time constant of activation and deactivation varies with the voltage in a bell-shaped manner, being maximal (about 80 ms) at about -45 mV, approaching 20 ms at -20 mV and -80 mV (Storm, unpublished). Unless the time constant becomes considerably shorter at more positive potentials, only a small fraction of I_K will be activated by an action potential. Still, it could contribute appreciably to spike repolarization if the total available I_K is very large at depolarized potentials, as suggested by voltage clamp data (culture: Segal and Barker, 1984; slice: Storm, unpublished). For example, a step to -35 mV already elicits about 9 nA of I_K (Segal and Barker, 1984).

I_K inactivates monoexponentially over several seconds ($\tau = 3-5$ s; Segal and Barker, 1984; Numann et al., 1987; Storm, 1988a, b and unpublished). Some, but not all, of the apparent inactivation recorded in slices can be attributed to extracellular K accumulation (Storm, unpublished).

I_K recovers from inactivation about 10 times as fast as I_D at highly negative membrane potentials (τ about 600 ms at -110 mV; Storm, unpublished). Both activation, inactivation and deactivation appear to be mono-exponential.

So far, a fairly consistent picture of I_K seems to emerge. However, Sah et al. (1988) report a fast-activating K current in acutely dissociated cells (τ, $1-7$ ms at $22-24°C$). This current also inactivates faster than I_K (τ, 450 ms), but it resembles I_K (and not I_D) in that it is resistant to 1 mM 4-AP and blocked by 30 mM TEA. Doerner et al. (1988), using acute dissociation and cultures, found a persistent K current which also seems to activate rapidly (their Fig. 1C). It is not clear how these fast K currents relate to the much slower I_K recorded previously (even with similar techniques; Numann et al., 1987).

(4–5) I_K persists when Ca-influx has been eliminated by Ca-free medium, or by the Ca-channel blockers Mn or Cd. It is blocked by relatively high concentrations of external TEA (partly by 5 mM, completely by $25-30$ mM), and is little affected by 4-AP ($0.1-5$ mM). I_K is also resistant to external caesium (Cs, 1 mM), which blocks I_Q. I_K is blocked by the psychotomimetic drug phencyclidine, but only at much higher concentrations ($IC_{50} = 17$ μM) than NMDA channels ($IC_{50} = 0.4$ μM), so I_K blockade is probably not responsible for the behavioural effects of the drug (ffrench-Mullen et al., 1988a, b).

(6) The exact function of I_K is not known.

Although quite slow, it may contribute to the repolarization of the action potential, because the peak of the spike is broadened by 5 mM TEA, which hardly affects I_A or I_D (Storm, 1988c). Voltage clamp measurements show that I_K becomes very large beyond -20 mV (Storm, unpublished), and this may allow it to contribute appreciably to the spike in spite of its relatively slow kinetics. I_K seems to contribute little or nothing to the after-hyperpolarizations (AHPs) following multiple spikes (which are dominated by I_{AHP}, I_M and I_C), but may cause a brief AHP after single spikes when I_C has been blocked (Storm, 1989).

(7) Modulation by transmitter substances have not been reported for I_K. The persistent K current studied by Doerner et al. (1988) was reduced by activators of protein kinase C (phorbol esters or 1-oleyl-2-acetylglycerol). This effect might explain why phorbol esters can enhance Ca spikes (Malenka et al., 1986) and broaden Na action potentials (Storm, 1987c, 1988d). However, the typical slowly activating I_K of CA1 cells in slices does not seem to be reduced by active phorbol esters (Storm, unpublished).

(8) Single K channels ($15-20$ pS) which may underlie I_K have been recorded in hippocampal cultures by Rogawsky (1986). They resembled the macroscopic I_K in that the probability of opening following a step depolarization increased exponentially with a time constant of about 100 ms. The channel openings were also independent of Ca, and were not observed in the presence of 20 mM TEA. Masukawa and Hansen (1987) found non-inactivating K channels (10 pS) in both somatic and dendritic patches. These channels were, however, considerably faster (ensemble averages showed peak current in 5 ms), more like the current reported by Sah et al. (1988) and Doerner et al. (1988).

I_M, the M-current (synonym: $I_{K(M)}$)

(1) I_M was one of the first hippocampal K currents to be recorded by voltage-clamp, in CA1 cells of rat hippocampal slices (Halliwell and Adams, 1982; reviewed by Adams and Galvan, 1986;

Brown, 1988a, b). It has later been recorded in CA3 and CA1 cells in fresh slices (Brown and Griffith, 1983; Madison et al., 1987; Storm, 1989) and in slice cultures (Gähwiler and Brown, 1985), but has so far not been clearly identified in dissociated cells in culture (Segal and Barker, 1984) or acutely dissociated cells (Numann et al., 1987; Sah et al., 1988).

(2) The hippocampal M current resembles closely the one in sympathetic ganglia (Brown and Adams, 1980; Adams et al., 1982), although I_M in the hippocampus is somewhat more sensitive to TEA (Storm, 1989). The TEA sensitivity is similar for I_M in olfactory cortex (Constanti and Sim, 1987).

(3) The M current is activated by depolarizations beyond about -60 mV. It activates and deactivates slowly and mono-exponentially (τ, about 50 ms) and does not inactivate. Thus, it behaves as if it is governed by a single voltage-sensitive gating particle, like in frog ganglia (Adams et al., 1982).

(4) I_M is Ca-independent; it persists in Ca-free medium with Mn or Cd. (5) It is blocked by bath-application of 1 mM Ba, or $5-10$ mM TEA, but not by 1 mM Cs, or $0.1-1$ mM 4-AP (Halliwell and Adams, 1982; Storm, 1989 and unpublished).

(6) The classical roles of I_M in frog ganglia are to stabilize the resting potential, to produce spike frequency adaptation, and to mediate muscarinic and peptidergic excitation (Brown and Adams, 1980; Adams et al., 1982; Adams and Brown, 1982; Jones et al., 1984; Jones, 1985; Adams et al., 1986; see, however, Jones, 1989). Thus, when the resting potential is within the activation range of I_M, any imposed depolarization will activate more M current, which will polarize the cell back towards the resting potential; and during an imposed hyperpolarization I_M will turn off and thus reduce the hyperpolarization. In this way, I_M can "clamp" the membrane potential at the resting level, and when I_M is blocked by acetylcholine and some peptides, the cell becomes more sensitive to other inputs, both because it depolarizes, *and* because the membrane resistance increases.

In hippocampal pyramidal cells, I_M underlies an early phase of spike frequency adaptation (Madison and Nicoll, 1984), and it seems to be the main factor in the medium AHP which follows a single spike or a spike burst (Storm, 1989). However, I_M does not seem to contribute much to the resting potential which seems to be negative (about -70 mV) to the activation threshold for I_M (about -60 mV) in these cells. Still, I_M will tend to attenuate depolarizing inputs, in particular those of long duration. Thus, the voltage response to injection of a subthreshold depolarizing current pulse typically shows a "sag" due to the delayed opening of M channels, and an undershoot (corresponding to the mAHP) after the pulse, due to the slow closing of M channels. Although I_M is partly activated by a single spike, it is too slow and small to contribute noticeably to spike repolarization (Storm, 1989). It has been estimated that a single spike will activate about 10% of the available I_M in a CA1 cell, in contrast to about 5% in frog ganglia (Pennefather, 1986; Storm, unpublished).

(7) In most cell types, I_M can be inhibited by acetylcholine and other *m*uscarinic agonists, hence the name *M* current. When this effect was first discovered in frog ganglia, it was the first example of modulation of a voltage-gated channel by a transmitter substance in a vertebrate neurone (Brown and Adams, 1980).

Gähwiler and Brown (1985), using co-cultured hippocampal and septal tissue, found that I_M is inhibited during a slow cholinergic EPSP elicited by stimulation of the septal explant. In slices, however, I_M does not seem to contribute much to the slow EPSP, unless an anti-cholinesterase drug is added (Madison et al., 1987). Instead, the slow EPSP in slices seems to be due mainly to blockade of a voltage- and time-independent "leak" K current (see below).

The M_2 subtype of muscarinic receptors seems to be involved in the cholinergic inhibition of I_M (Dutar and Nicoll, 1988). Only strong agonists of phosphoinositide (PI) turnover are effective, suggesting that this second messenger system is involved. However, the hippocampal M current is resistant to activators of protein kinase C (Malenka et al., 1986). Instead, it is reduced by intracellular application of inositol trisphosphate (IP_3) (Dutar and Nicoll, 1988), although different results have been obtained in other cell types (Higashida and Brown, 1986; Brown and Adams, 1987; Brown and Higashida, 1988; Pfaffinger et al., 1988). IP_3 does not seem to inhibit I_M by releasing Ca from internal stores, because the cholinergic effect was resistant to intracellular application of the Ca-buffers EGTA and BAPTA. In frog ganglia, a pertussis toxin-resistant G-protein seems to be involved (Jones, 1987; Lopez et al., 1987; Pfaffinger, 1988), and the cholinergic inhibition of the rat hippocampal I_M is also resistant to pertussis toxin (Dutar and Nicoll, 1988).

I_M may be modulated by other transmitter substances as well. Colino and Halliwell (1987) found that I_M is reduced by serotonin. However, Andrade and Nicoll (1986) found no effect on I_M. Instead, they saw a reduction of a voltage-independent "leak" K current which is distinct from I_M (see below). Somatostatin (Som 14 and Som 28, $0-1$ μM), on the other hand, seems to enhance I_M in rat CA1 cells (Moore et al., 1988; Watson and Pittman, 1988). This effect resembles the effect of noradrenaline in smooth muscle cells (Sims et al., 1988), but noradrenaline has no effect on the hippocampal M current (Gähwiler and Brown, 1985; Madison and Nicoll, 1986a).

(8) Single M channels have recently been recorded in frog ganglia (Gruner et al., 1989), but not yet in the hippocampus.

$I_{K(IR)}$, fast inward rectifier K current (synonym: $I_{f.i.r.}$)

$I_{K(IR)}$ has been reported in cultured hippocampal neurones (Owen, 1987), where it was partially activated at the resting potential (-60 mV), peaked within 5 ms, and inactivated at potentials more negative than -100 mV (τ, about 35 ms at -115 mV). In current clamp it produced non-sagging voltage-responses to hyperpolarizing current injection. Thus, it differs from the *slow* inward rectifier current, I_Q (see below). $I_{K(IR)}$ may correspond to

the classical fast inward (or "anomalous") rectifier K current e.g. in muscle and egg cells (Adrian, 1969; Hagiwara and Jaffe, 1979). A similar current has been recorded in pyramidal neurones of olfactory cortex (Constanti and Galvan, 1983), where it is activated by hyperpolarizations beyond the resting potential, and can be blocked by Cs and Ba ions.

I_Q, slow mixed Na/K inward rectifier current

I_Q is activated by hyperpolarization beyond -80 mV (Halliwell and Adams, 1982). Since it is not a pure K current (it is carried by both Na and K, and is an inward current throughout its activation range), it will not be discussed further here.

Calcium-dependent K-currents

The existence of a Ca-activated K conductance in hippocampal neurones was first revealed by current clamp experiments (Alger and Nicoll, 1980; Hotson and Prince, 1980; Schwartzkroin and Stafstrom, 1980). In the first voltage clamp study (Brown and Griffith, 1983a), the Ca-activated K current was designated I_C. Later, Lancaster and Adams (1986) found that there are actually *two* different Ca-dependent K currents in hippocampal pyramidal cells, a fast and TEA-sensitive one, now called I_C, and a slow and TEA-resistant one, called I_{AHP}. Current clamp experiments indicate that a fast TEA-sensitive Ca-dependent K current, thought to be I_C, is involved in spike repolarization and the fast AHP (Storm, 1985, 1987; Lancaster et al., 1986; Lancaster and Nicoll, 1987), whereas I_{AHP} generates the slow AHP (Lancaster and Adams, 1986).

I_C, the "fast" Ca-dependent K-current (synonym: $I_{K(C)}$)

(1 – 2) I_C is probably related to the C current in sympathetic ganglia (Adams et al., 1982b), and similar currents in other cells. I_C is thought to be mediated by the ubiquitous large-conductance "BK" channels, or related channels, which are both Ca- and voltage-dependent, non-inactivating,

and highly sensitive to external TEA (Marty, 1981; Barrett et al., 1982; Adams et al., 1982; Farley and Rudy, 1988; Reinhart et al., 1989). In invertebrates, the term I_C has also been applied to *slow* Ca-dependent K currents (Thompson, 1977; Adams et al., 1980) and a fast *transient* Ca-dependent K current (Elkins et al., 1986; Elkins and Ganetsky, 1988).

(3) I_C is activated by depolarization beyond about -40 mV. This corresponds to the activation range for the high-threshold Ca-current (Johnston et al., 1980; Brown and Griffith, 1983b). During depolarizing steps to about -30 mV or less, I_C grows slowly for more than a second (Brown and

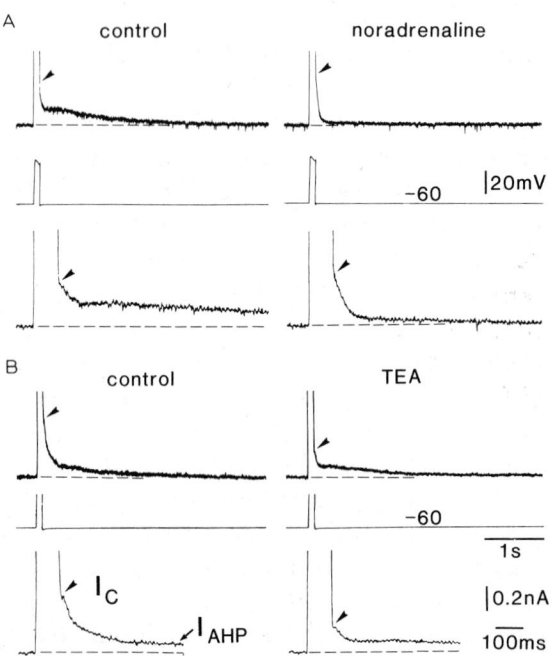

Fig. 4. Separation of the two Ca-dependent K currents, I_C and I_{AHP}, which are elicited by a brief depolarizing voltage clamp step. In this case the currents which flow after return to the holding current (tail currents) are studied. The outward tail current shows a fast and a slow component. The slow tail, I_{AHP}, is blocked by 5 μM noradrenaline (A), but not by 1.5 mM TEA. In contrast, a component of the fast tail, I_C, is blocked by TEA (B), but not by noradrenaline (A). The remaining part of the fast tail current consists mainly of I_M (which is also partly blocked by 1.5 mM TEA). TTX (1 μM) was present throughout. Note the different time scales in upper and lower traces. (Unpublished experiment.)

Griffith, 1983a; Lancaster and Adams, 1986). This sluggish behaviour seems to speak against a major role in spike repolarization. However, much faster voltage-dependent gating may become more important at depolarized potentials. The tail current has a time constant close to 50 ms at -60 mV (Brown and Griffith, 1983a; Lancaster and Adams, 1986; Madison et al., 1987; Storm, 1989). Brown and Griffith (1983a) found even slower tails, which may have contained a component of I_{AHP}.

However, tail currents following single action potentials or spike-like voltage-clamp steps have a faster component (time constant about 15 ms: Storm, unpublished), which also is sensitive to Cd, TEA and charybdotoxin (CTX). The faster component could represent direct voltage-gating of the channels, whereas the slow tail may reflect further closing due to the decline of $[Ca]_i$. Different phases of Ca sequestration may also give rise to different kinetic components of the I_C tails.

Since BK channels generally require both Ca influx and depolarization to be fully activated, this is likely to be true also for the hippocampal I_C. Thus, Brown and Griffith (1983a) found that the deactivation time constant was voltage-dependent (between -40 and -70 mV). Lancaster and Adams (1986), measuring the fast (I_C) and the slow (I_{AHP}) tail currents separately, did not see such an effect, but they suggested that this might be due to the limited voltage range tested (-65 to -50 mV).

(4) I_C is clearly dependent on influx of Ca ions, since it is eliminated by Ca-free medium and by adding the Ca-channel blockers Mn, Cd or Co, or by injection of the fast Ca chelator BAPTA. This has been inferred from current clamp recordings (Storm, 1985, 1987a; Lancaster et al., 1986; Lancaster and Nicoll, 1987) and shown in voltage clamp (Lancaster and Adams, 1986; Madison et al., 1987; Storm, 1989).

(5) I_C is also blocked by low concentrations of external TEA (5 mM: Brown and Griffith, 1983a; 2 mM: Lancaster and Adams, 1986; 0.5 – 1 mM: Lancaster and Nicoll, 1987; Storm, 1985, 1987a,

1989), and by CTX 1 (10–30 nM; current clamp: Lancaster et al., 1986; Lancaster and Nicoll, 1987; Storm, 1987a; voltage clamp: Storm, unpublished). CTX was first known as a potent blocker of BK channels from muscle (Miller et al., 1985), but is has later been shown to also block small Ca-dependent K channels, and even some Ca-independent K channels (Hermann and Erxleben, 1987; Farley and Rudy, 1988; MacKinnon et al., 1988; Reinhart et al., 1989).

(6) Like in frog sympathetic ganglia (Adams et al., 1982), I_C seems to be important for spike repolarization in the hippocampus (Storm, 1985; Lancaster et al., 1986). Thus, I_C seems to be mainly responsible for the last two thirds of the spike repolarization and the fast AHP. The spike broadens and the fast AHP disappears when I_C is blocked by external TEA (0.5–1 mM), CTX, or Ca-channel blockers, or by intracellular injection of the fast Ca chelator, BAPTA (Storm, 1985, 1987a, b; Lancaster et al., 1986; Lancaster and Nicoll, 1987). EGTA, however, does not broaden the spike, presumably because it binds Ca ions too slowly. Thus, it appears that I_C is triggered by Ca influx during the action potential, probably assisted by the depolarization itself.

I_C also contributes, along with I_M (Storm, 1989), to the medium AHP (50–100 ms duration; Gustafsson and Wigström, 1981), and to an early phase of spike frequency adaptation (Lancaster and Nicoll, 1987). During epileptiform activity, I_C seems to be important for the termination of the interictal spike (Alger and Williamson, 1988).

Why are the fast AHP and the Ca-dependent component of the medium AHP separate if they both are caused by I_C? One possibility is that most of I_C turns off shortly after the spike, due to fast voltage-dependent gating, and that the Ca-dependent mAHP is due to C channels which remain slightly active even after the cell has repolarized as long as $[Ca]_i$ is elevated. Alternatively, some C channels could be rapidly activated if they are located close to the Ca channels (Lancaster and Nicoll, 1987), whereas others may be more remote. In addition, if the I_C-dependent spike-repolarization is fastest at the soma, positive charge stored in the dendritic membrane capacitance may be redistributed from the dendrites to the soma after the spike, thus contributing to the after-depolarization which separates the fAHP and the mAHP (Storm et al., 1987). Alternatively, the fast AHP could be due to a fast transient Ca-dependent K current, I_{CT} (see below).

(7) In striking contrast to I_{AHP}, modulation of I_C by neurotransmitters has not been reported. Thus, I_C is resistant to both noradrenaline (2–10 μM; Lancaster and Adams, 1986) and muscarinic agonists (Madison et al., 1987).

(8) Currents through large-conductance (140–270 pS) Ca-dependent K channels, which may mediate I_C, have been recorded in patches from cultured and acutely dissociated hippocampal neurones (Brett and Lancaster, 1985; Brett et al., 1986; Franciolini, 1988; Ikemoto et al., 1989). The probability of opening increases both with the Ca concentration and with depolarization of the patch. At 0 mV, the channels begin to open at $[Ca]_i = 1$ μM, and are half activated at 4 μM. At a fixed $[Ca]_i = 10$ μM, the open probability is 0.5 at −15 mV and increases e-fold for each 14 mV depolarization (Franciolini, 1988). However, there was a considerable delay in the opening of the channels in response to an abrupt increase in $[Ca]_i$; at +40 mV the delay was 200 ms for 12 μM Ca, 113 ms for 100 μM Ca and 18 ms for 1000 μM Ca (Ikemoto et al., 1989). This speaks against a role for BK channels in spike repolarization, unless the channel kinetics had been altered during the isolation procedure. The channels can be blocked by application of TEA (5–30 mM), barium (1 mM), or the calmodulin inhibitors W-7 and W-5 to the cytoplasmic surface (Brett and Lancaster, 1985; Ikemoto et al., 1989).

It is possible that I_C is mediated by a family of related channels. It has recently been shown that rat brain membranes contain multiple voltage-sensitive, non-inactivating, Ca-activated K channels which are highly sensitive to TEA and CTX (Farley and Rudy, 1988; Reinhart et al., 1989).

I_{CT}, fast transient Ca-dependent K current (synonym: $I_{K(CT)}$)

In addition to I_C and I_{AHP}, a fast *transient* Ca-dependent K current (which here will be called I_{CT}) has been reported in CA3 cells in slices, and in cultured and acutely dissociated hippocampal pyramidal cells (Zbicz and Weight, 1985; Alger and Doerner, 1988). I_{CT} was found to activate rapidly above -45 mV, and to inactivate within about 20 ms. It was reduced by 10 mM TEA, cadmium, manganese and Ca-free medium, but resisted 0.5 mM 4-AP (Zbicz and Weight, 1985; Alger and Doerner, 1988).

A similar current has been observed in rat CA1 cells in slices, where it can be blocked by the same low TEA concentration (1 mM) that inhibits spike repolarization (Storm, 1987c). However, this current was only observed when high-resistance micro-electrodes were used, and the clamp voltage showed transient oscillations; it was not seen when a faster clamp was obtained with low-resistance electrodes (Storm, unpublished). Thus, it is not clear whether I_{CT} is actually a distinct current, or merely represents transient activation of I_C due to transient Ca influx or poor voltage control (Brown et al., 1982). It has also been suggested that I_{CT} could be identical to I_A (Numann et al., 1987), which may appear to be Ca-dependent due to the surface charge effects of divalent cations (Frankenhaeuser and Hodgkin, 1957; Gustafsson et al., 1982; Mayer and Sugiyama, 1988).

Although transient Ca-dependent K currents have also been reported in other vertebrate neurones (e.g. frog ganglia: MacDermott and Weight, 1982; neocortical pyramidal cells: Schwindt et al., 1988), it is still not clear whether they represent a distinct class of channels.

Recently, Ikemoto et al. (1989) observed transient openings of large K channels (BK channels) in 19% of patches from hippocampal neurones. Although the activation latency, following a step increase in the Ca concentration, appeared too long for the channels to be involved in spike repolarization, these observations support the idea of a transient Ca-dependent K current component.

I_{AHP}, slow Ca-dependent K current (synonym, $I_{K(AHP)}$)

(1 – 2) I_{AHP} resembles the AHP-current of frog sympathetic neurones in being slow, TEA-resistant, and with little or no intrinsic voltage-dependence (Pennefather et al., 1985; Lancaster and Adams, 1986). But it differs from the AHP-currents of frog ganglia and cat spinal motoneurones (Zhang and Krnjević, 1987) by being insensitive to the bee toxin *apamin* (Lancaster and Adams, 1986; Storm, 1989).

(3) I_{AHP} is activated by depolarizations which cause Ca influx. It activates slowly, over at least a second (Fig. 9 in Lancaster and Adams, 1986). Following a brief depolarizing step, the I_{AHP} tail current shows a distinct rising phase and peaks in 400 – 700 ms, like the slow AHP does in current clamp. The deactivation is even slower; the time constant (about 1.5 s at 30°C) is largely independent of the size of the current and the membrane potential (between -90 and -30 mV, Fig. 4C in Lancaster and Adams, 1986). It is not clear whether the slowness of I_{AHP} is partly intrinsic to the channels or whether it just reflects the time-course of the intracellular Ca concentration or subsequent biochemical steps. Diffusion of calcium from the Ca-channels to the AHP-channels, or release of Ca from internal stores, may also contribute to the time-course.

(4 – 5) I_{AHP} is clearly dependent on influx of Ca ions, as it is eliminated by Ca-free medium and Ca-channel blockers. It is, however, completely resistant to concentrations of TEA which wipes out I_C (1 – 5 mM; Lancaster and Adams, 1986). It is also resistant to 1 mM 4-AP in CA1 cells (Storm, unpublished). Kainic acid has been found to reduce the slow AHP (Ashwood et al., 1986; Gho et al., 1986), and this may contribute to the epileptogenic and excitotoxic effects of this drug. The slow AHP is also reduced by neuroleptics (Dinan et al., 1987).

(6) I_{AHP} provides a strong negative feedback control of the activity of the cell. Thus, I_{AHP} is activated by Ca influx during the action potentials, and it increases strongly with the number of spikes

(Lancaster and Adams, 1986). It generates the slow AHP which follows spike bursts and single spikes, and tends to suppress further discharge by hyperpolarizing the cell and shunting depolarizing inputs. Accordingly, I_{AHP} is mainly responsible for the strong spike frequency adaptation which is typical of pyramidal neurones (Madison and Nicoll, 1982, 1984). Still, an early phase of adaptation, which is mainly due to I_M and I_C, persists when I_{AHP} has been blocked (Madison and Nicoll, 1984; Lancaster and Nicoll, 1987; Jones and Heinemann, 1988). In contrast to I_C, I_{AHP} does not contribute to repolarization of single action potentials (Lancaster and Nicoll, 1987; Storm, 1987a).

(7) I_{AHP} can be regulated by several transmitter substances (acetylcholine, noradrenaline, histamine, serotonin, dopamine, adenosine, and corticotropin releasing factor). The regulation of I_{AHP} is probably one of the main effector mechanisms for some of these neuromodulators. The powerful dampening effect of I_{AHP} may render it a strategic target for modulatory control by signal substances. Similar mechanisms exist in several other neurones, including neocortical pyramidal cells (Schwindt et al., 1988).

(a) Acetylcholine and muscarinic agonists inhibit I_{AHP} (Benardo and Prince, 1982; Cole and Nicoll, 1983, 1984a, b; Madison et al., 1987). I_{AHP} is about 10-fold more sensitive to muscarinic agonists than I_M (with carbachol, IC_{50} is approximately 0.3 μM for I_{AHP} and 5 μM for I_M; Madison et al., 1987). Thus, I_{AHP} is suppressed during the slow cholinergic EPSP which follows stimulation of cholinergic fibers in stratum oriens, and this may be the main mechanism of cholinergic excitation (Cole and Nicoll, 1983, 1984a, b).

The effect on I_{AHP} seems to be mediated by M_1 receptors (Dutar and Nicoll, 1988; see however Muller and Misgeld, 1986). The signal pathway from the muscarinic receptors to the AHP channels is not known. It may involve PI turnover and activation of protein kinase C, since I_{AHP} is suppressed by active phorbol esters (Baraban et al., 1985; Malenka et al., 1986; Dutar and Nicoll,

1988). Although muscarine can inhibit the Ca current (Gähwiler and Brown, 1987), the suppression of I_{AHP} by muscarinic agonist is probably not due to a reduction in the Ca influx, since the Ca spikes which activate I_{AHP} were not attenuated (Cole and Nicoll, 1984a). Alternatively, cyclic GMP could be involved, since it can depress the slow AHP (Cole and Nicoll, 1984b).

(b) Noradrenaline (2 – 10 μM), acting via β_1 receptors and cyclic AMP, also blocks I_{AHP}, without reducing the Ca current (Madison and Nicoll, 1982, 1984 and 1986a, b; Haas and Konnerth, 1983; Lancaster and Adams, 1986; Storm, 1987a, 1989). It has been suggested that cyclic AMP-dependent protein kinase may phosphorylate the I_{AHP} channel itself (Nicoll, 1988). Although noradrenaline also affects the resting potential (see below), the suppression of I_{AHP} is probably the principal mechanism whereby the noradrenergic in put from the locus coeruleus can influence hippocampal excitability (Madison and Nicoll, 1986a). By both hyperpolarizing the cell and reducing the inhibition by I_{AHP}, noradrenaline may suppress the effects of small, just threshold depolarizations, while enhancing the response to strong depolarizations. Thus, it may increase the signal-to-noise ratio for excitatory inputs to the cell.

(c) Histamine, acting on H_2 receptors, also reduces I_{AHP}, probably through cyclic AMP, without attenuating the Ca spikes (Haas and Konnerth, 1983; Haas and Greene, 1986; Pellmar, 1986).

(d) Serotonin (5-HT) also reduces I_{AHP} without affecting Ca spikes (Andrade and Nicoll, 1987; Colino and Halliwell, 1987). This effect seems to depend on a previously unidentified receptor type, and a pertussis toxin-sensitive G-protein is not involved, unlike the hyperpolarizing effect of 5-HT (Andrade et al., 1986). Nor does cAMP seem to be involved (Andrade and Nicoll, 1987).

(e) Adenosine (10 μM) has been reported to increase the slow AHP and spike-frequency adaptation, without a similar increase in the Ca spikes, suggesting an enhancement of I_{AHP} (Haas and

Greene, 1984).

(f) Dopamine was first reported to enhance I_{AHP} in CA1 pyramidal cells (Benardo and Prince, 1982; Haas and Konnerth, 1983), but Malenka and Nicoll (1986) found that dopamine (1 – 100 μM) *reduced* I_{AHP} by acting on β-adrenergic receptors.

(g) Corticotropin-releasing factor (CRF) also reduces I_{AHP} in CA1 and CA3 pyramidal cells. Again, cyclic AMP is probably involved (Aldenhoff et al., 1983).

(8) Lancaster et al. (1987) found a class of small-conductance (19 pS) Ca-activated K channels which were activated by intracellular Ca (1 μM), remained active at hyperpolarized potentials (where the large Ca-activated K channels are closed) and were insensitive to apamine. Thus, I_{AHP} may be mediated by small voltage-independent channels and I_C by large voltage-dependent BK channels. Two similar classes of Ca-dependent K channels co-exist in muscle cells, but there the small channels are sensitive to apamine (Blatz and Magleby, 1986).

$I_{K1(Ca)}$ and $I_{K2(Ca)}$

In a study of acutely dissociated CA1 cells, Numann et al. (1987) found two slow Ca-dependent K currents, $I_{K1(Ca)}$ and $I_{K2(Ca)}$, which in some ways resemble and may correspond to I_C and I_{AHP}, respectively. $I_{K1(Ca)}$ is activated positive to -30 mV, does not inactivate, and deactivates slowly (τ, 190 ms). $I_{K2(Ca)}$ is activated by depolarizations beyond -60 mV and inactivates slowly (τ, about 2 s at -50 mV; complete inactivation at -55 mV). The tail current also decays slowly (τ, about 2 s). Both $I_{K1(Ca)}$ and $I_{K2(Ca)}$ are suppressed in Ca-free medium with 1.5 mM cobalt (Co). As pointed out by Numann et al. (1987), the kinetics of the currents may have been affected by the intracellular Ca-buffer which they used (10 mM EGTA).

Sodium-dependent K current?

Gustafsson and Wigström (1983) found evidence for a Na-dependent K current in hippocampal neurones, but suggested that it was actually due to Ca-dependent K channels activated by Na-dependent release of Ca. Thus, long-lasting tetanic activation or injection of Na ions elicited a ouabain-resistant hyperpolarization which reversed near E_K. However, the hyperpolarization disappeared when the cell was injected with the Ca buffer EGTA. Therefore, they concluded that it probably was due to Na-dependent release of Ca ions from intracellular stores, and subsequent activation of Ca-dependent K channels. More recent reports have suggested the existence of genuinely Na-dependent K currents in other vertebrate central neurones (Constanti and Sim, 1988; Dryer et al., 1988a, b; Schwindt et al., 1989). Since the current recorded in cat neocortex was not suppressed by EGTA injection (Schwindt et al., 1989), it may be mediated by Na-dependent K channels like those recorded in cardiac cells (Kameyama et al., 1984), although other explanations are possible, as pointed out by the authors.

Resting and receptor-operated K currents

The K channels which are active at the resting potential have not been extensively studied. Still, it may be helpful to list some K currents which have been suggested to contribute to the resting potential, and some receptor-operated K currents.

Resting K current inhibited by acetylcholine

Acetylcholine reduces the resting conductance of hippocampal pyramidal cells, apparently by inhibiting a "leak" K current via M_1 receptors and a pertussis toxin-resistant G-protein (Madison et al., 1987; Benson et al., 1988; Dutar and Nicoll, 1988; Brown et al., 1988). This effect appears to be mainly responsible for the slow EPSP which results from stimulation of cholinergic fibers (Cole and Nicoll, 1983, 1984a, b; Segal, 1988). The inhibition of I_{AHP}, this leak current, and I_M, may all contribute to the cholinergic excitation of these cells (Benardo and Prince, 1982; Halliwell and Adams, 1982; Segal, 1982; Gähwiler, 1984; Nicoll, 1985). It is more sensitive to muscarinic agonists than I_M, but less sensitive than I_{AHP} (Madison et al., 1987).

Resting K current inhibited by noradrenaline

Noradrenaline seems to suppress a resting K current, via β receptors, and to activate another K current, probably via α receptors (Madison and Nicoll, 1986a; see below), but little is known about the properties of these currents.

Resting K current inhibited by serotonin

Serotonin also seems to reduce a resting K current (Andrade and Nicoll, 1987), in addition to the activation of an inwardly rectifying K current (see below).

Resting K current ($K_{K,rest}$)

The resting potential seems to depend strongly on a barium-sensitive (1 mM) K current, dubbed $I_{K,rest}$ (Storm and Helliesen, 1989). This current persists in the presence of carbachol, noradrenaline, serotonin, Cs, TEA, 4-AP, Cd and Mn at concentrations which block I_M, I_D, I_A, I_C, I_{AHP}, I_Q, $I_{K(IR)}$ and the above transmitter-sensitive resting currents. However, it is possible that acetylcholine, noradrenaline and serotonin exert a *partial* inhibition of $I_{K,rest}$. It appears to be a largely voltage- and time-independent "leak" current, which is active over a wide voltage range (at least from -110 to -40 mV) and shows no inward rectification. Thus, it differs from $I_{K(IR)}$ and the

inwardly rectifying K current which is activated by GABA, serotonin or adenosine (see below). A similar current has recently been described in frog ganglia (Jones, 1989).

K current activated by GABA$_B$, serotonin, adenosine

This inwardly rectifying K current can be activated by GABA$_B$, serotonin or adenosine receptors via a G-protein, probably G_o (Jahnsen, 1980; Segal, 1980; Newberry and Nicoll, 1984; Gähwiler and Brown, 1985b; Andrade et al., 1986; Colino and Halliwell, 1987; Andrade and Nicoll, 1987; Nicoll, 1988; VanDongen et al., 1988; Zgombic et al., 1989). This current underlies the GABA$_B$-dependent slow inhibitory postsynaptic potential which can be elicited by stimulation of afferent fibers (Nicoll and Alger, 1981a; Alger and Nicoll, 1982; Alger et al., 1984; Newberry and Nicoll, 1984; Dutar and Nicoll, 1988b).

K current activated by noradrenaline

Noradrenaline seems to both inhibit a resting K current (see above), and to activate another K current, probably via α receptors (Madison and Nicoll, 1986a). The latter effect accounts for the hyperpolarizing response to noradrenaline (Langmoen et al., 1981; Madison and Nicoll, 1986a).

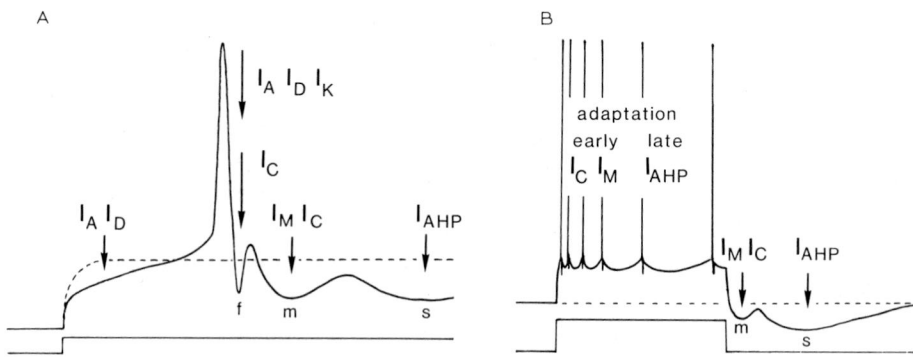

Fig. 5. Highly schematic drawing, indicating some suggested functional roles for K currents in hippocampal pyramidal cells, before, during and after a single action potential (A), and a train of spikes (B). Each response is elicited by injection of a square pulse of current (lower traces). f, the fast after-hyperpolarization (AHP); m, the medium AHP; s, the slow AHP. The dashed lines indicate the expected passive response in the absence of active currents (A), and the resting level (B). This working model is based on published and unpublished data.

ATP-sensitive K current ($I_{K(ATP)}$)

Depletion of oxygen, or glucose may activate a K current in hippocampal neurones. This current may be due to the opening of ATP-sensitive K channels (Hansen et al., 1982; Fujiwara et al., 1987; Krnjević and Leblond, 1988, 1989; Spuler et al., 1988; VanDongen et al., 1988; Leblond and Krnjević, 1989; Mourre et al., 1989).

Functions of hippocampal K currents

Figs. 5 and 6 summarize some of the functional roles which have been suggested for K currents in hippocampal pyramidal cells. K currents may be roughly divided into 3 functional groups: (1) those which determine the resting potential (resting K currents), (2) those which activate below the spike threshold and determine the initial excitability and spike latency (low-threshold K currents), and (3) those which are activated by the spike and mediate spike repolarization and feedback control of repetitive firing (high-threshold K currents).

The resting potential

The resting potential of hippocampal neurones appears to be mainly due to a resting K permeability, like in other neurones. Thus, the cells depolarize when the external K concentration is increased, but they maintain a highly negative resting potential even when E_{Cl} is shifted to a depolarized level, by loading the cell with chloride ions. The resting Cl permeability seems to be low (see e.g. Thompson and Gähwiler, 1989), although persistent Cl currents have been recorded (Madison et al., 1986; Segal et al., 1987; Franciolini and Nonner, 1988; Franciolini and Petris, 1988; Owen, 1988). The Na/K pump current may contribute to the resting potential, but it does not seem to be a major factor in the short term, since hippocampal neurones maintain a stable resting potential when the pump activity is temporarily inhibited (Gustafsson and Wigström, 1983; Thompson and Prince, 1986; McCarren and Alger, 1987).

However, it has been an open question *which* K

conductance dominates at the resting potential in these cells. As mentioned above, I_M does not seem to be involved, since the resting potential in healthy cells is below the activation threshold for I_M. An I_D "window current" may contribute (see above), but seems to be only a minor factor. In contrast to I_C and I_{AHP}, the resting K current does not seem to depend on influx of calcium ions, since Ca-free medium or Ca channel blockers has little effect on the resting potential (unlike in myenteric neurones; North and Tokimasa, 1987). I_Q can obviously not be the main resting current, since it is inward at rest. It does not even seem to contribute, since it activates negative to the apparent resting level in these cells, unlike in the neocortex (Schwindt et al., 1988). Although acetylcholine, serotonin and noradrenaline appear to block resting K channels (see above), this seems only to account for a fraction of the total resting conductance. However, recent data suggest that a barium-sensitive "leak" K current, $I_{K,rest}$ (see above), accounts for most of the remaining resting current.

Subthreshold responses

When the cell receives a depolarizing input (e.g. a square current pulse), I_A, I_D and I_M will start to turn on even before the membrane potential reaches the spike threshold (Fig. 6). I_A and I_D turn on rapidly and tend to counteract further depolarization until they have inactivated. When I_A and I_D are strong (due to a highly negative resting potential) compared to the stimulus current, they cause a ramp-like depolarization and a delayed onset of firing (Fig. 6B). In contrast, I_M turns on slowly and does not inactivate, thus causing a late sag in the depolarizing response (Fig. 6A).

In addition to the slow ramp-like depolarization caused by I_A and I_D, each spike is preceded by a slow Na-dependent prepotential (Lanthorn et al., 1984), which may be caused by a persistent Na current (I_{NaP} in Fig. 1; Hotson et al., 1979; Stafstrom et al., 1982; French and Gage, 1985). Thus, the prepotentials are eliminated by tetrodotoxin or Na-free medium (Storm, 1984; MacVicar, 1985).

Spike repolarization, AHP and adaptation

During the action potential, the 3 high-threshold K currents, I_K, I_C and I_{AHP} are also activated, along with further activation of I_A, I_D and I_M. Spike repolarization seems to consist of two phases: an early phase mediated by the voltage-gated currents I_A, I_D and I_K, and a late phase due to a fast Ca-dependent K current (I_C, or possibly I_{CT}) triggered by Ca influx and depolarization during the spike (Fig. 5A).

Although I_M and I_{AHP} are also substantially activated by the spike, they are too slow and small to contribute significantly to the repolarization. Instead, they generate the medium and slow AHPs respectively (I_C also contributes to the medium AHP), and during repetitive firing they cause spike-frequency adaptation (the early and the late phase, respectively; Fig. 5B).

The response pattern depends on the membrane potential prior to activation

Fig. 6 illustrates schematically some typical voltage responses to injected current pulses. At a slightly depolarized membrane potential (-60 mV, Fig. 6A), I_D is inactivated, so that the response pattern is dominated by other currents: I_M, I_C and I_{AHP} (I_A is disregarded in this example; see Fig. 5A). I_M turns on slowly and causes a sag in the voltage response to a subthreshold current. This pattern elicits an early spike when the injected current is increased (A2). A further increase in the stimulus current causes repetitive firing (A3). Now, the initial burst of spike strongly activates I_{AHP}, I_M and I_C, which cause spike-frequency adaptation and medium and slow AHPs after the spike train.

In contrast, at a highly negative membrane potential, I_D is deinactivated and ready to affect the response pattern. I_D turns on rapidly and inactivates slowly, causing a slow subthreshold ramp-like depolarization and a *delay* in the onset of firing (Fig. 6B 1 − 2). However, if the stimulus current pulse is increased further, it can overcome the inhibitory effect of I_D and elicit an initial high-frequency spike burst, which activates I_{AHP} sufficiently to cause spike-frequency adaptation, in spite of I_D (Fig. 6B 3).

Thus, variations in the membrane potential

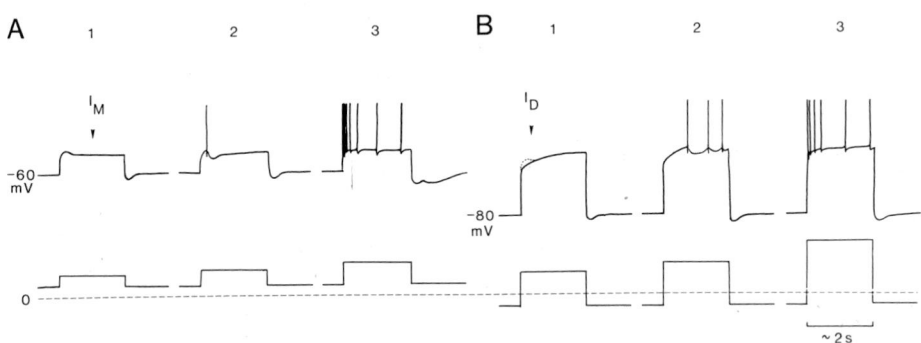

Fig. 6. The response pattern of CA1 hippocampal pyramidal cells depends on the membrane potential prior to activation. Schematic drawing of typical voltage responses (top traces) to injected current pulses (lower traces). A: at a depolarized membrane potential (-60 mV), I_D is inactivated and the response pattern is dominated by I_M, I_C and I_{AHP} (I_A is disregarded here). I_M turns on slowly and causes a sag in the voltage response (A1), favouring an early spike (A2). A further increase in the stimulus current causes repetitive firing (A3). Now, the initial burst of spike strongly activates I_{AHP} (and I_M and I_C), which causes spike frequency adaptation and AHPs after the spike train. B: at a highly negative membrane potential, I_D is available and can influence the response pattern. I_D turns on rapidly and inactivates slowly, causing a slow subthreshold ramp-like depolarization (B1) and a *delay* in the onset of firing (B2). However, a large stimulus current can overcome the inhibitory effect of I_D and elicit an initial high-frequency burst (B3), which activates enough I_{AHP} to cause adaptation in spite of I_D. I_Q, which is tonically activated at hyperpolarized potentials, can also cause an initial depolarizing hump (dotted outline in B1). (Based partly on Storm, 1984, 1988a and unpublished data.)

prior to activation can change the firing pattern of the cell, by varying the available D current. This effect can also influence how the depolarizing input is translated into spike frequency. Thus, the characteristic low gain in the initial firing frequency for low current intensities (the "primary range" of f/I plots; Lanthorn et al., 1984), disappears when I_D is inactivated by prior depolarization (Storm, 1984, 1988a).

Acknowledgements

Supported by a fellowship from the Norwegian Medical Research Council (RMT/NYCOMED). I thank Ole Paulsen for helping to correct the proofs. There are some journals that I have been unable to follow systematically. I apologize for any relevant papers that I may have missed. The original deadline was June 1, 1989, but a few more recent references have been included.

References

Adams, D.J., Smith, S.J. and Thompson, S.H. (1980) Ionic current in molluscan soma. *Ann. Rev. Neurosci.*, 3: 141–167.

Adams, P.R. and Brown, D.A. (1982) Synaptic inhibition of the M-current: slow excitatory post-synaptic potential mechanism in bullfrog sympathetic neurones. *J. Physiol. (Lond.)*, 332: 263–272.

Adams, P.R. and Galvan, M. (1986) Voltage-dependent currents of vertebrate neurons and their role in membrane excitability. In A. Delgado-Escueta, A.A. Ward, D.M. Woodbury and R. Porter (Eds.) *Advances in Neurology, Vol. 4, Basic Mechanisms of the Epilepsies*, New York, Raven Press, pp. 137–170.

Adams, P.R., Brown, D.A. and Constanti, A. (1982a) M-current and other potassium currents in bullfrog sympathetic neurones. *J. Physiol. (Lond.)*, 330: 537–572.

Adams, P.R., Brown, D.A. and Constanti, A. (1982b) Pharmacological inhibition of the M-current. *J. Physiol. (Lond.)*, 332: 223–262.

Adams, P.R., Constanti, A., Brown, D.A. and Clark, R.B. (1982c) Intracellular Ca^{2+} activates a fast voltage-sensitive K^+ current in vertebrate sympathetic neurones. *Nature (Lond.)*, 296: 746–749.

Adams, P.R., Jones, S.W., Pennefather, P., Brown, D.A., Koch, C. and Lancaster, B. (1986) Slow synaptic transmission in frog sympathetic ganglia. *J. Exp. Biol.*, 124: 259–285.

Adams, W.B. and Benson, J.A. (1985) The generation and modulation of endogenous rhytmicity in the Aplysia bursting pacemaker neurone R15. *Prog. Biophys. Mol. Biol.*, 46: 1–49.

Adrian, R.H. (1969) Rectification in muscle membrane. *Prog. Biophys. Mol. Biol.*, 19: 340–369.

Aghajanian, G.K. (1985) Modulation of a transient outward current in serotonergic neurones by alfa$_1$-adrenoceptors. *Nature (Lond.)*, 315: 501–503.

Aldenhoff, J.B., Gruol, D.L., Rivier, J., Vale, W. and Siggins, G.R. (1983). Corticotropin releasing factor decreases post-burst hyperpolarizations and excites hippocampal neurons. *Science*, 221: 875–877.

Alger, B.E. (1984) Characteristics of a slow hyperpolarizing synaptic potential in rat hippocampal pyramidal cells in vitro. *J. Neurophysiol.*, 52: 892–910.

Alger, B.E. and Doerner, D. (1988) Whole-cell voltage-clamp study of two distinct components of "A current" in hippocampal neurons. *Soc. Neurosci. Abstr.*, 14: 947.

Alger, B.E. and Nicoll, R.A. (1980) Epileptiform burst afterhyperpolarization: calcium-dependent potassium potential in hippocampal CA1 pyramidal cells. *Science*, 210: 1122–1124.

Alger, B.E. and Williamson, A. (1988) A transient calcium-dependent potassium component of the epileptiform burst after-hyperpolarization in rat hippocampus. *J. Physiol. (Lond.)*, 399: 191–205.

Andrade, R. and Nicoll, R.A. (1987) Pharmacologically distinct actions of serotonin on single pyramidal neurones of the rat hippocampus recorded *in vitro*. *J. Physiol. (Lond.)*, 394: 99–124.

Andrade, R., Malenka, R.C. and Nicoll, R.A. (1986) A G protein couples serotonin and GABA$_B$ receptors to the same channels in hippocampus. *Science*, 234: 1261–1265.

Ashwood, T.J., Lancaster, B. and Wheal, H. (1986) Intracellular electrophysiology of CA1 pyramidal neurones in slices of the kainic acid lesioned hippocampus of the rat. *Exp. Brain Res.*, 62: 189–198.

Baraban, J.M., Snyder, S.H. and Alger, B.E. (1985) Protein kinase C regulates ionic conductance in hippocampal pyramidal neurons: electrophysiological effects of phorbol esters. *Proc. Natl. Acad. Sci. U.S.A.*, 82: 2538–2542.

Barrett, E.F. and Barrett, J.N. (1976) Separation of two voltage-sensitive potassium currents and demonstration of a tetrodotoxin-resistant calcium-current in frog motoneurones. *J. Physiol. (Lond.)*, 255: 737–774.

Barrett, E.F., Barrett, J.N. and Crill, W.E. (1980) Voltage-sensitive outward currents in cat motoneurones. *J. Physiol. (Lond.)*, 304: 251–276.

Barrett, J.N. and Crill, W.E. (1972) Voltage clamp analysis of conductances underlying cat motoneuron action potentials. *Fed. Proc.*, 31: 305A.

Barrett, J.N., Magleby, K.L. and Pallotta, B.S. (1982) Properties of single calcium-activated potassium channels in cultured rat muscle. *J. Physiol. (Lond.)*, 331: 211 – 230.

Beluzzi, O. and Sacchi, O. (1988). The interaction between potassium and sodium currents in generating action potentials in the rat sympathetic neurone. *J. Physiol. (Lond.)*, 358: 127 – 147.

Beluzzi, O., Sacchi, O. and Wanke, E. (1985) A fast transient outward current in the rat sympathetic neurone studied under voltage clamp conditions. *J. Physiol. (Lond.)*, 358: 91 – 102.

Benoit, E. and Dubois, J.-M. (1986). Toxin I from the snake *Dendroaspis polyepis polyepis*: a highly specific blocker of one type of potassium channel in myelinated nerve fiber. *Brain Res.*, 377: 374 – 377.

Benardo, L.S. and Prince, D.A. (1982) Ionic mechanisms of cholinergic excitation in mammalian hippocampal pyramidal cells. *Brain Res.*, 249: 333 – 344.

Benson, D., Blitzer, R.D. and Landau, E.M. (1988) An analysis of the depolarization produced in guinea pig hippocampus by cholinergic receptor stimulation. *J. Physiol. (Lond.)*, 404: 479 – 496.

Bidard, J.-N., Gandolfo, G., Mourre, C., Gottesmann, C. and Lazdunski, M. (1987) The brain response to the bee venom peptide MCD. Activation and desensitization of a hippocampal target. *Brain Res.*, 418: 235 – 244.

Blatz, A.L. and Magleby, K.L. (1986) Single apamin-blocked Ca-activated K$^+$ channels of small conductance in cultured rat skeletal muscle. *Nature (Lond.)*, 323: 718 – 720.

Borg-Graham, L.J. (1987) *Modelling the Somatic Electrical Response of Hippocampal Pyramidal Neurons.* Thesis, Department of Electrical Engineering and Computer Science, Massachusetts Institute of Technology, Cambridge.

Brett, R.S. and Lancaster, B. (1985) Activation of potassium channels by rapid application of calcium to inside-out patches of cultured hippocampal neurons. *Soc. Neurosci. Abstr.*, 11: 954.

Brett, R.S., Dilger, J.P., Adams, P.R. and Lancaster, B. (1986) A method for rapid exchange of solutions bathing excised membrane patches. *Biophys. J.*, 50: 987 – 992.

Brown, D.A. (1988a) M-currents. In T. Narahashi (Ed.), *Ion Channels, Vol. 1*, Plenum, New York, pp. 55 – 94.

Brown, D.A. (1988b) M-currents: an update. *Trends Neurosci.*, 11: 294 – 299.

Brown, D.A. and Adams, P.R. (1980) Muscarinic suppression of a novel voltage-sensitive K$^+$ current in a vertebrate neurone. *Nature (Lond.)*, 283: 673 – 676.

Brown, D.A. and Adams, P.R. (1987) Effects of phorbol dibutyrate on M currents and M current inhibition in bullfrog sympathetic neurons. *Cell. Mol. Neurobiol.*, 7: 255 – 265.

Brown, D.A. and Griffith, W.H. (1983a) Calcium-activated outward current in voltage-clamped hippocampal neurones of the guinea-pig. *J. Physiol. (Lond.)*, 337: 287 – 301.

Brown, D.A. and Griffith, W.H. (1983b) Persistent slow inward calcium current in voltage-clamped hippocampal neurones of the guinea-pig. *J. Physiol. (Lond.)*, 337: 303 – 320.

Brown, D.A. and Higashida, H. (1988) Inositol 1,4,5-trisphosphate and diacylglycerol mimic bradykinin effects on mouse neuroblastoma × rat glioma hybrid cells. *J. Physiol. (Lond.)*, 397: 185 – 207.

Brown, D.A., Constanti, A. and Adams, P.R. (1982) Calcium-dependence of a component of transient outward current in bullfrog ganglion cells. *Soc. Neurosci. Abstr.*, 8: 252.

Brown, L.D., Nakajima, S. and Nakajima, Y (1988) Acetylcholine modulates resting K-current through a pertussis-toxin-resistant G-protein in hippocampal neurons. *Soc. Neurosci. Abstr.*, 14: 1328.

Brown, T.H., Fricke, R.A. and Perkel, D.H. (1981) Passive electrical constants in three classes of hippocampal neurones. *J. Neurophysiol.*, 46: 812 – 827.

Buckle, P.J. and Haas, H.L. (1982) Enhancement of synaptic transmission by 4-aminopyridine in hippocampal slices of the rat. *J. Physiol. (Lond.)*, 326: 109 – 122.

Byrne, J.H. (1980). Quantitative aspects of ionic conductance mechanisms contributing to firing pattern of motor cells mediating inking behavior in *Aplysia californica*. *J. Neurophysiol.*, 43: 651 – 668.

Carew, T.J. and Kandel, E.R. (1977) Inking in *Aplysia californica*. I. Neural circuit of an all-or-none behavioral response. *J. Neurophysiol.*, 40: 692 – 707.

Cherubini, E., Ben Ari, Y., Gho, M., Bidard, J.N. and Lazdunski, M. (1987) Long-term potentiation of synaptic transmission in the hippocampus induced by a bee venom peptide. *Nature (Lond.)*, 328: 70 – 73.

Cole, A.E. and Nicoll, R.A. (1983) Acetylcholine mediates a slow synaptic potential in hippocampal pyramidal cells. *Science*, 221: 1299 – 1301.

Cole, A.E. and Nicoll, R.A. (1984a) Characterization of a slow cholinergic postsynaptic potential recorded *in vitro* from rat hippocampal pyramidal cells. *J. Physiol. (Lond.)*, 352: 173 – 188.

Cole, A.E. and Nicoll, R.A. (1984b) The pharmacology of cholinergic excitatory responses in hippocampal pyramidal cells. *Brain Res.*, 305: 283 – 290.

Colino, A. and Halliwell, J.V. (1987) Differential modulation of three separate K-conductances in hippocampal CA1 neurons by serotonin. *Nature (Lond.)*, 328: 73 – 77.

Connor, J.A. and Stevens, C.F. (1971) Voltage clamp studies of a transient outward membrane current in gastropod neural somata. *J. Physiol. (Lond.)*, 213: 21 – 30.

Constanti, A. and Galvan, M. (1983) Fast inward-rectifying current accounts for anomalous rectification in olfactory cortex neurones. *J. Physiol. (Lond.)*, 385: 153 – 178.

Constanti, A. and Sim, J.A. (1987) Calcium-dependent potassium conductance in guinea-pig olfactory cortex neurones *in vitro*. *J. Physiol. (Lond.)*, 387: 173 – 194.

Dinan, T.G., Crunelli, V. and Kelly, J.S. (1987) Neuroleptics decrease calcium activated potassium conductance in hippocampal pyramidal cells. *Brain Res.*, 407: 159 – 162.

Docherty, R.J., Dolly, J.O., Halliwell, J.V. and Othman, I. (1983) Excitatory effects of dendrotoxin on the hippocampus in vitro. *J. Physiol. (Lond.)*, 336: 58P – 59P.

Doerner, D., Pitler, T.A. and Alger, B.E. (1988) Protein kinase C activators block specific calcium and potassium current components in isolated hippocampal neurons. *J. Neurosci.*, 8: 4069 – 4078.

Dolly, J.O., Halliwell, J.V., Black, J.D., Williams, R.S., Pelchen-Matthews, A., Breeze, A.L., Mehraban, F., Othman, I.B. and Black, A.R. (1984) Botulinum neurotoxin and dendrotoxin as probes for studies of transmitter release. *J. Physiol. (Paris)*, 79: 280 – 303.

Dreyfus, C.F., Gehrson, M.D. and Crain, S.M. (1979) Innervation of hippocampal explants by central catecholaminergic neurons in co-cultured fetal mouse brain stem explants. *Brain Res.*, 161: 431 – 445.

Dryer, S.E., Fuji, J. and Martin, A.R. (1988a) A sodium-activated potassium current in cultured brain stem neurones. *J. Physiol. (Lond.)*, 398: 12P.

Dryer, S.E., Fuji, J. and Martin, A.R. (1988b) A sodium-activated potassium current in brain stem neurons. *Biophys. J.*, 53: 552a.

Dubois, J.M. (1981) Evidence for the existence of three types of potassium channels in the frog ranvier node membrane. *J. Physiol. (Lond.)*, 318: 297 – 369.

Dubois, J.M. (1983) Potassium currents in the frog node of Ranvier. *Progr. Biophys. Mol. Biol.*, 42: 1 – 20.

Dubois, J.M. (1986) Toxin I from the snake *Dendroaspis polylepis polylepis*: a highly specific blocker of one type of potassum channel in myelinated nerve fiber. *Brain Res.*, 377: 374 – 377.

Dutar, P. and Nicoll, R.A. (1988a) Classification of muscarinic responses in hippocampus in terms of receptor subtypes and second messenger systems: electrophysiological studies *in vitro*. *J. Neurosci.*, 8: 4214 – 4224.

Dutar, P. and Nicoll, R.A. (1988b) A physiological role for $GABA_B$ receptors in the central nervous system. *Nature (Lond.)*, 332: 156 – 158.

Edwards, F.A., Konnerth, A. and Sakman, B. (1988) The patch clamp technique applied to synaptically connected cells in mammalian brain slices. GABA receptor mediated synaptic and single channel currents measured in rat hippocampal granule cells. *Eur. J. Neurosci.*, Suppl. 1: 342.

Edwards, F.A., Konnerth, A., Sakman, B. and Takahashi, T. (1989) A thin slice preparation for patch clamp recordings from synaptically connected neurones of the mammalian central nervous system. *Pflüg. Arch.*, in press.

Elkins, T. and Ganetzky, B. (1988) The roles of potassium currents in Drosophila flight muscle. *J. Neurosci.*, 8: 428 – 434.

Elkins, T., Ganetzky, B. and Wu, C.-F. (1986) A Drosophila mutation that eliminates a calcium-dependent potassium current. *Proc. Natl. Acad. Sci. U.S.A.*, 83: 8415 – 8419.

Farley, J. and Rudy, B. (1988) Multiple types of voltage-

dependent Ca^{2+}-activated K^+ channels of large conductance in rat brain synaptosomal membranes. *Biophys. J.*, 53: 919 – 934.

ffrench-Mullen, J.M.H., Rogawski, M.A. and Barker, J.L. (1988a) Phenyclidine at low concentrations selectively blocks the sustained but not the transient voltage-dependent potassium current in cultured hippocampal neurones. *Neurosci. Lett.*, 88: 325 – 330.

ffrench-Mullen, J.M.H., Suzuki, S., Barker, J.L. and Rogawski, M.A. (1988b) Phencyclidine: blockade of K^+ channels and NMDA receptor-coupled cation channels occurs at distinct sites in hippocampal neurons. *Biophys. J.*, 53: 544a.

Finkel, A.S. and Redman, S. (1984) Theory and operation of a single microelectrode voltage clamp. *J. Neurosci. Methods*, 11: 101 – 127.

Franciolini, F. (1988) Calcium and voltage dependence of single Ca^{2+}-activated K^+ channels from cultured hippocampal neurones of rat. *Biochim. Biophys. Acta*, 953: 419 – 427.

Franciolini, F. and Nonner, W. (1988) Anion and cation permeability of a chloride channel in rat hippocampal neurones. *J. Gen. Physiol.*, 90: 453 – 478.

Franciolini, F. and Petris, A. (1988) Single chloride channels in cultured rat neurones. *Arch. Biochem. Biophys.*, 261: 97 – 192.

Frankenhaeuser, B. and Hodgkin, A.L. (1957) The action of calcium on the electrical properties of squid axons. *J. Physiol. (Lond.)*, 137: 218 – 244.

French, C.R. and Gage, P.W. (1985) A threshold sodium current in pyramidal cells in rat hippocampus. *Neurosci. Lett.*, 56: 289 – 293.

Fujiwara, N., Higashi, H., Shimoji, K. and Yoshimura, M. (1987) Effects of hypoxia on rat hippocampal neurones in vitro. *J. Physiol. (Lond.)*, 384: 131 – 151.

Gähwiler, B.H. (1981) Organotypic monolayer cultures of nervous tissue. *J. Neurosci. Methods*, 4: 329 – 342.

Gähwiler, B.H. (1983) Facilitation by acetylcholine of tetrodoxin-resistant spikes in rat hippocampal pyramidal cells. *Neuroscience*, 11: 381 – 388.

Gähwiler, B. and Brown, D.A. (1985a) Functional innervation of cultured hippocampal neurones by cholinergic afferents from co-cultured septal explants. *Nature (Lond.)*, 313: 577 – 579.

Gähwiler, B. and Brown, D.A. (1985b) $GABA_B$-receptor-activated K^+ current in voltage-clamped CA3 pyramidal cells in hippocampal cultures. *Proc. Natl. Acad. Sci. U.S.A.*, 82: 1558 – 1562.

Gähwiler, B. and Brown, D.A. (1987) Muscarine affects calcium currents in rat hippocampal pyramidal cells *in vitro*. *Neurosci. Lett.*, 76: 301 – 306.

Galvan, M., Grafe, P. and Ten Bruggencate, G. (1982) Convulsant actions of 4-aminopyridine on the guinea pig olfactory cortex slice. *Brain Res.*, 241: 75 – 86.

Goh, M., King, A.E., Ben-Ari, Y. and Cherubini, E. (1986)

Kainate reduces two voltage-dependent potassium conductances in rat hippocampal neurons in vitro. *Brain Res.*, 385: 411–414.

Gray, R. and Johnston, D. (1985) Rectification of single GABA-gated chloride channels in adult hippocampal neurons. *J. Neurophysiol.*, 54: 134–144.

Gruner, W., Marrion, N.V. and Adams, P.R. (1989) Three kinetic components to M-currents in bullfrog sympathetic neurons. *Soc. Neurosci. Abstr.*, 15: 990.

Gustafsson, B. and Wigström, H. (1981) Evidence for two types of afterhypolarization in CA1 pyramidal cells in the hippocampus. *Brain Res.*, 206: 462–468.

Gustafsson, B. and Wigström, H. (1983) Hyperpolarization following long-lasting tetanic activation of hippocampal pyramidal cells. *Brain Res.*, 275: 159–163.

Gustafsson, B., Galvan, M., Grafe, P. and Wigström, H.A. (1982) Transient outward current in mammalian central neurone blocked by 4-aminopyridine. *Nature (Lond.)*, 299: 252–254.

Haas, H.L. and Greene, R.W. (1984) Adenosine enhances afterhyperpolarization and accommodation in hippocampal •pyramidal cells. *Pflüg. Arch.*, 402: 244–247.

Haas, H.L. and Greene, R.W. (1986) Effects of histamine on hippocampal pyramidal cells of the rat *in vitro*. *Exp. Brain Res.*, 62: 123–130.

Haas, H.L. and Konnerth, A. (1983) Histamine and noradrenaline decreases calcium-activated potassium conductance in hippocampal pyramidal cells. *Nature (Lond.)*, 302: 432–434.

Haas, H.L., Wieser, H.G. and Yasargil, M.G. (1983) 4-Aminopyridine and fiber potentials in rat and human hippocampal slices. *Experientia*, 39: 114–115.

Hagiwara, S. and Jaffe, L.A. (1979) Electrical properties of egg cell membranes. *Am. Rev. Biophys. Bioeng.*, 8: 385–416.

Halliwell, J.V. and Adams, P.R. (1982) Voltage clamp analysis of muscarinic excitation in hippocampal neurons. *Brain Res.*, 250: 71–92.

Halliwell, J.V., Othman, I.B., Pelchen-Matthews, A. and Dolly, J.O. (1986) Central actions of dendrotoxin: selective reduction of a transient K conductance in hippocampus and binding to localized acceptors. *Proc. Natl. Acad. Sci. U.S.A.*, 83: 493–497.

Hamill, O.P., Marty, A., Neher, E., Sakman, B. and Sigworth (1981) Improved patch-clamp techniques for high-resolution current recording from cells and cell-free membrane patches. *Pflüg. Arch.*, 391: 85–100.

Hansen, A.J., Hounsgaard, J. and Jahnsen, H. (1982) Anoxia increases potassium conductance in hippocampal nerve cells. *Acta Physiol. Scand.*, 115: 301–310.

Harvey, A.L. and Karlsson, E. (1980) Dendrotoxin from the venom of green mamba *Dendroaspis angusticeps*. A neurotoxin that enhances acetylcholine release at neuromuscular junctions. *Naunyn Schmiedeberg's Arch. Pharmacol.*, 312: 1–6.

Harvey, A.L. and Karlsson, E. (1982) Protease inhibitor homologues from mamba venoms: facilitation of acetylcholine release and interactions with prejunctional blocking toxins. *Br. J. Pharmacol.*, 77: 153–161.

Hermann, A. and Erxleben, C. (1987) Charybdotoxin selectively blocks small Ca-activated K channels in *Aplysia* neurons. *J. Gen. Physiol.*, 27–47.

Higashida, H. and Brown, D.A. (1986) Two polyphosphatidylinositide metabolites control two K^+ currents in a neuronal cell. *Nature (Lond.)*, 323: 333–335.

Hille, B. (1984) *Ionic Channels of Excitable Membranes*, Sinauer Associates Inc., Sunderland, MA.

Hodgkin, A.L. and Huxley, A.F. (1952) A quantitative description of membrane currents and its application to conduction and excitation in nerve. *J. Physiol. (Lond.)*, 117: 500–544.

Hotson, J.R. and Prince, D.A. (1980) A Ca-activated hyperpolarization follows repetitive firing in hippocampal neurons. *J. Neurophysiol.*, 43: 409–419.

Hotson, J.R., Prince, D.A. and Schwartzkroin, P.A. (1979) Anomalous inward rectification in hippocampal neurons. *J. Neurophysiol.*, 42: 889–895.

Hounsgaard, J. and Midtgaard, J. (1988) Intrinsic determinants of firing pattern in Purkinje cells of the turtle cerebellum *in vitro*. *J. Physiol. (Lond.)*, 402: 731–749.

Hounsgaard, J. and Midtgaard, J. (1989) Dendrite processing in more ways than one. *Trends Neurosci.*, 12: 313–315.

Ikemoto, Y., Ono, K., Yoshida, A. and Akaike, N. (1989) Delayed activation of large-conductance Ca^{2+}-activated K^+ channels in hippocampal neurons of the rat. *Biophys. J.*, 56: 207–212.

Jahnsen, H. (1980) The action of 5-hydroxytryptamine on neuronal membranes and synaptic transmission in area CA1 of the hippocampus in vitro. *Brain Res.*, 197: 83–94.

Johnston, D. (1981) Passive cable properties of hippocampal CA3 pyramidal neurons. *Cell. Mol. Neurobiol.*, 1: 41–55.

Johnston, D. and Brown, T.H. (1983) Interpretation of voltage clamp measurements in hippocampal neurons. *J. Neurophysiol.*, 50: 464–486.

Johnston, D., Hablitz, J.J. and Wilson, W.A. (1980) Voltage clamp discloses slow inward current in hippocampal burst-firing neurones. *Nature (Lond.)*, 286: 391–393.

Jones, R.S.G. and Heinemann, U. (1988) Verapamil blocks the afterhyperpolarization but not the spike frequency accommodation of rat CA1 pyramidal cells in vitro. *Brain Res.*, 462: 367–371.

Jones, S.W. (1985) Muscarinic and peptidergic excitation of bull-frog sympathetic neurones. *J. Physiol. (Lond.)*, 366: 63–87.

Jones, S.W. (1987) GTP-y-S inhibits the M-current of dissociated bullfrog sympathetic neurons. *Soc. Neurosci. Abstr.*, 13: p. 532.

Jones, S.W. (1988) Whole-cell and microelectrode voltage clamp. In C.H. Vanderwolf (Ed.), *Neurophysiological Methods*, Humana Press, Clifton, NJ.

Jones, S.W. (1989) On the resting potential of isolated frog sympathetic neurons. *Neuron,* 3: 153 – 161.

Jones, S.W., Adams, P.R., Brownstein, M. and Rievers, J.E. (1984) Teleost luteinizing hormone-releasing hormone: action in bullfrog sympathetic ganglia is consistent with a role as transmitter. *J. Neurosci.,* 4: 420 – 429.

Kameyama, M., Kakei, M., Sato, R., Shibasaki, T., Matsuda, H. and Irisawa, H. (1984) Intracellular Na^+ activates a K^+ channel in mammalian cardiac cells. *Nature (Lond.),* 309: 354 – 356.

Kay, A.R. and Wong, R.K.S. (1986) Isolation of neurons suitable for patch-clamping from adult mammalian central nervous systems. *J. Neurosci. Methods,* 16: 227 – 238.

Krnjević, K. and Leblond, J. (1988) Are there hippocampal ATP-sensitive K channels that are activated by anoxia? *Pflüg. Arch.,* 211: R145.

Krnjević, K. and Leblond, J. (1989) Changes in membrane currents of hippocampal neurons evoked by brief anoxia. *J. Neurophysiol.,* 62: 15 – 30.

Lancaster, B. and Adams, P.R. (1986) Calcium-dependent current generating the after-hyperpolarization of hippocampal neurons. *J. Neurophysiol.,* 55: 1268 – 1282.

Lancaster, B. and Nicoll, R.A. (1987) Properties of two calcium-activated hyperpolarizations in rat hippocampal neurones. *J. Physiol. (Lond.),* 389: 187 – 204.

Lancaster, B., Madison, D.V. and Nicoll, R.A. (1986) Charybdotoxin selectively blocks a fast, Ca-dependent afterhyperpolarization (AHP) in hippocampal pyramidal cells. *Soc. Neurosci. Abstr.,* 12: p. 560.

Lancaster, B., Perkel, D.J. and Nicoll, R.A. (1987) Small conductance Ca^{2+}-activated K^+ channels in hippocampal neurons. *Soc. Neurosci. Abstr.,* 13: p. 176.

Langmoen, I.A., Segal, M. and Andersen, P. (1981) Mechanisms of norepinephrine actions in hippocampal pyramidal cells in vitro. *Brain Res.,* 208: 349 – 362.

Lanthorn, T., Storm, J. and Andersen, P. (1984) Current-to-frequency transduction in CA1 hippocampal pyramidal cells. *Exp. Brain Res.,* 53: 431 – 443.

Leblond, J. and Krnjević, K. (1989) Hypoxic changes in hippocampal neurons. *J. Neurophysiol.,* 62: 1 – 14.

Llano, I., Marty, A., Johnson, J.W., Asher, P. and Gähwiler, B.H. (1988). Patch-clamp recording of amino acid-activated responses in "organotypic" slice cultures. *Proc. Natl. Acad. Sci. U.S.A.,* 85: 3221 – 3225.

Lopez, H., Brown, D. and Adams, P.R. (1987) Possible involvement of GTP-binding proteins in coupling of muscarinic receptors to M-current in bullfrog ganglion cells. *Soc. Neurosci. Abstr.,* 13: p. 533.

MacDermott, A.B. and Weight, F.F. (1982) Action potential repolarization may involve a transient Ca-sensitive outward current in a vertebrate neurone. *Nature (Lond.),* 300: 185 – 188.

MacKinnon, R., Reinhart, P. and White, M.M. (1988) Charybdotoxin block of *Shaker* K^+ channels suggests that different types of K^+ channels share common structural features. *Neuron,* 1: 997 – 1001.

MacVicar, B.A. (1985) Depolarizing prepotentials are Na^+-dependent in CA1 pyramidal neurons. *Brain Res.,* 333: 378 – 381.

Madison, D.V. and Nicoll, R.A. (1982) Noradrenaline blocks accommodation of pyramidal cell discharge in the hippocampus. *Nature (Lond.),* 299: 636 – 638.

Madison, D.V. and Nicoll, R.A. (1984) Control of repetitive discharge of rat CA1 pyramidal neurones *in vitro.* *J. Physiol. (Lond.),* 354: 319 – 331.

Madison, D.V. and Nicoll, R.A. (1986a) Actions of noradrenaline recorded intra-cellularly in CA1 pyramidal neurones *in vitro.* *J. Physiol. (Lond.),* 372: 221 – 244.

Madison, D.V. and Nicoll, R.A. (1986b) Cyclic adenosine 3′,5′-monophosphate mediates beta-receptor actions of noradrenaline in rat hippocampal pyramidal cells. *J. Physiol. (Lond.),* 372: 245 – 259.

Madison, D.V., Malenka, R.C. and Nicoll, R.A. (1986) Phorbol esters block a voltage-sensitive chloride current in hippocampal pyramidal cells. *Nature (Lond.),* 321: 695 – 697.

Madison, D.V., Lancaster, B. and Nicoll, R.A. (1987) Voltage clamp analysis of cholinergic action in the hippocampus. *J. Neurosci.,* 7: 733 – 741.

Malenka, R.C. and Nicoll, R.A. (1986) Dopamine decreases the calcium-activated afterhyperpolarization in hippocampal CA1 pyramidal cells. *Brain Res.,* 379: 210 – 215.

Malenka, R.C., Madison, D.V., Andrade, R. and Nicoll, R.A. (1986) Phorbol esters mimic some cholinergic actions in hippocampal pyramidal neurons. *J. Neurosci.,* 6: 475 – 480.

Marty, A. (1981) Ca-dependent K channels with large unitary conductance in chromaffin cell membranes, *Nature (Lond.),* 291: 497 – 500.

Masukawa, L.M. and Hansen, A. (1987) Regional distribution of voltage-dependent single channel conductances in cultured hippocampal neurons from the rat. *Soc. Neurosci. Abstr.,* 13: 1442.

Mayer, M. and Sugiyama, K. (1988) A modulatory action of divalent cations on transient outward current in cultured rat sensory neurones. *J. Physiol. (Lond.),* 396: 417 – 433.

McCarren, M. and Alger, B.E. (1987) Sodium-potassium pump inhibitors increase neuronal excitability in the rat hippocampal slice: role of a Ca-dependent conductance. *J. Neurophysiol.,* 57: 496 – 509.

Miller, C., Moczydlowsky, E., Latorre, R. and Phillips, M. (1985) Charybdotoxin, a protein inhibitor of single Ca^{2+}-activated K^+ channels from mammalian skeletal muscle. *Nature (Lond.),* 331: 316 – 318.

Moore, S.D., Madamba, S.G., Joels, M. and Siggins, G.R. (1988) Somatostatin augments the M-current in hippocampal neurons. *Science,* 239: 278 – 280.

Mourre, C., Ben-Ari, Y., Benardi, H., Fosset, M. and Lazdunski, M. (1989) Antidiabetic sulfonylureas: localization of binding sites in the brain and effect on the hyperpolarization induced by anoxia in hippocampal slices. *Brain Res.*, 486: 159–164.

Muller, W. and Misgeld, U. (1986) Slow cholinergic excitation of guinea pig hippocampal neurons is mediated by two muscarinic receptor subtypes. *Neurosci. Lett.*, 67: 107–112.

Nakajima, Y., Nakajima, S., Leonard, R.J. and Yamaguchi, K. (1986) Acetylcholine raises the excitability by inhibiting the fast transient outward current in cultured hippocampal neurons. *Proc. Natl. Acad. Sci. U.S.A.*, 83: 3022–3026.

Newberry, N. and Nicoll, R.A. (1985) Comparison of the action of baclofen with gamma-aminobutyric acid on rat hippocampal pyramidal cells *in vitro*. *J. Physiol. (Lond.)*, 348: 239–254.

Nicoll, R.A. (1985) The septo-hippocampal projection: a model cholinergic pathway. *Trends Neurosci.*, 8: 533–536.

Nicoll, R.A. (1988). The coupling of neurotransmitter receptors to ion channels in the brain. *Science,* 241: 545–551.

North, R.A. and Tokimasa, T. (1987) Persistent calcium-sensitive potassium current and the resting properties of guinea pig myenteric neurones. *J. Physiol. (Lond.)*, 386: 333–353.

Numann, R.E., Wadman, W.J. and Wong, R.K.S. (1987) Outward currents of single hippocampal cells obtained from the adult guinea-pig. *J. Physiol. (Lond.)*, 393: 331–353.

Othman, I.B., Spokes, J.W. and Dolly, O.J. (1982) Preparation of neurotoxic ^{3}H-β-bungarotoxin: demonstration of a saturable binding to brain synapses and its inhibition by toxin I. *Eur. J. Biochem.*, 128: 267–276.

Owen, D.G. (1987) Three types of inward rectifier currents in cultured hippocampal neurones. *Neurosci. Lett.*, Suppl. 29: 518.

Owen, D.G. (1988) Three types of chloride channels in cultured rat hippocampal neurones. *Soc. Neurosci. Abstr.*, 14: 1203.

Peacock, J.H. (1979) Electrophysiology of dissociated hippocampal cultures from fetal mice. *Brain Res.*, 169: 247–260.

Pellmar, T.C. (1986) Histamine decreases calcium-mediated potassium current in guinea-pig hippocampal CA1 pyramidal cells. *J. Neurophysiol.*, 55: 727–738.

Pfaffinger, P. (1988) Muscarine and t-LHRH suppress M-current by activating an IAP-insensitive G-protein. *J. Neurosci.*, 8: 3343–3353.

Pfaffinger, P., Leibowitz, M.D., Subers, E.M., Nathanson, N.M., Almers, W. and Hille, B. (1988) Agonists that suppress M-current elicit phosphoinositide turnover and Ca^{2+}-transients, but these events do not explain M-current suppression. *Neuron*, 1: 477–484.

Pennefather, P. (1986) The rate of activation of M current at positive potentials in bullfrog sympathetic ganglion cells. *Biophys. J.*, 49: 166a.

Pennefather, P., Lancaster, B., Adams, P.A. and Nicoll, R.A. (1985) Two distinct Ca-dependent K currents in bullfrog sympathetic ganglion cells. *Proc. Natl. Acad. Sci. U.S.A.*, 82: 3040–3044.

Penner, R., Petersen, M., Pierau, F.-K. and Dreyer, F. (1986) Dendrotoxin: a selective blocker of a non-inactivating potassium current in guinea-pig dorsal root ganglion neurones. *Pflüg. Arch.*, 407: 365–369.

Pfaffinger, P.J., Leibowitz, M.D., Bosma, M., Almers, W. and Hille, B. (1988) M-current suppression by agonists: the role of the phospholipase C pathway. *Biophys. J.*, 53: 637a.

Rehm, H. and Betz, H. (1982) Binding of β-bungarotoxin to synaptic membrane fractions of chick brain. *J. Biol. Chem.*, 257: 10015–10022.

Rehm, H. and Betz, H. (1984) Solubilization and characterization of the β-bungarotoxin-binding protein of chick brain membranes. *J. Biol. Chem.*, 259: 6865–6869.

Rehm, H. and Lazdunski, M. (1988a) Purification and subunit structure of a putative K^+-channel protein identified by its binding properties for dendrotoxin I. *Proc. Natl. Acad. Sci. U.S.A.*, 85: 4919–4923.

Rehm, H. and Lazdunski, M. (1988b) Existence of different populations of the dendrotoxin I binding protein associated with neuronal K^+-channels. *Biochem. Biophys. Res. Comm.*, 153: 231–240.

Reinhart, P.H., Chung, S. and Lewitan, I.B. (1989) A family of calcium-dependent potassium channels from rat brain. *Neuron*, 2: 1031–1041.

Rogawsky, M. (1985) The A-current: how ubiquitous a feature of excitable cells is it? *Trends Neurosci.*, 8: 214–219.

Rogawsky, M. (1986) Single voltage-dependent potassium channels in cultured rat hippocampal neurons. *J. Neurophysiol.*, 56: 481–493.

Rudy, B. (1988) Diversity and ubiquity of K channels. *Neuroscience*, 25: 729–749.

Rutecki, P., Lebeda, F.J. and Johnston, D. (1987) 4-Aminopyridine produces epileptiform activity in hippocampus and enhances synaptic excitation and inhibition. *J. Neurophysiol.*, 57: 1911–1924.

Sah, P., Gibb, A.J. and Gage, P.W. (1988) Potassium current activated by depolarization of dissociated neurons from adult guinea-pig hippocampus. *J. Gen. Physiol.*, 92: 263–278.

Salkoff, L.B. and Wyman, R.J. (1983) Ion currents in Drosophila flight muscles. *J. Physiol. (Lond.)*, 337: 687–709.

Schmidt, R.R., Betz, H. and Rehm, H. (1988) Inhibition of β-bungarotoxin binding to membranes by mast-cell degranulating peptide, toxin I and ethylene glycol bis (β-aminoethyl ether)-*N,N,N',N'*-tetraacetic acid. *Biochemistry*, 27: 963–967.

Schwarz, J.R. and Vogel, W. (1971) Potassium inactivation in single myelinated nerve fibers of *Xenopus laevis*. *Pflüg. Arch.*, 330: 60–73.

Schwartzkroin, P.A. and Stafstrom, C.E. (1980) Effects of EGTA on the calcium-activated afterhyperpolarization in hippocampal CA3 pyramidal cells. *Science*, 210: 1125–1126.

Schwindt, P. and Crill, W.E. (1977) A persistent negative

186

resistance in cat lumbar motoneurons. *Brain Res.*, 120: 173–178.

Schwindt, P.C., Spain, W.J., Foehring, R.C., Stafstrom, C.E., Chubb, M.C. and Crill, W.E. (1988) Multiple potassium conductances and their functions in neurons from cat sensorimotor cortex in vitro. *J. Neurophysiol.*, 59: 424–449.

Schwindt, P.C., Spain, W.J. and Crill, W.E. (1989) Long-lasting reduction of excitability by a sodium-dependent potassium current in cat neocortical neurons. *J. Neurophysiol.*, 61: 233–244.

Segal, M. (1980) The action of serotonin in the rat hippocampal slice preparation. *J. Physiol. (Lond.)*, 303: 432–439.

Segal, M. (1982) Multiple actions of acetylcholine at a muscarinic receptor studied in the rat hippocampal slice. *Brain Res.*, 246: 77–87.

Segal, M. (1983) Rat hippocampal neurons in culture: responses to electrical and chemical stimuli. *J. Neurophysiol.*, 50: 1249–1264.

Segal, M. (1988) Synaptic activation of a cholinergic receptor in rat hippocampus. *Brain Res.*, 452: 79–86.

Segal, M. and Barker, J.L. (1984) Rat hippocampal neurons in culture: potassium conductances. *J. Neurophysiol.*, 51: 1409–1433.

Segal, M. and Barker, J.L. (1986) Rat hippocampal neurons in culture: Ca^{2+} and Ca^{2+}-dependent K^+ conductances. *J. Neurophysiol.*, 55: 751–766.

Segal, M., Barker, J.L. and Owen, D.G. (1987) Chloride conductances in central neurons. *Israel J. Med. Sci.*, 23: 95–100.

Segal, M., Rogawsky, M.A. and Barker, J.L. (1984) A transient potassium conductance regulates the excitability of cultured hippocampal and spinal neurons. *J. Neurosci.*, 4: 604–609.

Sims, S.M., Singer, J.J. and Walsh, J.V. (1988) Antagonistic adrenergic-muscarinic regulation of M current in smooth muscle cells. *Science*, 239: 190–193.

Shimahara, T. (1983) Presynaptic modulation of transmitter release by the early outward potassium current in *Aplysia*. *Brain Res.*, 263: 51–56.

Spain, W.J., Schwindt, P.C. and Crill, W.E. (1988) Repetitive firing patterns in cat neocortical neurons depend on preceding subthreshold membrane potential. *Soc. Neurosci. Abstr.*, 14: 298.

Spuler, A., Endres, W. and Grafe, P. (1988) Glucose depletion hyperpolarizes guinea pig hippocampal neurons by an increase in potassium conductance. *Exp. Neurol.*, 100: 248–252.

Stafstrom, C.E., Schwindt, P.C. and Crill, W.E. (1982) Negative slope conductance due to a persistent subthreshold sodium current in cat neocortical neurons in vitro. *Brain Res.*, 236: 221–226.

Stansfeld, C.E. and Feltz, A. (1988) Dendrotoxin-sensitive K channels in dorsal rat ganglion cells. *Neurosci. Lett.*, 93: 49–55.

Stansfeld, C.E., March, S.J., Halliwell, J.V. and Brown, D.A. (1986) 4-amino-pyridine and dendrotoxin induce repetitive firing in rat visceral sensory neurones by blocking a slowly inactivating outward current. *Neurosci. Lett.*, 64: 299–304.

Stansfeld, C.E., March, S.J., Parcej, D.N., Dolly, J.O. and Brown, D.A. (1987) Mast cell degranulating peptide and dendrotoxin selectively inhibit a fast-activating potassium current and bind to common neuronal proteins. *Neuroscience*, 23: 893–902.

Storm, J.F. (1984) Two components of slow prepotentials in CA1 hippocampal pyramidal cells. *Acta Physiol. Scand.*, 120: 15A.

Storm, J.F. (1985) Calcium-dependent spike repolarization, and three kinds of afterhyperpolarization (AHP) in hippocampal pyramidal cells. *Soc. Neurosci. Abstr.*, 11: 1183.

Storm, J.F. (1986a) A-current and Ca-dependent transient outward current control the intial repetitive firing in hippocampal neurons. *Biophys. J.*, 49: 369a.

Storm, J.F. (1987a) Action potential repolarization and a fast after-hyperpolarization in rat hippocampal pyramidal cells. *J. Physiol. (Lond.)*, 385: 733–759.

Storm, J.F. (1987b) Intracellular injection of a Ca^{2+} chelator inhibits spike repolarization in hippocampal neurons. *Brain Res.*, 345: 387–392.

Storm, J.F. (1987c) Potassium currents underlying afterhyperpolarizations (AHPs) and spike repolarization in rat hippocampal pyramidal cells (CA1). *Neurosci. Abstr.*, 13: 176.

Storm, J.F. (1987d) Phorbol esters (PEs) broaden the action potential in CA1 hippocampal pyramidal cells. *Neurosci. Lett.*, 75: 71–74.

Storm, J.F. (1988a) Temporal integration by a slowly inactivating K^+ current in hippocampal neurons. *Nature (Lond.)*, 336: 379–381.

Storm, J.F. (1988b) Four voltage-dependent potassium currents in adult hippocampal pyramidal cells. *Biophys. J.*, 53: 148a.

Storm, J.F. (1988c) Evidence that two 4-aminopyridine (4-AP)-sensitive potassium currents, I_A and I_D, contribute to spike repolarization in rat hippocampal pyramidal cells. *Eur. J. Neurosci.*, Suppl. 1: 42.

Storm, J.F. (1988d) Modulation of spike repolarization in hippocampal neurones by tumor-promoting phorbol esters. In H.L. Haas and G. Buzaki (Eds.), *Synaptic Plasticity in the Hippocampus*, Springer-Verlag, Berlin, Heidelberg.

Storm, J.F. (1989) An after-hyperpolarization of medium duration in rat hippocampal pyramidal cells. *J. Physiol. (Lond.)*, 409: 171–190.

Storm, J.F., Borg-Graham, L. and Adams, P.R. (1987) A passive component of the afterdepolarization (ADP) in rat hippocampal pyramidal cells. *Biophys. J.*, 51: 65a.

Storm, J.F. and Helliesen, M. (1989) Evidence that a barium-sensitive potassium current contributes to the resting potential and spike repolarization in rat hippocampal neurons. *Soc. Neurosci. Abstr.*, 15: 77.

Strong, J.A. (1984) Modulation of potassium current kinetics in bag cell neurons of Aplysia by an activator of adenyl cyclase. *J. Neurosci.*, 4: 2772 – 2783.

Thesleff, S. (1980) Aminopyridines and synaptic transmission. *Neuroscience*, 5: 1413 – 1419.

Thompson, S.H. (1977) Three pharmacologically distinct potassium channels in molluscan neurones. *J. Physiol. (Lond.)*, 265: 465 – 488.

Thompson, S.M. (1989) Activity-dependent disinhibition. II. Effects of extracellular potassium, furosemide and membrane potential on E_{Cl^-} in hippocampal CA3 neurons. *J. Neurophysiol.*, 61: 512 – 523.

Tsuji, S. and Kuba, K. (1988) Muscarinic regulation of two ionic currents in the bullfrog sympathetic neurone. *Pflügers Arch.*, 411: 361 – 370.

Turner, D.A. and Schwartzkroin, P.A. (1980) Steady-state electrotonic analysis of intracellularly-stained hippocampal neurons. *J. Neurophysiol.*, 44: 184 – 189.

Turner, D.A. and Schwartzkroin, P.A. (1984) Passive electrotonic structure and dendritic properties of hippocampal neurons. In R. Dingledine (Ed.), *Brain Slices*, Plenum, New York.

VanDongen, A.M.J., Codina, J., Olate, J., Mattera, R., Joho, R., Birnbaumer, L. and Brown, A.M. (1988) Newly identified brain potassium channels gated by the guanine nucleotide binding protein G_o. *Science*, 242: 1433 – 1437.

Watson, T.W.J. and Pittman, Q.J. (1988) Pharmacological evidence that somatostatin activates the M-current in hippocampal pyramidal neurons. *Neurosci. Lett.*, 91: 172 – 176.

Williamson, A. and Alger, B.E. (1987) A transient Ca-dependent K potential follows a brief spike train in hippocampus. *Soc. Neurosci. Abstr.*, 13: 156.

Wilson, W.A. and Goldner, M.A. (1975) Voltage clamping with a single microelectrode. *J. Neurobiol.*, 6: 411 – 422.

Yamamoto, C. and McIlwain, H. (1966) Electrical activities in thin sections from the mammalian brain maintained in chemically defined media in vitro. *J. Neurochem.*, 13: 1333 – 1343.

Yarom, Y. and Llinas, R. (1987) Long-term modifiability of anomalous and delayed rectification in guinea pig inferior olivary neurons. *J. Neurosci.*, 7: 1166 – 1177.

Zbicz, K.L. and Weight, F.F. (1985) Transient voltage and calcium-dependent outward currents in hippocampal CA3 pyramidal neurons. *J. Neurophysiol.*, 53: 1038 – 1058.

Zhang, L. and Krnjević, K. (1987) Apamin depresses selectively the after-hyperpolarization of cat spinal motoneurons. *Neurosci. Lett.*, 74: 58 – 62.

Zgombic, J.M., Beck, S.G. Mahle, C.D., Craddock-Royal, B. and Maayani, S. (1989) Pertussis-toxin sensitive guanine nucleotide binding protein(s) couple adenosine A1 and 5-hydroxytryptamine$_{A1}$ receptors to the same effector systems in rat hippocampus: biochemical and electrophysiological studies. *Mol. Pharmacol.*, 35: 484 – 494.

J. Storm-Mathisen, J. Zimmer and O.P. Ottersen (Eds.)
Progress in Brain Research, Vol. 83
© 1990 Elsevier Science Publishers B.V. (Biomedical Division)

CHAPTER 13

Cytosolic free calcium in hippocampal CA3 pyramidal cells

Thomas Knöpfel[1], Serge Charpak[1], David A. Brown[2] and Beat H. Gähwiler[1]

[1] *Brain Research Institute, University of Zürich, August Forel Strasse 1, CH-8029 Zürich, Switzerland and*
[2] *Department of Pharmacology, University College, Gower Street, London WC1E 6BT, U.K.*

The dynamics of cytosolic free Ca^{2+} ($[Ca^{2+}]_i$) of single voltage-clamped CA3 pyramidal cells in hippocampal slice cultures is reviewed. $[Ca^{2+}]_i$ amounts to about 30 nM at resting membrane potential and increases slowly when the membrane potential is clamped at more positive values (up to 500 nM at -30 mV). Short lasting depolarizations (40–100 ms) induce a transient rise in $[Ca^{2+}]_i$ which activates a slow aftercurrent (I_{AHP}). The muscarinic or β-adrenergic depression of I_{AHP} is not accompanied by any change in the dynamics of Ca^{2+} and appears, therefore, to result primarily from an inhibition of the K^+-current itself or of the ability of Ca^{2+} to activate the current. At higher concentrations than those required to inhibit I_{AHP}, muscarine produces a pronounced inward current and this is accompanied by a rise in resting $[Ca^{2+}]_i$ concentration.

Introduction and methods

Calcium ions serve as an intracellular messenger for numerous neuronal functions. In the past few years powerful Ca^{2+} indicators have been developed which allow us to monitor cytosolic free Ca^{2+} of individual central neurons (Grynkiewicz et al., 1985). This paper reports on measurements of cytosolic Ca^{2+} by means of the fluorescent calcium indicator fura-2 in single voltage-clamped CA3 pyramidal cells in hippocampal slice cultures. This in vitro preparation of the hippocampus is thin enough to allow experimental manipulations, such as fast changes of the extracellular solution, and visualization of individual cells, but on the other hand keeps an organotypic organization of the original tissue (Gähwiler, 1981; Gähwiler and Knöpfel, 1989).

For electrophysiological studies, cultures were transferred to a perfused temperature-controlled (32°C) chamber which was mounted on the stage of an inverted microscope. The composition of the perfusate was (mM): Na^+ 148.9; K^+ 2.7; Cl^- 145.9; Ca^{2+} 3.8; Mg^{2+} 2.5; HCO_3^- 11.6; $H_2PO_4^-$ 0.4; D-glucose 5.6. Neurons of the hippocampal CA3 region were impaled with thin-walled microelectrodes which contained the calcium indicator fura-2. After microiontophoretic injection of fura-2 into CA3 pyramidal cells, they were morphologically identified and recorded using switched single electrode voltage-clamp techniques. To measure cytosolic Ca^{2+} concentrations, the intensity of fura-2 fluorescence was recorded by means of a photodiode and low-noise electronics. The calculation of the cytosolic Ca^{2+} concentration ($[Ca^{2+}]_i$) from fura-2 fluorescence intensity takes advantage of the difference in the excitation spectra of fura-2 in the free and Ca^{2+}-bound form. The measurements of intensity obtained at two excitation wavelengths allows the $[Ca^{2+}]_i$ to be calculated (Grynkiewicz et al., 1985).

Cytosolic Ca^{2+} increases upon depolarization

Fig. 1 shows combined voltage-clamp and optical

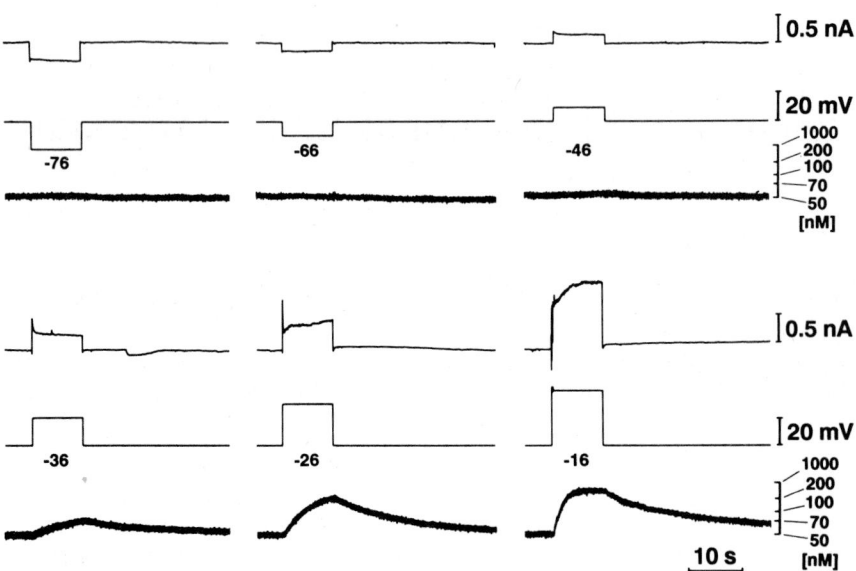

Fig. 1. Combined intracellular recordings and microfluorometric measurements of cytosolic free Ca^{2+} in a hippocampal CA3 pyramidal cell. The cell was voltage-clamped at a holding potential of -56 mV and subjected to a family of voltage steps of varying amplitudes. Clamp-current, voltage and cytosolic free Ca^{2+} are shown on the upper, middle and lower trace, respectively. Depolarization to -36 mV or more positive values results in a progressive rise in $[Ca^{2+}]_i$. Note non-linear scaling of Ca^{2+}-signal.

recordings from a CA3 pyramidal cell injected with fura-2. Cytosolic free Ca^{2+}, which amounts to around 30 nM at the holding membrane potential of -50 mV increases slowly when the membrane potential is clamped at more positive values. Notably, $[Ca^{2+}]_i$ could increase to values as large as 500 nM at -30 mV. This large increase in $[Ca^{2+}]_i$ has to be taken into account when cells are clamped at depolarized holding potentials to study voltage-dependent conductances. Even more important is to note that Ca^{2+} might rise to similar high levels in vivo as a consequence of processes leading to pronounced long lasting depolarizations such as paroxysmal depolarization shifts (Ayala et al., 1973).

What is the source of this Ca^{2+}? Hippocampal pyramidal cells possess at least 3 types of voltage-gated calcium channels. The depolarization induced Ca^{2+}-increase results at least in part from the activation of some of these (or other) voltage-gated Ca^{2+} conductances, since the Ca^{2+} increase is abolished after changing the recording solution to one containing no Ca^{2+} and a high Mg^{2+} concen-

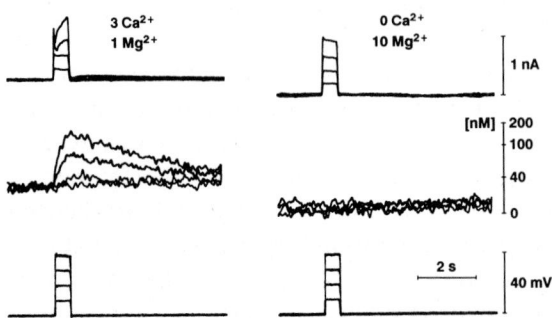

Fig. 2. Depolarization-induced increase in cytosolic free Ca^{2+} is abolished by removing external Ca^{2+}. A CA3 pyramidal cell superfused with a solution containing 1 μM TTX was voltage-clamped at a holding potential of -58 mV and subjected to 500 ms voltage steps to -48, -38, -28 and -18 mV. Commands to -28 and -18 mV trigger a rise in cytosolic Ca^{2+}. After switching from the recording solution containing 3 mM Ca^{2+} and 1 mM Mg^{2+} (left panel) to one containing zero Ca^{2+} and 10 mM Mg^{2+} (right panel), the Ca^{2+} transients disappear, resting $[Ca^{2+}]_i$ drops close to zero and an inward current develops.

tration (Fig. 2). This observation does not exclude the possibility that part of the Ca^{2+} increase might stem from intracellular stores, release from which is triggered by Ca^{2+} inflow.

Short-lasting depolarizations induce Ca^{2+} transients and slow AHPs

Short-lasting depolarizations (40 – 100 ms) induce a transient rise in Ca^{2+} as well. Fig. 3A1 shows the progressive increase in $[Ca^{2+}]_i$ during a train of action potentials. Ca^{2+} stays up after the depolarization and slowly falls; this is accompanied by a slow after-hyperpolarization (AHP). This slow AHP has previously been studied in hippocampal pyramidal cells using the acute slice preparation (Hotson and Prince, 1980; Alger and Nicoll, 1980; Schwartzkroin and Stafstrom, 1980; Gustafsson and Wigström, 1981). It is blocked by removing external Ca^{2+} or by adding a divalent Ca^{2+}-channel blocker, and hence has been attributed to the depolarization induced rise in cytosolic Ca^{2+} concentration. The slow AHP could also be blocked by intracellular injection of Ca^{2+} chelators (Alger and Nicoll, 1980; Schwartzkroin and Stafstrom, 1980; Storm, 1987). Since it can still be recorded in our fura-2 loaded cells, the amounts of fura-2 injected are sufficiently low as not to buffer the Ca^{2+} transient and so inhibit the AHP.

The slow AHP is generated by a potassium current which has been termed I_{AHP} (Lancaster and Adams, 1986). Under voltage clamp conditions I_{AHP} can be induced by applying a short (40 – 100 ms) depolarizing voltage step (Fig. 3B). I_{AHP} is then seen as a slow outward after-current, of similar time-course to the after-hyperpolarization following an action potential train. The induction of I_{AHP} is accompanied by a rise in cytosolic Ca^{2+}, peaking slightly earlier and lasting somewhat longer than the outward current. Increasing the amplitude of the voltage steps is followed by both an after-current and a Ca^{2+} transient of increasing amplitude. Parallel changes in Ca^{2+} transients and I_{AHP} can be elicited as well

by changes in extracellular Ca^{2+} (Fig. 4A). The after-current appears to be caused by the Ca^{2+} transient since the relation between the after-current and the Ca^{2+} signal is unaffected by a

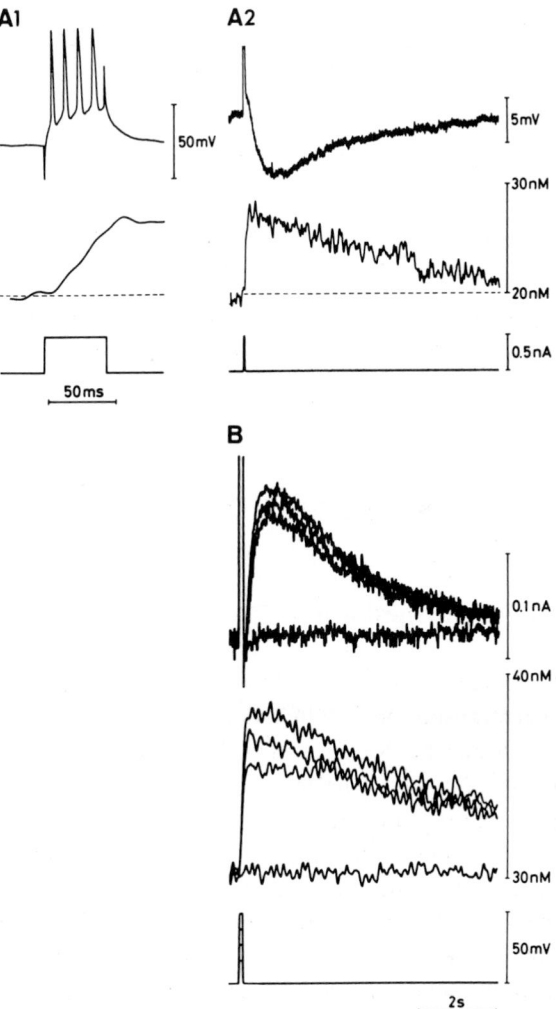

Fig. 3. Induction of Ca^{2+} transients and of a slow afterhyperpolarization by short-lasting depolarizations. A1, A2: action potentials evoked by injection of a current pulse are followed by a slowly decaying AHP and induce a transient increase in cytosolic $[Ca^{2+}]$. Reproduction at fast (A1) and slow (A2) time scale of membrane potential (upper trace), $[Ca^{2+}]_i$ (middle trace) and injected current (lower trace). B: in the presence of 1 μM TTX the cell shown in A was voltage-clamped at a holding potential of -55 mV and subjected to 100-ms voltage steps to -35, -25, -15 and -5 mV. Voltage steps to -25 mV or more positive values induce an outward after-current (upper records) and a transient rise in $[Ca^{2+}]_i$ (lower records).

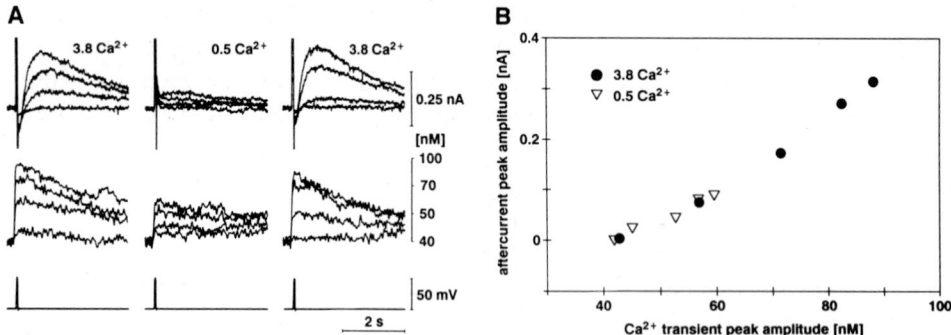

Fig. 4. Dependence of the slow after-hyperpolarization on the Ca^{2+} load. A: a CA3 pyramidal cell superfused with a solution containing 1 μM TTX, voltage clamped at -53 mV and submitted to 100-ms voltage steps of increasing amplitude. Records of clamp current (upper traces), Ca^{2+} transient (middle traces) and voltage (lower traces) were obtained in control recording solution containing 3.8 mM Ca^{2+} (left panel), in the presence of 0.5 mM Ca^{2+} (middle panel) and again in control solution (right panel). The slow after-current and the depolarization-induced calcium transient are markly reduced when decreasing the extracellular concentration of Ca^{2+}, though induced by the same voltage steps (note the non-linear scaling for the Ca^{2+} recording). B: the after-current peak amplitude as a function of Ca^{2+} transient peak amplitude. Note that the relationship is linear and is unaffected by the change of the extracellular Ca^{2+} concentration.

change of the extracellular Ca^{2+} concentration (Fig. 4B).

Adrenergic depression of I_{AHP}

I_{AHP} can be readily inhibited by several neurotransmitters including noradrenaline (Madison and Nicoll, 1982; Haas and Konnerth, 1983) and acetylcholine (Benardo and Prince, 1982; Cole and Nicoll, 1983, 1984a; Gähwiler, 1984; Madison et al., 1987). The action of noradrenaline is mediated by a β-adrenoceptor. Based on their observation that noradrenaline did not depress Ca^{2+} spikes in CA1 pyramidal neurons, Madison and Nicoll (1986) suggested that the adrenergic depression of Ca^{2+}-activated AHP is not the result of a decreased Ca^{2+}-inflow. This suggestion is in line with evidence that activation of β-adrenoceptors even enhances the activity of voltage-dependent calcium channels in granule cells of the dentate gyrus (Gray and Johnston, 1987).

On the other hand, effects on Ca^{2+} currents are difficult to separate from those on potassium currents and the lack of an effect on calcium currents does not exclude other transmitter actions resulting

in an alteration of depolarization induced cytosolic Ca^{2+} transients. For instance, it is conceivable that alterations of the Ca^{2+} sequestration mechanism would affect depolarization-induced Ca^{2+} transients without having any effect on Ca^{2+} currents as evaluated by means of microelectrode recording techniques. To test this possibility, we have measured the cytosolic Ca^{2+} transients accompanying I_{AHP} before, during and after adrenergic depression of I_{AHP}. Bath application of the selective β-adrenoceptor agonist isoproterenol (1–2.5 μM) for 1–2 min reversibly depresses the I_{AHP} without affecting the evoked calcium transient or the resting calcium concentration (Fig. 5A). This substantiates the initial suggestion of Madison and Nicoll that the adrenergic inhibition of I_{AHP} does not result from a change in Ca^{2+} influx.

Muscarinic depression of I_{AHP}

The effect of acetylcholine on hippocampal pyramidal cells is mediated by muscarinic receptors. Initial experiments suggested that acetylcholine does not inhibit Ca^{2+} currents (as measured from the Ca^{2+} spike recorded in tetrodotoxin/tetra-ethylammonium solution: Cole and Nicoll, 1984b) but some subsequent observations have shown that Ca^{2+} currents in hippocampal pyramidal neurons recorded under voltage-clamp can be inhibited by muscarinic agonists (Gähwiler and Brown, 1987; Toselli and Lux, 1989). Thus the mechanism of I_{AHP} inhibition by muscarine is not clear: muscarine might modify Ca^{2+} entry, intracellular Ca^{2+} homeostasis or the K^+ current itself. Again, these possibilities were tested by combined microfluorometric and microelectrode measurements.

Distinct effects of muscarine can be separated by the concentration of muscarine which was bath-applied. Low concentrations of muscarine

$(0.25 - 1 \ \mu M$ for $30 - 60$ s) can fully abolish I_{AHP} without affecting the calcium transient or the resting cytosolic free Ca^{2+} concentration (Fig. 5B). We conclude, therefore, that the depression of I_{AHP} produced by muscarine results primarily from an inhibition of the K^+ current itself or of the ability of Ca^{2+} to activate the current, rather than from a change in Ca^{2+} influx or sequestration.

Higher concentrations of muscarine $(1 - 100 \ \mu M)$, not only depress I_{AHP} but also induce a pro-

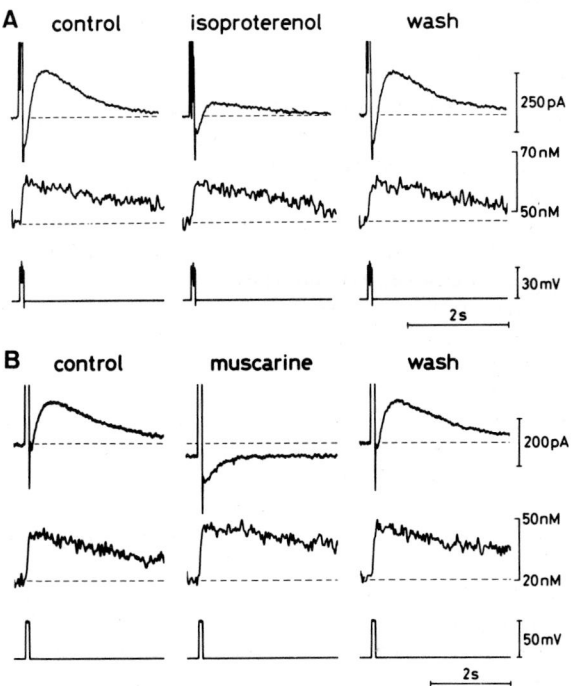

Fig. 5. Effect of isoproterenol and muscarine on I_{AHP} and on cytosolic $[Ca^{2+}]$. CA3 pyramidal cells were superfused with a solution containing 1 μM TTX and voltage-clamped at about -55 mV. Voltage jumps of 100 ms duration to about 0 mV induce slow outward after-currents and Ca^{2+} transients. Clamp-current (upper traces), $[Ca^{2+}]_i$ (middle traces) and voltage (lower traces) before (control), during, and 20 min (A) respectively 5 min (B) after (wash) application of 1.25 μM isoproterenol (A), and 0.25 μM of muscarine (B).

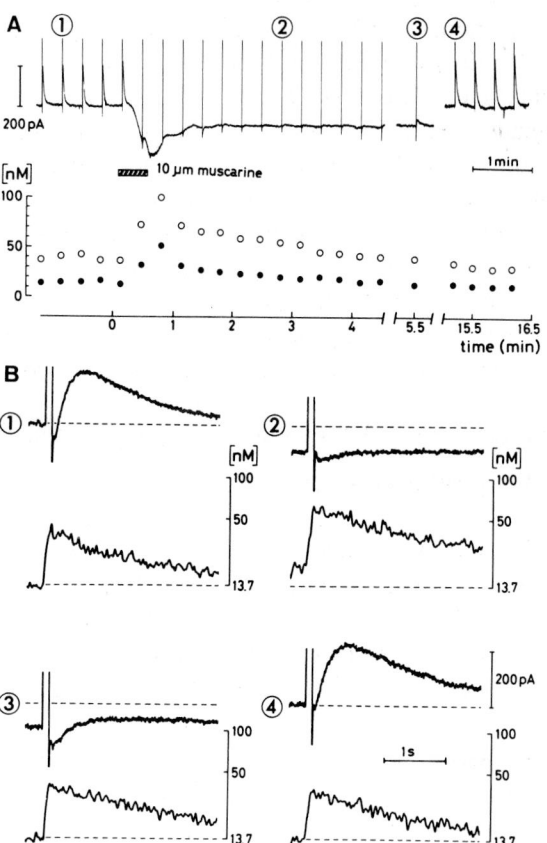

Fig. 6. Effect of higher concentrations of muscarine on $[Ca^{2+}]_i$. Slow outward after-currents were induced by 100-ms voltage jumps from a holding potential of -50 mV to 0 mV at 0.05 Hz in a CA3 pyramidal cell bathed in 1 μM TTX. A: recording of clamp-current (upper trace), time-course of $[Ca^{2+}]_i$ ($\bullet$) and time-course of peak amplitudes of Ca^{2+} transients ($\circ$). B: records of clamp-currents, cytosolic Ca^{2+} transients and voltage obtained at times $1 - 4$ as indicated in A.

nounced inward current amounting up to 0.5 nA. This inward current has been attributed to inhibition of at least two species of K^+ current: the voltage-dependent M-current (Halliwell and Adams, 1982; Gähwiler and Brown, 1985) and a voltage-independent leak current (Madison et al., 1987; Benson et al., 1988). It appears immediately after the onset of the muscarine application and typically exhibits a biphasic time course consisting of a larger fast component and a smaller slow component (cf. Pitler et al., 1988). During this inward current, $[Ca^{2+}]_i$ dynamics are significantly altered. A typical experiment is illustrated in Fig. 6. In parallel with the inward current, cytosolic Ca^{2+} rises and the Ca^{2+} transients increase in amplitude. The inward current and the Ca^{2+} signals drop to initial values after a wash of about 5 min while I_{AHP} recovers only after about 15 min. The time course of the inward current and $[Ca^{2+}]_i$ rise are strikingly similar but differed from that of the AHP depression. We conclude therefore that both the inward current and the accompanying change in $[Ca^{2+}]_i$ are effects of muscarine distinct from its action on the slow AHP.

Acknowledgements

This study was supported by the Swiss National Science Foundation (Grant No. 31 – 8885.86) and a grant of the U.K. Medical Research Council (D.A.B.). We thank L. Rietschin, R. Emch, and R. Schoeb for excellent technical assistance.

References

Alger, B.E. and Nicoll, R.A. (1980) Epileptiform burst after hyperpolarization; calcium-dependent potassium potential in hippocampal CA1 pyramidal cells. Science, 210: 1122 – 1124.

Ayala, G.F., Dichter, M., Gumnit, R.J., Matsumoto, H. and Spencer, W.A. (1973) Genesis of epileptic interictal spikes. New knowledge of cortical feedback systems suggests a neurophysiological explanation of brief paroxysms. Brain Res., 52: 1 – 17.

Benardo, L.S. and Prince, D.A. (1982) Ionic mechanisms of cholinergic excitation in mammalian hippocampal pyramidal cells. Brain Res., 249: 333 – 344.

Benson, D.M., Blitzer, R.D. and Landau, E.M. (1988) An analysis of the depolarization produced in guinea-pig hippocampus by cholinergic receptor stimulation. J. Physiol. (Lond.), 404: 479 – 496.

Cole, A.E. and Nicoll, R.A. (1983) Acetylcholine mediates a slow synaptic potential in hippocampal pyramidal cells. Science, 221: 1299 – 1301.

Cole, A.E. and Nicoll, R.A. (1984a) Characterization of a slow cholinergic postsynaptic potential recorded in vitro from rat hippocampal pyramidal cells. J. Physiol. (Lond.), 352: 173 – 188.

Cole, A.E. and Nicoll, R.A. (1984b) The pharmacology of cholinergic excitatory responses in hippocampal pyramidal cells. Brain Res., 305: 283 – 290.

Gray, R. and Johnston, D. (1987) Noradrenaline and β-adrenoceptor agonists increase activity of voltage-dependent calcium channels in hippocampal neurons. Nature (Lond.), 327: 620 – 622.

Grynkiewicz, G., Poenie, M. and Tsien, R.Y. (1985) A new generation of Ca^{2+} indicators with greatly improved fluorescence properties. J. Biol. Chem., 260: 3440 – 3450.

Gustafsson, B. and Wigström, H. (1981) Evidence for two types of afterhyperpolarization in CA1 pyramidal cells in the hippocampus. Brain Res., 206: 462 – 468.

Gähwiler, B.H. (1981) Organotypic monolayer cultures of nervous tissue. J. Neurosci. Methods, 4: 329 – 342.

Gähwiler, B.H. (1984) Facilitation by acetylcholine of tetrodotoxin-resistant spikes in rat hippocampal pyramidal cells. Neuroscience, 11: 381 – 388.

Gähwiler, B.H. and Brown, D.A. (1985) Functional innervation of cultured hippocampal neurones by cholinergic afferents from co-cultured septal explants. Nature (Lond.), 313: 577 – 579.

Gähwiler, B.H. and Brown, D.A. (1987) Muscarine affects calcium-currents in rat hippocampal pyramidal cells in vitro. Neurosci. Lett., 76: 301 – 306.

Gähwiler, B.H. and Knöpfel, T. (1990) Cultures of brain slices. In H. Jahnsen (Ed.), In vitro Preparations from Vertebrate Nervous Systems, John Wiley and Sons.

Haas, H.L. and Konnerth, A. (1983) Histamine and noradrenaline decrease calcium-activated potassium conductance in hippocampal pyramidal cells. Nature (Lond.), 302: 432 – 434.

Halliwell, J.V. and Adams, P.R. (1982) Voltage-clamp analysis of muscarinic excitation in hippocampal neurons. Brain Res., 250: 71 – 92.

Hotson, J.R. and Prince, D.A. (1980) A Ca-activated hyperpolarization follows repetitive firing in hippocampal neurons. J. Neurophysiol., 43: 409 – 419.

Lancaster, B. and Adams, P.R. (1986) Calcium-dependent current generating the after-hyperpolarization of hippocampal neurons. J. Neurophysiol., 55: 1268 – 1282.

Madison, D.V. and Nicoll, R.A. (1982) Noradrenaline blocks

accommodation of pyramidal cell discharge in the hippocampus. *Nature (Lond.)*, 299: 636 – 638.

Madison, D.V. and Nicoll, R.A. (1986) Actions of noradrenaline recorded intracellularly in rat hippocampal CA1 pyramidal neurones, in vitro. *J. Physiol. (Lond.)*, 372: 221 – 244.

Madison, D.V., Lancaster, B. and Nicoll, R.A. (1987) Voltage clamp analysis of cholinergic action in the hippocampus. *J. Neurosci.*, 7: 733 – 741.

Pitler, T.A., McCarren, M. and Alger, B.E. (1988) Calcium-dependent pirenzepine-sensitive muscarinic response in the rat hippocampal slice. *Neurosci. Lett.*, 91: 177 – 182.

Schwartzkroin, P.A. and Stafstrom, C.E. (1980) Effects of EGTA on the calcium-activated afterhyperpolarization in hippocampal CA3 pyramidal cells. *Science*, 210: 1125 – 1126.

Storm, J.F. (1987) Intracellular injection of a Ca^{2+} chelator inhibits spike repolarization in hippocampal neurons. *Brain Res.*, 435: 387 – 392.

Toselli, M. and Lux, H.D. (1989) GTP-binding proteins mediate acetylcholine inhibition of voltage dependent calcium channels in hippocampal neurons. *Pflügers Arch.*, 413: 319 – 321.

J. Storm-Mathisen, J. Zimmer and O.P. Ottersen (Eds.)
Progress in Brain Research, Vol. 83
© 1990 Elsevier Science Publishers B.V. (Biomedical Division)

CHAPTER 14

Activity-dependent ionic changes and neuronal plasticity in rat hippocampus

Uwe Heinemann, Jasmine Stabel and Günther Rausche

Institut für Neurophysiologie, Zentrum Physiologie und Pathophysiologie, Universität zu Köln, Robert Kochstr. 39, D-5000 Köln 41, F.R.G.

We describe here the ionic changes which occur during repetitive stimulation of a type which will induce long-term potentiation and kindling plasticity. The causes of these ionic changes, particularly of changes in $[Ca^{2+}]_o$, are discussed. Evidence will be presented which shows that only a fraction of the decreases in $[Ca^{2+}]_o$ is due to movement through N-methyl-D-aspartate (NMDA)-operated channels. Since NMDA-receptor activation is critical in many synapses for induction of long-term potentiation (LTP) and since the initial response to a stimulus in hippocampus is a long-lasting slow inhibitory postsynaptic potential (IPSP), mechanisms must be defined which ultimately permit activation of NMDA receptors. We conclude that increases in $[K^+]_o$ and reductions in $[Ca^{2+}]_o$ and $[Mg^{2+}]_o$, together with a K^+-dependent reduction of slow IPSP promote the activation of NMDA receptors during a stimulus train and help to overcome the blocking effect which the long-lasting hyperpolarizations exert on NMDA receptors. Preliminary evidence derived from analysis of quisqualate and NMDA-induced changes in $[Ca^{2+}]_o$ suggests that NMDA-receptor activation slows the extrusion of Ca^{2+} from cells. This mechanism may be important for induction of long-term changes. Finally, we document that a number of long-term changes in neuronal excitability are associated with alterations of stimulus and excitatory amino acid (EAA)-induced changes in the ionic microenvironment, which give some insight into the mechanisms underlying stimulus-induced plasticity and, perhaps, progression of temporal lobe epilepsy.

Introduction

The hippocampus is unique not only with respect to its anatomical organization and its plastic properties but also for its involvement in seizure generation, often with chronic progression. The hippocampus receives a major input from the medial and lateral entorhinal cortex (EC) and provides feedback to the subiculum and entorhinal cortex (Andersen et al., 1971). Probably, the EC has less plastic properties than the hippocampus, suggesting that plastic alterations within the hippocampal formation account for progressive aspects of temporal lobe epilepsies.

Fig. 1 illustrates some of the basic features of epileptogenesis in a slice preparation of the hippocampal formation containing the rhinal, perirhinal and entorhinal cortex as well as the den-

tate gyrus (DG) and the CA subfields (Dreier, Köhr and Heinemann, in preparation). The epileptiform activity in this preparation was induced by lowering $[Mg^{2+}]_o$ (Walther et al., 1986; Avoli et al., 1987; Heinemann, 1987; Mody et al., 1987; Stanton et al., 1987; Köhr and Heinemann, 1989). In the rhinal cortex (i.e. the cortex neighboring the perirhinal cortex around the rhinal fissure) both ictal and interictal activity do occur while in the entorhinal cortex ictal-like events are observed (Jones and Heinemann, 1988). In spite of heavy synaptic bombardment from the EC via the medial and lateral perforant path the DG is not recruited into the seizure-like events (Walther et al., 1986; Lambert and Jones, 1988). Hence the areas CA3 and CA1 develop independent interictal-like activity with a mean frequency of 20/min (Walther et al., 1986). Some of the seizure-like events are transferred directly to area CA1 and to some degree also to area CA3 presumably through the subiculum and the alvear path. This afferent input also does not recruit these areas into seizure activity.

The failure of the DG to actively participate in seizure events is also noted when seizure-like activity is induced in such preparations by application of GABA antagonists such as bicuculline (Heinemann and Jones, 1989). Thus the DG normally prevents spread of seizure activity from the EC to the hippocampal formation. The filter function of the DG may be related to the behavior of synaptic responses during repetitive stimulation of the medial and lateral perforant path. This leads to frequency habituation, (i.e. a decrease in postsynaptic responses) which only later turns into frequency potentiation. Frequency potentiation is characteristic of postsynaptic responses in the rest of the hippocampus (Alger and Teyler, 1976; Collingridge et al., 1983; Harris and Cotman, 1985).

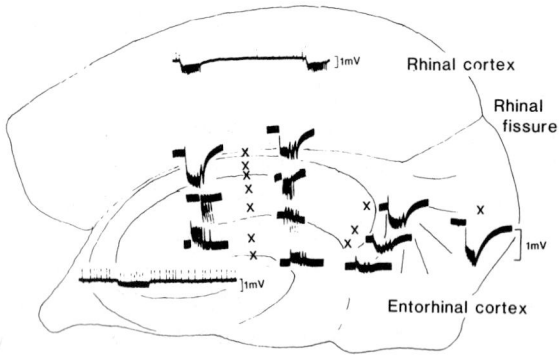

Fig. 1. Epileptiform activity induced by lowering extracellular magnesium concentration in temporal cortex slices including rhinal, perirhinal, entorhinal, subicular and frontal hippocampal areas. Composite figure from 3 different experiments in which Mg^{2+} was lowered for about 45 – 60 min. Note interictal and ictal activity in temporal neocortex, interictal activity in CA3 which is not affected by the propagated activity from EC and subiculum and the accommodating activity in dentate gyrus. Positive going slow field potentials are typical for sites with little active participation in seizures. Seizure-like events lasted between 10 and 60 s in 8 experiments.

Since a number of conditions exist where the DG actively participates in seizure generation, its filter capabilities must be adjustable. Indeed, the filter function of the hippocampus can be changed acutely by synaptic mechanisms. Baclofen, a $GABA_B$ receptor agonist (Dutar and Nicoll, 1988) with stronger effects on inhibitory neurons in this area than on granule cells can disinhibit the DG by inhibiting the hilar inhibitory neurons (Misgeld et al., 1984, 1986, 1989; Misgeld and Frotscher, 1986; Mott et al., 1989). Also norepinephrine (NE) can reverse frequency habituation into frequency potentiation (Stanton et al., 1989a).

In chronic epilepsies, such as the kindling epilepsy, it is likely that the DG loses some of its filter capabilities in spite of augmented GABAergic inhibition and in spite of loss of effects of NE on the synaptic responses. The kindling epilepsy is usually induced by repetitive stimulation of a type which normally induces long-term potentiation (LTP) (Bliss and Lømo, 1973). When such repetitive stimulation is repeated within some hours to a day (kindling) to the perforant path or other pathways in the EC-hippocampal formation, it will eventually induce generalized seizures (Goddard et al., 1969).

The fact that hippocampal cells are initially hyperpolarized during a stimulus train raises the question, how activation of NMDA receptors and accumulation of intracellular Ca^{2+} is accomplished (Nowak et al., 1984) which appear to be prerequisites for the induction of LTP and perhaps of kindling plasticity. Since these stimulus conditions are associated with changes in the extracellular microenvironment, this review will describe the types of ionic changes observed during repetitive stimulation. We will then proceed to document some of the causes and consequences of such ionic changes. Subsequently, we will discuss the role such ionic changes play in frequency potentiation and frequency habituation. More specifically, we will demonstrate that slow IPSPs underlie frequency habituation in the DG. Finally, we will relate these ionic changes to the development of LTP and kindling plasticity.

Stimulus-induced ionic changes in rat hippocampus

The ionic changes in the CA1 subfield, evoked by repetitive stimulation to the Schaffer collateral/commissural pathways, are illustrated in Fig. 2. Such repetitive stimulation leads to increases in $[K^+]_o$ and to decreases in $[Ca^{2+}]_o$ and in $[Na^+]_o$. These alterations are accompanied by decreases in $[Cl^-]_o$ and $[Mg^{2+}]_o$. More prolonged stimuli will also cause a reduction in the extracellular space (ES) (Heinemann et al., 1983). All these ionic changes are associated with negative slow field potentials (fp). These changes are strongly dependent on both train duration and stimulus intensity and frequency. $[K^+]_o$ can increase by 9 mM (Benninger et al., 1980; Krnjević

et al., 1982; Heinemann et al., 1986c; Lux et al., 1986), $[Na^+]_o$ can decrease by 28 mM (Köhr and Heinemann, 1988), $[Ca^{2+}]_o$ by 0.6 mM (Krnjević et al., 1982; Köhr and Heinemann, 1989) and $[Mg^{2+}]_o$ by 0.3 mM (Arens and Heinemann, in preparation). Extracellular $[Cl^-]_o$ can decrease by 6 mM (Müller et al., 1989) and the extracellular space by more than 10% (Heinemann et al., 1983). Associated negative slow fp can be as large as 6 mV (Benninger et al., 1980; Heinemann and Pumain, unpublished).

For the functional consequences of changes in the minor ion concentrations, the baseline levels from which these ionic changes occur are important. Physiologically, the baseline $[K^+]_o$ is near 3 mM and baseline $[Ca^{2+}]_o$ near 1.2 mM (Heinemann et al., 1977). In the presence of a bicarbonate buffer about one quarter of the extracellularly available Ca^{2+} is in a chelated form. Thus, if one adds 1.2 mM to a bicarbonate-buffered solution the available $[Ca^{2+}]_o$ is only in the order of 0.9 mM. The baseline $[Mg^{2+}]_o$ was not determined in rat hippocampus but recent measurements by Pumain (in preparation) in rat neocortex have revealed that the baseline $[Mg^{2+}]_o$ is near 2 mM. Thus, many in vivo slice experiments are carried out in physiologically abnormal conditions with $[K^+]_o$ and $[Ca^{2+}]_o$ slightly elevated. Unfortunately, a number of more recent studies which try to take account of "physiological baseline levels" work with $[Ca^{2+}]_o$ and $[Mg^{2+}]_o$ levels which are too low.

Regional variations in alterations of the ionic microenvironment

In the different subfields of the hippocampus stimulus-induced changes in $[Na^+]_o$ and $[K^+]_o$ are, in contrast to changes in $[Ca^{2+}]_o$, well comparable. The largest decreases in $[Ca^{2+}]_o$ are observed in area CA1 followed by area CA3 and the dentate gyrus. However, this relationship does not necessarily result from a much larger cellular Ca^{2+} load in area CA1 than in the DG. Studies on the volume fraction of the ES have revealed that

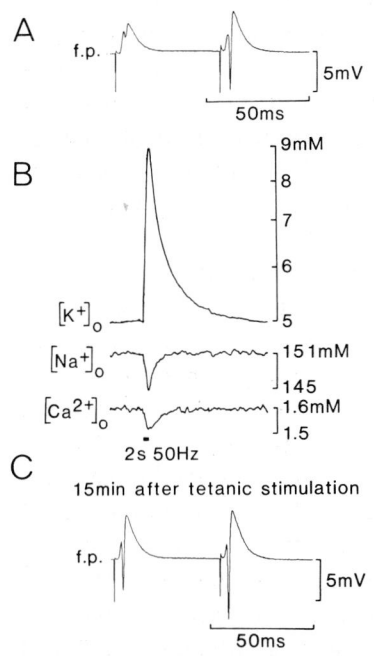

Fig. 2. Changes in extracellular potassium, calcium and sodium concentration (B) during a stimulus (2 s, 50 Hz, ca 100 μA applied to stratum radiatum of area CA1) used to potentiate the control response in A to that in C. Recording in stratum pyramidale of area CA1. Measurements performed with a combined electrode ensemble consisting of different ion-selective/reference electrode pairs glued together with tip separations of less than 50 μm.

the packing density is particularly high in stratum pyramidale (SP) of area CA1 with volume fractions of approximately 7% (Heinemann et al., 1983; Holsheimer, 1987). In the DG and area CA3, the volume fraction is larger (approximately 16%). Hence, the cellular Ca^{2+} load during repetitive stimulation and seizures might actually be larger in the DG than in area CA1.

Apart from stimulus intensity, frequency, and train duration, ionic changes are predominantly dependent on the layer in which they are recorded. Largest decreases in $[Na^+]_o$ and $[Ca^{2+}]_o$ and increases in $[K^+]_o$ are usually observed in the principal relay layers of the hippocampal subfields: i.e. in SP of areas CA3 and CA1 and in stratum granulare (SG) of the DG (Benninger et al., 1980, Mody and Heinemann, 1986). There is a considerable decay in the amplitude of the ionic signals towards apical dendritic layers of the DG (Mody and Heinemann, 1986) and towards apical and basal dendritic layers in areas CA1 and CA3. This decay is somewhat dependent on stimulation site. For example, in area CA1 the decay is flatter in stratum radiatum (SR) and in stratum lacunosum moleculare (SLM) when the Schaffer collaterals are stimulated while it is steeper when the alveus is activated. All ionic changes in the hilus are negligible except changes in $[K^+]_o$.

Regional and laminar differences have also been observed for changes in $[Cl^-]_o$. Decreases in $[Cl^-]_o$ occur in SP of areas CA1 and CA3, while increases in $[Cl^-]_o$ are observed in stratum granulare of the DG and in all dendritic input layers of the different hippocampal subfields (Müller et al., 1989). This discrepancy likely depends on differences of the Cl^- transport mechanism. The transport is inwardly directed in dendrites of hippocampal pyramidal cells and in somata and dendrites of granule cells resulting in depolarizing $GABA_A$ responses. At such sites blockade of GABA receptors will reduce the probability of NMDA receptor activation. This could explain why application of $GABA_A$ antagonists produces, in spite of prolonged EPSPs, often only weak NMDA-dependent potentials (Dingledine et al., 1983; Köhr and Heinemann, 1989).

Excitatory amino acid induced ionic changes

The study of excitatory amino acid (EAA)-induced ionic changes gives some insight into mechanisms involved in stimulus-induced ionic changes. The main EAA transmitters in the hippocampus are Glu(tamate) and Asp(artate). Glu and Asp can bind to at least 4 different types of receptors which can be classified as NMDA, Quis(qualate), and low- and high-affinity kainate (L-Kain, H-Kain) (Watkins and Evans, 1981; Cotman et al., 1987). While H-Kain receptors may act by blocking K^+ and Ca^{2+} channels, the other receptors appear to mediate depolarizing events by opening channels permeable to Na^+ and K^+ (Mayer and Westbrook, 1987). Studies of Glu, Asp and DL-homocysteic acid (DLH)-induced ionic changes in area CA1 of rat hippocampus and in cat and rat neocortex have revealed that these EAAs produce large dose-dependent decreases in $[Na^+]_o$, $[Ca^{2+}]_o$ and $[Cl^-]_o$ as well as increases in $[K^+]_o$ (Pumain and Heinemann, 1985; Heinemann et al., 1986c; Pumain et al., 1987; Heinemann and Pumain, unpublished). These ionic changes are associated with negative slow fp of sometimes more than 10 mV. The kinetics of ionic changes induced by these different EAAs are all comparable with the exception that decreases in $[Ca^{2+}]_o$ associated with DLH application are larger than those associated with Glu and Asp application. Since DLH prefers NMDA receptors over non-NMDA receptors this finding is in line with the notion that NMDA receptor activated channels possess a larger Ca^{2+} permeability than non-NMDA receptor associated channels (MacDermott et al., 1986).

This was confirmed by studies with the more specific agonists NMDA, Quis and Kain (Lambert and Heinemann, 1986a, b and unpublished). While NMDA, Quis and Kain all induce similar changes in $[Na^+]_o$ and $[K^+]_o$, they differ with respect to changes in $[Ca^{2+}]_o$ (Fig. 3). NMDA can produce decreases in $[Ca^{2+}]_o$ and cellular uptake at threshold concentrations which only depolarize nearby cells by a few mV (MacDermott et al., 1986; Lambert and Heinemann, unpublished). On the other hand, Quis and Kain elicit decreases in

$[Ca^{2+}]_o$ only when nearby cells are depolarized by at least 30 mV (Lambert and Heinemann, unpublished).

Does NMDA reduce calcium extrusion from cells?

Interestingly, the recovery of $[Ca^{2+}]_o$ is quite different following application of NMDA and non-NMDA receptor agonists (Fig. 3) (Hamon and Heinemann, 1986; Lambert and Heinemann, unpublished). After application of DLH and NMDA the $[Ca^{2+}]_o$ recovers directly to baseline while it overshoots baseline after application of Quis and Kain. $[Ca^{2+}]_o$ could increase to levels above 2.5 mM. These increases are not simply a consequence of different degrees of cell swelling which is well comparable for the different EAAs (Lambert and Heinemann, unpublished). Since the mixed agonists Glu and Asp which activate both NMDA and non-NMDA receptors do not produce overshooting responses it appears as if activation of NMDA receptors would delay or inhibit the process underlying the overshoots (Arens and Heinemann, in preparation; Stabel, Lambert and Heinemann, in preparation). Four findings suggest that the overshoots are due to Ca^{2+} extrusion via the Na^+/Ca^{2+} exchanger. The overshooting responses disappear and the $[Ca^{2+}]_o$ decreases are greater when $[Na^+]_o$ is lowered below 90 mM. The overshoots also disappear when $[Na^+]_i$ is increased due to blockade of the Na/K-ATPase, either by reducing $[K^+]_o$ to levels below 1 mM or by application of ouabain. Finally Li^+ also prevents the overshoot, which according to previous observations slows down Ca^{2+} extrusion from cells. Interestingly, substances which block Ca^{2+} uptake into cells (i.e. Ni^{2+}, verapamil and amiloride) all enhance the Ca^{2+} overshoots, when applied for short periods. This would suggest that part of the overshoots stem from intracellular Ca^{2+} stores. Since Quis stimulates IP3 production in neurons which in turn may cause Ca^{2+} release from intracellular stores (Recasens et al., 1987) some part of the overshoots may stem from such a source. This hypothesis gets support by the finding that ryanodine, which depletes intracellular Ca^{2+} stores in other tissues, also reduces the Quis-induced Ca^{2+} overshoots (Arens and Heinemann, in preparation). Thus it appears that the relatively long-lasting increases in intracellular $[Ca^{2+}]$ after Glu and NMDA application (Connor et al., 1988), result mostly from a slowed Ca^{2+} extrusion under the influence of NMDA receptor activation.

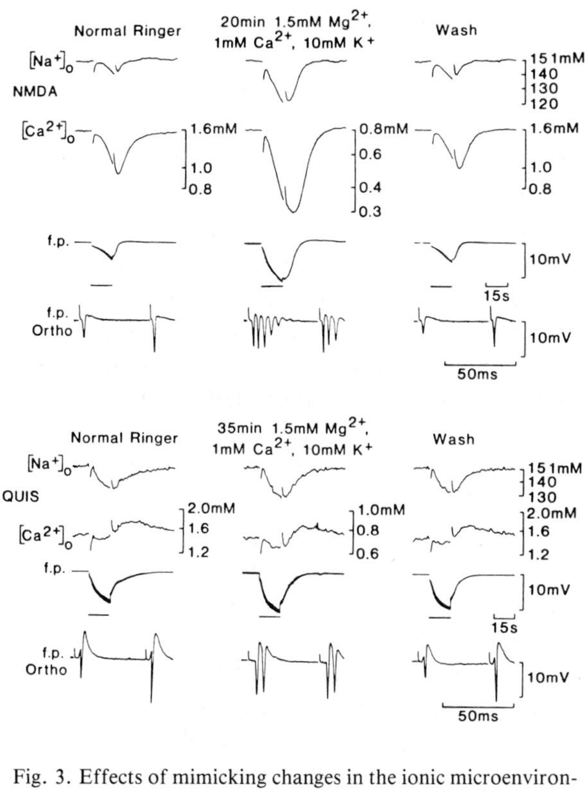

Fig. 3. Effects of mimicking changes in the ionic microenvironment as they occur during repetitive stimulation in area CA1 on paired pulse stimulus induced responses and on NMDA and quisqualate induced ionic changes. Note augmentation of NMDA and quisqualate responses. Bars indicate time of iontophoretic application of the excitatory amino acids. Note also differences in recovery kinetics of $[Ca^{2+}]_o$ following application of Quis and NMDA. Recordings were performed in stratum pyramidale of area CA1. The iontophoresis electrode tip was about 30 μm from the site of recording. Horizontal bars mark the time of application of the agonists. NMDA was applied with 15 nA, Quis with about 30 nA. Recordings from two different experiments.

Distribution of functional glutamate receptors in hippocampal tissue

The classical way to estimate the receptor distribution for the different subtypes of glutamate receptors are autoradiographic methods (Monaghan et al., 1984; Monaghan and Cotman, 1985). These display the density of binding sites including sometimes sites which would not necessarily mediate excitation. Indeed, increasing evidence suggests that intracellular phosphorylation is a prerequisite for receptors to be in a functional state (Mody et al., 1988b).

The ionic changes induced by the various glutamate receptor agonists can be used for such an estimate of functional receptor distribution. Most suitable are the agonist-induced decreases in $[Na^+]_o$ produced by iontophoretically applied Quis and NMDA ejected at different positions within the hippocampal slice. Such studies suggest that the density of Quis and NMDA receptors is largest in the middle of stratum radiatum and stratum oriens of area CA1. Similarly, the density is greatest in stratum moleculare of the dentate gyrus at a distance of roughly 50 μm from stratum granulare. The laminar profiles of the Na^+ signals in all hippocampal areas are similar in the presence of tetrodotoxin, a blocking agent for voltage-regulated Na^+ channels. It is of interest that the laminar profiles of NMDA-induced ionic changes are not constant. Thus, NMDA induced $[Ca^{2+}]_o$ changes are enhanced in stratum radiatum in slices from young animals (Hamon and Heinemann, 1988) with maximal responses in SR at about day 10 – 15 after birth.

Effects of other neurotransmitters on ionic changes

GABA, apart from effects on $[Cl^-]_o$ may also alter the $[K^+]_o$. GABA, like baclofen, has further a depressing effect on stimulus and EAA-induced reductions in $[Ca^{2+}]_o$, particularly when applied with large concentrations (Heinemann et al., 1984; Hamon and Heinemann, 1986). Bicuculline and picrotoxin, on the other hand, enhance stimulus and amino acid-induced ionic changes and shift the maximum decrease from SP towards SR (Hamon and Heinemann, 1986).

This illustrates that application of EAAs causes release of GABA from interneurons which in turn influences the uptake of Ca^{2+} into cells. There are a number of other neurotransmitters which affect these ionic changes. Of particular interest are the catecholamines. Norepinephrine (NE) and its β agonists enhance stimulus and NMDA-induced $[Ca^{2+}]_o$ changes (Stanton and Heinemann, 1986; Stanton et al., 1989a). This effect is particularly prominent in the DG. In the presence of β receptor antagonists the $[Ca^{2+}]_o$ decreases are reduced, an effect mimicked by α receptor agonists. This effect is also exerted by NE, when 2-aminophosphono-valerate (2-APV) is present. Thus, the NE effects on $[Ca^{2+}]_o$ changes are dependent on the relative expression of α and β receptors. In the EC the depressant effects dominate over the enhancement effect (Stanton et al., 1987). In area CA1 the net effect of NE is small. Acetylcholine and carbachol have, like NE, no effect on baseline ionic concentration but enhance strongly stimulus-induced Ca^{2+} and K^+ concentration changes (Müller et al., 1988). Another substance which can modulate ionic changes is adenosine. A_1 receptor antagonists enhance stimulus-induced $[Ca^{2+}]_o$ changes while adenosine itself and some of its agonists, in high doses, depress $[Ca^{2+}]_o$ changes. The order of efficacy of these agonists is such that the depressant effect is likely mediated via A_1 receptors (Schubert et al., 1986; Schubert and Heinemann, 1988).

Drug effects on changes in extracellular calcium concentration

Inorganic Ca^{2+} entry blockers such as Ni^{2+} strongly reduce stimulus-induced changes in $[Ca^{2+}]_o$ (Marciani et al., 1982). The organic Ca^{2+} entry blockers have much less effect, reducing these signals only by approximately 30%. This applies to verapamil and its derivatives, to nifedipine and to fendilline (Louvel et al., 1986; Jones and Heinemann, 1987a). ω-Conotoxin also has a depressant effect on $[Ca^{2+}]_o$ decreases, again in the order of 30% (Igelmund and Heinemann, in preparation). Recently it has been shown that the petit mal anticonvulsants may act by blocking transient Ca^{2+} currents. These agents also block part of the Ca^{2+} signals. Again, this effect is only in the order of 30% (Heinemann et al., 1988). Since Ca^{2+} may leave the ES via NMDA receptor channels it was of interest to study the effects of ketamine and 2-APV on stimulus-induced $[Ca^{2+}]_o$ changes. In SP of area CA1 and in SG of the DG, stimulus-induced changes in $[Ca^{2+}]_o$ are hardly affected by the NMDA receptor antagonists (Köhr and Heinemann, 1989). This applies both to or-thodromically and antidromically induced changes in $[Ca^{2+}]_o$. Only when convulsants are applied or when Mg^{2+} is lowered, do the enhanced $[Ca^{2+}]_o$ changes exhibit a component which is sensitive to NMDA antagonists such as ketamine and 2-APV. Thus, it appears that the major fraction of Ca^{2+} uptake into cells is mediated by voltage-sensitive channels. Since overshoots do not appear after stimulus-induced $[Ca^{2+}]_o$ decreases, at sites where NMDA receptors become activated, the possibility exists that NMDA receptors reduce Ca^{2+} extru-sion from cells irrespective of the way in which Ca^{2+} enters the cells and thereby causes a pro-longed Ca^{2+} load within cells. Indeed, Ca^{2+} recordings in the stratum moleculare of the cerebellar cortex, where NMDA receptors are minimally activated, during parallel fiber stimula-tion display a considerable overshoot following stimulation.

Elements which take up calcium

Glia, postsynaptic elements and presynaptic en-dings could all take up the Ca^{2+} which leaves the ES. However, it is not very likely that glia takes up Ca^{2+} under pysiological conditions since the max-imal depolarization of glial cells during repetitive stimulation is approximately 30 mV from a resting membrane potential of about -90 mV (Rausche,

Albrecht and Heinemann, in preparation). The threshold for activation of L-type Ca^{2+} currents lies near -30 mV. T-type Ca^{2+} currents are not activatable during sustained depolarizations (Car-bone and Lux, 1984a, b) and hence are not able to

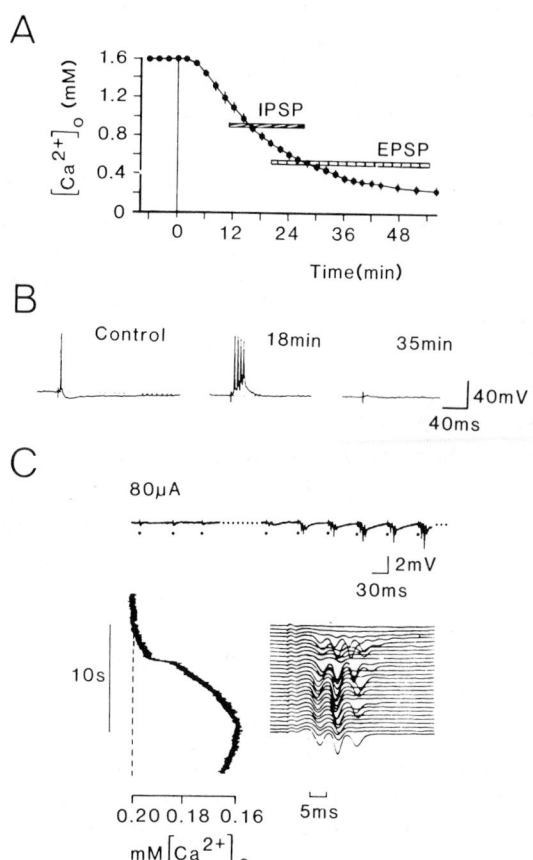

Fig. 4. Effects of lowering extracellular calcium concentration on synaptically evoked responses in area CA1. A: washout curve of $[Ca^{2+}]_o$ during bath application of 0.1 mM Ca^{2+} con-taining medium. Hatched bars represent the time when for a given stimulus block of synaptic responses was noted. B: obser-vations during washout of Ca^{2+}. Note the disappearance of IPSPs (both early and late) 18 min after onset of low Ca^{2+} per-fusion. C: recovery of synaptic transmission from block of synaptic transmission during repetitive stimulation (20/s, 100 μA). Note the initially small decay in $[Ca^{2+}]_o$ plotted in vertical direction and its acceleration when synaptic transmission is recovered. The horizontal displays are the fp recordings follow-ing single stimuli during the stimulus train. Each 5th response is shown.

mediate much Ca^{2+} uptake during the prolonged stimulus induced glial depolarizations. This leaves the neuronal elements as the main sink for extracellular Ca^{2+} (Krnjević et al., 1986).

Studies on the proportion of pre- vs postsynaptic Ca^{2+} uptake (reviewed elsewhere (Heinemann et al., 1988)) showed that between 60 and 80% of extracellular Ca^{2+} loss can be attributed to Ca^{2+} entry into postsynaptic elements. This conclusion is based on the following findings:

(1) Lowering of extracellular Ca^{2+} blocks synaptic transmission (Fig. 4). Recordings in SR and SM during orthodromic stimulation reveal a small decrease in $[Ca^{2+}]_o$ attributed to presynaptic Ca^{2+} uptake. Application of K^+ channel blocking agents, changes in ionic constitution, and, under suitable conditions, also repetitive stimulation (Konnerth and Heinemann, 1983a, b) lead to an enhancement of presynaptic Ca^{2+} entry and eventually to recovery of synaptic transmission. At the moment when synaptic transmission is recovered, an additional component of extracellular Ca^{2+} loss appears which is more than twice as great as that prior to synaptic transmission recovery (Fig. 4).

(2) When high doses of kainate are used to destroy the postsynaptic elements in the CA1 and CA3 subfield, stimulation of afferent fibers will still induce a small component of $[Ca^{2+}]_o$ decrease, provided afferent fiber function is preserved as judged by the presence of afferent fiber volleys. This component is again equivalent to about 20 to 30% of the original $[Ca^{2+}]_o$ decreases observed under control conditions (Walther and Heinemann, in preparation). Since the presynaptic Ca^{2+} uptake shows little sensitivity to organic Ca^{2+} entry blockers and surprisingly also to ω-conotoxin, the nature of the presynaptic Ca^{2+} channels appears to be still uncertain.

Mechanisms involved in frequency habituation

At many synapses in the hippocampus, activation of NMDA receptors is apparently required for the induction of LTP. As can be seen in Figs. 4 and 5,

the initial response to a stimulus is a prolonged hyperpolarization, which can last for 200 – 800 ms (Thalmann and Ayala, 1982). This hyperpolarization can even summate during repetitive stimulation. During such a hyperpolarization NMDA receptors are more difficult to activate (Nowak et al., 1984). In the DG the situation is even more complex since frequency habituation is the usual

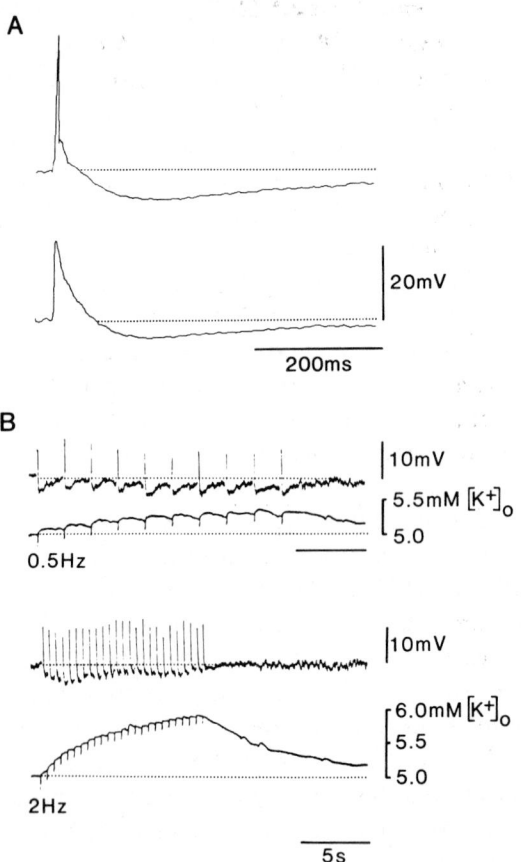

Fig. 5. A: slow IPSPs recorded from a dentate gyrus granule cell during lateral perforant path stimulation with suprathreshold (upper panel) and subthreshold stimulation (lower panel). The fact that slow IPSPs can be induced by stimulation subthreshold for population spike generation and intracellular action potential generation suggests that part of the slow IPSP represents a feed forward inhibition. B: behavior of slow IPSPs during repeated stimulation. Note that slow IPSPs can follow frequent stimulation but become reduced parallel to extracellular potassium accumulation; potassium concentration was measured with a nearby ion selective microelectrode (tip intervals less than 100 μm).

response after stimulation of the perforant path.

It appears that slow IPSPs underlie this frequency habituation since frequency habituation reverses into frequency potentiation when the slow IPSP is reduced to about 50% of its original amplitude. This can be achieved by the $GABA_B$ receptor antagonist phaclofen or by reducing Ca^{2+} entry into presynaptic endings. Thus, we observed during Ca^{2+} washout experiments that the IPSPs disappear much earlier than the EPSPs (Fig. 4). Similarly, application of Ni^{2+}, Mn^{2+} and Mg^{2+} can all transiently reduce the fast as well as the late slow IPSP and reverse frequency habituation into frequency potentiation. This then suggests that the slow IPSP imposes the filter function on the DG (Rausche et al., 1988, 1989). Interestingly, the slow IPSP does not have that function in areas CA1 and CA3. However, also in these areas frequency potentiation can be augmented when the slow IPSP is blocked (Rausche et al., 1989).

The reason for the earlier blocking of IPSPs than of EPSPs during Ca^{2+} washout lies presumably in the fact that a disynaptic pathway is more sensitive to lowering of $[Ca^{2+}]_o$ than a monosynaptic excitatory pathway (Jones and Heinemann, 1987b). As the decreases are particularly large near the somata of pyramidal cells it may well be that $[Ca^{2+}]_o$ reductions, due to Ca^{2+} uptake into pyramidal cells and granule cells, contribute to disinhibition. Since frequency potentiation is uncovered once the slow IPSP is blocked, frequency potentiation is obviously the natural response to synapses in the hippocampus. The degree to which this happens is modified by the strength of the slow IPSP and presumably also by other inhibitory processes. The slow IPSP largely results from a G-protein dependent activation of a K^+ conductance (Hablitz and Thalmann, 1987; Thalmann, 1988) and thereby is very sensitive to extracellular K^+ accumulation. Indeed, extracellular $[K^+]_o$ elevation reverses frequency habituation into frequency potentiation (Rausche et al., 1989).

Mechanisms underlying frequency potentiation

The question then can be asked of the mechanism mediating frequency potentiation. During experiments where recovery of synaptic transmission was studied, we noted that frequency potentiation occurs immediately after recovery from block of synaptic transmission (Konnerth and Heinemann, 1983b). The finding that enhanced presynaptic Ca^{2+} entry recovers presynaptic transmitter release, also suggests that presynaptic Ca^{2+} accumulation is an important factor in the generation of frequency potentiation (Fig. 4).

However, there may be additional postsynaptic mechanisms contributing to frequency potentiation and to the reversal of frequency habituation into frequency potentiation during prolonged stimulation in the dentate gyrus. These factors might well involve changes in the ionic environment. We therefore tested the effects of changes in $[Ca^{2+}]_o$, $[Mg^{2+}]_o$, and $[K^+]_o$ on cellular and synaptic properties.

Effects of lowering extracellular calcium concentration

As mentioned above, lowering of $[Ca^{2+}]_o$ leads ultimately to blocking of synaptic transmission. During Ca^{2+} washout, stimulus induced ortho- and antidromic responses can become epileptiform (Fig. 4B). This effect is due to reduced surface charge screening (McLaughlin et al., 1971) and a reduction in the efficacy of Ca^{2+}-dependent K^+ currents (Rausche and Heinemann, in preparation). As stated above, lowering of $[Ca^{2+}]_o$ reduces IPSPs more readily than EPSPs, thus contributing to the increase in excitation (Fig. 4B). Finally, lowering of $[Ca^{2+}]_o$ also facilitates the activation of NMDA receptors (Köhr and Heinemann, 1988). Therefore, it is not surprising that moderate decreases in $[Ca^{2+}]_o$ facilitate excitatory synaptic coupling.

Effects of lowering extracellular magnesium concentration

Lowering $[Mg^{2+}]_o$ likewise has net excitatory effects. The activation of NMDA receptors is facilitated strongly at concentrations below 1 mM (Albrecht and Heinemann, in preparation). An activatory function of inward currents can also be noted during Mg^{2+} washout. Thus, the threshold for action potential generation is lowered by about 5 mV when Mg^{2+} is lowered from 2 mM to levels near 50 μM (Mody et al., 1987, 1988a). Finally, and perhaps most important is the effect on presynaptic transmitter release. Thus an NMDA receptor independent augmentation of synaptic responses is noted when Mg^{2+} is lowered from 2 to 1 mM (Hamon et al., 1987).

Effects of elevating extracellular potassium concentration

Elevating $[K^+]_o$ has a multitude of effects. On the cellular level, the cells become depolarized. Synaptically and intrinsically generated K^+ currents become reduced, leading to an increase in excitability (Schwindt and Crill, 1981). On the presynaptic level, moderate $[K^+]_o$ increases facilitate transmitter release (Rausche et al., 1989). Thus, the level of $[Ca^{2+}]_o$ at which synaptic transmission is blocked is strongly K^+ dependent. With larger elevations of $[K^+]_o$ (at levels above 8 mM), however, some of this facilitating effect is reversed. This is probably due to depolarization-dependent inactivation of transient Na^+ and Ca^{2+} currents with a subsequently reduced presynaptic Ca^{2+} uptake. Increasing $[K^+]_o$ has finally also pronounced effects on NMDA receptor mediated postsynaptic responses which can be more than doubled when $[K^+]_o$ is increased from 5 to 10 mM. Even Quis responses show some augmentation with elevation of $[K^+]_o$ due to the reduced outward driving force for K^+ (Stabel and Heinemann, in preparation). Finally, $[K^+]_o$ eleva-

tion might reduce the transmembrane Cl^- concentration gradients (Chamberlin and Dingledine, 1988). This ultimately leads to a reduced efficacy of fast IPSPs.

Combined effects of changes in the ionic microenvironment as observed during repetitive stimulation

In view of the multitude of effects, during repetitive stimulation, it is a useful exercise to investigate the effects of the alterations in the minor cation concentrations. Such an experiment is illustrated in Fig. 3 where the baseline medium was exchanged with a medium containing 10 mM K^+, 1 mM Ca^{2+} and 1.5 mM Mg^{2+}. Such a medium strongly augments NMDA-mediated responses. Evoked field potentials display prolonged bursts of epileptiform activity. In many slices even spontaneous convulsant behavior develops which displays both periods of tonic-like activity and prolonged periods of clonic-like after-discharges (Traynelis and Dingledine, 1989). This behavior can be blocked only partially by ketamine which indicates that a multitude of factors contribute to this type of epileptiform activity (Stabel and Heinemann, in preparation). These data show that the extracellular ionic responses modulate profoundly the neuronal activity.

However, in physiological conditions the ionic changes are the result of transmembrane ion fluxes. The intracellular consequences of ionic changes also modify the cell excitability. These are largely anticonvulsant and involve the activation of an electrogenic sodium potassium pump and of Ca^{2+}-dependent K^+ conductances (Krnjević and Lisiewic, 1972; Alger and Williamson, 1988). Therefore the increase in excitability during repetitive stimulation is weaker than during passive alterations of the ionic environment. Indeed, late during the prolonged period of stimulation, initially augmented synaptic responses decline in amplitude.

Frequency potentiation and the role of calcium in inducing LTP

In general, these findings give us an idea how frequency potentiation develops during repetitive stimulation. Presynaptic Ca^{2+} accumulation, leading to augmented transmitter release, is involved initially. Postsynaptic Ca^{2+} uptake may reduce GABA receptor mediated responses (Behrends et al., 1988). Slow negative field potentials develop in SG and SP which reverse into positive fp in SR and SM. These are due, in part, to spatial K^+ buffering through glial cells (Albrecht and Heinemann, 1989; Albrecht et al., 1989; Dietzel et al., 1980, 1982; Dietzel and Heinemann, 1986; Orkand et al., 1966). The voltage gradient in area CA1 is in the order of 40 mV/mm. Such gradients are sufficient to excite nerve cells by imposing an additional depolarization onto soma potentials (Jefferys, 1981; Chan and Nicholson, 1986; Heinemann and Pumain, unpublished).

K^+ accumulation will eventually reverse the slow IPSP into a depolarizing response (Fig. 5). The combination of ionic changes and postsynaptic depolarization will help to activate NMDA receptors. These will enhance Ca^{2+} entry into cells and by blocking of Ca^{2+} extrusion will delay the removal of Ca^{2+} from the cell, thereby prolonging intracellular Ca^{2+} elevations. This, together with the Ca^{2+} release mediated by IP3 (Recasens et al., 1987) and perhaps Ca^{2+} itself (Mody, personal communication), and the Ca^{2+} which enters the cells through voltage-dependent channels may provide one of the key signals for the translation of short-term potentiation into long-term changes of excitability.

The intracellular Ca^{2+} increase may, however, be only one of the necessary conditions. Thus we have noted that alvear stimulation in spite of considerable Ca^{2+} entry into cells does not induce LTP (Stanton and Sejnowski, 1989). The synaptic potentials induced by alvear stimulation also contain an NMDA component as they become augmented during washout of Mg^{2+}, an effect which is partially reversed by ketamine and 2-APV

(Köhr and Heinemann, 1989).

This would suggest that the development of LTP requires another co-factor for its induction. One such co-factor could be norepinephrine. Noradrenergic fibers are widely distributed in the hippocampus. It is likely that release of NE is enhanced under many stimulus conditions. The availability of NE appears to be necessary for a tissue to develop LTP. The induction of LTP can be prevented in DG after destruction of the locus coeruleus (Stanton and Sarvey, 1985). When the expression of NE receptors is slowed during ontogenesis as is the case during the foetal alcohol syndrome, the induction of LTP is also reduced (Stanton et al., 1987). When cells lose NE receptors as is the case after kindling (Stanton et al., 1989a) the capability of the tissue to induce LTP is lost. Finally, an interplay between NMDA receptors and NE is required for NE to induce the NE-dependent 2-APV-sensitive long-lasting potentiation (Stanton et al., 1989a).

Changes in the ionic microenvironment during long-term potentiation

Surprisingly the alterations in hippocampal cells following induction of long-term potentiation are much more impressive in extracellular recordings than in intracellular recordings. Apparently they are relatively small and difficult to catch. This may indicate a population effect based on relatively small alterations in individual cells and synaptic contacts. The anatomical organization of the pathways in the hippocampus is such that a "beam" of cells is simultaneously activated within the hippocampus and then projects back to rather circumscribed areas in the EC.

Taking these considerations into account it is useful to record ionic changes in the hippocampus which result from transmembrane ion fluxes in a population of cellular elements in the immediate surrounding of the electrode. Recordings with Ca^{2+} selective electrodes have shown that stimulus-induced decreases in $[Ca^{2+}]_o$ recorded from SP and SR become enhanced during development of LTP (Heinemann et al., 1986a, b). Interestingly, the enhanced Ca^{2+} signals in SR are reversed by NMDA receptor antagonists while in SP they are almost unaffected. This would suggest alterations in intrinsic membrane currents and perhaps also in presynaptic transmitter release (Bliss et al., 1986; Errington et al., 1987; Kauer et al., 1988; Lynch et al., 1989) which would increase both NMDA and non-NMDA dependent synaptic transmission.

That alterations in membrane characteristics may be associated with long-term potentiation is supported by observations with the NE-induced long-lasting potentiation of perforant path induced synaptic responses in DG (Stanton et al., 1989a). This type of long-lasting potentiation can be prevented by 2-APV. Extracellular Ca^{2+} signals are not significantly altered after application of NE. The increase in postsynaptic responses is insensitive to 2-APV. Intracellular recordings revealed that NE-induced long-lasting potentiation is associated with a moderate depolarization of DG granule cells and a marked increase in input resistance. This could be due to reduced K^+ currents.

Alterations of cellular and synaptic properties in the kindled hippocampus

We compared various conditions of kindling: namely kindling of area CA1, kindling of the commissural fibers and kindling of the amygdala. While in all these conditions a number of alterations is found in the hippocampal formation, no changes have been detected after pentylenetetrazole kindling (Walther and Heinemann, in preparation). Data from the laboratory of M. Gutnick suggest, however, alterations in the neocortex with this kindling model, some of which resemble the alterations observed with the other kindling models in the hippocampus. All 3 kindling models affecting the hippocampus had in common that stimulus-induced changes in $[Ca^{2+}]_o$ were augmented particularly in the synaptic input layers of the hippocampus (Fig. 6). This effect is most prominent in area CA1 after CA1 kindling, while the effects are more drastic in dentate gyrus during kindling of the amygdala and commissural fibers.

Studies on Asp and DLH-induced $[Ca^{2+}]_o$ changes after CA1 kindling had suggested that changes in the laminar distribution of EAA-induced Ca^{2+} signals were associated with this kindling model (Wadman and Heinemann, 1985). Laminar profiles of NMDA- and Quis-induced $[Ca^{2+}]_o$ changes showed that cellular Ca^{2+} uptake mediated through NMDA receptor activated ionophores is strongly augmented while the laminar profiles of Quis-induced ionic changes are unaltered on a long-term scale (Heinemann et al., 1986b,c). This suggests some enhancement in the utilization of NMDA receptors.

The possibility that GABAergic disinhibition in kindled area CA1 (Kamphuis et al., 1987 – 1989) accounts for the alteration of NMDA-induced laminar profiles is unlikely since application of bicuculline affected similarly laminar profiles of Quis- or NMDA-induced decreases in $[Ca^{2+}]_o$, unlike the situation in kindling where only the NMDA-induced ionic signals were augmented. Indeed, kindling leads in the DG both to an augmentation of the early and the late IPSP (King et al., 1985; Oliver and Miller, 1985). Nevertheless, stimulus-induced changes in $[Ca^{2+}]_o$ are augmented in DG (Fig. 6). Intracellular recordings revealed that following lateral perforant path stimulation, NMDA receptors contribute little to EPSPs in control recordings while they contribute strongly after kindling (Mody and Heinemann, 1987; Mody et al., 1988a).

This statement needs some qualification. Recently, reports appeared indicating an NMDA component in mediating synaptic transmission from the perforant path (Lambert et al., 1989). The determination of laminar profiles of functional NMDA receptors in the DG indicated that the density of NMDA receptors is largest at a distance of $50 - 100$ μm from SG with a steep decline in receptor density towards outer SM. We subsequently investigated the effects of lowering $[Mg^{2+}]_o$ on synaptic responses evoked by lateral and medial perforant path and by commissural fiber stimulation and antidromic stimulation. While antidromic responses are affected little by lowering $[Mg^{2+}]_o$, commissural and medial perforant path fiber evoked responses are strongly enhanced. These effects are very sensitive to ketamine (20 μM). Lateral perforant path evoked responses also show some, although weaker, enhancement. It always appears later during Mg^{2+} washout and it is less sensitive to NMDA antagonists (Clusmann, Stabel and Heinemann, in preparation).

In kindled animals this is markedly different. There, stimulation of the lateral perforant path results in EPSPs which are strongly augmented soon after onset of Mg^{2+} washout (Mody and Heinemann, 1987; Mody et al., 1988a). This effect is readily reversed by 2-APV. As expected for NMDA-dependent signals the amplitude of the EPSPs increases with depolarization (Fig. 6), an effect which is reversed to the control situation by 2-APV. Thus we conclude that in a preparation with enhanced inhibition, there can nevertheless be enhancement of NMDA receptor utilization. Since

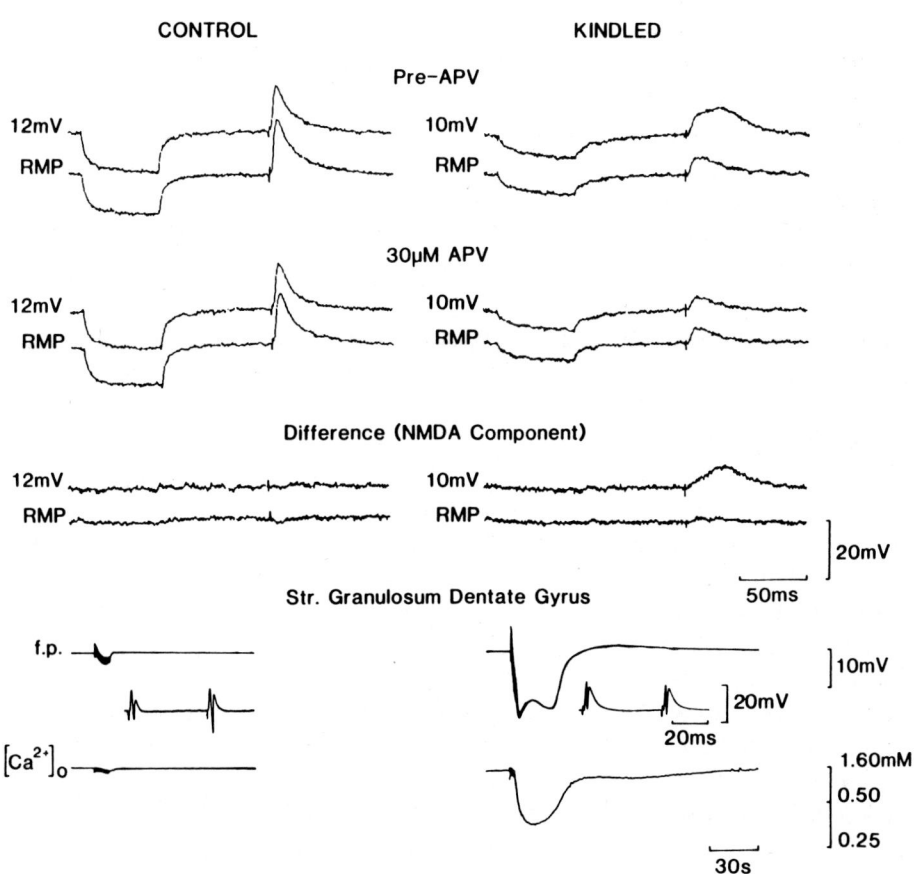

Fig. 6. Alterations of input resistance, synaptic responses and extracellularly recorded changes in $[Ca^{2+}]_o$ in normal and kindled rats. Recordings in dentate gyrus. Intracellular responses from dentate gyrus granule cells were obtained in the current clamp mode at two different membrane potentials: resting membrane potential (RMP) and current depolarized membrane. Note that EPSPs decrease upon depolarization in control granule cells but increase in granule cells from kindled animals. Note also differences in membrane time constant in granule cells from control and kindled animals. Note that 2-APV reduced the EPSPs in kindled but not in control animals as revealed by digital subtraction.

autoradiographic studies show no enhancement of binding sites (Okazaki et al., 1989) it appears that other mechanisms must account for the augmented NMDA receptor utilization. This could be due to receptor phosphorylation but other mechanisms might contribute as well (Mody et al., 1988b; MacDonald et al., 1989).

One such mechanism could be the enhanced input resistance of kindled cells (Mody et al., 1988a). It would augment synaptic responses and thereby increase contribution of NMDA receptors to synaptic transmission. Sprouting of perforant path fibers and consequently enhanced transmitter release with subsequent activation of extrasynaptic NMDA receptors is another possibility presently being investigated in our laboratory (Mody et al., 1988a; Represa et al., 1989). We have so far studied the possibility that the Ca^{2+} dependence of transmitter release is altered by measuring the level at which synaptic transmission is blocked. The statistical evaluation of the data in area CA1 suggests no statistical significant difference.

It should be noted that these are not the sole differences in the kindling model. The observation that LTP is much more difficult to elicit led us to study typical NE receptor mediated responses. We found that block of after-hyperpolarizations and frequency accommodation mediated by β receptor agonists was lost in cells from kindled animals. Also the α receptor dependent reduction of changes in $[Ca^{2+}]_o$ disappeared after kindling, thus indicating a reduction in the number of NE receptors (Stanton et al., 1989b). Meanwhile there is also evidence for a change in proopioid peptides defined on the level of the mRNA (Morris et al., 1988). This means that many cellular and synaptic properties change following kindling. It remains to be seen which of them are underlying stimulus-induced synaptic plasticity.

In conclusion, particularly the data on dentate gyrus granule cells suggest that this normally habituating synaptic connection can change its coupling behavior profoundly. We suggest that such alterations are important in the chronic progression of temporal lobe epilepsies which are often difficult to treat. It is well possible, although far from proven, that similar alterations in synaptic connections also underlie processes of memory formation in this area.

Acknowledgement

This research was supported by the SFB 200/C8 and a grant from the DFG (He 1128/2 – 4). We are grateful to M. Groenenwald and G. Heske for technical assistance in the experiments and in preparation of the manuscript.

References

Albrecht, D. and Heinemann, U. (1989) Low calcium-induced epileptiform activity in hippocampal slices from infant rats. Dev. Brain Res., 48: 316–320.

Albrecht, D., Rausche, G. and Heinemann, U. (1989) Reflections of low calcium epileptiform activity from area CA1 into dentate gyrus in the rat hippocampal slice. Brain Res., 480: 393–396.

Alger, B.E. and Teyler, T.J. (1976) Long-term and short-term plasticity in CA1, CA3 and dentate region of the rat hippocampal slice. Brain Res., 110: 463–480.

Alger, B.E. and Williamson, A. (1988) A transient calcium-dependent potassium component of the epileptiform burst after-hyperpolarization in rat hippocampus. J. Physiol. (Lond.), 399: 191–205.

Andersen, P., Bliss, T.V.P. and Skrede, K.K. (1971) Lamellar organization of hippocampal excitatory pathways. Exp. Brain Res., 13: 222–238.

Avoli, M., Louvel, J., Pumain, R. and Olivier, A. (1987) Seizure-like discharges induced by lowering $[Mg^{2+}]_o$ in the human epileptogenic neocortex maintained in vitro. Brain Res., 417: 199–203.

Behrends, J.C., Maruyama, T., Tokutomi, N. and Akaike, N. (1988) Ca^{2+}-mediated suppression of the GABA-response through modulation of chloride channel gating in frog sensory neurones. Neurosci. Lett., 86: 311–316.

Benninger, C., Kadis, J.L. and Prince, D.A. (1980) Extracellular calcium and potassium changes in hippocampal slices. Brain Res., 221: 299–305.

Bliss, T.V.P. and Lømo, T. (1973) Long-lasting potentiation of synaptic transmission in the dentate area of the anaesthetized rabbit following stimulation of the perforant path. J. Physiol. (Lond.), 232: 331–356.

Bliss, T.V.P., Douglas, R.M., Errington, M.L. and Lynch, M.A. (1986) Correlation between long-term potentiation and release of endogenous amino acids from dentate gyrus of anaesthetized rats. J. Physiol. (Lond.), 377: 391–408.

Carbone, E. and Lux, H.D. (1984a) A low voltage-activated, fully inactivating Ca channel in vertebrate sensory neurones. *Nature (Lond.)*, 310: 501–502.

Carbone, E. and Lux, H.D. (1984b) A low voltage-activated calcium conductance in embryonic chick sensory neurons. *Biophys. J.*, 46: 413–418.

Carbone, E. and Lux, H.D. (1987) Kinetics and selectivity of a low-voltage-activated calcium current in chick and rat sensory neurones. *J. Physiol. (Lond.)*, 386: 547–570.

Chamberlin, N.L. and Dingledine, R. (1988) GABAergic inhibition and the induction of spontaneous epileptiform activity by low chloride and high potassium in the hippocampal slice. *Brain Res.*, 445: 12–18.

Chan, C.Y. and Nicholson, C. (1986) Modulation by applied electrical fields of Purkinje and stellate cell activity in the isolated turtle cerebellum. *J. Physiol. (Lond.)*, 371: 89–114.

Collingridge, G.L., Kehl, S.J. and McLennan, H. (1983) Excitatory amino acids in synaptic transmission in the Schaffer collateral-commissural pathway of the rat hippocampus. *J. Physiol. (Lond.)*, 334: 33–46.

Connor, J.A., Wadman, W.J., Hockberger, P.E. and Wong, R.K. (1988) Sustained dendritic gradients of Ca^{2+} induced by excitatory amino acids in CA1 hippocampal neurons. *Science*, 240: 649–653.

Cotman, C.W., Monaghan, D.T., Ottersen, P.O. and Storm-Mathisen, J. (1987) Anatomical organization of excitatory amino acid receptors and their pathways. *Trends Neurosci.*, 10: 273–280.

Dietzel, I. and Heineman, U. (1986) Dynamic variations of the brain cell microenvironment in relation to neuronal hyperactivity. *Ann. N.Y. Acad. Sci.*, 481: 72–86.

Dietzel, I., Heinemann, U., Hofmeier, G. and Lux, H.D. (1980) Transient changes in the size of the extracellular space in the sensorimotor cortex of cats in relation to stimulus induced changes in potassium concentration. *Exp. Brain Res.*, 40: 432–439.

Dietzel, I., Heinemann, U., Hofmeier, G. and Lux, H.D. (1982) Stimulus-induced changes in extracellular Na^+ and Cl^- concentration in relation to changes in the size of the extracellular space. *Exp. Brain Res.*, 46: 73–84.

Dingledine, R., Hynes, M.A. and King, G.L. (1983) Involvement of N-methyl-D-aspartate receptors in epileptiform bursting in the rat hippocampal slice. *J. Physiol. (Lond.)*, 380: 175–190.

Dutar, P. and Nicoll, R.A. (1988) A physiological role for $GABA_B$ receptors in the central nervous system. *Nature (Lond.)*, 332: 156–158.

Errington, M.L., Lynch, M.A. and Bliss, T.V.P. (1987) Long-term potentiation in the dentate gyrus: induction and increased glutamate release are blocked by D-(–)-aminophosphonovalerate. *Neuroscience*, 20: 279–284.

Goddard, G.V., McIntyre, D.C. and Leech, C.K. (1969) A permanent change in brain function resulting from daily electrical stimulation. *Exp. Neurol.*, 25: 295–330.

Hablitz, J.J. and Thalmann, R.H. (1987) Conductance changes underlying a late synaptic hyperpolarization in hippocampal CA3 neurons. *J. Neurophysiol.*, 58: 160–179.

Hamon, B. and Heinemann, U. (1986) Effects of GABA and bicuculline on N-methyl-D-aspartate- and quisqualate-induced reductions in extracellular free calcium in area CA1 of the hippocampal slice. *Exp. Brain Res.*, 64: 27–36.

Hamon, B., Stanton, P.K. and Heinemann, U. (1987) An N-methyl-D-aspartate receptor-independent excitatory action of partial reduction of extracellular $[Mg^{2+}]_o$ in CA1 region of rat hippocampal slices. *Neurosci. Lett.*, 75: 240–245.

Hamon, B. and Heinemann, U. (1988) Developmental changes in neuronal sensitivity to excitatory amino acids in area CA1 of the rat hippocampus. *Dev. Brain Res.*, 38: 286–290.

Harris, E.W. and Cotman, C.W. (1985) Effects of synaptic antagonists on perforant path paired-pulse plasticity: differentiation of pre- and post-synaptic antagonism. *Brain Res.*, 334: 348–353.

Heinemann, U. (1987) Basic mechanisms of the epilepsies. In A.M. Halliday, S.R. Butler and R. Paul (Eds.), *A. Textbook of Clinical Neurophysiology,* John Wiley and Sons, Chichester, pp. 497–534.

Heinemann, U. and Jones, R.S.G. (1989) Neurophysiology of epilepsy. In L. Gram and M. Dam (Eds.), *Perspectives of Epilepsy,* Raven Press, New York, in press.

Heinemann, U., Lux, H.D. and Gutnick, M.J. (1977) Extracellular free calcium and potassium during paroxysmal activity in the cerebral cortex of the cat. *Exp. Brain Res.*, 27: 237–243.

Heinemann, U., Neuhaus, S. and Dietzel, I (1983) Aspects of potassium regulation in normal and gliotic brain tissue. In M. Baldy-Moulinier, D.-H. Ingvar, and B.S. Meldrum, (Eds.), *Current Problems in Epilepsy/Cerebral Blood Flow, Metabolism and Epilepsy,* John Libbey Eurotext, London, pp. 271–277.

Heinemann, U., Hamon, B. and Konnerth, A. (1984) GABA and baclofen reduce changes in extracellular free calcium in area CA1 of rat hippocampal slices. *Neurosci. Lett.*, 47: 295–300.

Heinemann, U., Hamon, B., Jones, R.S.G. et al. (1986a) Stimulus-induced plasticity in area CA1 of rat hippocampus. In E.-J. Speckmann, H. Schulze and J. Walden (Eds.), *Epilepsy and Calcium,* Urban and Schwarzenberg, Munich, pp. 1–16.

Heinemann, U., Hamon, B., Konnerth, A. and Wadman, W.J. (1986b) Stimulus-dependent synaptic plasticity in area CA1 of the in vitro hippocampal slice of rats. *Exp. Brain Res.*, 14: 291–299.

Heinemann, U., Konnerth, A., Pumain, R. and Wadman, W.J. (1986c) Extracellular calcium and potassium concentration changes in chronic epileptic brain tissue. In A.V. Delgado-Escueta, A.A. Ward, D.M. Woodbury and R.J. Porter, *Advances in Neurology/Basic Mechanisms of the Epilepsies,* Raven Press, New York, pp. 641–661.

Heinemann, U., Igelmund, P., Jones, R.S.G., Köhr, G. and Walther, H. (1988) Effects of organic calcium-entry blockers on stimulus-induced changes in extracellular calcium concentration in area CA1 of rat hippocampal slices. In M. Morad, W. Nayler, S. Kazda and M. Schramm, (Eds.), *The Calcium Channel: Structure, Function and Implications*, Springer Verlag, Berlin pp. 528 – 540.

Hirning, L.D., Fox, A.P., McClesky, E.W., Olivera, B.M., Thayer, S.A., Miller, R.J. and Tsien, R.W. (1988) Dominant role of N-type Ca channels in evoked release of norepinephrine from sympathetic neurons. *Science*, 239: 57 – 61.

Holsheimer, J. (1987) Electrical conductivity of the hippocampal CA1 layers and application to current source density analysis. *Exp. Brain Res.*, 67: 402 – 410.

Jefferys, J.G.R. (1981) Influence of electric fields on the excitability of granule cells in guinea-pig hippocampal slices. *J. Physiol. (Lond.)*, 319: 143 – 152.

Jones, R.S.G. and Heinemann, U. (1987a) Abolition of the orthodromically evoked IPSP of CA1 pyramidal cells before the EPSP during washout of calcium from hippocampal slices. *Exp. Brain Res.*, 65: 676 – 680.

Jones, R.S.G. and Heinemann, U. (1987b) Differential effects of calcium entry blockers on pre- and postsynaptic influx of calcium in the rat hippocampus in vitro. *Brain Res.*, 416: 257 – 266.

Jones, R.S.G. and Heinemann, U. (1988) Synaptic and intrinsic responses of medial entorhinal cortical cells in normal and magnesium-free medium in vitro. *J. Neurophysiol.*, 59: 1476 – 1497.

Kamphuis, W., Wadman, W.J., Buijs, R.M. and Lopes da Silva, F.H. (1987) The development of changes in hippocampal GABA immunoreactivity in the rat kindling model of epilepsy: a light microscopic study with GABA antibodies. *Neuroscience*, 23: 433 – 446.

Kamphuis, W., Lopes da Silva, F.H. and Wadman, W.J. (1988) Changes in local evoked potentials in the rat hippocampus (CA1) during kindling epileptogenesis. *Brain Res.*, 440: 205 – 215.

Kamphuis, W., Huisman, E., Wadman, W.J. and Lopes da Silva, F.H. (1989) Decrease in GABA immunoreactivity and alteration of GABA metabolism after kindling in the rat hippocampus. *Exp. Brain Res.*, 74: 375 – 386.

Kauer, J.A., Malenka, R.C. and Nicoll, R.A. (1988) NMDA application potentiates synaptic transmission in the hippocampus. *Nature (Lond.)*, 334: 250 – 252.

King, G.L., Dingledine, R., Giacchino, J.L. and McNamara, J.O. (1985) Abnormal neuronal excitability in hippocampal slices from kindled rats. *J. Neurosphysiol.*, 54: 1295 – 1304.

Köhr, G. and Heinemann, U. (1988) Differences in magnesium and calcium effects on N-methyl-D-aspartate- and quisqualate-induced decreases in extracellular sodium concentration in rat hippocampal slices. *Exp. Brain Res.*, 71: 425 – 430.

Köhr, G. and Heinemann, U. (1989) Effects of NMDA-antagonists on picrotoxin-, low Mg^{2+}- and low Ca^{2+}-induced epileptogenesis and on evoked changes in extracellular Na^+- and Ca^{2+}-concentrations in rat hippocampal slices. *Epilepsy Res.*, 4: 187 – 200.

Konnerth, A. and Heinemann, U. (1983a) Presynaptic involvement in frequency facilitation in the hippocampal slice. *Neurosci. Lett.*, 42: 255 – 260.

Konnerth, A. and Heinemann, U. (1983b) Effects of GABA on presumed presynaptic Ca^{2+} entry in hippocampal slices. *Brain Res.*, 270: 185 – 189.

Krnjević, K. and Lisiewic, A. (1972) Injections of calcium ions into spinal motoneurones. *J. Physiol. (Lond.)*, 225: 363 – 390.

Krnjević, K., Morris, M.E. and Reiffenstein, R.J. (1982) Stimulation-evoked changes in extracellular K^+ and Ca^{2+} in pyramidal layers of the rat's hippocampus. *Can. J. Physiol. Pharmacol.*, 60: 1643 – 1657.

Krnjević, K., Morris, M.E. and Ropert, N. (1986) Changes in free calcium ion concentration recorded inside hippocampal pyramidal cells in situ. *Brain Res.*, 374: 1 – 11.

Lambert, J.D.C. and Heinemann, U. (1986a) Aspects of the action of excitatory amino acids on hippocampal CA1 neurons. In U. Heinemann, M. Klee, E. Neher and W. Singer (Eds.), *Calcium Electrogenesis and Neuronal Functioning*, Springer-Verlag, Heidelberg, pp. 279 – 290.

Lambert, J.D.C. and Heinemann, U. (1986b) Extracellular calcium changes accompanying the action of excitatory amino acids in area CA1 of the hippocampus. Possible implications for the initiation and spread of epileptic discharges. In E.-J. Speckmann, H. Schulze and J. Walden (Eds.), *Epilepsy and Calcium*, Urban and Schwarzenberg, Munich, pp. 35 – 61.

Lambert, J.D.C. and Jones, R.S.G. (1988) Both NMDA and non-NMDA receptors participate in transmission at perforant path synapses in the rat dentate gyrus. *Exp. Brain Res.*, in press.

Lambert, J.D.C., Jones, R.S.G., Andreasen, M., Jensen, M.S. and Heinemann, U. (1989) The role of excitatory amino acids in synaptic transmission in the hippocampus. *Comp. Biochem. Physiol. A*, 93A: 195 – 201.

Louvel, J., Abbes, S., Godfraind, J.M. and Pumain, R. (1986) The action of various organic calcium channel blockers on epileptic phenomena in hippocampal slices. In E.-J. Speckmann, H. Schulze and J. Walden (Eds.), *Epilepsy and Calcium*, Urban and Schwarzenberg, Munich, pp. 277 – 299.

Lux, H.D., Heinemann, U. and Dietzel, I. (1986) Ionic changes and alterations in the size of the extracellular space during epileptic activity. In A.V. Delgado-Escueta, A.A. Ward, D.M. Woodbury and R.J. Porter (Eds.), *Advances in Neurology, Vol. 44: Basic Mechanisms of Epilepsies: Molecular and Cellular Approaches*, Raven Press, New York, pp. 619 – 639.

Lynch, M.A., Errington, M.L. and Bliss, T.V.P. (1989) Nordihydroguaiaretic acid blocks the synaptic component of long-term potentiation and the associated increases in release of glutamate and arachidonate: an *in vivo* study in the dentate gyrus of the rat. *Neuroscience*, 30: 693–701.

MacDermott, A.B., Mayer, M.L., Westbrook, G.L., Smith, S.J. and Barker, J.L. (1986) NMDA-receptor activation increases cytoplasmic calcium concentration in cultured spinal cord neurones. *Nature (Lond.)*, 321: 519–522.

MacDonald, J.F., Mody, I. and Salter, M.W. (1989) Regulation of N-methyl-D-aspartate receptors revealed by intracellular dialysis. *J. Physiol. (Lond.)*, 414: 17–34.

Marciani, M.G., Louvel, J. and Heinemann, U. (1982) Aspartate-induced changes in extracellular free calcium in "in vitro" hippocampal slices of rats. *Brain Res.*, 238: 272–277.

Mayer, M.L. and Westbrook, G.L. (1987) The physiology of excitatory amino acids in the vertebrate central nervous system. *Prog. Neurobiol.*, 28: 197–276.

McLaughlin, S.G., Szabo, G. and Eisenman, G. (1971) Divalent ions and the surface potential of charged phospholipid membranes. *J. Gen. Physiol.*, 58: 667–687.

Misgeld, U., Klee, M.R. and Zeise, M.L. (1984) Differences in baclofen-sensitivity between CA3 neurons and granule cells of the guinea pig hippocampus in vitro. *Neurosci. Lett.*, 47: 307–311.

Misgeld, U. and Frotscher, M. (1986) Postsynaptic-GABAergic inhibition of non-pyramidal neurons in the guinea-pig hippocampus. *Neuroscience*, 19: 193–206.

Misgeld, U., Klee, M.R. and Zeise, M.L. (1986) Blockade of hippocampal GABA-ergic inhibition by baclofen. In E.-J. Speckmann, H. Schulze and J. Walden (Eds.), *Epilepsy and Calcium*, Urban and Schwarzenberg, Munich, pp. 17–33.

Misgeld, U., Müller, W. and Brunner, H. (1989) Effects of (–)baclofen on inhibitory neurons in the guinea pig hippocampal slice. *Pflügers Arch.*, in press.

Mody, I. and Heinemann, U. (1986) Laminar profiles of the changes in extracellular calcium concentration induced by repetitive stimulation and excitatory amino acids in the rat dentate gyrus. *Neurosci. Lett.*, 69: 137–142.

Mody, I. and Heinemann, U. (1987) NMDA receptors of dentate gyrus granule cells participate in synaptic transmission following kindling. *Nature (Lond.)*, 326: 701–704.

Mody, I., Lambert, J.D.C. and Heinemann, U. (1987) Low extracellular magnesium induces epileptiform activity and spreading depression in rat hippocampal slices. *J. Neurophysiol.*, 57: 869–888.

Mody, I., Stanton, P.K. and Heinemann, U. (1988a) Activation of N-methyl-D-aspartate receptors parallels changes in cellular and synaptic properties of dentate gyrus granule cells after kindling. *J. Neurophysiol.*, 59: 1033–1054.

Mody, I., Salter, M.W. and MacDonald, J.F. (1988b) Requirement of NMDA receptor/channels for intracellular high energy phosphates and the extent of intraneuronal calcium buffering in cultured mouse hippocampal neurons. *Neurosci.*

Lett., 93: 73–78.

Monaghan, D.T., Yao, D. and Cotman, C.W. (1984) Distribution of [³H]AMPA binding sites in the rat brain as determined by quantitative autoradiography. *Brain Res.*, 324: 160–164.

Monaghan, D.T. and Cotman, C.W. (1985) Distribution of N-methyl-D-aspartate-sensitive [L-³H]glutamate binding sites in rat brain as determined by quantitative autoradiography. *J. Neuroscience*, 5: 2909–2919.

Morris, B.J., Feasey, K.J., ten Bruggencate, G., Herz, A. and Höllt, V. (1988) Electrical stimulation in vivo increases the expression of prodynorphin mRNA in rat hippocampal granule cells. *Proc. Natl. Acad. Sci. U.S.A.*, 85: 3226–3230.

Mott, D.D., Bragdon, A.C., Lewis, D.V. and Wilson, W.A. (1989) Baclofen has a proepileptic effect in the rat dentate gyrus. *J. Pharmacol. Exp. Ther.*, 249: 721–725.

Müller, W., Misgeld, U and Heinemann, U. (1988) Carbachol effects on hippocampal neurons in vitro: dependence on the rate of rise of carbachol tissue concentration. *Exp. Brain Res.*, 72: 287–298.

Müller, W., Misgeld, U. and Lux, H.D. (1989) Gamma-aminobutyric acid-induced ion movements in the guinea pig hippocampal slice. *Brain Res.*, 484: 184–191.

Nowak, L., Bregestovski, P., Ascher, P., Herbet, A. and Prochiantz, A. (1984) Magnesium gates glutamate-activated channels in mouse central neurons. *Nature (Lond.)*, 307: 462–465.

Numann, R.E., Wadman, W.J. and Wong, R.K.S. (1987) Outward currents of single hippocampal cell obtained from the adult guinea-pig. *J. Physiol. (Lond.)*, 393: 331–353.

Okazaki, M.M., McNamara, J.O. and Nadler, J.V. (1989) N-Methyl-D-aspartate receptor autoradiography in rat brain after angular bundle kindling. *Brain Res.*, in press.

Oliver, M.W. and Miller, J.J. (1985) Alterations of inhibitory processes in the dentate gyrus following kindling-induced epilepsy. *Exp. Brain Res.*, 57: 443–447.

Orkand, R.K., Nicholls, J.G. and Kuffler, S.W. (1966) Effects of nerve impulses on the membrane potential of glial cells in the central nervous system of amphibia. *J. Neurophysiol.*, 29: 788–806.

Pumain, R. and Heinemann, U. (1985) Stimulus- and amino acid-induced calcium and potassium changes in the rat neocortex. *J. Neurophysiol.*, 53: 1–16.

Pumain, R., Kurcewicz, I. and Louvel, J. (1987) Ionic changes induced by excitatory amino acids in the rat cerebral cortex. *Can J. Physiol. Pharmacol.*, 65: 1067–1077.

Rausche, G., Sarvey, J.M. and Heinemann, U. (1988) Lowering extracellular calcium reverses paired pulse habituation into facilitation in dentate granule cells and removes a late IPSP. *Neurosci. Lett.*, 88: 275–280.

Rausche, G., Igelmund, P. and Heinemann, U. (1989) Effects of changes in extracellular potassium, magnesium and calcium concentration on synaptic transmission in area CA1 and the dentate gyrus of rat hippocampal slices. *Pflügers*

Arch., in press.

Recasens, M., Sassetti, I., Nourigat, A., Sladezcek, F. and Bockaert, J. (1987) Characterization of subtypes of excitatory amino acid receptors involved in the stimulation of inositol phosphate synthesis in rat brain synaptoneurosomes. *Eur. J. Pharmacol.*, 141: 87–93.

Represa, A., Le Gall La Salle, G. and Ben-Ari, Y. (1989) Hippocampal plasticity in the kindling model of epilepsy in rats. *Neurosci. Lett.*, 99: 345–350.

Schubert, P., Heinemann, U. and Kolb, R. (1986) Differential effects of adenosine on pre- and postsynaptic calcium fluxes. *Brain Res.*, 376: 382–386.

Schubert, P. and Heinemann, U. (1988) Adenosine antagonists combined with 4-aminopyridine cause partial recovery of synaptic transmission in low Ca media. *Exp. Brain Res.*, 70: 539–549.

Schwindt, P.C. and Crill, W.E. (1981) Differential effects of TEA and cations on outward ionic currents of cat motoneurons. *J. Neurophysiol.*, 46: 1–16.

Stanton, P.K. and Sarvey, J.M. (1985) Depletion of norepinephrine, but not serotonin, reduces long-term potentiation in the dentate gyrus of rat hippocampal slices. *J. Neurosci.*, 5: 2169–2176.

Stanton, P.K. and Heinemann, U. (1986) Norepinephrine enhances stimulus-evoked calcium and potassium concentration changes in dentate granule cell layer. *Neurosci. Lett.*, 67: 233–238.

Stanton, P.K., Bommer, M., Heinemann, U. and Noble, E.P. (1987) In utero alcohol exposure impairs postnatal development of hippocampal noradrenergic sensitivity. *Neurosci. Res. Commun.*, 1: 145–152.

Stanton, P.K., Jones, R.S.G., Mody, I. and Heinemann, U. (1987) Epileptiform activity induced by lowering extracellular $[Mg^{2+}]$ in combined hippocampal-entorhinal cortex slices: modulation by receptors for norephinephrine and *N*-methyl-L-aspartate. *Epilepsy Res.*, 1: 53–62.

Stanton, P.K., Mody, I. and Heinemann, U. (1989a) Downregulation of noradrenaline receptors during kindling. *Brain Res.*, 476: 367–372.

Stanton, P.K., Mody, I. and Heinemann, U. (1989b) Mechanisms of action of norepinephrine in dentate gyrus granule cells: implications for long-term neuronal plasticity. *Exp. Brain Res.*, 77: 517–530.

Stanton, P.K. and Sejnowski, T.J. (1989c) Associative long-term depression in the hippocampus induced by hebbian covariance. *Nature (Lond.)*, 339: 215–218.

Thalmann, R.H. and Ayala, G.F. (1982) A late increase in potassium conductance follows synaptic stimulation of granule neurons of the dentate gyrus. *Neurosci. Lett.*, 29: 243–284.

Thalmann, R.H. (1988) Evidence that guanosine triphosphate (GTP)-binding proteins control a synaptic response in brain: effect of pertussis toxin and GTPgammaS on the late inhibitory postsynaptic potential of hippocampal CA3 neurons. *J. Neurosci.*, 8: 4589–4602.

Traynelis, S.F. and Dingledine, R. (1989) Modification of potassium-induced interictal bursts and electrographic seizures by divalent cations. *Neurosci. Lett.*, 98: 194–199.

Wadman, W.J. and Heinemann, U. (1985) Laminar profiles of $(K^+)_o$ and $(Ca^{2+})_o$ in region CA1 of the hippocampus of kindled rats. In M. Kessler et al. (Eds.), *Ion Measurements in Physiology and Medicine*. Springer-Verlag, Berlin, pp. 221–228.

Walther, H., Lambert, J.D.C., Jones, R.S.G., Heinemann, U and Hamon, B. (1986) Epileptiform activity in combined slices of the hippocampus, subiculum and entorhinal cortex during perfusion with low magnesium medium. *Neurosci. Lett.*, 69: 156–161.

Watkins, J.C. and Evans, R.H. (1981) Excitatory amino acid transmitters. *Annu. Rev. Pharmacol. Toxicol.*, 21: 165–204.

Yaari, Y., Hamon, B. and Lux, H.D. (1987) Development of two types of calcium channels in cultured mammalian hippocampal neurons. *Science*, 235: 680–682.

Zucker, R.S. and Stockbridge, N. (1983) Presynaptic calcium diffusion and the time course of transmitter release and synaptic facilitation in the squid giant synapse. *J. Neurosci.*, 3: 1263–1269.

J. Storm-Mathisen, J. Zimmer and O.P. Ottersen (Eds.)
Progress in Brain Research, Vol. 83
© 1990 Elsevier Science Publishers B.V. (Biomedical Division)

CHAPTER 15

Synaptic integration in hippocampal CA1 pyramids

Per Andersen

Institute of Neurophysiology, University of Oslo, Karl Johans gate 47, 0162 Oslo 1, Norway

Excitatory synapses on hippocampal pyramids are exclusively located to dendritic spines, usually in a 1 : 1 proportion. The number of spines indicates a convergence of as many as 25,000 – 30,000 excitatory boutons per CA1 pyramidal cell in rats. Activation of a single afferent fibre produces a unitary excitatory postsynaptic potential (EPSP) of about 150 μV, probably produced by a single quantum of transmitter. The release probability is normally low, but may be increased by facilitatory processes. On the average, each afferent fibre has few boutons (mostly 1, but up to 5) in contact with a given CA1 pyramid. Surprisingly, in view of the large synaptic convergence, only 100 – 300 synchronously active excitatory synapses seem necessary to make the cell discharge. Synapses in various parts of the dendritic tree are nearly equally effective in this regard. Excitatory postsynaptic potentials produced by neighbouring synapses sum linearly, both with each other and with hyperpolarizing, inhibitory potentials. Cable theoretical considerations suggest that the summation effect will be greater for synapses contacting the same secondary dendrite than for more distributed dendritic contacts. Three types of inhibitory neurones provide different classes of interference. The chandelier cells (axo-axonic cells) terminate upon the initial axons of a large number of pyramidal cells, and are thus capable of producing a wide-spread and effective inhibition. By hyperpolarizing the somata of a smaller number of cells, basket cells counteract all excitatory inputs to these cells, irrespective of synaptic location. In contrast to these two forms of global inhibition, stellate cells may cause a shunting form of inhibition at specific dendritic sites. Such local inhibition effectively removes the influence of synapses lying further distally on the same dendritic branch, while it either has no effect, or even a certain facilitatory influence on more centrally placed inputs. After-hypolarization also reduces the efficiency of an excitatory synaptic drive, but only for discharging neurones. Finally, synaptic efficiency, and thereby integration, depends heavily on several activity-dependent plastic changes: facilitation, augmentation, post-tetanic potentiation and long-term potentiation, named in order of increasing duration. The large number of factors which influence the synaptic interplay makes an individual pyramidal cell a quite complicated calculating machine, far more intricate than a simple switching device.

Degree of convergence

Pyramidal cells receive a large convergence of excitatory synapses, suggesting that a main task of these cells is to integrate signals coming from a variety of sources. Essential information to understand this integration are the size of the contribution from each participating excitatory synapse, and the rules for the interaction. In this context, synaptic strength is defined as the efficiency with which the synapse contributes to bringing the membrane potential to the discharge threshold. The wealth of data which recently has accumulated in this area has made it evident that a single cortical pyramid is a far more complex unit than we

thought a few years ago. For this reason it may be of interest to survey some of the major factors that influence the strength, or efficiency, of cortical excitatory synapses, and their interaction. Because so much work has been aimed at hippocampal neurones, the CA1 pyramidal cell will be the target of this review.

Spine synapses

Virtually all excitatory contacts are found on spines (Andersen et al., 1966), and most CA1 spines are contacted by a single bouton only (Westrum and Blackstad, 1962). Based upon a three-dimensional reconstruction of two Golgi-impregnated guinea pig CA1 cells, Blackstad (1985) calculated the total length of their dendrites to 11,130 and 10,170 μm, respectively. If the conservative estimate of 1 spine per μm dendritic length (Wenzel et al., 1973; Andersen et al., 1987) is used, the number of spines on one cell will also be just over 10,000. A similar number (between 10,500 and 16,200 spines) was found by counting the number of dendritic spines in a representative sample of rat CA1 pyramidal cells filled with horseradish peroxidase (HRP) (Andersen, unpublished observations). Consequently, hippocampal pyramidal cells may be thought to receive the same number of boutons. With both techniques, however, longitudinal sections were used which leads to a serious underestimation of the spine number due to the difficulty of finding spines with the neck oriented transversely to the plane of section. Based upon dendritic cross-sections, in which most of the spines can be found (M. Trommald, G. Hulleberg, J. Line Vaaland, T. Blackstad and P. Andersen, in preparation), a spine density of 2.5 – 3 per μm length appears a more realistic figure, raising the total spine number per cell to about 25,000 – 30,000.

Contribution by a single excitatory synapse

Size of the single fibre EPSP

An estimation of the amplitude of the depolarization produced in CA1 pyramidal cells by an impulse in a single afferent fibre is not easily obtained. The main difficulty is the large amplitude of the synaptic noise which drowns the small unitary EPSPs. An attempt to arrive at an estimate for this unit was made by stimulation of a very small number of afferent fibres and deconvolution of the amplitude histogram produced by a large number of trials (Sayer et al., 1989). With this technique a value of about 200 μV was found for the unitary EPSP. A higher estimate was made by Hess et al. (1987). The reason for the latter finding may lie in the relatively small sample used to construct their amplitude histograms. This adds to the difficulty of applying the methods of failures and variance due to the high spontaneous synaptic noise level in the CA1 cells in standard recording conditions in slices.

Recently, Sayer (1988) succeeded in measuring the amplitude of a single fibre EPSP by penetra-

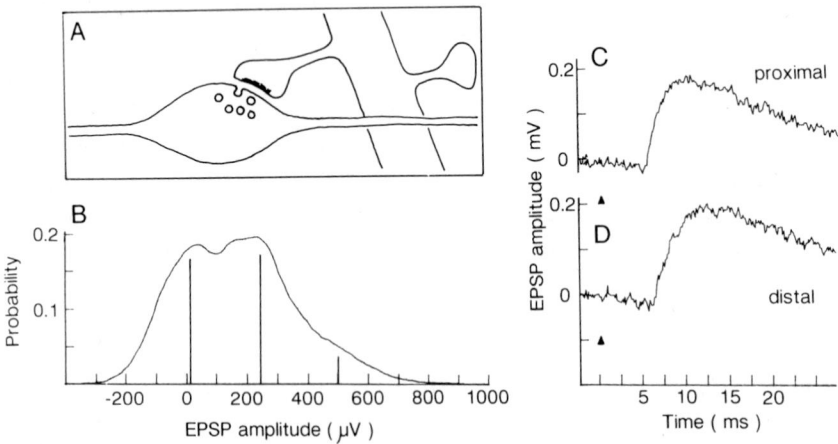

Fig. 1. Diagram of a single spine synapse in which A shows a single release site, with one vesicle just emptying its content into the synaptic cleft with another somewhat removed from the release position. B: smoothed amplitude histogram (full line) of EPSPs recorded from a CA1 pyramidal cell and evoked by minimal strength stimulation of proximal radiatum fibres. Vertical lines give best fit for amplitudes and probability of occurrence of unitary EPSPs. C and D give average EPSPs from a proximal and a distal dendritic input to the same cell (n = 200). (Sayer et al., unpublished observations).

tion of pairs of connected CA3 and CA1 cells in slices from guinea pig hippocampus. By stimulating the CA3 neurone with intracellular pulses, and recording a large number of responses from the CA1 neurone, the average unitary EPSP measured 131 μV (range 30 – 665 μV). This value has the same order of magnitude as an earlier estimate of single fibre EPSPs in dentate granule cells (between 180 and 320 μV), based upon minimal amplitude steps (McNaughton et al., 1981).

Number of quanta released per bouton

Studies of single Ia fibre activation of cat motoneurones have shown such a low variance of the amplitude fluctuations of the unitary EPSPs, that a single release site with full saturation of the subsynaptic receptors appears likely (Jack et al., 1981; Redman and Walmsley, 1983a). In addition, by filling both the presynaptic fibre and the postsynaptic cell with HRP, the identified Ia fibres had as many terminals on the target cell as the estimated number of released quanta, suggesting that only one quantum is released per bouton per impulse (Redman and Walmsley, 1983b).

In an attempt on a similar analysis of hippocampal synapses, Sayer et al. (1989) found that the high spontaneous synaptic noise level in CA1 pyramids prevents a valid estimate of the coefficient of variation (CV). However, analysing the data from the quantal analysis of CA3/CA1 pairs (Sayer, 1988) with assumptions of either a low CV (about 0.05 as in Ia/motoneuronal synapses) or with a CV of 0.3 (as in the neuromuscular junction) makes it likely that the radiatum/CA1 synapses release less than one quantum per release site per impulse. With 1.3 bouton per fibre (see below), and a low probability of release (around 0.2 – 0.4 for one quantum, and 0.05 – 0.2 for two quanta (Sayer, 1988)), the contribution of one impulse in a single fibre may range from 0.3 to 1.0 quanta of about 130 μV each. For a functional assessment, we also need to know the average number of release sites at each bouton and the probability of release at these sites.

An estimation of the longitudinal resistance of the spine neck was made from three-dimensional reconstructions from serial electron micrographs, assuming the same internal specific resistivity of 70 $\Omega \cdot$ cm as found in motoneurones, gave values from 3 to 20 MΩ (Andersen et al., 1987). If all receptors are saturated by a single quantum, an interesting consequence of such a high spine neck resistance is that a spine head may be fully depolarized by a single transmitter quantum (Redman, 1976), causing a digitization of the input. Consequently, the variation of the strength of a single fibre input will then be given exclusively by the probability of release *(P)* of a quantum. The fact that release of more than one quantum per spine per impulse would not give additional depolarization may explain why these synapses have developed into a low quantal type.

Number of boutons per fibre

The single fibre EPSP may conceivably be produced by the release of transmitter at several of the en passage boutons through which the fibre synapses with the impaled cell. After filling of radiatum fibres in rat hippocampal slices with HRP, I measured the average distance between boutons in the CA1 area. Assuming a fixation shrinkage of 15%, the average inter-bouton distance was 7.8 ± 1.8 μm (S.D., n = 620). There was no significant difference at different somatofugal levels of the CA1 dendritic field. For an assessment of the number of contacts per cell, the double conical dendritic tree of each CA1 pyramidal cell (Fig. 2A) was imagined to have collapsed into an equally wide cylinder in a unicellular palisade structure (Fig. 2B). The diameter of one of these cylinders represents the width of the "private" territory of a single CA1 pyramid for its exclusive reception of afferent fibres. Taking the average soma diameter to be 20 μm, and 4 layers of equally sized ellipsoid somata in the pyramidal layer, the average diameter of a cylinder into which all dendritic branches of a CA1 cell could be fit, would measure $20/\sqrt{4} = 10 \ \mu$m. Thus, on average, the most likely number of contacts between a single radiatum fibre and a CA1 cell is $10/7.8 = 1.3$.

Hippocampal cells have multiple axons

Intracellular staining of CA3 and CA1 pyramidal cells have revealed a large number of axon collaterals. In addition to the numerous short-term collaterals which branch profusely in the immediate vicinity of the cell of origin ($< 200 \ \mu$m), both cell types also have a number of longer projecting branches, often forming a bundle of parallel axons (Finch and Babb, 1981; Sayer and Andersen, unpublished observations). Well stained CA3 neurones may have up to 8 axon collaterals projecting over long distances, often into CA1 or another CA3 subfield. In all properly filled CA3 cells the axon traversed the stratum oriens, sending off a number (up to 6) of collaterals which we could not follow longer than about 100 μm. Close to the alveus/oriens border a relatively thick collateral branched off and ran through stratum oriens and pyramidale to enter str. radiatum where it curved to proceed parallel to the pyramidal layer through CA1 in a subicular direction. This is the classical Schaffer collateral (Schaffer, 1892). However, just inside str. radiatum, several side-branches were seen to emerge from the stem of the Schaffer collateral at various distances from the pyramidal layer, and later running parallel to it. Initially, these branches were extremely thin, but became thicker after $50 - 100 \ \mu$m when they started to show boutons, at first scattered but later with the same frequency as along the standard radiatum fibre. These collaterals were at least 100 μm apart vertically.

We have noted up to 4 such Schaffer-type collaterals coming from a single CA3 cell. Consequently, a CA3 neurone may have up to $1.3 \times 4 = 5$ boutons in contact with a CA1 target cell. Because of the long distance between the collaterals along the dendritic axis, the synapses are likely to be located at different secondary dendrites. These multiple axonal patterns may perhaps explain some of the multiple peaks in the single fibre EPSP amplitude histograms and also some of the higher values for unitary EPSPs.

Naturally, the synaptic contacts made by a single fibre need not be randomly distributed. A much more powerful coupling would be the result if a fibre makes several contacts with a given target cell. At a level where the width of the dendritic tree is 100 μm, for example, the inter-bouton distance would allow the fibre to have about 13 contacting boutons (Fig. 2A). With an average quantal EPSP of 130 μV, and a release probability around 0.4, each fibre would then contribute about 0.7 mV, and only $15 - 20$ co-active fibres would be required to discharge the cell. Such an arrangement would, however, demand a mechanism for attracting all, or most, boutons of an afferent fibre to the spines of a single target cell. One possibility for such a solution could be a co-activation situation, in which simultaneous pre- and postsynaptic depolarization initiated a process of attraction between the co-active elements.

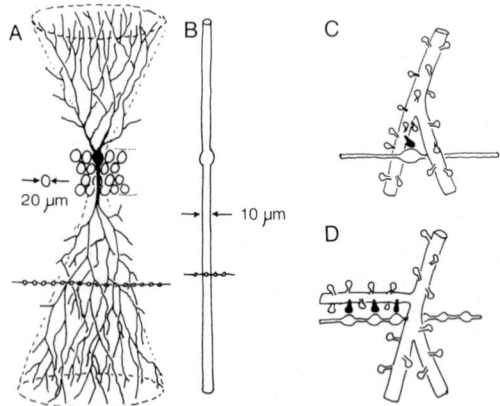

Fig. 2. Diagram of density of connections in CA1. A: a single radiatum fibre makes only one contact (black bouton) with the dendrites of a given CA1 pyramid. The other boutons contact different cells. B shows the dendritic tree collapsed into a narrow cylinder indicating the size of the "private" dendritic territory of this cell. C: diagram of the likely type of connections in CA1 with a single contact per dendritic tree (black spine), whereas D illustrates a situation with multiple contacts. This is less likely, but, if present, would give a more efficient transmission from the fibre in question.

Efficient patterns of convergence

Minimal number of excitatory synapses

Two methods have been employed in an attempt to give an estimate of the number of excitatory synapses that must be synchronously active to raise the membrane potential from the resting level to the discharge threshold for a CA1 cell. First, by making progressively larger lesions of afferent fibres in str. radiatum, the smallest remaining tissue bridge that gave effective activation of all cells when stimulated contained about 1 – 3% of the total amount of radiatum fibres (Andersen et al., 1980b). Assuming first a 1.3 : 1 fibre-to-cell coupling and second that 2/3 of all 30,000 synapses contact the apical dendrites, the required number of activated synapses should lie between 250 and 750. However, because of the low probability of transmitter release the number of releasing boutons is much lower, probably under half this figure.

With an alternative method, Sayer et al. (1989) divided the average amplitude of an EPSP which gave a 50% discharge rate with the size of the minimal EPSP. With a liminal EPSP of about 15 mV, and a unitary EPSP of 200 μV, an estimate of 75 synapses may be made. Thus, both methods give an estimate of around 100 – 300 synapses, which is only 3‰ of the total number of excitatory synapses. Naturally, this is an upper figure. The more the membrane is depolarized by other influences, the smaller is the required number of synapses.

Effect of synaptic position in the dendritic tree

Equally strong synaptic inputs to restricted parts of the dendritic tree show a surprisingly similar ability to discharge CA1 neurones (Andersen et al., 1980b). The input strength (number of excited fibres) was judged from the size of the field potential recorded from the appropriate area. Surprisingly, just suprathreshold EPSPs elicited by stimulation of proximal and distal inputs were nearly similar in shape. However, with smaller EPSPs, Turner (1988) found that EPSPs in response to distally located synapses were appreciably slower than those elicited by proximally located synapses on the same cell, as expected from cable theory. With an input separation of about 400 μm, the 10 – 90% rising time of the proximal EPSP was 0.43 times that of the distal one. The results with the larger, just threshold size EPSPs could either be due to some spread of fibres away from the zone of stimulation and/or the assistance of active processes from the dendritic membrane.

Summation of EPSPs

When two synaptic conductances are generated simultaneously and near each other on the same target cell, they may interfere with each other (Kuno, 1964; Martin, 1966; Jack et al., 1975). When the consequent membrane voltage change is less than the algebraic sum of the individual synaptic potentials, the synaptic potentials have summed non-linearly. The reason is the reduced driving voltage for the second EPSP when elicited on the summit of the first EPSP. In addition, the conductance produced by the first EPSP acts as a shunt for the second synaptic current. Because of the large synaptic convergence on CA1 pyramidal cells, it is conceivable that non-linear interaction might occur, and thereby reduce the apparent effect of the participating synapses. However, when spatially restricted synaptic inputs were activated simultaneously, EPSPs up to 2.5 mV summed perfectly linearly (Langmoen and Andersen, 1983). The apparent deficit in the summed records that was observed with larger EPSPs could be explained by an addition of inhibitory potentials. After blockade of inhibition by penicillin or moving the membrane potential to the equilibrium potential for the IPSP, the summation of larger EPSPs was linear as well. However, for technical reasons inputs closer than 75 μm could not be tested, leaving the possibility open that local non-linear summation may occur.

Influence of inhibitory processes

Needless to say, inhibition profoundly changes the efficiency of an excitatory synaptic input. The various types of inhibition have different properties and possible roles, however.

In the CA1 area 4 types of inhibitory cells mediate inhibition by way of *GABA$_A$ receptors*. Although not verified physiologically, the morphology of the *chandelier cells,* terminating on the initial axon of a large number of cells, particularly densely near the start of the myelination (Somogyi et al., 1983), suggests that it may hyperpolarize the initial axons, and thus cast a total veto on the discharges, irrespective of the source or location of the excitatory synaptic input. *Basket cells* also effectively inhibit pyramidal cells by hyperpolarization due to a bicuculline-sensitive inward chloride current. The synapses lie around the axonal pole of the soma and the nearest part of the axon, but affect fewer cells than the former type does (Andersen et al., 1964). *One type of stellate cells* hyperpolarizes a sector of the dendritic tree by GABA-containing shaft synapses (Alger and Nicoll, 1982), thereby reducing the effectiveness of excitatory currents in the same part of the dendritic tree. *Another category of stellate cells* acts by creating a local shunt, also mediated through GABA$_A$ receptors (Andersen et al., 1980a; Alger and Nicoll, 1982). This type of inhibition is extremely powerful, effectively negating the currents produced by excitatory synapses located in that dendritic area or distal to it. Both the hyperpolarizing and the shunting type of dendritic inhibition is blocked by bicuculline. Finally, a *GABA$_B$-mediated* inhibition of long duration and caused by potassium efflux is seen in the soma of CA1 pyramids (Newberry and Nicoll, 1984). Whether this effect is mediated by the basket cells or a special type of interneurone is not known.

After-potentials

When the cell is brought to discharge, 3 different forms of *after-hyperpolarization* (AHP) counteract all further excitatory synaptic action (Storm, 1988 and this volume). The size of both the medium and slow AHPs are particularly prominent after a repetitive discharge. The mAHP is partly due to the activation of the muscarinic K$^+$ current I_M, and thus under cholinergic control. The amplitude and duration of the slow AHP depends heavily upon the number of spikes and the frequency of the preceding discharges.

Importance of spatial pattern of convergence

Topological constraints for summation of excitatory synaptic potentials

Excitatory synapses are predominantly located on spines on secondary dendrites and to a smaller extent on spines on the peripheral parts of the primary apical and basal dendrites. Non-linear summation would be much more likely to occur if the co-activated synapses contact neighbouring spines on the same secondary dendrite as compared with contacts on different secondary dendrites (Fig. 2C,D). With the afferent fibres running largely parallel to the pyramidal layer and crossing the dendritic tree orthogonally, multiple synapses between a single fibre and spines on the same dendritic branch are probably a rare occurrence (Fig. 2D).

Only when a stretch of secondary dendrite runs parallel to the alvear surface will an afferent fibre get an opportunity to make such contacts. Even in this case, a separation of about 8 μm between boutons would reduce the chance for non-linear interaction. However, non-linear summation between synapses made by separate fibres on two neighbouring spines is possible, although the thin neck of the spine with its high longitudinal resistance would effectively shield the neighbouring spine from the conductance change. The latter is likely to last less than a millisecond (Redman, 1976; Jack et al., 1981) and the charging time constant would probably significantly delay the voltage change in the next-door spine.

Activity-dependent synaptic changes

There is a whole range of processes related to repetitive activation of synapses that greatly influences their effectiveness. The number, frequency and pattern of the afferent impulse traffic are important, and both presynaptic and postsynaptic mechanisms are involved.

At *low repetition rates* each EPSP stands alone, as it were. It is probably the result of glutamate binding to the quisqualate (QA) receptor (Kauer et al., 1988; Muller et al., 1988). When a *train of impulses* is delivered, however, the standing depolarization caused by the summating EPSPs allows the NMDA receptor to be activated as well. This mechanism adds an amount of inward current, carried by sodium and calcium ions, to the QA receptor mediated responses, representing a boosting of the synaptic effect and may also initiate Ca^{2+}-dependent intracellular processes.

Facilitation appears as an increased EPSP to the second of two identical stimuli. While facilitation in the frog neuromuscular junction (at 20°C; Magleby, 1973) and the lateral perforant path/dentate granule cell synapse (at 33°C; McNaughton, 1982) both had a time constant of decay around 100 ms, the corresponding figure for radiatum fibre/CA1 synapses is around 5 s (Andersen et al., 1984). A major difference is likely to be a smaller degree of transmitter depletion in the CA1 as compared to the dentate synapses. Following a relatively weak train of impulses an additional enhancement of the EPSP appears and is called *augmentation* (Magleby and Zengel, 1976). This process is relatively weaker in the CA1/radiatum synapses compared to those of the perforant path, but the time course of decay is about 4 s for both. The augmentation is followed by the more durable process of *posttetanic potentiation* which has a time constant of decay of 90 s in perforant synapses (McNaughton, 1982), and a very similar value for CA1 radiatum synapses (Andersen et al., 1984). All 3 facilitatory processes seem related to the presynaptic concentration of Ca^{2+} ions. The duration of the 3 facilitatory processes in question is likely to depend upon the amount of calcium ion that remains after the previous activation. From their time-courses, it is likely that different types of calcium sequestration (Blaustein, 1988) could regulate the decay. Candidates are various Ca^{2+}-binding proteins for facilitation, the Ca^{2+}/Na^+ exchange mechanism for the augmentation and Ca^{2+}-pumping devices for posttetanic potentiation.

Finally the powerful process of *long-term potentiation* (Bliss and Lømo, 1973) will have a profound effect on the synaptic efficiency. Because of its strength and very long time-course it is probably the most important of the activity-dependent processes for synaptic efficiency control (Collingridge and Bliss, 1987)

References

Alger, B.E. and Nicoll, R.A. (1982) Feed-forward dendritic inhibition in rat hippocampal pyramidal cells studied *in vitro. J. Physiol. (Lond.),* 328: 105 – 123.

Andersen, P., Eccles, J.C. and Løyning, Y. (1964). Location of postsynaptic inhibitory synapses on hippocampal pyramids. *J. Neurophysiol.,* 27: 592 – 607.

Andersen, P., Blackstad, T.W. and Lømo, T. (1966) Location and identification of excitatory synapses on hippocampal pyramidal cells. *Exp. Brain Res.,* 1: 236 – 248.

Andersen, P., Dingledine, R., Gjerstad, L., Langmoen, I.A. and Mosfeldt Laursen, A. (1980a) Two different responses of hippocampal pyramidal cells to application of gamma-amino-butyric acid (GABA). *J. Physiol. (Lond.),* 305: 279 – 296.

Andersen, P., Silfvenius, H., Sundberg, S.H. and Sveen, O. (1980b) A comparison of distal and proximal dendritic synapses on CA1 pyramids in hippocampal slices *in vitro. J. Physiol. (Lond.),* 307: 273 – 299.

Andersen, P., Anfinsen, I.-L. and Hvalby, Ø. (1984) Frequency potentiation of synaptic transmission in the hippocampus at low rates of stimulation. *Acta Physiol. Scand.,* 120: 23A.

Andersen, P., Blackstad, T., Hulleberg, G., Vaaland, J.L. and Trommald, M. (1987) Dimensions of dendritic spines of rat dentate granule cells during long-term potentiation (LTP). *J. Physiol. (Lond.),* 390: 264P.

Blackstad, T.W. (1985) Laminar specificity of dendritic morphology: examples from the guinea pig hippocampal region. In L.F. Agnati and K. Fuxe (Eds.), *Quantitative Neuroanatomy in Transmitter Research,* Macmillan, London, 1985, pp. 55 – 69.

Blaustein, M. (1988) Calcium transport and buffering in

222

neurons. *Trends Neurosci.,* 11: 438 – 443.

Bliss, T.V.P. and Lømo, T. (1973) Long-lasting potentiation of synaptic transmission in the dentate area of the anaesthetized rabbit following stimulation of the perforant path. *J. Physiol. (Lond.),* 232: 331 – 356.

Collingridge, G.L. and Bliss, T.V.P. (1987) NMDA receptors – their role in long-term potentiation. *Trends Neurosci.,* 10: 288 – 293.

Finch, D.M. and Babb, T.L. (1981) Demonstration of caudally directed hippocampal efferents in the rat by intracellular injection of horseradish peroxidase. *Brain Res.,* 214: 405 – 410.

Hess, G., Kuhnt, U. and Voronin, L.L. (1987) Quantal analysis of paired-pulse facilitation in guinea pig hippocampal slices. *Neurosci. Lett.,* 77: 187 – 192.

Jack, J.J.B., Noble, D. and Tsien, R.W. (1975) *Electric Current Flow in Excitable Cells,* Clarendon Press, Oxford, 182 pp.

Jack, J.J.B., Redman, S.J. and Wong, K. (1981) The components of synaptic potentials evoked in cat spinal motoneurones by impulses in single group Ia afferents. *J. Physiol. (Lond.),* 321: 65 – 96.

Kauer, J.A., Malenka, R.C. and Nicoll, R.A. (1988). A persistent postsynaptic modification mediates long-term potentiation in the hippocampus. *Neuron,* 1: 911 – 917.

Kuno, M. (1964) Quantal components of excitatory synaptic potentials in spinal motoneurones. *J. Physiol. (Lond.),* 175: 81 – 99.

Langmoen, I.A. and Andersen, P. (1983) Summation of excitatory postsynaptic potentials in hippocampal pyramidal cells. *J. Neurophysiol.,* 50: 1320 – 1329.

Martin, A.R. (1966) Quantal nature of synaptic transmission. *Physiol. Rev.,* 46: 51 – 66.

McNaughton, B.L. (1982) Long-term synaptic enhancement and short-term potentiation in rat fascia dentata act through different mechanisms. *J. Physiol. (Lond.),* 324: 249 – 262.

McNaughton, B.L., Barnes, C.A. and Andersen, P. (1981) Synaptic efficacy and EPSP summation in granule cells of rat fascia dentata studies *in vitro. J. Neurophysiol.,* 46: 952 – 966.

Magleby, K.L. (1973) The effect of repetitive stimulation on facilitation of transmitter release at the frog neuromuscular junction. *J. Physiol. (Lond.),* 234: 327 – 352.

Magleby, K.L. and Zengel, J.E. (1976) Augmentation: a process that acts to increase transmitter release at the frog neuromuscular junction. *J. Physiol. (Lond.),* 257: 449 – 470.

Muller, D., Joly, M. and Lynch, G. (1988) Contribution of quisqualate and NMDA receptors to the induction and expression of LTP. *Science,* 242: 1694 – 1697.

Newberry, N.R. and Nicoll, R.A. (1984) A bicuculline-resistant inhibitory post-synaptic potential in rat hippocampal pyramidal cells *in vitro. J. Physiol. (Lond.),* 348: 239 – 254.

Redman, S.J. (1976) A quantitative approach to the integrative function of dendrites. In R. Porter (Ed.), *Int. Rev. Physiol., Neurophysiology II, Vol. 10,* University Park Press, Baltimore, MD, pp. 1 – 36.

Redman, S. and Walmsley, B. (1983a) The time course of synaptic potentials evoked in cat spinal motoneurones at identified group Ia synapses. *J. Physiol. (Lond.),* 343: 117 – 133.

Redman, S. and Walmsley, B. (1983b) Amplitude fluctuations in synaptic potentials evoked in cat spinal motoneurones at identified group Ia synapses. *J. Physiol. (Lond.),* 343: 135 – 145.

Sayer, R.J. (1988) *Synaptic Transmission between CA3 and CA1 Neurones in the Guinea Pig Hippocampal Slice,* Thesis, Australian National University, Canberra.

Sayer, R.J., Redman, S.J. and Andersen, P. (1989) Amplitude fluctuations in small EPSPs recorded from CA1 pyramidal cells in the guinea pig hippocampal slice. *J. Neurosci.,* 9: 840 – 850.

Schaffer, K. (1892) Beitrag zur Histologie der Ammonshornformation. *Arch. Mikr. Anat.,* 39: 611 – 632.

Somogyi, P., Nunzi, M.G., Gorio, A. and Smith, A.D. (1983) A new type of specific interneuron in the monkey hippocampus forming synapses exclusively with the axon initial segment of pyramidal cells. *Brain Res.,* 259: 137 – 142.

Storm, J.S. (1988) An after-hyperpolarization of medium duration in rat hippocampal pyramidal cells. *J. Physiol. (Lond.),* 409: 171 – 190.

Turner, D. (1988) Waveform and amplitude characteristics of evoked responses to dendritic stimulation of CA1 guinea-pig pyramidal cells. *J. Physiol. (Lond.),* 395: 419 – 439.

Wenzel, J., Kirsche, W., Kunz, G., Neumann, H., Wenzel, M. and Winkelmann, E. (1973) Licht- und elektronenmikroskopische Untersuchungen über die Dendritenspines an Pyramiden-Neuronen des Hippocampus (CA1) bei der Ratte. *J. Hirnforsch.,* 13: 387 – 408.

Westrum, L.E. and Blackstad, T.W. (1962) An electron microscopic study of the stratum radiatum of the rat hippocampus (regio superior, CA_1) with particular emphasis on synaptology. *J. Comp. Neurol.,* 119: 281 – 292.

J. Storm-Mathisen, J. Zimmer and O.P. Ottersen (Eds.)
Progress in Brain Research, Vol. 83
© 1990 Elsevier Science Publishers B.V. (Biomedical Division)

CHAPTER 16

Long-term potentiation in the hippocampal CA1 region: its induction and early temporal development

Bengt Gustafsson[1] and Holger Wigström[2]

Departments of [1] Physiology and [2] Medical Physics, University of Göteborg, S-400 33 Göteborg, Sweden

Long-term potentiation (LTP) is a process that due to its prolonged time course and associative nature of induction is believed to be involved in learning and memory in the mammalian brain. In this chapter the experimental evidence for the view that LTP is initiated by an influx of calcium ions through synaptically controlled *N*-methyl-D-aspartate (NMDA) receptor channels is discussed. It will also be described how LTP develops following its induction. It will be shown that there is a considerable delay, about $2-3$ s, between a tetanus and the initiation of LTP, and that additional $20-30$ s are needed for the potentiation to reach peak levels. The potentiation subsequently decays to a degree which depends primarily on tetanus length. It will be argued that this early phase of tetanus-induced LTP is of the same nature as that present a few hours later.

Introduction

Learning and memory have since long been considered to be related to changes in synaptic efficacy, and long-term potentiation (LTP) is a major candidate for such a role (see e.g. Teyler and Discenna, 1984). In the last few years there has been a rapid advance in the understanding of LTP, especially with regard to its induction mechanisms. This advance has been based mainly on work performed on pathways in the hippocampal formation but, as discussed e.g. by Bear et al. (1987), similar induction mechanisms for long-term synaptic potentiation might operate for neocortical synapses as well (see also Bindman et al., 1988). For the CA1 region of the hippocampus it has been demonstrated that LTP requires both pre- and postsynaptic activity for its induction, i.e., that these hippocampal synapses operate as Hebb synapses (Kelso et al., 1986; Malinow and Miller, 1986; Wigström et al., 1986b). The basis for the dependence on both pre- and postsynaptic activity is also likely revealed; there is much evidence implicating a key role for the postsynaptically located

N-methyl-D-aspartate (NMDA) receptor channel (see e.g. Collingridge and Bliss, 1987; Gustafsson and Wigström, 1988). This channel is able to sense the simultaneous occurrence of transmitter release and postsynaptic membrane depolarization, and will allow calcium influx, assumed to trigger LTP, only when there is combined pre- and postsynaptic activity. In the first part of this chapter experimental evidence for this induction model will be discussed.

While the events that occur during a tetanus and that constitute the trigger for LTP are now at least partly understood, the question as to what kind of biochemical processes are initiated by the trigger signal(s) and what kinds of modification these processes give rise to still remains unanswered. In this context it seems of interest to know in some detail how LTP develops with time, how its development depends on induction conditions, and how it may be affected by substances interfering with biochemical processes assumed to participate in the production of LTP. In the second part of this chapter some recent results concerning these questions will be taken up.

How to define LTP

Throughout the years the term LTP has been used to denote practically any potentiation lasting more than 15 min (measured as increase in synaptic potential or population spike) that is evoked by tetanization, by certain drugs (Neuman and Harley, 1983; Malenka et al., 1986; Cherubini et al., 1987), or by changes in extracellular calcium concentration (Turner et al., 1982). In this chapter we will deal only with a potentiation that satisfies the following two criteria: (a) it is associated with an increase in the initial slope of the synaptic potential and (b) its induction depends on association between the activated pre- and postsynaptic elements. These criteria focus on induction requirements that may be considered to be necessary for learning and memory. They also restrict LTP to processes that concern only changes in the synaptic potential itself (implying a local synaptic modification), and that does not involve unspecific changes in inhibitory circuits or cell excitability (since the initial slope of the synaptic potential will be unaffected by such changes). With respect to the criteria concerning the durability of the potentiation it seems intuitively most reasonable that the term LTP should be restricted to a potentiation process lasting at least for weeks, as the potentiation evidenced while using chronically implanted electrodes. On the other hand, analysis of LTP has most often been performed with the in vitro slice technique, the potentiation measured for at most one or a few hours after the induction. Whether the potentiation observed in slice experiments is equivalent to that seen using chronically implanted electrodes is then uncertain. Recent work by Staubli and Lynch (1987) suggests that stimulus parameters that are effective in inducing LTP in slice experiments also produce a stable potentiation lasting for weeks. Thus, it seems possible that the LTP analysed in the slice preparation represents the initial stage of a potentiation process that will last for a considerable time.

Induction of LTP

While LTP has in common with other more short-lasting potentiation processes that it is restricted to the activated synapses, it requires for its induction a simultaneous activation of a considerable number of afferent fibres (Bliss and Gardner-Medwin, 1973; McNaughton et al., 1978; Levy and Steward, 1979; Lee, 1983). The latter requirement could be related either to the number of activated presynaptic fibres per se, or to the postsynaptic activity mediated by the activity of these fibres. The finding that LTP induction is greatly facilitated after blockade of postsynaptic inhibition and the resulting increase in the postsynaptic activity produced by a given afferent tetanus (Wigström and Gustafsson, 1983, 1985b), has been the first one to clearly favour the latter alternative. On the basis of this finding and the observation that the induction of LTP is blocked following the application of an antagonist to the NMDA receptor (Collingridge et al., 1983), it was hypothesized a few years ago (Wigström and Gustafsson, 1985a) that LTP is induced via the opening of synaptically controlled NMDA receptor channels that coexist with non-NMDA receptor channels in the postsynaptic spine membrane. The synaptic control of the NMDA receptor channels would ensure that calcium influx which is assumed to trigger the modification of the non-NMDA excitatory postsynaptic potential (EPSP) only takes place at active synapses, while the voltage dependence of the NMDA receptor channel would ensure the dependence on postsynaptic depolarization. The experimental data that have been gathered since this proposal was made have unequivocally strengthened this idea, even though some queries still remain. In the following we shall discuss the status of this proposal.

The hypothesis first predicted the existence of a dual synaptic potential at each spine, an early one due to the opening of non-NMDA receptor channels and a somewhat later and slower one mediated via NMDA receptor channels. At the time of the proposal it was known that a tetanus inducing LTP is associated with current flowing through NMDA receptor channels, as indicated by a decrease of the field potential by NMDA receptor antagonists during a tetanus (Wigström and Gustafsson, 1984; see also Herron et al., 1985). However, to agree with the proposal it had to be demonstrated that such an NMDA-mediated potential follows also single afferent volleys. It had also to be excluded that the second component was caused by opening of extrasynaptic NMDA receptor channels (ligated by circulating glutamate) secondary to the depolarization produced via the non-NMDA receptor channels. There is now good evidence that single volleys do indeed give rise to a dual EPSP, as postulated. This has first been demonstrated by showing that EPSPs that were reversed in polarity, by keeping the membrane potential at positive membrane potentials, consisted both of a non-NMDA and an NMDA component (Wigström and Gustafsson, 1986). In this case, the NMDA component could not be secondary to the non-NMDA EPSP. In more recent studies in which specific antagonists to the non-NMDA receptor were used, the NMDA component has also been shown to occur in isolation (Muller et al., 1988). The question still remains, however, whether these NMDA EPSPs are generated at the same synapses as the non-NMDA ones. The parallel growth of the two components of the reversed EPSPs with increasing stimulus strength (recruiting additional afferents) indicates that they are mediated by the same afferents (Wigström and Gustafsson, 1986). There also appears to be a rather strict quantitative relation between the amplitudes of the non-NMDA and NMDA EPSPs when examined for various inputs in different slices and experiments (Muller et al., 1988). However, further evidence for this essential point seems to be needed. If these EPSPs are not localized to the same spines, some other factor than a local calcium influx must account for the fact that only activated synapses potentiate (see also below).

The second point of the original hypothesis was

that LTP induction is controlled by the postsynaptic membrane potential (via its effect on the opening of NMDA receptor channels). The control of LTP induction by postsynaptic depolarization has since then been directly proven. With the use of intracellular recording, the amount of depolarization during a tetanus has been controlled by injecting either depolarizing or hyperpolarizing current through the intracellular microelectrode, producing the postulated facilitation and inhibition of LTP induction, respectively (Kelso et al., 1986; Malinow and Miller, 1986). By injecting local anaesthetics into the cell and thereby blocking the appearance of action potentials, it has been shown that the critical conditioning factor is postsynaptic depolarization rather than action potentials per se (Kelso et al., 1986; Gustafsson et al., 1987). By pairing single volley EPSPs with intracellularly injected depolarizing current pulses it has also been demonstrated that the depolarization only induces LTP when timed to coincide with the synaptic NMDA component (Gustafsson et al., 1987). When the applied depolarization ended just before the onset of the synaptic potential no LTP was induced. It did on the other hand develop when the depolarizing pulse was positioned during the NMDA component but after the end of the synaptic non-NMDA component, as was expected if the induction were to be controlled by a direct interaction between the depolarization and the synaptically controlled NMDA receptor channels (see also Gustafsson and Wigström, 1986).

The third point of our hypothesis was that the event that actually triggers LTP is the influx of calcium ions through the NMDA receptor channels. In keeping with this hypothesis, it has been demonstrated that the NMDA receptor channel, in contrast to the non-NMDA receptor channel, has a high permeability to calcium ions (MacDermott et al., 1986). A number of studies have also indicated that LTP is related to calcium ions, however only few of these provide evidence for the essential role of calcium influx. The demonstration that EGTA (a calcium chelator) injected into the postsynaptic cell prevents the induction of LTP strongly suggests that LTP requires a certain intracellular concentration of calcium ions (Lynch et al., 1983). However, it does not discriminate between calcium ions entering from the extracellular space or from the intracellular compartments, nor does it indicate whether the requirement for calcium ions is related to the induction or to the expression of LTP. In more recent studies calcium was injected intracellularly in combination with a calcium chelator and was photo-released from this chelator, the resulting increase in postsynaptic calcium ion concentration leading to a long-lasting synaptic potentiation (Malenka et al., 1988). However, this result does not prove either that calcium influx plays any specific role. Moreover, it was not shown in this case that the synaptic potentiation induced by calcium was indeed LTP (i.e. interacted with tetanus-induced LTP).

That extracellular calcium, and by implication, calcium influx is important for LTP, has been suggested by results obtained several years ago. Thus, reduction of extracellular calcium ion concentration to 1 mM combined with an increase in extracellular magnesium ion concentration greatly diminished the capacity for a given tetanus to evoke LTP, despite the fact that the synaptic transmission was still functional (Dunwiddie and Lynch, 1979). However, this effect could have been related to a reduction in postsynaptic activity rather than to an effect on calcium influx per se. Later studies have however shown that increased extracellular calcium ion concentration enhances the LTP produced by a given tetanus, in a manner which did not seem to be related either to a presynaptic action or to changes in the postsynaptic activity during the tetanus (Huang et al., 1988). More recently it has been demonstrated, using intracellular recording, that pairing of single volley EPSPs with depolarizing current pulses which were large enough to displace the membrane potential to levels which suppressed the influx of calcium ions, produced no or less LTP than in the case where the EPSPs were paired with weaker current pulses (Malenka et al., 1988). This result is most easily explained by LTP being actually triggered by the influx of calcium; it constitutes so far the best evidence for a critical role for a calcium influx.

Are NMDA receptor channels of direct importance for LTP induction?

That NMDA receptor channels are involved in LTP induction was first indicated by the finding that LTP is not generated in the presence of NMDA receptor antagonists (Collingridge et al., 1983). However, this in itself did not indicate whether their role was pre- or postsynaptic, direct or indirect. As discussed above, the evidence that postsynaptic depolarization controls LTP induction has been linked to the need for depolarization in order to open postsynaptically located NMDA receptor channels. However, the postsynaptic depolarization could be a critical variable by being linked to some other controlling factors. The NMDA receptor activation might then be necessary only to provide a sufficient depolarization. In other words, NMDA receptor antagonists might block LTP induction by reducing the postsynaptic depolarization during a tetanus rather than by reducing calcium influx through NMDA receptor channels. The critical factor could instead be the need for sufficient depolarization to activate extrasynaptic voltage-operated calcium channels (see below). One might also imagine a membrane-bound enzyme that is triggered by the transmitter and whose induction is controlled by the level of membrane potential reached during a tetanus.

While there is no absolute proof against the indirect role of NMDA receptor activation, a number of results suggest that NMDA receptor activation rather than postsynaptic depolarization is the critical factor. For example, in low extracellular magnesium solution in which NMDA receptor channels open with less postsynaptic depolarization, LTP induction is facilitated in the presence of low levels of postsynaptic activity during the tetani (Huang et al., 1987). Recently, with the use of non-NMDA receptor antagonists it has also been demonstrated that NMDA receptor activation by itself induces LTP (Muller et al., 1988).

Since it is unlikely that tetanization with only NMDA receptor channels available produces more postsynaptic depolarization during a tetanus than in the case of only non-NMDA receptor activation, this result suggests a specific effect of NMDA receptor activation on LTP induction in a manner unrelated to depolarization. It should be clear however that these results suffer from one limitation. Since the NMDA EPSP is more prolonged than the non-NMDA EPSP, it may possibly provide for a more sustained depolarization and the latter may be of critical importance for the LTP induction.

Are voltage-operated extrasynaptic calcium channels of direct importance for LTP induction?

While the results discussed above strongly suggest a role for calcium influx through NMDA receptor channels as the first step in LTP induction, the question still remains as to whether calcium influx through extrasynaptic voltage-operated channels may contribute to LTP induction in the CA1 region, as might be the case for LTP in the mossy fibre synapse on CA3 pyramidal cells (Harris and Cotman, 1986). In the CA1 region the finding that LTP induction is greatly enhanced in the presence of the calcium agonist BAY K8644 has been taken to suggest a certain involvement of calcium inflow through voltage-operated calcium channels in LTP (Mulkeen et al., 1987). A similar enhancement following application of 4-aminopyridine, which might increase calcium influx by blocking of potassium channels, was also reported (Lee et al., 1986). While these results may be compatible with the finding that calcium influx through extrasynaptic calcium channels may partake in the induction of LTP, they do not constitute any definitive evidence. For instance presynaptic actions of these drugs might influence the amount of transmitter released which could be primarily responsible for the observed effects. The LTP evoked in 4-aminopyridine-treated slices was reported to be blocked by NMDA antagonists, as

if it were mediated via NMDA receptor activation. Moreover, since the same test was not performed in the case of BAY K8644-treated slices one cannot exclude that the action of BAY K8644 was actually mediated by enhanced entry of calcium ions through NMDA receptor channels; the latter could for instance be due to an increase in postsynaptic depolarization during tetanization in the presence of BAY K8644. It may be noted in this context that if calcium influx through extrasynaptic channels induces LTP, other factors than a local calcium influx have to account for the fact that only active synapses potentiate; for a proposed solution to this problem, see e.g. Bliss and Lynch, 1988. On the other hand, it was not actually demonstrated by Mulkeen at al. (1988) that the potentiation observed in the presence of BAY K8644 is specific for the tetanized input and thus equivalent to LTP (as discussed here).

While the available data seem to indicate that LTP is primarily induced by calcium influx through NMDA receptor channels, the question remains as to what kind of biochemical processes are triggered by this influx and are responsible for the EPSP enhancement. A description of the temporal development of LTP under various induction conditions presented in the next section might give some indication for such processes.

Early temporal development of LTP

Since a tetanus gives rise to LTP as well as to potentiation directly related to presynaptic activity (such as augmentation and posttetanic potentiation), and to an unspecific depression, the early development of LTP has not been defined with any certainty (see e.g. Teyler and Discenna, 1984). Thus, there are several questions with respect to LTP that have remained unanswered. For example, it is not known whether there is a delay between the tetanization and the onset of LTP, and whether this delay is dependent on the induction strength. It is not known how fast the peak level is reached and whether this time course is dependent on induction conditions, and whether the potentiation established early on is the same as the potentiation observed hours later etc. Calcium entering into the spine during a tetanus could in principle initiate a number of different biochemical processes leading to a number of modifications with varying onset and duration. LTP may thus be dependent not on a single but several not necessarily coupled processes, and not all might involve a sustained modification.

Experiments in which LTP was elicited by brief tetani, before and after blockade of postsynaptic inhibition or of NMDA receptors, have shown that tetanus-induced LTP is not inherently stable. For example, following a 10-impulse tetanus there is a considerable decay during the first 5 – 10 min that is not accounted for by the decay of augmentation or posttetanic potentiation (Wigström and Gustafsson, 1985b; Wigström et al., 1986) (see also Fig. 1A). Such a decay is also observed when LTP is evoked by pairing single volley EPSPs with brief tetani to separate afferents or with depolarizing current pulses, i.e., without any presynaptic tetanic activity (Gustafsson and Wigström, 1986a; Gustafsson et al., 1987). By pairing single volleys with weak depolarizing pulses the potentiation can fully decay within a few minutes (Gustafsson et al., 1987). There may thus exist at least two separate components of LTP, an early one that decays rather rapidly and a later one that is more stable. As recently shown by Kauer et al. (1988) iontophoretic application of NMDA results in a potentiation lasting only about 30 min or less that appears separate from the later phase of LTP since the NMDA-induced potentiation is not affected when it is evoked on top of a stable tetanus-induced LTP about 50 min following tetanization. However, the potentiation induced by iontophoretic application of NMDA seems less associated with changes in the initial slope than with changes in the later parts of the EPSP (see e.g. Fig. 2, Kauer et al., 1988). In contrast to the NMDA-induced potentiation, the early phase of LTP induced by tetanization recovers only to a minor extent after 1 h (Gustafsson et al., 1989) or even after 2 h (unpublished observations) follow-

ing tetanization. Thus, our data suggest a single process that is initially in an unstable state instead of an early phase of tetanus-induced LTP that is separate from the later one (see further below).

The temporal development of the early phase of LTP has only recently been studied in some detail

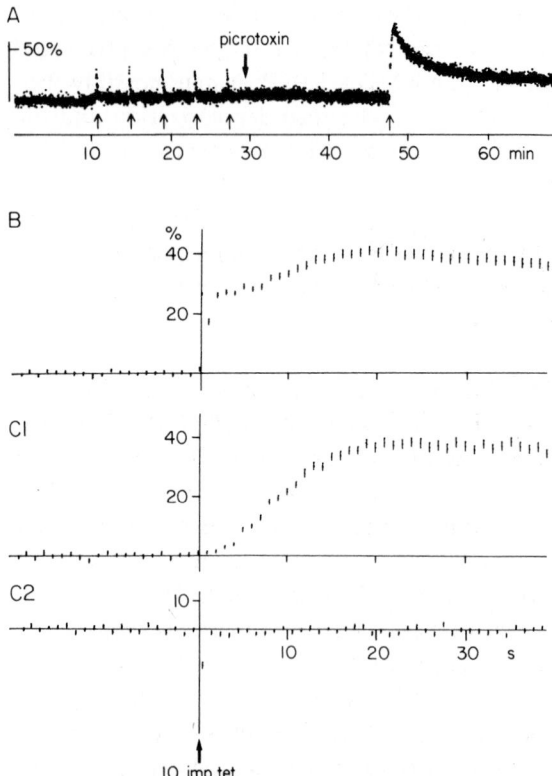

Fig. 1. LTP early time course obtained using picrotoxin application. A: measurements of the initial slope of the field EPSP are shown from one experiment for a series of test responses evoked at 1 Hz. The values are plotted as percentage of the baseline preceding the first tetanus. The potentiations following 6 successive 10-impulse tetani (arrows) (at 50 Hz, using the test strength) are shown. At the time indicated in the graph, picrotoxin (0.1 mM) was added to the bath solution. B – C: average values (± S.E.M.) of potentiation, expressed in percent of the average value obtained during the 20 s immediately preceding each tetanus, are plotted in each graph. B shows the potentiation following 10-impulse tetani evoked in picrotoxin solution (n = 50 tetani). C1: same as in B but after each potentiation had been divided by the averaged potentiation obtained for that input before the application of picrotoxin. C2: same as in C1, but for the control input activated 0.5 s out of phase with respect to the test input. Adapted from Gustafsson et al., 1989.

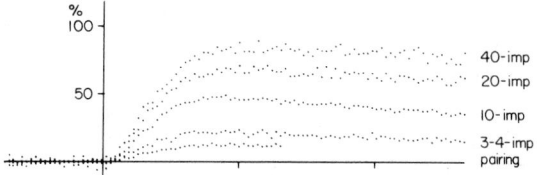

Fig. 2. LTP time course following single volley conjunction and homosynaptic tetanization. Average values of potentiation following pairing and the various homosynaptic tetani (after division by LTP-unrelated potentiation) are plotted as indicated in the figure. Time scale is 30 s between marks. (Adapted from Gustafsson et al., 1989.)

under various induction conditions (Gustafsson et al., 1989). The results show that there exists a delay of 2 – 3 s before any significant potentiation is observed and that it is followed by an almost linear development of LTP for 15 – 20 s (at 30°C) (Fig. 1, C1). Such a time course has been found to be independent of induction conditions (Fig. 2), whether LTP is induced by pairing, by brief (3 – 4 impulse) tetani or by long (20 – 40 impulse) tetani producing varying degrees of potentiation; it was true for increases of EPSP initial slope from about 5% (pairing) to more than 100% (40-impulse tetani) for a single induction event. Since in most cases the tetanus (during which calcium ions could enter the cell) lasted less than a fraction of a second there is a considerable delay between the calcium influx assumed to trigger LTP and the actual start of the potentiation, implying a more complicated process for the EPSP increase than a simple calcium-activated phosphorylation of some key proteins. There must exist a rate-limiting process for the initiation and rate of rise of LTP that requires a considerable time and that is independent of the amount of calcium ions that enter during the tetanus. Since the time course of LTP was the same under different induction conditions it likely represents that at each individual synapse. However, whether there is a gradual change at each synapse, or an all or none switch to a potentiated state with a probability distribution (independent of induction conditions) resembling the overall time course, cannot be decided from these results.

After the early linear rise, LTP increases somewhat slower towards a peak value which is reached 20 – 25 s after the tetanus. Subsequently it starts to decay, e.g. to half of its peak value within 3 min and to one third within 8 min following a 10-impulse tetanus (cf. Fig. 1A and Fig. 3, A1). In contrast to the rising phase, the decay phase is affected by the induction conditions, tending to be slower after longer than after shorter tetani (Fig. 3A), though independently of the induction strength, or of the degree of LTP following a given tetanus length (Gustafsson et al., 1989).

Role of protein kinase C (PKC) activity in LTP maintenance

Several studies have recently drawn the attention to a role of PKC activation for maintenance of LTP. For example, tetanization in the presence of PKC inhibitors produces only a short-lasting LTP component (Kauer et al., 1988; Malinow et al., 1988) and phorbol esters, activators of PKC, slow the decay of tetanus-induced LTP, simulating the effect of a prolongation of train duration (Lovinger and Routtenberg, 1988). Fig. 3 shows such a result. Illustrated in this figure are potentiations following single 10- and 40-impulse tetani, and the algebraical difference between their normalized (see legend to Fig. 3) time courses. The figure includes also examples of potentiations following a single 10-impulse tetanus before and after application of phorbol ester (1 μM), and the algebraical difference between their normalized time courses. It can be noted that both after prolongation of tetanus duration and after phorbol ester application, there is a slowing of the decay of the potentiation, appearing as a component with a delay of about 20 s and a time to peak of 1 – 2 min (Fig. 3, A3, B3). The onset of the phorbol ester effect (and of the expected PKC activation) on LTP revealed by this type of experiment is quite fast. It seems to directly affect the stabilization of the earliest phase of LTP rather than to represent an additional potentiation process.

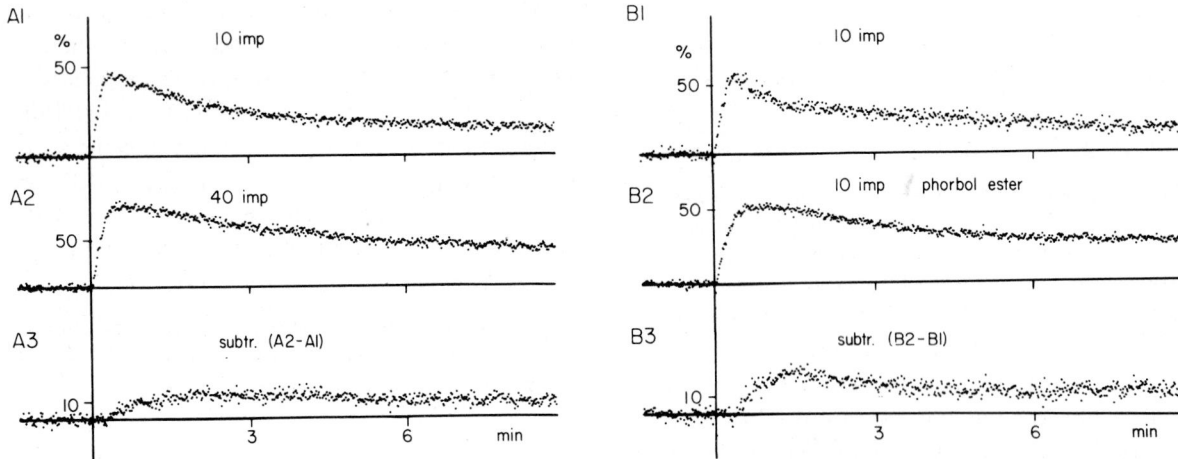

Fig. 3. Effect of tetanus duration and of phorbol ester on the early time course of LTP. A: average values of potentiation following 10-impulse tetani (A1, $n = 51$) and 40-impulse tetani (A2, $n = 8$) in picrotoxin solution after division by that found in normal solution or after application of amino-phosphonovalerate (50 μM). In A3 is shown the algebraical difference between these two curves after adjustment to allow for a matching of their rising phases. (Adapted from Gustafsson et al., 1989.) B: average values of potentiation following 10-impulse tetani in picrotoxin solution without (B1, $n = 6$) and with 1 μM phorbol-12,13-diacetate (B2, $n = 13$) in the bath solution (after division by the potentiation found after application of aminophosphonovalerate (50 μM)). B3, same as in A3 but for the curves shown in B1 and B2. For the experiments shown in B, the extracellular concentrations of calcium and magnesium were 2 and 6 mM, respectively, to counteract the enhancement of transmitter release produced by the phorbol ester application. (Adapted from F. Asztely, E. Hanse, B. Gustafsson and H. Wigström, in preparation).

On the basis of the considerable occlusion between the early phase of LTP and the LTP present 1 − 2 h later, discussed above, and of the results shown in Fig. 3, our tentative conclusion is that LTP (at least within the first few hours) is caused by a single type of modification that is initiated by calcium influx a few seconds after a tetanus and the stabilization of which is somehow controlled by PKC activity. Whether the PKC activation is a consequence of the calcium influx (see Eberhard and Holz, 1988), longer tetani producing a more prolonged period of calcium influx more efficiently activating PKC, or requires activation of some other receptor by the presynaptic release of glutamate, is not answered by these studies. It should, however, be noted that quite prolonged LTP can be evoked by pairing single volleys with depolarizing current pulses (Gustafsson et al., 1987), indicating that tetanic presynaptic activity may not be a necessary requirement for the stabilization. As discussed above, the conclusion that a single process underlies both the early and later phase of LTP is at variance with the results emerging from NMDA application. It is also at variance with the recent finding of a slowly developing change in postsynaptic sensitivity to quisqualate following LTP-inducing tetanization which is taken to suggest an early presynaptic and a later postsynaptic modification underlying LTP (Davies et al., 1989). However, as described by Muller et al. (1988), the NMDA EPSP shows practically no increase at any time after tetanization, a finding which also is at variance with an early presynaptic modification involving increase in transmitter release, at least from a fixed population of terminals projecting to spines containing both non-NMDA and NMDA receptor channels. It is thus clear that further studies will be needed to reconcile, or to resolve these apparently conflicting experimental data.

Acknowledgements

The work described above, such as it pertains to original work by the authors, has been supported by the Swedish Medical Research Council (Projects 05180 and 05954) and the Magnus Bergvall Foundation.

References

Bear, M.F., Cooper, L.N. and Ebner, F.F. (1987) A physiological basis for a theory of synapse modification. *Science,* 237: 42 – 48.

Bindman, L.J., Murphy, K.P.S.J. and Pockett, S. (1988) Postsynaptic control of the induction of long-term changes in efficacy of transmission at neocortical synapses in slices of rat brain. *J. Nerurophysiol.,* 60: 1053 – 1065.

Bliss, T.V.P. and Gardner-Medwin, A.R. (1973) Long-lasting potentiation of synaptic transmission in the dentate area of the unanaesthetized rabbit following stimulation of the perforant path. *J. Physiol. (Lond.),* 232: 357 – 374.

Cherubini, E., Ben Ari, Y., Gho, M., Bidard, J.N. and Lazdunski, M. (1987) Long-term potentiation of synaptic transmission in the hippocampus induced by a bee venom peptide. *Nature (Lond.),* 328: 70 – 73.

Collingridge, G.L. and Bliss, T.V.P. (1987) NMDA receptors – their role in long-term potentiation. *Trends Neurosci.,* 10: 288 – 293.

Collingridge, G.L., Kehl, S.J. and McLennan, H. (1983) Excitatory amino acids in synaptic transmission in the Schaffer collateral-commissural pathway of the rat hippocampus. *J. Physiol. (Lond.),* 334: 33 – 46.

Davies, S.N., Lester, R.A.J., Reymann, K.G. and Collingridge, G.L. (1989) Temporally distinct pre- and postsynaptic mechanisms maintain long-term potentiation. *Nature (Lond.),* 338: 500 – 503.

Dunwiddie, T. and Lynch, G. (1979) The relationship between extracellular calcium concentrations and the induction of hippocampal long-term potentiation. *Brain Res.,* 169: 103 – 110.

Eberhard, D.A. and Holz, R.W. (1988) Intracellular Ca^{2+} activates phospholipase C. *Trends Neurosci.,* 11: 517 – 520.

Gustafsson, B. and Wigström, H. (1986) Hippocampal longlasting potentiation produced by pairing single volleys and brief conditioning tetani evoked in separate afferents. *J. Neurosci.,* 6: 1575 – 1582.

Gustafsson, B. and Wigström, H. (1989) Physiological mechanisms underlying long-term potentiation. *Trends Neurosci.,* 11: 156 – 162.

Gustafsson, B., Wigström, H., Abraham, W.C. and Huang, Y.-Y. (1987) Long-term potentiation in the hippocampus using depolarizing current pulses as the conditioning stimulus to single volley synaptic potentials. *J. Neurosci.,* 7: 774 – 780.

Gustafsson, B., Asztely, F., Hanse, E. and Wigström, H. (1989) Onset characteristics of long-term potentiation in the guinea pig hippocampal CA1 region in vitro. *Eur. J. Neurosci.,* 1: 382 – 394.

Harris, E.W. and Cotman, C.W. (1986) Long-term potentiation of guinea pig mossy fibre responses is not blocked by N-methyl-D-aspartate antagonists. *Neurosci. Lett.,* 70: 132 – 137.

Herron, C.E., Lester, R.A.J., Coan, E.J. and Collingridge, G.L. (1985) Intracellular demonstration of an N-methyl-D-aspartate receptor mediated component of synaptic transmission in the rat hippocampus. *Neurosci. Lett.,* 60: 19 – 23.

Huang, Y.-Y., Wigström, H. and Gustafsson, B. (1987) Facilitated induction of hippocampal long-term potentiation in slices perfused with low concentrations of magnesium. *Neuroscience,* 22: 9 – 16.

Huang, Y.-Y., Gustafsson, B. and Wigström, H. (1988) Facilitation of hippocampal long-term potentiation in slices perfused with high concentrations of calcium. *Brain Res.,* 456: 88 – 94.

Kauer, J.A., Malenka, R.C. and Nicoll, R.A. (1988) NMDA application potentiates synaptic transmission in the hippocampus. *Nature (Lond.),* 334: 250 – 252.

Kelso, S.R., Ganong, A.H. and Brown, T.H. (1986) Hebbian synapses in hippocampus. *Proc. Natl. Acad. Sci. U.S.A.,* 83: 5326 – 5330.

Lee, K.S. (1983) Cooperativity among afferents for the induction of long-term potentiation in the CA1 region of the hippocampus. *J. Neurosci.,* 3: 1369 – 1372.

Lee, W.-L., Anwyl, R. and Rowan, M.J. (1986) 4-aminopyridine-mediated increase in long-term potentiation in CA1 of the rat hippocampus. *Neurosci. Lett.,* 70: 106 – 109.

Levy, W.B. and Steward, O. (1979) Synapses as associative memory elements in the hippocampal formation. *Brain Res.,* 175: 233 – 245.

Lovinger, D. and Routtenberg, A. (1988) Synapse-specific protein kinase C activation enhances maintenance of long-term potentiation in rat hippocampus. *J. Physiol. (Lond.),* 400: 321 – 333.

Lynch, G., Larson, J., Kelso, S., Barrionuevo, G. and Schottler, F. (1983) Intracellular injections of EGTA block induction of hippocampal long-term potentiation. *Nature (Lond.),* 305: 719 – 721.

MacDermott, A.B., Mayer, M.L., Westbrook, G.L., Smith, S.J. and Barker, J.L. (1986) NMDA receptor activation increases cytoplasmic calcium concentration in cultured spinal cord neurones. *Nature (Lond.),* 321: 519 – 522.

Malenka, R.C., Madison, D.V. and Nicoll, R.A. (1986) Potentiation of synaptic transmission in the hippocampus by phorbol esters. *Nature (Lond.),* 321: 175 – 177.

Malenka, R.C., Kauer, J.A., Zucker, R.S. and Nicoll, R.A.

232

(1988) Postsynaptic calcium is sufficient for potentiation of hippocampal synaptic transmission. *Science,* 242: 81 – 84.

Malinow, R. and Miller, J.P. (1986) Postsynaptic hyperpolarization during conditioning reversibly blocks induction of long-term potentiation. *Nature (Lond.),* 320: 529 – 530.

Malinow, R., Madison, D.V. and Tsien, R.W. (1988) Persistent protein kinase activity underlying long-term potentiation. *Nature (Lond.),* 335: 820 – 824.

McNaughton, B.L., Douglas, R.M. and Goddard, G.V. (1978) Synaptic enhancement in fascia dentata: cooperativity among coactive afferents. *Brain Res.,* 157: 277 – 293.

Mulkeen, D., Anwyl, R. and Rowan, M.J. (1987) Enhancement of long-term potentiation by the calcium channel agonist Bayer K8644 in CA1 of the rat hippocampus in vitro. *Neurosci. Lett.,* 80: 351 – 355.

Muller, D., Joly, M. and Lynch, G. (1988) Contributions of quisqualate and NMDA receptors to the induction and expression of LTP. *Science,* 242: 1694 – 1697.

Neuman, R.S. and Harley, C.W. (1983) Long-lasting potentiation of the dentate gyrus population spike by norepinephrine. *Brain Res.,* 273: 162 – 165.

Staubli, U. and Lynch, G. (1987) Stable hippocampal long-term potentiation elicited by "theta" pattern stimulation. *Brain Res.,* 435: 227 – 234.

Teyler, T.J. and Discenna, P. (1984) Long-term potentiation as a candidate mnemonic device. *Brain Res. Rev.,* 7: 15 – 28.

Turner, R.W., Baimbridge, K.G. and Miller, J.J. (1982) Calcium-induced long-term potentiation in the hippocampus. *Neuroscience,* 7: 1411 – 1416.

Wigström, H. and Gustafsson, B. (1983) Facilitated induction of hippocampal long-lasting potentiation during blockade of inhibition. *Nature (Lond.),* 301: 603 – 604.

Wigström, H. and Gustafsson, B. (1984) A possible correlate of the postsynaptic condition for long-lasting potentiation in the guinea pig hippocampus in vitro. *Neurosci. Lett.,* 44: 327 – 332.

Wigström, H. and Gustafsson, B. (1985a) On long-lasting potentiation in the hippocampus: a proposed mechanism for its dependence on coincident pre- and postsynaptic activity. *Acta Physiol. Scand.,* 123: 519 – 522.

Wigström, H. and Gustafsson, B. (1985b) Facilitation of hippocampal long-lasting potentiation by GABA antagonists. *Acta Physiol. Scand.,* 125: 159 – 172.

Wigström, H. and Gustafsson, B. (1986) Postsynaptic control of hippocampal long-term potentiation. *J.Physiol. (Paris),* 81: 228 – 236.

Wigström, H., Gustafsson, B. and Huang, Y.-Y. (1986a) Mode of action of excitatory amino acid receptor antagonists on hippocampal long-lasting potentiation. *Neuroscience,* 17: 1105 – 1115.

Wigström, H., Gustafsson, B., Huang, Y.-Y. and Abraham, W.C. (1986b) Hippocampal long-term potentiation is induced by pairing single afferent volleys with intracellularly injected depolarizing current pulses. *Acta Physiol. Scand.,* 126: 317 – 319.

J. Storm-Mathisen, J. Zimmer and O.P. Ottersen (Eds.)
Progress in Brain Research, Vol. 83
© 1990 Elsevier Science Publishers B.V. (Biomedical Division)

CHAPTER 17

The nature and causes of hippocampal long-term potentiation

Gary Lynch, Markus Kessler, Amy Arai and John Larson

Bonney Center for the Neurobiology of Learning and Memory, University of California, Irvine, CA 92717, U.S.A.

One of the most fascinating features of the hippocampus is its capacity for plasticity. Long-term potentiation (LTP), a stable facilitation of synaptic potentials after high-frequency synaptic activity, is very prominent in hippocampus and is a leading candidate memory storage mechanism. Here, we discuss the nature and causes of LTP and relate them to endogenous rhythmic neuronal activity patterns and their potential roles in memory. Anatomical studies indicate that LTP is accompanied by postsynaptic structural modifications while pharmacological studies strongly suggest that LTP is not due to an increase in presynaptic transmitter release. In field CA1, LTP induction appears to be triggered by a postsynaptic influx of calcium through NMDA receptor-linked channels. Possible roles of several calcium-sensitive enzyme systems in LTP are discussed and it is argued that activation of a calcium-dependent protease (calpain) could produce the structural changes linked to LTP. Rhythmic bursting activity is highly effective in inducing LTP and it is argued that the endogenous hippocampal theta rhythm plays a role in LTP induction in vivo. Finally, studies indicate that LTP and certain types of memory share a common pharmacology and the use of electrical brain stimulation as a sensory cue suggests that LTP develops when the significance of that cue is learned.

Introduction

The hippocampus has figured prominently in studies of synaptic plasticity and memory. While these two phenomena are presumably closely related, it is somewhat ironic that hippocampal work on the one has not been greatly influenced by studies of the other. Analysis of synaptic changes is most easily carried out on brain structures with relatively simple and stratified anatomies and it is these properties of hippocampus that have led to its being so widely used in studies of plasticity. The commonly held assumption that hippocampus plays a critical role in memory encoding and/or processing arose from clinical observations of brain-damaged patients and has had little direct influence on neurobiological investigations. We can expect that the behavioral and biological lines of investigation will eventually begin to converge and recent studies of one form of plasticity associated with hippocampus suggest that progress is being made towards this goal. These findings constitute the subject of the present chapter.

Both anatomical and physiological plasticity are very much in evidence in the adult hippocampus. Axon sprouting and synaptogenesis provide a conspicuous example of the former. When the dense perforant path inputs to the middle and outer molecular layers of the dentate gyrus are removed, the septal projections to that region increase the density of their projections (Lynch et al., 1972) and the associational afferents from the hilar polymorph neurons sprout outwards into the denervated territory (Lynch et al., 1976). Electron microscopic studies indicate that the sprouted endings form spine synapses (Lee et al., 1977) that are very probably functional (Lynch et al., 1973; West et al., 1975). The sprouting paradigm provides us with a measure of the capacity of hippocampus to remodel its microanatomy and the manner in which this changes with development (Gall et al., 1980; McWilliams and Lynch, 1983) and aging (McWilliams and Lynch, 1984) but it is not likely that the phenomenon itself is directly involved in memory storage. Sprouting requires 5 days to begin (Lynch et al., 1977b; McWilliams and Lynch, 1979) and is preceded and perhaps triggered by dramatic glial reactions (Rose et al., 1976; Gall et al., 1978) – phenomena that are not likely to occur during normal behavior. However, as will be shown, the capacity for anatomical reorganization revealed by the sprouting studies may be exploited in a more modest fashion in a type of plasticity that could be involved in memory.

Physiological studies have uncovered an example of synaptic plasticity that in many ways is more remarkable than the sprouting effect. Specifically, high-frequency afferent stimulation produces a potentiation of synaptic potentials that can persist for weeks (Bliss and Lømo, 1973). Certain characteristics of the long-term potentiation (LTP) effect make it an excellent candidate for a storage process; i.e., it develops quickly and lasts for a long period, two properties that are necessary ingredients for memory. Research on LTP first sought to define the nature of the effect (e.g. where the changes occur that express the potentiation) and to identify its causes (e.g. second messenger chemistries involved in its induction). More recently, some experimental attention has been directed to questions concerning the relationship of LTP to physiological activity occurring during learning and to memory itself. We shall discuss each of these issues in turn.

The nature of long-term potentiation

An illustration of the LTP effect, as exhibited by the Schaffer/commissural synapses on CA1 neurons, is provided in Fig. 1. High-frequency stimulation induces an initial decremental short-term potentiation (STP) that stabilizes in 10 – 20 min to a stable LTP that does not detectably decay thereafter. Several lines of evidence indicate that stable LTP is due to a modification of the synapses between the stimulated afferents and their target dendrites (Fig. 2). Induction of LTP in one input does not affect the responses to other inputs to the same dendritic field, indicating that dendrite-wide changes are not responsible for potentiation (McNaughton and Barnes, 1977; Lynch et al., 1977a; Dunwiddie and Lynch, 1978; Andersen et al., 1977). Moreover, injections of calcium chelating agents (Lynch et al., 1983) or hyperpolarizing currents (Malinow and Miller, 1986) into a target neuron block LTP in that cell without affecting its occurrence in neighboring neurons, a result which rules out widespread modifications of the axons that received high-frequency stimulation (Fig. 2B).

Whether the stable synaptic changes responsible for LTP are located in the axon terminal or dendritic spine has been much debated. Bliss and co-

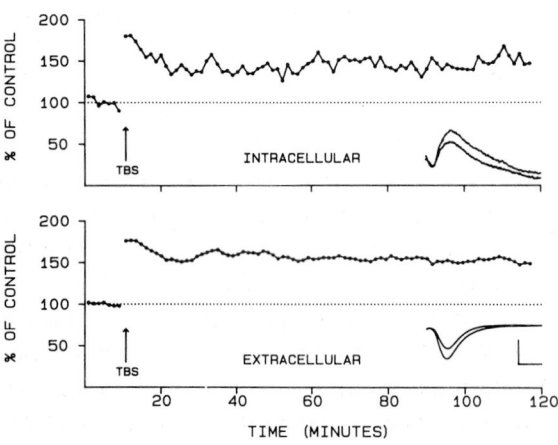

Fig. 1. Long-term potentiation on the hippocampal slice. Plot of intracellular EPSP amplitude and initial slope of the extracellularly recorded population EPSP in the apical dendritic field before and after theta burst stimulation (TBS). Each point is an average of 4 consecutive responses. TBS consisted of 4-pulse bursts (100 Hz) repeated 10 times at 5 Hz. Responses showed a decremental short-term potentiation (STP) effect for about 10 min and then stabilized at a potentiated level that did not decrement for the duration of the experiment. Inset shows records (averages of 4 responses each) obtained before and during LTP. Calibration bars: 5 mV and 5 ms for intracellular, 2 mV and 5 ms for extracellular.

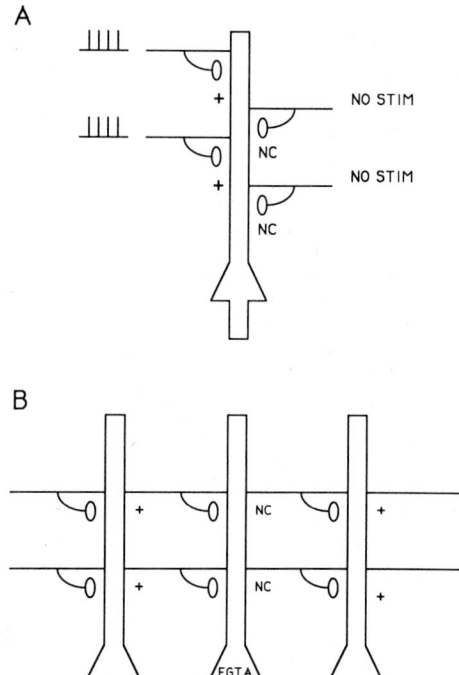

Fig. 2. Specificity of LTP. A: postsynaptic selectivity. Schematic illustrates 4 synapses on one pyramidal cell. Two of these are given burst stimulation and exhibit LTP (+); the non-stimulated synapses show no change (NC). B: presynaptic selectivity. Two axons are shown making en passant synapses with 3 pyramidal cells. Injection of EGTA into the middle cell prevents induction of LTP at its synapses. This indicates that LTP is not due to changes in the entire axon since synapses on the EGTA-filled cell are not changed but other synapses are potentiated.

workers (see Bliss and Lynch, 1988, for a review) reported evidence for increased release of glutamate, the likely transmitter, in the perforant path after induction of LTP but these results are open to a variety of criticisms which cannot be elaborated here (see Lynch et al., 1988, for a discussion). Two types of argument pointed to a postsynaptic location (Lynch et al., 1983). First, as noted above, the triggering mechanism for LTP is located postsynaptically and it seemed only reasonable to assume that the processes that express the effect are located proximal to the events that induce it. Second, electron microscopic studies have identified changes in spines and synapses that accompany LTP (Lee et al., 1980, 1981; Chang and Greenough, 1984; Desmond and Levy, 1986) and it would be surprising if such structural alterations did not have functional consequences. These arguments are of course quite indirect and there are in fact several ways in which the morphological correlates of LTP might relate to potentiation of synaptic strength: (1) the anatomical changes are an epiphenomenon associated with the changes that actually express LTP, (2) new synapses are formed (in which case LTP would be *both* a pre- and a postsynaptic effect), (3) modifications of postsynaptic morphology disturb the presynaptic terminals and thereby increase release, (4) alterations in spine morphology change the biophysics of spine to dendrite coupling (Rall, 1978), or (5) the morphological effects alter the surface chemistry of the spine producing a larger synaptic current for a given amount of released transmitter (see Lynch and Baudry, 1984).

The discovery of pharmacological agents that selectively block the various subclasses of transmitter receptors found in hippocampal synapses provided a more direct means for testing between pre- and postsynaptic mechanisms. It is widely accepted that these connections contain at least two classes of glutamate receptors which have come to be known as the NMDA and AMPA (or quisqualate) subtypes. Under most circumstances, the NMDA group contributes little to transmission because its associated ion channel is blocked in a voltage-dependent manner by magnesium ions (Nowak et al., 1984; Mayer et al., 1984). However, when extracellular magnesium is reduced, the postsynaptic response contains a sizeable component that is mediated by the NMDA receptor in addition to the normally present AMPA current (Muller and Lynch, 1988b). (This effect is probably due to increased transmitter release — and hence increased depolarization — and a partial relaxation of the magnesium blockade of the NMDA receptor ionophore.)

Increased release of transmitter from a fixed population of terminals would be expected to increase the synaptic currents generated by both the NMDA and the AMPA receptors and this has been confirmed experimentally. Thus, paired pulse facilitation (Muller and Lynch, 1988a) and frequency facilitation (Muller et al., 1989), as well as posttetanic potentiation (Kauer et al., 1988), all transient forms of synaptic facilitation that involve increased release, cause large increases in the responses generated by both classes of receptors. LTP, on the other hand, has little effect on the NMDA receptor currents but instead selectively increases the currents produced by the AMPA receptors (Muller and Lynch, 1988a; Muller et al., 1988a). Figure 3A illustrates one of several experiments that led to this conclusion. Two pathways with overlapping terminal fields were used, one designated to serve as the potentiated pathway, and the other as a control. The hippocampal slices were maintained in low magnesium to augment the NMDA receptor potentials; DNQX, an antagonist of the AMPA sites, was added to the bath *after* inducing LTP in one of the two pathways. As can be seen in the figure, the drug reduced both potentiated and control responses to the same absolute values; thus when the AMPA receptors were blocked and the responses consisted solely of an NMDA-mediated component, the difference between potentiated and control responses was eliminated. From this result we concluded that induction of LTP does not affect the synaptic currents generated by the NMDA receptors. This point was also made by an experiment that is the reverse of the above (Fig. 3B). That is, when we administered LTP inducing stimulation *in the presence of DNQX* we found that the NMDA-dependent potentials were unchanged, again pointing to the conclusion that the pertinent receptors do not express LTP. However, when the drug was washed out of the slice and the AMPA receptors exposed, then normal LTP was present in the pathway that received the high-frequency stimulation. This tells us that the NMDA receptors by themselves can induce LTP but that expression of the potentiation effect is accomplished by the AMPA sites (Muller et al.,

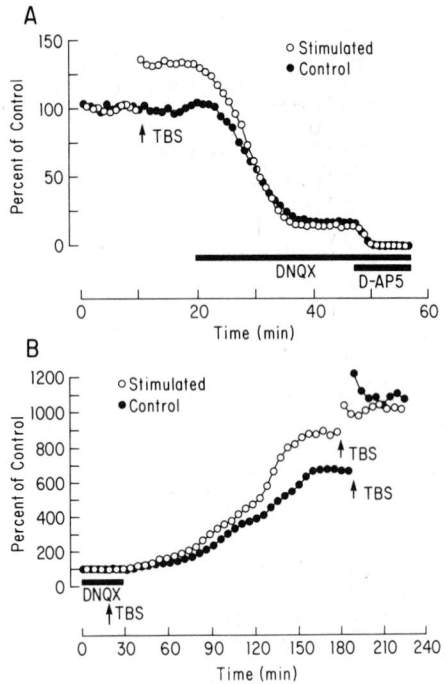

Fig. 3. NMDA receptors induce LTP but AMPA receptors express it. A: LTP is not expressed when AMPA receptors are blocked with DNQX. Amplitude of population EPSPs evoked by two independent sets of Schaffer/commissural fibers in CA1 are shown; one pathway (open circles) was given theta burst stimulation (TBS arrow), the other (filled circles) served as a control. After LTP induction, application of DNQX reduced both potentiated and control responses to the same absolute magnitude. These resultant responses were mediated by NMDA receptors as indicated by their abolition with the NMDA antagonist D-AP5. B: LTP can be induced by NMDA receptor activation when AMPA receptors are blocked but can only be expressed when AMPA receptors are exposed. NMDA receptor responses in the presence of DNQX were unaffected by TBS but after DNQX washout the responses to the stimulated pathway were increased above control levels. Further TBS had little effect on this potentiated pathway although TBS of the control pathway induced robust LTP (data from Muller et al., 1988a).

1988a; Kauer et al., 1988, also reached this conclusion using a different experimental paradigm).

These results are clearly incompatible with the hypothesis that LTP is due to an increase in release from a constant population of terminals but can they be explained by the ultrastructural correlates of potentiation? Note that for an increased number of effective synapses to explain the selective nature of LTP it would be necessary that such contacts lack NMDA receptors, a perhaps unlikely circumstance. Changes in the shapes of existing spines might produce the observed results in one of two ways. First, the processes that produce shape change could modify the surface geometry and hence chemistry of the synaptic region and thereby expose previously inaccessible AMPA receptors. This would not be unprecedented: blood platelets upon activation change their shape and add or expose membrane proteins, in this case fibrinogen receptors, on their surface (Marguerie et al., 1979; Jennings et al., 1981). Second, morphological alterations could affect the biophysics of the dendritic spine in such a way as to facilitate AMPA receptor currents without markedly changing those associated with NMDA receptors. This type of biophysical selectivity may seem at first to be unlikely but it will be recalled that the NMDA receptor-generated responses are somewhat slower than the AMPA-produced responses. Models of dendritic spines have stressed the point that a reduction in the linear resistance of the spine would have much greater effects on fast synaptic currents than on slower ones (Fig. 4; see Wilson, 1984, and the references therein).

Unfortunately, the two possibilities just noted are not easy subjects for experimental testing. Changes in receptors might be expected to be reflected in altered responses to ionophoretically applied glutamate (or AMPA) but it is no easy matter to establish that exogenous compounds are in fact operating via synaptic receptors and in particular those receptors found in potentiated contacts. Beyond that, since the synaptic receptor may exhibit desensitization (Tang et al., 1989), it is not at all clear that seconds-long stimulation of receptors in any meaningful way reproduces the millisecond-long events occurring during transmission. The first studies attempting to use the ionophoretic approach found that induction of LTP sometimes produced a depression of responses to brief pulses of glutamate (Lynch et al., 1976). While this might be taken as evidence for a change in receptor function it is perhaps more

likely that it was related to a heterosynaptic depression of responses that sometimes accompanied LTP (Lynch et al., 1977a; Abraham and Goddard, 1983; Levy and Steward, 1983). More recently, Collingridge and co-workers (Davies et al., 1989) reported that 20-s applications of AMPA produce greater responses following induction of LTP; however, these effects did not develop until well after the period in which stable LTP appears, a point that calls into question any relationship between the ionophoretic changes and physiological potentiation. Further research along these lines is needed.

Ligand binding offers another approach for testing the effects of LTP on receptor function. A major difficulty here lies in potentiating a sufficient number and proportion of synapses within a sample so that a modification can be detected in a biochemical assay. One experiment of this type used approximately 30 stimulation sites in field CA1 and then measured binding of radio-labelled glutamate to crude synaptic membranes prepared from dissected samples of the target dendritic field

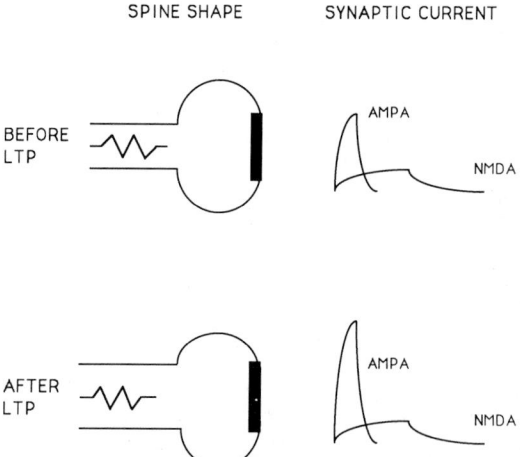

Fig. 4. Potential consequences of spine shape change for AMPA- and NMDA-mediated synaptic currents. Widening of the spine neck would decrease its longitudinal resistance. Modelling studies indicate that this would have a greater impact on fast vs slow synaptic currents. Such a mechanism might account for the finding that the fast AMPA receptor-generated currents express LTP but the slow NMDA receptor-generated currents do not.

(Lynch et al., 1982). A positive effect was reliably obtained but subsequent work revealed that most of the labelled glutamate, rather than being bound to receptors, was being sequestered into small vesicles created during subcellular fractionation (Pin et al., 1984; Kessler et al., 1987). It is of interest that a comparable result was obtained in hippocampus following induction of kindling (Savage et al., 1982). The origins of this effect are unknown but one possibility is that LTP and kindling change the manner in which synaptic membranes behave during subcellular fractionation. We have recently repeated the ligand-binding experiments using assay conditions that more reliably measure AMPA and NMDA receptor numbers and affinities. As is evident from Table I, induction of LTP at many sites in field CA1 did not significantly affect binding to either receptor class.

It would be surprising if sizeable shifts in the number of the AMPA sites would have escaped detection in binding assays. However, if changes were to occur primarily in the receptor channel kinetics then any associated changes in agonist binding parameters may be too subtle to be observed and might be further obscured by alterations incurred during the membrane preparation. In all, while there is no clear evidence that receptors change with LTP, experimental and interpretative difficulties preclude firm conclusions in this regard.

Evaluation of the possibility that LTP is due to biophysical changes in spines (e.g. decreased neck resistance) requires a more accurate description of the structural changes mentioned above. More specifically, we need to determine if these effects are predominantly due to the transformation of existing spines into new synaptic configurations as

---

TABLE I

Changes in AMPA and NMDA receptor binding after LTP induction

Ligand		Average change in binding (in %)	n
[³H]AMPA	10 nM	+3.8 ± 10.0	(3)
[³H]AMPA	50 nM	−4.6 ± 3.0	(5)
[³H]AMPA	100 nM	+5.7 ± 7.0 (S.D.)	(2)
[³H]AMPA	100 nM		
(0 KSCN)		+8.2 ± 2.0 (S.D.)	(2)
[³H]Glutamate 50 nM			
(total binding)		+0.94 ± 3.5	(5)
[³H]Glutamate 50 nM			
(AP5-displaceable binding)		−4.1 ± 7.5	(3)

Hippocampal slices were stimulated at one stimulating electrode position in the stratum radiatum of the CA1 field. If the resulting increase in the EPSP exceeded 40% of the prestimulation EPSP and remained stable for at least 10 min, the slice was subsequently exposed to extensive theta-patterned stimulation by positioning the stimulating electrode sequentially in at least 16 positions in both the stratum radiatum and oriens of the CA1 field. Stimulation intensity was adjusted to produce cell spiking. One hour after stimulation, the treated slice was removed from the chamber together with a control slice. CA1 fields were then dissected and frozen. Four each of the stimulated and control CA1 slices were pooled and processed in parallel to prepare membranes according to a standard procedure, which involves differential centrifugation, osmotic lysis and extensive washing by several cycles of centrifugation and resuspending in the assay buffer (100 mM HEPES/Tris, 50 µM EGTA, pH 7.4). Membrane aliquots containing 3–5.5 µg protein were incubated at 0°C with [³H]glutamate for 30 min or with [³H]AMPA for 45 min and then filtered through GF/C filters. For [³H]AMPA binding, 50 mM KSCN was included in the assay medium and the stop solution (filtration time including filter washing was < 4 s; binding loss during filtration was less than 20% and was smaller than the loss incurred with centrifugation assays during the washing of the pellet). [³H]Glutamate binding was measured both in presence or absence or 100 µM AP5. The difference between the two measures represents binding to NMDA receptors. Specific binding was in general calculated from triplicate or quadruplicate determinations (typical values for both ligands: 1.5–2.5 pmoles/mg protein at a concentration of 50 nM). The percent difference in binding was determined for each pair of samples processed in parallel. The data shown represent the average change after LTP stimulation (mean and S.E.M., or S.D. where indicated) of the indicated number of experiments. Limitations in the amount of material precluded the determination of saturation curves. [³H]AMPA binding was instead determined at 3 ligand concentrations chosen to preferentially reveal high affinity (10 nM) or low affinity (50–100 nM) sites. KSCN was omitted in some assays since binding activation by SCN ions might occlude changes in the functional status of the receptors.

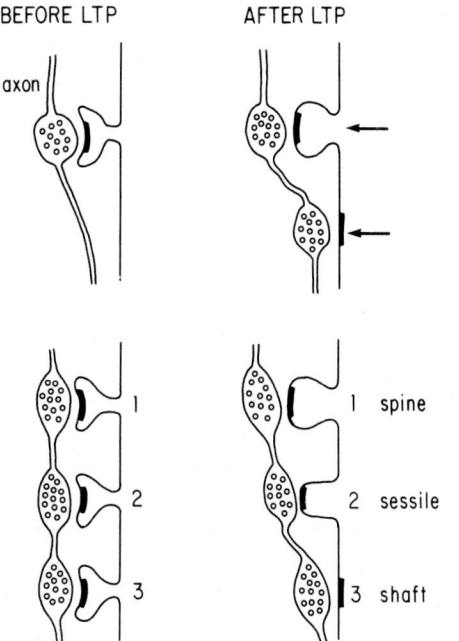

BEFORE LTP   AFTER LTP

axon

1 spine

2 sessile

3 shaft

Fig. 5. Interpretations of anatomical changes associated with LTP. Top panel shows the formation of a new synapse on a dendritic shaft and also a change in the shape of the existing spine. Bottom panel illustrates the transformation of spine synapses to "sessile" spine or shaft configurations.

opposed to the addition of new profiles (Fig. 5). The hippocampus clearly possesses the capacity for synaptic growth as indicated by studies on axon sprouting (Lynch et al., 1973) but it is far more difficult to establish such effects in the LTP paradigm. Moreover, as noted above, the growth argument carries with it the cumbersome corollary that the added contacts would be likely to lack NMDA receptors. Spine transformation could in principle be detected as a reduction in the numbers of one type of contact and a gain in another. The former has not been observed but there are formidable problems which might explain this. Specifically, small changes in the total spine population might be sufficient to account for the percentage increases seen in unusual synaptic types (shaft synapses and sessile spines, see Fig. 5); thus, gains may be more obvious than losses. Studies in which spines are grouped into categories will help to evaluate the transformation argument.

But even if a satisfactory description of the structural correlates of LTP were at hand, there would remain the problem of evaluating their significance to the biophysics of postsynaptic responses. Perhaps the most obvious approach to this would be to use computer simulations but the experimental validation of spine models poses its own set of problems (see Wilson, 1984, for a discussion).

To summarize, physiological and pharmacological experiments strongly suggest that LTP reflects a modification occurring in dendritic spines with the most likely possibilities being a change in receptor physiology or spine biophysics. Ligand-binding studies have not provided evidence for receptor changes and the results of ionophoretic experiments are ambiguous. Electron microscopic experiments indicate that structural modifications do occur in spines and in principle these could account for the selective nature of LTP indicated by pharmacological experiments; however, the anatomical changes are not sufficiently defined to allow for computer modelling, an enterprise that itself is still in the early stages of development. In all, much has been learned about the nature of LTP but there is still a considerable distance to travel before satisfactory answers are obtained; it should not be surprising, given the history of the field, if the journey takes some unexpected turns.

The causes of long-term potentiation

It now appears well established that the initial events that induce LTP involve activation of NMDA receptor currents (Collingridge et al., 1983; Harris et al., 1984; Morris et al., 1986) and increases in postsynaptic calcium levels (Lynch et al., 1983; Malenka et al., 1988). These two points are nicely connected by the observation that the NMDA receptor ionophore passes extracellular calcium into the target cells (MacDermott et al., 1986; Mayer and Westbrook, 1987). However, the events that follow upon calcium entry, or occur in parallel with it, are very much disputed. It need not be emphasized that the processes triggered by calcium or that participate in its regulation encompass a great deal of cell biology and therefore that a host of factors are in one way or another going to be involved in the production of LTP. However, the issue can be usefully focussed by asking which of these many factors are most directly linked to the production of stable modifications that augment postsynaptic responses. It should also be possible to constrain the list of candidate mechanisms by considering two aspects of LTP that have received surprisingly little attention: how long in fact does it last and how quickly is it formed. Taking these in order, Barnes (1979) reported that LTP in the perforant path projections to dentate gyrus declines over a period of several days while Racine and co-workers (Racine et al., 1983) obtained evidence that two forms of potentiation exist with half-lives of several hours and several days respectively. However, a recent chronic recording study from our laboratory using the two-input paradigm described above found that LTP can persist without decrement for weeks (Staubli and Lynch, 1987). With regard to the time required to produce stable potentiation, we have recently discovered that hypoxia reverses LTP without affecting control responses if applied within one to two min after high-frequency stimulation but is without effect if administered beyond this time period (Arai et al., 1990). Thus, if we restrict our discussions to field CA1, it would appear that LTP develops within a minute or so and once formed is stable for weeks. It would seem that the list of cellular processes that satisfy these constraints cannot be overly long.

Some have argued that phosphorylation could be the event that expresses LTP (Akers et al., 1985; Lovinger et al., 1987; Malinow et al., 1988; Reymann et al., 1988a) but this seems extremely unlikely given the extraordinary stability of the potentiation effect; a more likely possibility is that phosphorylation is one step in the minute or so long sequence that yields LTP, but the evidence for this is unclear.

Protein kinase C has received considerable at-

tention with regard to LTP. It is calcium-dependent and is reported to be activated by high-frequency stimulation of the dentate gyrus (Akers et al., 1985). Certainly the most striking evidence that PKC plays a pivotal role came with a report that phorbol esters, drugs that activate the enzyme, potentiate synapses in CA1 in an LTP-like fashion (Malenka et al., 1986). However, we found that the effects of phorbol esters are fully reversible upon washout and that the potentiation they produce is qualitatively different from LTP (Muller et al., 1988b; see also Gustafsson et al., 1988). It has also been claimed that H-7, a drug that, among many other actions, suppresses PKC activity, selectivity reverses already established LTP (Malinow et al., 1988) but we have been unable to replicate this; that is, in our hands, the drug is equally likely to depress control responses as it is to reduce potentiated ones (Arai et al., in preparation). In all, the role of PKC in long-term potentiation remains to be clarified.

Activation of the Ca^{2+}/calmodulin-dependent protein kinase type II (CaM kinase) provides a second and in many ways plausible candidate for a step in the production of LTP. This enzyme is calcium-dependent and has the additional attractive feature of being concentrated in the postsynaptic density (Kennedy et al., 1983), a region in which the changes responsible for LTP might well be located. Work in our laboratory indicated that inhibitors of calmodulin interfere with the development of LTP (Finn et al., 1980) and this result has also been obtained by other groups (Mody et al., 1984; Reymann et al., 1988b). However, the drugs used in these various experiments are not sufficiently selective to allow for firm conclusions, and suppression of calmodulin can be expected to produce a variety of very generalized effects. It will be of interest to repeat the above experiments using recently developed stimulation paradigms that permit easy measurements of NMDA receptor mediated postsynaptic responses (Larson and Lynch, 1988; Muller and Lynch, 1988b; Muller et al., 1989). If it could be shown that these events antecedent to

LTP induction are not affected by the calmodulin antagonists, then the argument that calmodulin-dependent processes participate in the development of LTP would be noticeably strengthened.

Work in our laboratory has focussed on calcium-stimulated mechanisms that could rapidly produce the types of structural changes that correlate with LTP. Structural changes provide a logical explanation for the extreme persistence of LTP and therefore cellular mechanisms that produce such effects are a priori candidates for the intermediary events that result in potentiation. In a series of early studies, we found that activation of a calcium-sensitive protease (calpain) in crude synaptic membrane fractions reproduced the changes in glutamate sequestration elicited by LTP (Baudry and Lynch, 1980); the enzyme appeared to cause these effects by partially degrading spectrin, a primary constituent of postsynaptic densities and of the membrane cytoskeleton (Siman et al., 1984, 1985). This led to the hypothesis that LTP results from a calpain-triggered disassembly-reassembly of the membrane cytoskeleton, an event that would be expected to alter the morphology of dendritic spines (Lynch and Baudry, 1984).

Recent experiments have provided some support for the above idea. First, synaptosomal fractions contain unusually high levels of calpain activity (Baudry et al., 1987) while immunoelectron-microscopy has localized the enzyme to spines and postsynaptic densities (Perlmutter et al., 1988). Spectrin is found in high concentrations in highly purified postsynaptic densities along with the breakdown product (Carlin et al., 1983) that results when the native protein is co-incubated with calpain (Siman et al., 1984; Seubert et al., 1987). Second, stimulation of NMDA receptors causes a marked increase in the spectrin breakdown product produced by calpain (Seubert et al., 1988). This effect is not reproduced by simply depolarizing slices. Third, an inhibitor of calpain blocks the development of LTP both in chronic recording studies (Staubli et al., 1988) and in hippocampal slices (Oliver et al., 1990). In the latter experiments, it was possible to show that the calpain

antagonist did not interfere with the within burst synaptic facilitation that triggers LTP (Larson and Lynch, 1988) and therefore presumably exerted its effects on events that normally follow NMDA receptor currents and calcium influx. Each of the above lines of work needs to be extended. Thus, while pharmacological stimulation of NMDA receptors produces spectrin breakdown, it is not known if the much briefer activation occurring during repetitive synaptic stimulation causes a similar effect. The experiments showing that an inhibitor of calpain blocks development of LTP need to be repeated using recently developed, more selective antagonists of the enzyme.

Figure 6 summarizes several of the points made above. A synapse is shown containing NMDA and AMPA receptors and their associated ion channels. Structural proteins including membrane-anchoring sites, spectrin, and actin filaments are also illustrated. Finally, 3 classes of calcium-sensitive enzymes are illustrated: phospholipases, CaM kinase, and calpain. Stimulation of the NMDA receptor under conditions of intense depolarization causes an elevation of calcium in the dendritic spine resulting in the activation of the 3 enzyme systems. These produce effects at successively deeper levels of the spine. The lipases (in the schematic), by cleaving phospholipids, change the fluid characteristics of the local membrane opening the way for conformational changes in integral membrane proteins such as receptors and ion channels. The interactions of these entities with each other as well as with the structural skeleton lying beneath the synapse would be further influenced by phosphorylation. Still more pronounced changes in the chemistry of the postsynaptic zone could be produced by partial disassembly and rearrangement of the membrane cytoskeleton itself. Calpain is postulated to produce localized breakup of the skeleton by partially digesting spectrin (and possibly other structural proteins associated with it); the reorganization stage would involve still other enzymatic systems. Amplification of postsynaptic responses results from these enzymatic actions either by an effect on the AMPA

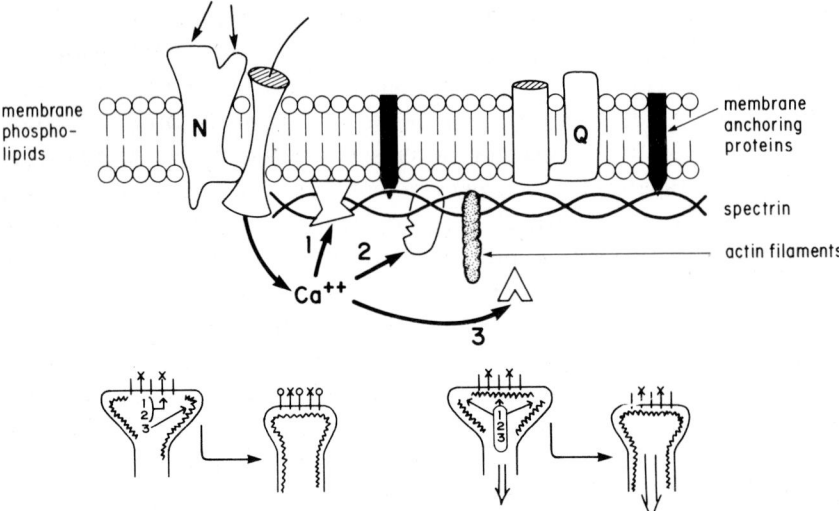

Fig. 6. Potential consequences of LTP-triggering postsynaptic calcium influx on membrane organization. AMPA/quisqualate receptors (Q) and associated ion channels mediate normal synaptic transmission. NMDA receptors (N) are activated during bursting and calcium enters through the NMDA channel. Intracellular Ca^{2+} can activate phospholipases (1), CaM kinase (2), and calpain (3). These can alter the functional characteristics and inter-relationships between membrane proteins, phosphorylate channels or structural elements, or cleave cytoskeletal proteins such as spectrin. Two possible long-lasting outcomes of these events are shown below. At left, membrane reorganization exposes occult AMPA/quisqualate receptors and cytoskeletal proteolysis stabilizes these changes but the associated shape change does not itself impact on transmission. At right, membrane and cytoskeletal reorganization results in a change in spine shape that enhances current flow from the spine to the dendrite. In this case, the spine neck resistance limits the current through the spine.

receptor complex (binding sites, interaction with channels, or the channel itself) or via a more global change involving reconfiguration of the entire spine. Note that these two possibilities are not mutually exclusive.

While it is perhaps simpler to imagine that the 3 calcium-dependent enzymes act in sequence with the final step producing the expression of LTP, it is also possible that they are responsible for different aspects of LTP. Thus, for example, we might imagine that lipases and kinases alter the lipid and protein environment of the AMPA receptor such that it produces larger synaptic currents while cytoskeletal changes wrought by calpain anchor or stabilize the changes. An attractive feature of this idea is that it might account for the potentiations of different durations that appear to be triggered by the NMDA receptor system. It is not uncommon in LTP experiments to obtain potentiated responses that decline for 10–15 min (short-term potentiation or STP) before reaching a stable

(potentiated) level (Fig. 7). Using a stimulation paradigm that involves very brief bursts of pulses and that is extremely well suited for inducing LTP, it was found that antagonists of the NMDA receptor block all forms of potentiation lasting more than 5 s (Larson and Lynch, 1988). Indirect evidence has also been obtained indicating that the optimal conditions for eliciting the decremental STP are detectably different from those for LTP itself (Larson et al., 1986). The work of Racine and co-workers (Racine et al., 1983) showing that a form of potentiation exists in hippocampus (and elsewhere) which lasts for several hours should also be noted in this context; interestingly enough, prior induction of kindling prevented expression of the LTP that lasts for days without affecting the hours-long effect (Racine et al., 1983). The possibility thus exists that at least 3 forms of NMDA receptor- and calcium-dependent synaptic facilitation can be induced by brief periods of high-frequency stimulation. It is tempting to

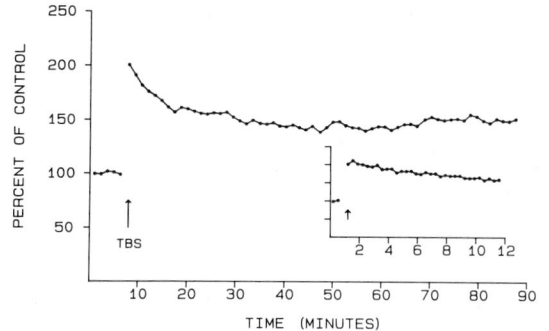

Fig. 7. STP and LTP induced by theta burst stimulation (TBS). Plot of initial slope of the population EPSP before and after TBS (4 pulses at 100 Hz per burst, repeated 10 times at 5 Hz). Each point is the average of 4 consecutive responses. The initial STP stabilized to a non-decremental LTP. Inset: plot of individual responses evoked at 20-s intervals for the first 11 min after TBS (arrow). The *y*-axis scale is the same as for the main graph.

hypothesize that the multiple calcium-dependent processes described in the schematic operate upon a common target and contribute changes that persist for varying durations. Nevertheless, it is important to note that, with certain stimulation conditions, the LTP present 10 – 15 min after stimulation remains non-decremental for hours (Fig. 1) and in chronic preparations can be shown to persist unchanged for weeks (Staubli and Lynch, 1987).

It bears repeating that the model described here is only one of several possibilities and that more evidence is needed to establish links between the 3 enzymes and LTP. Note also that the schematic ignores the second messengers generated by the phospholipases and does not consider possible interactions between the enzymes. It may be useful to consider how these calcium-dependent systems work together in simpler systems. Blood platelets contain all of the intracellular machinery described in the model and there is growing evidence that lipases, kinases, and calpain work together to produce the characteristic response of these cells to external stimuli (Bennett et al., 1979; Fox et al., 1987; Verhallen et al., 1987; Kramer et al., 1989). This response includes structural transformation and alterations in surface receptors (Marguerie et

al., 1979; Jennings et al., 1981), two features that were discussed in terms of how spines might express LTP. Given the opportunistic nature of evolutionary adaptation, it would not be surprising if much that lies beneath LTP were to be found performing quite different functions outside the brain; there may be much to be gained from a careful examination of how stable alterations in function are achieved in contexts far simpler than those found in hippocampus.

Rhythmic hippocampal activity and long-term potentiation

Recent studies have led to the conclusion that the 4 – 7 Hz theta rhythm, which is one of the most characteristic features of hippocampal physiological activity, is linked to the cellular events that induce LTP. Theta appears in the hippocampal EEG during a wide variety of behaviors, one of the most intriguing of which is the sampling of odors. Rats and other small mammals sniff (inhale – exhale) significant odors at the theta frequency and hippocampal theta becomes entrained to the sniffing pattern (Macrides, 1975; Macrides et al., 1982); moreover, during olfactory learning, pyramidal cells fire in short, high-frequency bursts which themselves are phase-locked to theta and hence to the sniffing cycle (Eichenbaum et al., 1987, for a description). This is not unique to olfactory learning; theta bursting has also been recorded in rats exploring a new environment (Hill, 1978).

Tests of the effects of theta burst activity on synaptic responses were carried out using in vitro slices. Stimulation was delivered in short high-frequency bursts (4 pulses in 30 ms) somewhat like the above-described bursts recorded from pyramidal cells. A single burst of this type produced a potentiation lasting for only several seconds but when 5 bursts per second (i.e. the theta rhythm) were administered, then robust LTP appeared. If the interval between the bursts was shortened or lengthened, progressively less LTP was induced; the optimal interburst interval in fact

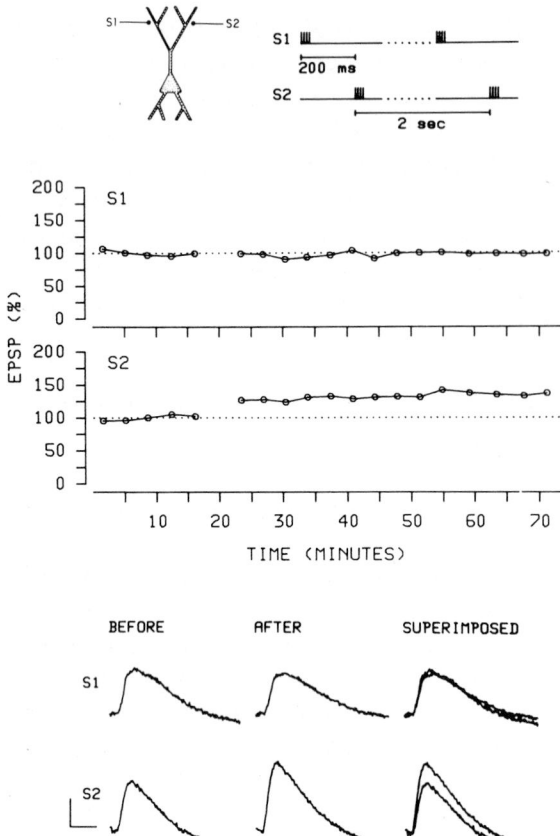

Fig. 8. Heterosynaptic priming of LTP induction. Top: schematic of the stimulation paradigm. Two separate collections of Schaffer/commissural inputs (S1, S2) onto a single CA1 pyramidal neuron were used. S1 received 10 bursts at 2-s intervals; S2 was stimulated 200 ms after each S1 burst. Middle: plot of EPSP amplitude (as percent of baseline) for single pulse stimulation of S1 and S2 before and after patterned burst stimulation (gap). S2 exhibited stable LTP after burst stimulation, but S1 was unchanged. Bottom: records of EPSPs evoked 5 min before and 40 min after burst stimulation. Calibration bars: 5 mV and 5 ms. (Data from Larson and Lynch, 1986).

corresponded to the period of the theta wave (~ 200 ms) (Larson et al., 1986).

Why should theta be so effective in eliciting LTP? This was answered in a series of experiments using the two-input paradigm described earlier with single bursts applied to each electrode in sequence (see Fig. 8). Under these conditions the second (delayed) input exhibited robust LTP after several pairings while the initial input was un-

changed; again the optimal interval proved to be 200 ms (Larson and Lynch, 1986). This procedure allowed us to ask how the burst responses to the second input differed from those to the first. The answer was clear; the EPSPs to the initial input were shortened by a fast feedforward IPSP while those to the second member of the pair were not and as a result generated a much greater degree of depolarization (Larson and Lynch, 1986). Not surprisingly, the burst responses to the delayed input included a sizeable component that was blocked by NMDA receptor antagonists (see Fig. 9), indicating that the enhanced depolarization obtained in the absence of the IPSP was sufficient to activate the trigger for LTP (Larson and Lynch, 1988).

Intracellular recording indicated that the IPSPs lasting for 50 – 100 ms cannot be reactivated for an additional 500 ms with the peak of their refractoriness falling at the theta period (i.e. 150 – 250 ms after onset) (Larson and Lynch, 1986). The

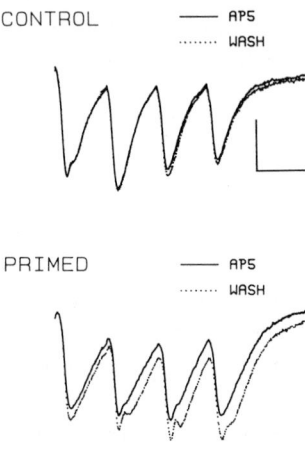

Fig. 9. Effects of the NMDA receptor antagonist AP5 on postsynaptic responses to theta burst stimulation in field CA1. Control records show the response to a single 4-pulse burst (100 Hz) in the presence of 100 μM DL-AP5 and after washout of the drug from the slice. AP5 only slightly reduced the field potential. Primed records show responses to burst stimulation 200 ms after burst stimulation of a separate input. AP5 considerably reduced the response enhancement associated with priming. Calibration bars: 2 mV and 10 ms. (Data from Larson and Lynch, 1988).

origin of this peculiar refractory period is unknown but we suspect it occurs at the synapses between the inhibitory interneurons and pyramidal cells (see also McCarren and Alger, 1985; Thompson and Gähwiler, 1989).

In all, by transiently blocking IPSPs, theta burst stimulation permits a degree of temporal summation to occur within a series of burst responses that is of sufficient degree and duration to unblock the NMDA receptor channel (see Larson and Lynch, 1988, for a discussion). These observations provide a first connection between cue sampling patterns, brain rhythms, and cellular mechanisms that produce enduring changes in the strength of synapses.

They also raise the intriguing question of whether the physiological and biochemical triggers for LTP evolved in hippocampus (and elsewhere) in response to repetitive behaviors that maximize cue sampling or if the sampling patterns emerged to exploit an already present plasticity mechanism. That the relationship between the NMDA receptor system and rhythmic behavior goes back to the very beginnings of vertebrate evolution is strongly suggested by Grillner's elegant studies of the lamprey spinal cord (see Grillner et al., 1987, for a review). Perhaps then the receptor complex served timing functions in the telencephalon of the early reptiles as well and became modified into a plasticity device with the rise of the mammals. The links between theta and LTP thus would reflect pressures generated by the need to encode the increased information made available by the explosive growth of the inherently rhythmic olfactory system in the earliest mammals (see Lynch, 1986, for a discussion).

Finally, it should be noted that the analysis of how the spatio-temporal patterns of physiological activity associated with learning relate to the LTP effect is still in its earliest stages. Studies subsequent to those described above have already established that patterns occurring *within* a single theta period have pronounced effects on whether or not potentiation will occur (Larson and Lynch, 1989; Lynch and Larson, 1988, for a review). As more is learned of these relationships, it should become possible to construct learning rules that describe how sequentially arriving inputs are translated into spatial patterns of encoding.

Memory and long-term potentiation

The discovery that brain activity patterns occurring during at least some types of learning are optimal for inducing LTP certainly encourages the hypothesis that the potentiation effect participates in memory encoding. More direct examination of the LTP : memory relationship leads naturally to the question of whether particular instances of behavioral memory can be attributed to an LTP-like process. Two quite different types of experiments are pertinent to this.

Psychopharmacological studies have shown that NMDA receptor antagonists and calpain inhibitors interfere with the acquisition of spatial and olfactory memory without affecting avoidance conditioning (Staubli et al., 1985, 1989; Morris et al., 1986). This selectivity suggests that the drugs do not produce behaviorally disabling side-effects but it is of course possible that spatial and olfactory learning are for some reason more easily disrupted than conditioning. However, it was also found that protein synthesis inhibitors impair avoidance conditioning but do not affect olfactory learning (Staubli et al., 1985).

Correlational evidence implicating LTP in memory has also been obtained. The goal of these studies was to ask if synapses processing central representations of a peripheral cue would exhibit LTP as an animal learned that cue. The evident difficulty in such an effort lies in finding and testing the presumably small percentage of synapses in any given region of the brain that might be involved in processing a particular environmental signal. This problem led us to develop a paradigm in which electrical stimulation of the lateral olfactory tract (LOT), the primary input to the olfactory cortex, was substituted for natural odors in a successive cue discrimination problem. The LOT-cortex projections exhibit very little topography and we assumed that any adequately sized subpopulation of the tract could potentially serve as the representation of an odor. As noted, rats sniff at the theta frequency, suggesting that the cortex receives its inputs at this rhythm as well; accordingly, we used theta burst stimulation as "electric odors". In the experiments, the rats were first trained on a series of two-odor discrimination problems before being tested with the electric odors. We found that the animals would quickly learn to approach or avoid the artificial cues depending upon their reward valence. This held true when they were asked to discriminate electric odors from natural odors or from each other. The electrical cues were not only learned quickly but their significance was recognized in tests given days later.

Having established a known and testable population of synapses that carried a significant signal into the cortex, we were able to ask if these same connections exhibited LTP-like effects as behavioral learning occurred. Recording electrodes were placed in the terminal field of the LOT and monosynaptic field EPSPs collected before, during, and after a discrimination was acquired. A robust and stable potentiation occurred over the course of several acquisition trials; this appeared to be synapse-specific since responses to control electrodes were unchanged. Finally, the effect was behaviorally dependent since theta burst stimulation administered to rats not engaged in learning did not produce potentiation (Roman et al., 1987); other authors have noted that high-frequency stimulation of the LOT-synapses does not produce LTP in naive rats (Racine et al., 1983; Stripling et al., 1988).

If something like LTP is in fact an encoding process then we may be justified in assuming that the neurobiological study of learning and memory has reached the threshold of an entirely new period. To this point biological work has been directed at finding cellular processes and anatomical systems that could account for particular behavioral phenomena. Now, however, we can begin to ask how the many neurobiological features that describe the induction and expression of synaptic

potentiation might be manifested in behavior. Some steps in this direction have already been taken using computer simulations of specific cortical networks. These suggest the unexpected conclusion that LTP, coupled with repetitive sampling, organizes the cue world into information hierarchies such that early responses of the network produce categorical representations while later ones yield outputs that are specific to the cue now present (Lynch and Granger, 1989; Granger et al., 1989). Hopefully, future efforts using the still being discovered spatio-temporal synaptic learning rules mentioned earlier will produce insights and formal theories about memory that would not have been evident from behavioral studies alone.

References

Abraham, W.C. and Goddard, G.V. (1983) Asymmetric relationships between homosynaptic long-term potentiation and heterosynaptic long-term depression. *Nature (Lond.)*, 305: 717–719.

Akers, R.F., Lovinger, D.M., Colley, P.A., Linden, D.J. and Routtenberg, A. (1985) Translocation of protein kinase C activity may mediate hippocampal long-term potentiation. *Science*, 231: 587–589.

Andersen, P., Sundberg, S.H., Sveen, O. and Wigström, H. (1977) Specific long-lasting potentiation of synaptic transmission in hippocampal slices. *Nature (Lond.)*, 266: 736–737.

Arai, A., Larson, J. and Lynch, G. (1990) Anoxia reveals a vulnerable period in the development of long-term potentiation. *Brain Res.*, in press.

Barnes, C.A. (1979) Memory deficits associated with senescence: a neurophysiological and behavioral study in the rat. *J. Comp. Physiol. Psychol.*, 93: 74–104.

Baudry, M. and Lynch, G. (1980) Regulation of hippocampal glutamate receptors: evidence for the involvement of a calcium-activated protease. *Proc. Natl. Acad. Sci. U.S.A.*, 77: 2298–2302.

Baudry, M., Dubrin, R. and Lynch, G. (1987) Subcellular compartmentalization of calcium-dependent and calcium-independent proteases in brain. *Synapse*, 1: 506–511.

Bennett, W.F., Belville, J.S. and Lynch, G. (1979) A study of protein phosphorylation in shape change and Ca^{++}-dependent serotonin release by blood platelets. *Cell*, 18: 1015–1023.

Bliss, T.V.P. and Lømo, T. (1973) Long-lasting potentiation of synaptic transmission in the dentate area of the anaesthetized rabbit following stimulation of the perforant path. *J.*

Physiol. (Lond.), 232: 334–356.

Bliss, T.V.P. and Lynch, M.A. (1988) Long-term potentiation of synaptic transmission in the hippocampus: properties and mechanisms. In P.W. Landfield and S.A. Deadwyler (Eds.), *Long-Term Potentiation: From Biophysics to Behavior.* Alan R. Liss, New York; pp. 3–72.

Carlin, R.K., Bartelt, D.C. and Siekevitz, P. (1983) Identification of fodrin as a major calmodulin-binding protein in postsynaptic density preparations. *J. Cell Biol.,* 96: 443–448.

Chang, F.-L.F. and Greenough, W.T. (1984) Transient and enduring morphological correlates of synaptic activity and efficacy change in the rat hippocampal slice. *Brain Res.,* 309: 35–46.

Collingridge, G.L., Kehl, S.J. and McLennan, H. (1983) Excitatory amino acids in synaptic transmission in the Schaffer-commissural pathway of the rat hippocampus. *J. Physiol. (Lond.),* 334: 33–46.

Davies, S.N., Lester, R.A.J., Reymann, K.G. and Collingridge, G.L. (1989) Temporally distinct pre- and post-synaptic mechanisms maintain long-term potentiation. *Nature (Lond.),* 338: 500–503.

Desmond, N.L. and Levy, W.B. (1986) Changes in the postsynaptic density with long-term potentiation in the dentate gyrus. *J. Comp. Neurol.,* 253: 476–482.

Dunwiddie, T. and Lynch, G. (1978) Long-term potentiation and depression of synaptic responses in the rat hippocampus: localization and frequency dependency *J. Physiol. (Lond.),* 276: 353–367.

Eichenbaum, H., Kuperstein, M., Fagan, A. and Nagode, J. (1987) Cue-sampling and goal-approach correlates of hippocampal unit activity in rats performing an odor-discrimination task. *J. Neurosci.,* 7: 716–732.

Finn, R.C., Browning, M. and Lynch, G. (1980) Trifluoperazine inhibits hippocampal long-term potentiation and the phosphorylation of a 40,000 dalton protein. *Neurosci. Lett.,* 19: 103–108.

Fox, J.E.B., Reynolds, C.C., Morrow, J.S. and Phillips, D.R. (1987) Spectrin is associated with membrane-bound actin filaments in platelets and is hydrolyzed by the Ca^{2+}-dependent protease during platelet activation. *Blood,* 2: 537–545.

Gall, C., Rose, G. and Lynch, G. (1978) Proliferative and migratory activity of glial cells in the deafferented hippocampus. *J. Comp. Neurol.,* 183: 539–550.

Gall, C., McWilliams, R. and Lynch, G. (1980) Accelerated rates of synaptogenesis by "sprouting" afferents in the immature hippocampal formation. *J. Comp. Neurol.,* 193: 1047–1062.

Granger, R., Ambros-Ingerson, J. and Lynch, G. (1989) Derivation of encoding characteristics of layer II cerebral cortex. *J. Cog. Neurosci.,* 1: 52–78.

Grillner, S., Wallen, P., Dale, N., Brodin, L., Buchanan, J. and Hill, R. (1987) Transmitters, membrane properties and network circuitry in the control of locomotion in lamprey. *Trends Neurosci.,* 10: 34–41.

Gustaffson, H., Huang, Y.-Y. and Wigström, H. (1988) Phorbol ester-induced synaptic potentiation differs from long-term potentiation in the guinea pig hippocampus *in vitro. Neurosci. Lett.,* 85: 77–81.

Harris, E.W., Ganong, A.H. and Cotman, C.W. (1984) Long-term potentiation in the hippocampus involves activation of *N*-methyl-D-aspartate receptors. *Brain Res.,* 323: 132–137.

Hill, A.J. (1978) First occurrence of hippocampal spatial firing in a new environment. *Exp. Neurol.,* 62: 282–297.

Jennings, L.K., Fox, J.E.B., Edwards, H.H. and Phillips, D.R. (1981) Changes in the cytoskeletal structure of human platelets following thrombin activation. *J. Biol. Chem.,* 256: 6927–6932.

Kauer, J.A., Malenka, R.C. and Nicoll, R.A. (1988) A persistent postsynaptic modification mediates long-term potentiation in the hippocampus. *Neuron,* 1: 911–917.

Kennedy, M.B., Bennett, M.K. and Erondu, N.E. (1983) Biochemical and immunochemical evidence that the "major postsynaptic density protein" is a subunit of a calmodulin-dependent protein kinase. *Proc. Natl. Acad. Sci. U.S.A.,* 80: 7357–7361.

Kessler, M., Petersen, G., Vu, H.M., Baudry, M. and Lynch, G. (1987) L-phenylalanyl-L-glutamate-stimulated, chloride-dependent glutamate binding represents glutamate sequestration mediated by an exchange system. *J. Neurochem.,* 49: 1191–1200.

Kramer, R.M., Hession, C., Johansen, B., Hayes, G., McGray, P., Chow, E.P., Tizard, R. and Pepinsky, R.B. (1989) Structure and properties of a human non-pancreatic phospholipase A_2. *J. Biol. Chem.,* 264: 5768–5775.

Larson, J. and Lynch, G. (1986) Induction of synaptic potentiation in hippocampus by patterned stimulation involves two events. *Science,* 232: 985–988.

Larson, J. and Lynch, G. (1988) Role of *N*-methyl-D-aspartate receptors in the induction of synaptic potentiation by burst stimulation patterned after the hippocampal theta rhythm. *Brain Res.,* 441: 111–118.

Larson, J. and Lynch, G. (1989) Theta pattern stimulation and the induction of LTP: the sequence in which synapses are stimulated determines the degree to which they potentiate. *Brain Res.,* 489: 49–58.

Larson, J., Wong, D. and Lynch, G. (1986) Patterned stimulation at the theta frequency is optimal for the induction of hippocampal long-term potentiation. *Brain Res.,* 368: 347–350.

Lee, K., Stanford, E., Cotman, C.W. and Lynch, G. (1977) Ultrastructural evidence of bouton proliferation in the partially deafferented dentate gyrus of the adult rat. *Exp. Brain Res.,* 9: 475–485.

Lee, K., Schottler, F., Oliver, M. and Lynch, G. (1980) Brief bursts of high frequency stimulation produce two types of structural changes in rat hippocampus. *J. Neurophysiol.,* 44:

247 – 258.

Lee, K., Oliver, M., Schottler, F. and Lynch, G. (1981) Electron microscopic studies of brain slices: the effects of high frequency stimulation on dendritic ultrastructure. In G. Kerkut and H.V. Wheal (Eds.), *Electrical Activity in Isolated Mammalian C.N.S. Preparations,* Academic Press, New York, pp. 189 – 212.

Levy, W.B. and Steward, O. (1983) Temporal contiguity requirements for long-term associative potentiation/depression in the hippocampus. *Neuroscience,* 8: 791 – 797.

Lovinger, D.M., Wong, K.L., Murakami, K. and Routtenberg, A. (1987) Protein kinase C inhibitors eliminate hippocampal long-term potentiation. *Brain Res.,* 436: 177 – 183.

Lynch, G. (1986) *Synapses, Circuits, and the Beginnings of Memory.* MIT Press, Cambridge, MA. 124 pp.

Lynch, G. and Baudry, M. (1984) The biochemistry of memory: a new and specific hypothesis. *Science,* 224: 1057 – 1063.

Lynch, G. and Granger, R. (1989) Simulation and analysis of a simple cortical network. *Psychol. Learning Motiv.,* 23: 205 – 237.

Lynch, G. and Larson, J. (1988) Rhythmic activity, synaptic changes, and the "how and what" of memory storage in simple cortical networks. In J.L. Davis, R.W. Newburgh and E.J. Wegman (Eds.), *Brain Structure, Learning and Memory,* Westview Press, Boulder, CO, pp. 33 – 68.

Lynch, G., Matthews, D., Mosko, S., Parks, T. and Cotman, C.W. (1972) Induced acetylcholinesterase-rich layer in rat dentate gyrus following entorhinal lesions. *Brain Res.,* 42: 311 – 318.

Lynch, G., Deadwyler, S. and Cotman, C. (1973) Postlesion axonal growth produces permanent functional connections. *Science,* 180: 1364 – 1366.

Lynch, G., Gribkoff, V.K. and Deadwyler, S.A. (1976) Long term potentiation is accompanied by a reduction in dendritic responsiveness to glutamic acid. *Nature (Lond.),* 263: 151 – 153.

Lynch, G., Dunwiddie, T. and Gribkoff, V. (1977a) Heterosynaptic depression: a postsynaptic correlate of long term potentiation. *Nature (Lond.),* 266: 737 – 739.

Lynch, G., Gall, C. and Cotman, C.W. (1977b) Temporal parameters of axon "sprouting" in the brain of the adult rat. *Exp. Neurol.,* 54: 179 – 183.

Lynch, G., Halpain, S. and Baudry, M. (1982) Effects of high frequency synaptic stimulation on glutamate receptor binding studied with a modified *in vitro* hippocampal slice preparation. *Brain Res.,* 244: 101 – 111.

Lynch, G., Larson, J., Kelso, S., Barrionuevo, G. and Schottler, F. (1983) Intracellular injections of EGTA block induction of hippocampal long-term potentiation. *Nature (Lond.),* 305: 719 – 721.

Lynch, G., Muller, D., Seubert, P. and Larson, J. (1988) Long-term potentiation: persisting problems and recent results. *Brain Res. Bull.,* 21: 363 – 372.

MacDermott, A.B., Mayer, M.L., Westbrook, G.L., Smith, S.J. and Barker, J.L. (1986) NMDA-receptor activation increases cytoplasmic calcium concentration in cultured spinal cord neurones. *Nature (Lond.),* 321: 519 – 522.

Macrides, F. (1975) Temporal relationships between hippocampal slow waves and exploratory sniffing in hamsters. *Behav. Biol.,* 14: 295 – 308.

Macrides, F. Eichenbaum, H.B. and Forbes, W.B. (1982) Temporal relationship between sniffing and the limbic theta rhythm during odor discrimination reversal learning. *J. Neurosci.,* 2: 1705 – 1717.

Malenka, R.C., Madison, D.V. and Nicoll, R.A. (1986) Potentiation of synaptic transmission in the hippocampus by phorbol esters. *Nature (Lond.),* 321: 175 – 177.

Malenka, R.C., Kauer, J.A, Zucker, R.S. and Nicoll, R.A. (1988) Postsynaptic calcium is sufficient for potentiation of hippocampal synaptic transmission. *Science,* 242: 81 – 84.

Malinow, R. and Miller, J.P. (1986) Postsynaptic hyperpolarization during conditioning reversibly blocks induction of long-term potentiation. *Nature (Lond.),* 320: 529 – 530.

Malinow, R., Madison, D.V. and Tsien, R.W. (1988) Persistent protein kinase activity underlying long-term potentiation. *Nature (Lond.),* 335: 820 – 824.

Marguerie, G.A., Plow, E.F. and Edgington, T.S. (1979) Human platelets possess an inducible and saturable receptor specific for fibrinogen. *J. Biol. Chem.,* 254: 5357 – 5363.

Mayer, M.L. and Westbrook, G.L. (1987) Permeation and block of N-methyl-D-aspartic acid receptor channels by divalent cations in mouse cultured central neurones. *J. Physiol. (Lond.),* 394: 501 – 527.

Mayer, M.L., Westbrook, G.L. and Guthrie, P.B. (1984) Voltage-dependent block by Mg^{2+} of NMDA responses in spinal cord neurons. *Nature (Lond.),* 309: 261 – 263.

McCarren, M. and Alger, B.E. (1985) Use-dependent depression of IPSPs in rat hippocampal pyramidal cells *in vitro*. *J. Neurophysiol.,* 53: 557 – 571.

McNaughton, B.L. and Barnes, C.A. (1977) Physiological identification and analysis of dentate granule cell responses to stimulation of the medial and lateral perforant pathways in the rat. *J. Comp. Neurol.,* 175: 439 – 454.

McWilliams, J.R. and Lynch, G. (1979) Terminal proliferation in the partially deafferented dentate gyrus: time courses for the appearance and removal of degeneration and the replacement of lost terminals. *J. Comp. Neurol.,* 187: 191 – 198.

McWilliams, J.R. and Lynch, G. (1983) Rate of synaptic replacement in denervated rat hippocampus declines precipitously from the juvenile period to adulthood. *Science,* 221: 572 – 574.

McWilliams, J.R. and Lynch, G. (1984) Synaptic density and axonal sprouting in rat hippocampus: stability in adulthood and decline in late adulthood. *Brain Res.,* 294: 152 – 156.

Mody, I., Baimbridge, K.G. and Miller, J.J. (1984) Blockade of tetanic- and calcium-induced potentiation in the hippocampal slice preparation by neuroleptics. *Neuropharmacology,* 23: 625 – 631.

Morris, R.G.M., Anderson, E., Lynch, G.S. and Baudry, M. (1986) Selective impairment of learning and blockade of long-term potentiation by an *N*-methyl-D-aspartate receptor antagonist, AP5. *Nature (Lond.)*, 319: 774 – 776.

Muller, D. and Lynch, G. (1988a) Long-term potentiation differentially affects two components of synaptic responses in hippocampus. *Proc. Natl. Acad. Sci. U.S.A.*, 85: 9346 – 9350.

Muller, D. and Lynch, G. (1988b) *N*-methyl-D-aspartate receptor-mediated component of synaptic responses to single-pulse stimulation in rat hippocampal slices. *Synapse*, 2: 666 – 668.

Muller, D., Joly, M. and Lynch, G. (1988a) Contributions of quisqualate and NMDA receptors to the induction and expression of LTP. *Science*, 242: 1694 – 1697.

Muller, D., Turnbull, J., Baudry, M. and Lynch, G. (1988b) Phorbol ester-induced synaptic facilitation is different than long-term potentiation. *Proc. Natl. Acad. Sci. U.S.A.*, 85: 6997 – 7000.

Muller, D., Larson, J. and Lynch, G. (1989) The NMDA receptor mediated components of responses evoked by patterned stimulation are not increased by long-term potentiation. *Brain Res.*, 477: 369 – 399.

Nowak, L., Bregestovski, P., Ascher, P., Herbet, A. and Prochiantz, A. (1984) Magnesium gates glutamate-activated channels in mouse central neurones. *Nature (Lond.)*, 307: 462 – 465.

Oliver, M., Baudry, M. and Lynch, G. (1990) The protease inhibitor leupeptin interferes with the development of LTP in hippocampal slices. *Brain Res.*, 505: 233 – 238.

Perlmutter, L.S., Siman, R., Gall, C., Seubert, P., Baudry, M. and Lynch, G. (1988) The ultrastructural localization of calcium-activated protease "calpain" in rat brain. *Synapse*, 2: 79 – 88.

Pin, J.P., Bockaert, J. and Recasens, M. (1984) The Ca^{++}/Cl-dependent L-^{3}H-glutamate binding: a new receptor or a particular transport process? *FEBS Lett.*, 175: 31 – 36.

Racine, R.J., Milgram, N.W. and Hafner, S. (1983) Long-term potentiation phenomena in the rat limbic forebrain. *Brain Res.*, 260: 217 – 231.

Rall, W. (1978) Dendritic spines and synaptic potency. In R. Porter (Ed.), *Studies in Neurophysiology*, Cambridge University Press, Cambridge, pp. 203 – 209.

Reymann, K.G., Frey, U., Jork, R. and Matthies, H. (1988a) Polymyxin B, an inhibitor of protein kinase C, prevents the maintenance of synaptic long-term potentiation in hippocampal CA1 neurons. *Brain Res.*, 440: 305 – 314.

Reymann, K.G., Brodemann, R., Kase, H. and Matthies, H. (1988b) Inhibitors of calmodulin and protein kinase C block different phases of hippocampal long-term potentiation. *Brain Res.*, 461: 388 – 392.

Roman, F., Staubli, U. and Lynch, G. (1987) Evidence for synaptic potentiation in a cortical network during learning.

Brain Res., 418: 221 – 226.

Rose, G., Lynch, G. and Cotman, C.W. (1976) Hypertrophy and redistribution of astrocytes in the deafferented hippocampus. *Brain Res. Bull.*, 1: 87 – 92.

Savage, D.D., Werling, L.L., Nadler, J.V. and McNamara, J.O. (1982) Selective increase in L-[^{3}H]-glutamate binding to a quisqualate-sensitive site on hippocampal synaptic membranes after angular bundle kindling. *Eur. J. Pharmacol.*, 85: 255 – 256.

Seubert, P., Baudry, M., Dudek, S. and Lynch, G. (1987) Calmodulin stimulates the degradation of brain spectrin by calpain. *Synapse*, 1: 20 – 24.

Seubert, P., Larson, J., Oliver, M., Jung, M.W., Baudry, M. and Lynch, G. (1988) Stimulation of NMDA receptors induces proteolysis of spectrin in hippocampus. *Brain Res.*, 460: 189 – 194.

Siman, R., Baudry, M. and Lynch, G. (1984) Brain fodrin: substrate for the endogenous calcium-activated protease, calpain I. *Proc. Natl. Acad. Sci. U.S.A.*, 81: 3276 – 3280.

Siman, R., Baudry, M. and Lynch, G. (1985) Glutamate receptor regulation by proteolysis of the cytoskeletal protein fodrin. *Nature (Lond.)*, 315: 225 – 227.

Staubli, U. and Lynch, G. (1987) Stable hippocampal long-term potentiation elicited by "theta" pattern stimulation. *Brain Res.*, 435: 227 – 234.

Staubli, U., Faraday, R. and Lynch, G. (1985) Pharmacological dissociation of memory: anisomycin, a protein synthesis inhibitor, and leupeptin, a protease inhibitor, block different learning tasks. *Behav. Neurol. Biol.*, 43: 287 – 297.

Staubli, U., Larson, J., Baudry, M., Thibault, O. and Lynch, G. (1988) Chronic administration of a thiol-proteinase inhibitor blocks long-term potentiation of synaptic responses. *Brain Res.*, 444: 153 – 158.

Staubli, U., Thibault, O., DiLorenzo, M. and Lynch, G. (1989) Antagonism of NMDA receptors impairs acquisition but not retention of olfactory memory. *Behav. Neurosci.*, 103: 54 – 60.

Stripling, J.S., Patneau, D.K. and Gramlich, C.A. (1988) Selective long-term potentiation in the pyriform cortex. *Brain Res.*, 441: 281 – 291.

Tang, C.-M., Dichter, M. and Morad, M. (1989) Quisqualate activates a rapidly inactivating high conductance ionic channel in hippocampal neurons. *Science*, 243: 1474 – 1477.

Thompson, S.M. and Gähwiler, B.H. (1989) Activity-dependent disinhibition: I. Repetitive stimulation reduces IPSP driving force and conductance in the hippocampus *in vitro*. *J. Neurophysiol.*, 61: 501 – 511.

Verhallen, P.F.J., Bevers, E.M., Comfurius, P. and Zwaal, R.F.A. (1987) Correlation between calpain-mediated cytoskeletal degradation and expression of platelet procoagulant activity. A role for the platelet membrane-skeleton in the regulation of membrane lipid asymmetry? *Biochim. Biophys. Acta*, 903: 206 – 217.

West, J.R., Deadwyler, S.A., Cotman, C.W. and Lynch, G.

(1975) Time dependent changes in the dentate gyrus following lesions of the entorhinal cortex in adult rats: a
neurophysiological study of axon sprouting. *Brain Res.*, 97:
215 – 233.

Wilson, C.J. (1984) Passive cable properties of dendritic spines
and spiny neurons. *J. Neurosci.*, 4: 281 – 297.

J. Storm-Mathisen, J. Zimmer and O.P. Ottersen (Eds.)
Progress in Brain Research, Vol. 83
© 1990 Elsevier Science Publishers B.V. (Biomedical Division)

CHAPTER 18

Increases in glutamate release and phosphoinositide metabolism associated with long-term potentiation and classical conditioning

M.A. Lynch[1], M.L. Errington[1], M.P. Clements[1], T.V.P. Bliss[1], C. Rédini-Del Negro[2] and S. Laroche[2]

[1]*Division of Neurophysiology and Neuropharmacology, National Institute for Medical Research, Mill Hill, London NW7 1AA, U.K. and* [2]*Département de Psychophysiologie, LPN2, Centre National de la Recherche Scientifique, 91198 Gif-sur-Yvette, France*

Long-term potentiation (LTP) is a widely studied model of the kind of activity-dependent modulation of synaptic efficacy which is assumed to provide the physical basis for learning. Whether LTP, in the hippocampus or elsewhere in the brain, does in fact serve such a role is still a matter for debate. One approach to answering this question is to identify physiological or biochemical changes which are common to both learning and LTP; in the hippocampus, for example, one can ask whether the biochemical changes associated with LTP are also associated with learning. In this chapter we summarize the results which we have obtained in a study of glutamate release and phosphoinositide turnover in the dentate gyrus of rats trained in a classical conditioning task. The similarity between the changes occurring after classical conditioning and those associated with LTP is consistent with the hypothesis that LTP is one of the mechanisms by which a neural trace of the learned association is formed. We discuss this interpretation in the light of the observation that classical conditioning does not appear to affect synaptic responses in the hippocampus.

Over the last few years we have found, using a number of in vivo and in vitro methods, that LTP in the dentate gyrus is correlated with a sustained increase in the release of glutamate, the putative transmitter for this pathway; procedures or drugs which block the induction of LTP also block the increase in glutamate release, suggesting that LTP is maintained, at least in part, by presynaptic mechanisms leading to increased transmitter release (Dolphin et al., 1982; Bliss et al., 1986; Errington et al., 1987; Lynch et al., 1989a). Of the techniques we have used for the study of transmitter release in LTP, the one most easily adapted to behavioural experiments is the so-called ex vivo method, in which the dentate gyrus is removed from the trained (or potentiated) animal, chopped, and incubated in radiolabelled glutamate. Release is stimulated by depolarization in high potassium, in the presence and absence of calcium. The calcium-dependent component of potassium-stimulated release is taken as a measure of the ability of terminals to release glutamate from the vesicular pool of transmitter (Collins et al., 1981). Glutamate release estimated in this way is significantly greater in slices obtained from potentiated tissue than it is from contralateral control tissue, whether measurements are made in slices from anaesthetized animals killed 2.5 min, 45 min (Fig. 1a) or 3 h after the induction of LTP (Lynch et al., 1989a), or from animals with implanted electrodes, killed 72 h after induction (Bliss et al., 1987; Fig. 1b). Similar increases in calcium-

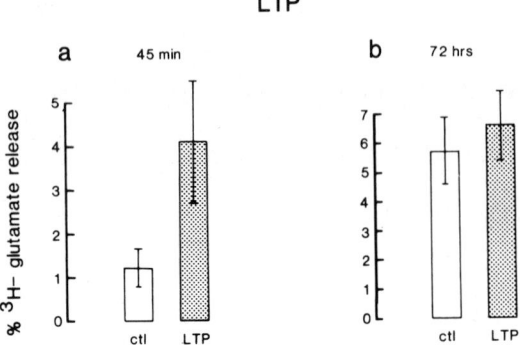

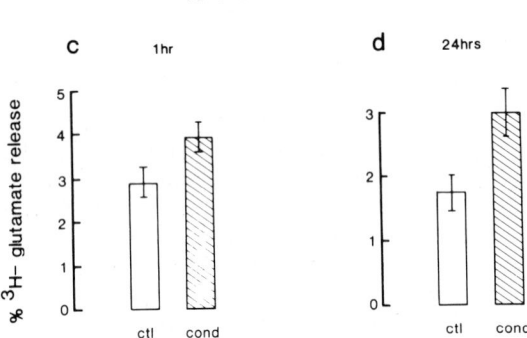

Fig. 1. In vitro analysis of radiolabelled glutamate in the dentate gyrus following the induction of LTP (a,b) or classical conditioning (c,d). Values are mean fractional release ± S.E.M. obtained in slices of dentate gyrus prepared from control (ctl) tissue (open bars) and potentiated (LTP) tissue (dotted bars). Potassium-stimulated, Ca^{2+}-dependent release of [^{3}H]glutamate was significantly increased ($P < 0.05$, paired t-test) in potentiated tissue taken 45 min (a) and 72 h (b) after the induction of LTP in vivo, compared to control tissue. Significant increases in K^+-stimulated, Ca^{2+}-dependent release of [^{3}H]glutamate are also seen in slices of dentate tissue obtained 1 h (c), or in synaptosomes obtained 24 h (d), after classical conditioning (hatched bars) relative to control dentate (ctl) taken at the same time intervals after pseudoconditioning (open bars).

dependent potassium-stimulated release of labelled glutamate are seen in dentate tissue obtained from rats which have learned a classical conditioning task. Animals were first trained to press a lever for food reward in a variable interval schedule of reinforcement. During training, a tone (the conditioned stimulus, or CS) is repeatedly paired with the

footshock (the unconditioned stimulus or US). This procedure results in a robust suppression of lever pressing to the CS (see Laroche et al. (1987) for full details of the training procedure). In the first experiment, animals were killed one hour after the last of a series of 4 training sessions given over a period of 4 days. The dentate gyrus was removed for in vitro analysis of glutamate release. Measurements were also made on slices obtained from pseudo-conditioned animals in which the relationship during training between the CS and the US was explicitly unpaired. As can be seen in Fig. 1c, the release of [^{3}H]glutamate was significantly greater in the conditioned group than in the pseudo-conditioned group. A similar result was obtained in a second experiment in which synaptosomes (consisting predominantly of resealed synaptic terminals) were prepared from the dentate gyrus of animals killed 24 h after conditioning (Fig. 1d).

We can conclude that these two very different procedures – on the one hand, the induction of long-term potentiation by tetanic stimulation in the anaesthetized or unanaesthetized animal, and on the other, the learning of a simple associative task by the intact animal, are both associated with a rapid and sustained increase in the ability of glutamatergic terminals in the dentate gyrus to release transmitter in a calcium-dependent manner. We have also observed broadly similar changes in transmitter release in conditioning and in LTP in the pyramidal cell regions of the hippocampus (Laroche et al., 1987; Bliss and Lynch, 1988).

An increase in the hydrolysis of the membrane phospholipid (PIP$_2$) phosphatidylinositol-4,5-bisphosphate (PIP$_2$) has been reported in tissue obtained from area CA3 of potentiated animals (Bär et al., 1984; Lynch et al., 1988). The two products of PIP$_2$ hydrolysis, inositol-1,4,5-trisphosphate (IP$_3$) and diacylglycerol (DAG) both play second messenger roles – IP$_3$ releases calcium from a non-mitochondrial store, and DAG is an activator of protein kinase C. Both calcium and protein kinase C (Kaczmarek, 1987; Nichols et al., 1987;

Shapira et al., 1987; Lynch et al., 1988) are potent activators of transmitter release, and sustained changes in the rate of hydrolysis of PIP_2 therefore provide one mechanism by which the changes in transmitter release seen in LTP and conditioning might be mediated. With this in mind, we have extended our observations on PI turnover in LTP to the dentate gyrus, and to animals trained in the conditioned suppression task described above.

To measure PIP_2 turnover in the dentate gyrus, slices were incubated in radiolabelled inositol, and the incorporation of radiolabel into membrane-bound inositol phospholipids and into cytosolic inositol phosphates is counted (see Lynch et al., 1988, for full details). The histograms shown in Fig. 2a,b compare the uptake of label into phosphoinositides and inositol phosphates in synaptosomes prepared from the dentate gyrus of animals in which LTP was induced in one hemisphere; the other hemisphere provided control tissue. [3H]Inositol labelling of inositol phosphates was significantly higher in the potentiated hemisphere of animals killed 45 min after the unilateral induction of LTP; similar results were obtained at 2.5 min and 3 h postinduction. Changes in labelling of the membrane-bound phosphoinositol fraction were not significant at any of the 3 time intervals, a result which implies that increase in inositol phosphate labelling is due to an increase in the rate of hydrolysis of PIP_2, rather than to an increase in the concentration of substrate. We have made similar measurements on synaptosomes prepared from the dentate gyrus of animals killed 24 h after learning the tone-footshock association described above. There is an increase in the incorporation of labelled inositol into both inositol phosphates and, in contrast to LTP, into phosphoinositides. This result suggests that the increase in inositol phosphate labelling may occur through an increase in the availability of the substrate phosphoinositides, rather than through an increase in the rate of hydrolysis of PIP_2 by phospholipase C. In any event, the significantly increased labelling of inositol phosphates suggests that both in LTP and in con-

ditioning, the increase in glutamate release may at least in part be explained by an increase in second messenger activity. Further evidence for this conclusion comes from the finding that incorporation of labelled arachidonic acid into diacylglycerol is increased in tissue obtained from conditioned (Laroche et al., 1990b) and potentiated animals (Clements et al., 1988). Moreover, LTP in the den-

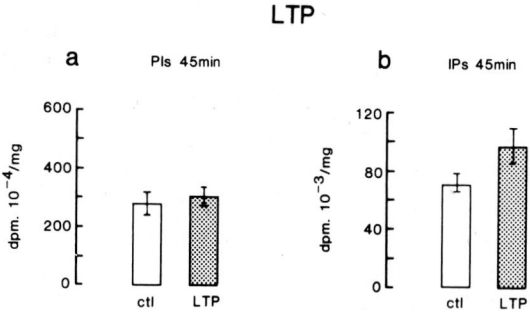

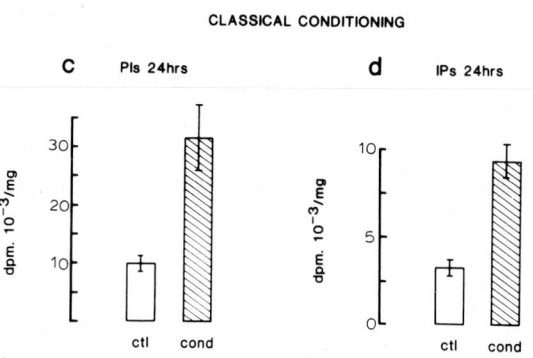

Fig. 2. In vitro analysis of total labelling of phosphoinositides (a,c) and inositol phosphates (b,d) in synaptosomes prepared from the dentate gyrus 45 min after the induction of LTP (a,b), or 24 h after classical conditioning (c,d). Values are expressed as d.p.m./mg protein ± S.E.M. In LTP experiments, there was a significant increase in inositol phosphates (IPs) labelling by [3H]inositol, but no significant changes in phosphoinositides (PIs), in potentiated tissue (dotted bars) compared to control tissue (open bars). In classical conditioning experiments, there was a significant increase in the incorporation of labelled inositol into both inositol phosphates (d) and phosphoinositides (c) in synaptosomes prepared from conditioned (hatched bars) relative to pseudo-conditioned (open bars) animals.

tate gyrus of the rat is associated with a translocation of protein kinase C from the cytosol to its active site in the membrane (Akers et al., 1986), an effect which has also been found in area CA1 following eyelid conditioning in the rabbit (Bank et al., 1988).

Conclusions

The biochemical data summarized above indicates a considerable degree of similarity in the changes associated with classical conditioning and LTP. It is tempting to regard these results as evidence for what we shall call the LTP hypothesis, which asserts that LTP is at least partly responsible for the hippocampal component of the neural trace established during classical conditioning. However, there is a major obstacle for this hypothesis: although classical conditioning of the nictitating membrane is associated with a potentiation of the population spike in the dentate gyrus (Weisz et al., 1984), and a similar result has been reported for an operant conditioning task (Skelton et al., 1987), there has as yet been no convincing demonstration for any hippocampal subfield that conditioning produces an increase in the amplitude of the synaptic component of the evoked response. This insensitivity of the evoked response to conditioning raises two problems for the LTP hypothesis. First, how can classical conditioning be mediated by LTP if there is no apparent increase in synaptic efficacy; and second, what is the explanation for the apparent dissociation between the increase in potassium-evoked transmitter release and the lack of effect on the evoked response? There is no immediately compelling answer to the first question. However, in our view it would be premature to conclude that the hypothesis is false on the basis of the rather meagre data currently available. In our own studies, for example, we only measured evoked potentials immediately after each trial, and again 48 h after the end of conditioning (Laroche et al., 1989); clearly, many more measurements at different time intervals are required before we can conclude that no changes occur. Furthermore, it is by no means obvious that with field potential recording it will be possible to detect what may be small individual changes in synaptic weight widely distributed over the relevant hippocampal network. Another approach to the question would be to monitor evoked potentials while an animal is learning a task which is known to be sensitive to drugs which block LTP.

With regard to the second problem, although responses evoked by single shocks are not affected by conditioning, increases in the amplitude of the EPSP have been reported both during (LoTurco et al., 1988) and after (Laroche et al., 1983a) a period of tetanic stimulation. Thus, as we have argued elsewhere "the training procedure may endow synaptic terminals with a potential for increased release which is only realized under conditions of strong depolarization such as may be presumed to occur during a high-frequency train, or on exposure to high concentrations of potassium" (Laroche et al., 1987). If this explanation is correct, conditioning would not be expected to be accompanied by any increase in the release of glutamate into push – pull perfusates, a prediction which it should be possible to examine experimentally.

Experiments on cellular changes in the hippocampus associated with nictitating membrane conditioning in the rabbit have revealed widespread changes in unit activity (Berger et al., 1976, 1983) and in the calcium-dependent potassium current responsible for the long-duration after-hyperpolarization in CA1 cells (Disterhoft et al., 1986); in both cases, over 50% of cells are affected. Tone-footshock conditioning in the rat is also associated with widespread increases in cellular activity in the dentate gyrus and hippocampus (Bloch and Laroche, 1981; Laroche et al., 1983b). These changes in postsynaptic excitability may be compared with the substantial presynaptic changes in transmitter release and phosphoinositide turnover documented in this chapter for the dentate gyrus following classical conditioning, changes which for the most part mirror those occurring in LTP. It seems probable that in classical conditioning, as for LTP, both sides of the synapse have a part to play.

References

Akers, R.F., Lovinger, D.M., Colley, P.A., Linden, D.J. and Routtenberg, A. (1986) Translocation of protein kinase C may mediate hippocampal long-term potentiation. *Science*, 231: 587 – 589.

Bank, B., DeWeer, A., Kuzirian, A.M., Rasmussen, H. and Alkon, D.L. (1988) Classical conditioning induces long-term translocation of protein kinase C in rabbit hippocampal CA1 cells. *Proc. Natl. Acad. Sci. U.S.A.*, 85: 1988 – 1992.

Bär, P.R., Wiegant, F., Lopes da Silva, F.H. and Gispen, W.H. (1984) Tetanic stimulation affects the metabolism of phosphoinositides in hippocampal slices. *Brain Res.*, 321: 381 – 385.

Berger, T.W., Alger, B. and Thompson, R.F. (1976) Neuronal substrate of classical conditioning in the hippocampus. *Science*, 192: 483 – 485.

Berger, T.W., Rinaldi, P.C., Weisz, D.J. and Thompson, R.F. (1983) Single-unit analysis of different hippocampal cell types during classical conditioning of the rabbit nictitating membrane response. *J. Neurophysiol.*, 50: 1197 – 1219.

Bliss, T.V.P. and Lynch, M.A. (1988) Long-term potentiation of synaptic transmission in the hippocampus: properties and mechanisms. In P.W. Landfield and S.A. Deadwyler (Eds.), *Long-Term Potentiation: From Biophysics to Behavior*, Alan R. Liss, New York, pp. 3 – 72.

Bliss, T.V.P., Douglas, R.M., Errington, M.L. and Lynch, M.A. (1986) Correlation between long-term potentiation and release of endogenous amino acids from dentate gyrus of anaesthetized rats. *J. Physiol. (Lond.)*, 377: 391 – 408.

Bliss, T.V.P., Errington, M.L., Laroche, S. and Lynch, M.A. (1987) Increase in K^+-stimulated, Ca^{2+}-dependent release of ^{3}H-glutamate from rat dentate gyrus three days after induction of long-term potentiation. *Neurosci. Lett.*, 83: 107 – 112.

Bloch, V. and Laroche, S. (1981) Conditioning of hippocampal cells: its acceleration and long-term facilitation by post-trial reticular stimulation. *Behav. Brain Res.*, 3: 23 – 42.

Clements, M.P., Lynch, M.A. and Bliss, T.V.P. (1988) The increase in phosphoinositide turnover associated with long-term potentiation may be mediated through a GTP binding protein. *Neurosci. Res. Commun.*, 3: 11 – 19.

Collins, G.G.S., Anson, J. and Probett, G.A. (1981) Pattern of endogenous amino acid release from slices of rat and guinea pig olfactory cortex. *Brain Res.*, 204: 103 – 120.

Disterhoft, J.F., Coulter, D.A. and Alkon, D.L. (1986) Conditioning-specific membrane changes of rabbit hippocampal neurons measured in vitro. *Proc. Natl. Acad. Sci. U.S.A.*, 83: 2733 – 2737.

Dolphin, A.C., Errington, M.L. and Bliss, T.V.P. (1982) Long-term potentiation in the perforant path in vivo is associated with increased glutamate release. *Nature (Lond.)*, 297: 496 – 498.

Errington, M.L., Lynch, M.A. and Bliss, T.V.P. (1987) Long-term potentiation in the dentate gyrus: induction and increased glutamate release are blocked by D(–)aminophosphonovalerate. *Neuroscience*, 20: 279 – 284.

Kaczmarek, L.K. (1987) The role of protein kinase C in the regulation of ion channels and neurotransmitter release. *Trends Neurosci.*, 10: 30 – 34.

Laroche, S., Bergis, O.E. and Bloch, V. (1983a) Posttrial reticular facilitation of dentate multiunit conditioning is followed by an increased long-term potentiation. *Soc. Neurosci. Abstr.*, 9: 645.

Laroche, S., Falcou, R. and Bloch, V. (1983b) Post-trial reticular facilitation of associative changes in multiunit activity: comparison between dentate gyrus and entorhinal cortex. *Behav. Brain Res.*, 9: 381 – 387.

Laroche, S., Errington, M.L., Lynch, M.A. and Bliss, T.V.P. (1987) Increase in ^{3}H-glutamate release from slices of dentate gyrus and hippocampus following classical conditioning in the rat. *Behav. Brain Res.*, 25: 23 – 29.

Laroche, S., Bloch, V., Doyère, V. and Rédini-Del Negro, C. (1990a) The significance of long-term potentiation for learning and memory. In F. Morrell (Ed.), *Kindling and Synaptic Plasticity: The Legacy of Graham Goddard*, Birkhäuser, Boston, in press.

Laroche, S., Rédini-Del Negro, C., Clements, M.P. and Lynch, M.A. (1990b) Long-term activation of phosphoinositide turnover associated with increased release of amino acids in the dentate gyrus and hippocampus following classical conditioning in the rat. *Eur. J. Neurosci.*, in press.

LoTurco, J.J., Coulter, D.A. and Alkon, D.L. (1988) Enhancement of synaptic potentials in rabbit CA1 pyramidal neurons following classical conditioning. *Proc. Natl. Acad. Sci. U.S.A.*, 85: 1672 – 1676.

Lynch, M.A., Clements, M.P., Errington, M.L. and Bliss, T.V.P. (1988) Increased hydrolysis of phosphatidylinositol-4,5-bisphosphate in long-term potentiation. *Neurosci. Lett.*, 84: 291 – 296.

Lynch, M.A., Errington, M.L. and Bliss, T.V.P. (1989a) Nordihydroguaiaretic acid blocks the synaptic component of long-term potentiation and the associated increases in release of glutamate and arachidonate: an *in vivo* study in the dentate gyrus of the rat. *Neuroscience*, 30: 693 – 705.

Lynch, M.A., Errington, M.L. and Bliss, T.V.P. (1989b) The increase in ^{3}H-glutamate release associated with long-term potentiation in the dentate gyrus is blocked by commissural stimulation. *Neurosci. Lett.*, 103: 191 – 196.

Nichols, R.A., Haycock, J.W., Wang, J.K.T. and Greengard, P. (1987) Phorbol ester enhancement of neurotransmitter release from rat brain synaptosomes. *J. Neurochem.*, 48: 615 – 621.

Shapira, R., Silberberg, S.D., Ginsburg, S. and Rahamimoff, R. (1987) Activation of protein kinase C augments evoked transmitter release. *Nature (Lond.),* 325: 58 – 60.

Skelton, R.W., Scarth, A.S., Wilkie, D.M., Miller, J.J. and Phillips, A.G. (1987) Long-term increases in dentate granule cell responsivity accompany operant conditioning. *J.*

Neurosci., 7: 3081 – 3087.

Weisz, D.J., Clark, G.A. and Thompson, R.F. (1984) Increased responsivity of dentate granule cells during nictitating membrane response conditioning in rabbit. *Behav. Brain Res.,* 12: 145 – 154.

J. Storm-Mathisen, J. Zimmer and O.P. Ottersen (Eds.)
Progress in Brain Research, Vol. 83
© 1990 Elsevier Science Publishers B.V. (Biomedical Division)

CHAPTER 19

Spatial organization of physiological activity in the hippocampal region: relevance to memory formation

György Buzsáki, Lan S. Chen and Fred H. Gage

Department of Neurosciences, M-024, University of California at San Diego, La Jolla, CA 92093, U.S.A.

Based on a review of anatomical and physiological findings, we suggest that the hippocampus may be viewed as a positive feedback device (autoassociator), which is capable of modifying the activity of the neocortical neurons. We examine the three-dimensional organization of evoked and spontaneous physiological patterns of the hippocampus and suggest rules how these patterns emerge during different behaviors from a hard-wired structural network. The high spatial coherence of theta activity is due to an external pacemaker, while the high synchrony of population bursts underlying hippocampal sharp waves is explained by the similar probability of recruitment of neurons by the burst-initiator cells along the whole extent of the hippocampus. We suggest that the burst-initiator cells are a group of CA3 neurons whose excitability is increased by a transient potentiation action of the neocortical activity during theta-concurrent exploratory behaviors. We hypothesize that sharp wave-concurrent population bursts result in a highly synchronous hippocampal output, converging preferentially on those entorhinal neurons which were instrumental in the creation of the burst-initiator neurons. The feedback action of population activity thus provides a selective mechanism for potentiation of connections between information-carrying neurons in the hippocampus and entorhinal cortex. The state-dependent operations of the anatomical hardware also point to the importance and advantage of studying the physiological activity of the intact brain.

Introduction

The hippocampal formation consists of a series of unidirectionally coupled feedback circuitries. The information fed into the hippocampal circuitry may or may not return to the neocortex, depending on the status of the subcortical inputs (Winson and Abzug, 1978; Buzsáki et al., 1981; Buzsáki, 1984). A key issue in understanding the function of the hippocampal circuitry is therefore to reveal the conditions and mechanisms that govern the reverberation of neuronal impulses in the entorhinal cortex – hippocampus – entorhinal cortex circuitries.

What could be the function of a neuronal network which is simply attached to the neocortical mantle as an "appendage" and feeds back its output to the origin of its inputs and which resides several synapses away from both the sensory afferents and motor effectors of the brain? Intuitively, we surmise that such an architectural organization may serve to modify the activity of its target structures. The thesis of this chapter is that the hippocampus feeds back the afferent copy to the same entorhinal cells which originated the input. The high fidelity of this feedback process takes place despite the enormous convergence and divergence of the anatomical organization within the hippocampal formation (see chapter by Amaral et al., this volume), and may be subserved by the rules of population bursting of the hippocampal pyramidal cells. We also point out that knowledge of anatomical connectivity is prerequisite but not sufficient to account for the mechanisms of operation of neuronal networks.

The trisynaptic circuitry

The efficacy of the spread of neuronal activity in a multisynaptic system can be tested by delivering a test volley and observing the magnitude of the electrical responses throughout successive neuronal populations. When the perforant path is stimulated, evoked neuronal activity can be tested at each subregion of the hippocampal formation (Fig. 1). Based on stimulation studies of the intrahippocampal circuitry a hypothesis was put forward that neuronal impulses travel along a relatively narrow slice or lamella perpendicular to the long axis of the hippocampus, and that these lamellae may operate as relatively independent functional units (Andersen et al., 1971). As discussed in a recent paper by Amaral and Witter (1989), the organization of the trisynaptic circuitry of the hippocampus does not provide a direct "hardware" verification of the lamellar hypothesis

of hippocampal function, mainly because the intrahippocampal excitatory connections are as extensively organized in the septotemporal axis of the hippocampus as in the medio-lateral axis. As we will point out, however, spatially organized physiological patterns emerge in the CA1 region even when the dentate gyrus is activated relatively homogeneously.

In the freely moving animal the evoked response method can be used to obtain "snapshots" about the excitability states of the hippocampus during different behaviors and to infer which afferent systems are responsible for the modification of the intrahippocampal flow of information (Winson and Abzug, 1978; Buzsáki et al., 1981). Based on these experiments, it was hypothesized that the cholinergic and aminergic afferents to the hippocampus are responsible for the behavior-dependent gating of the hippocampal circuitry.

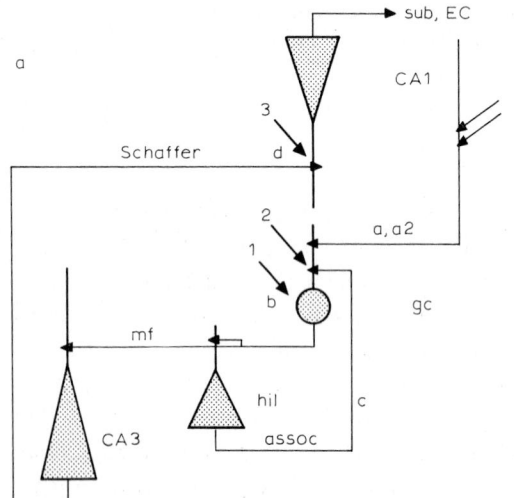
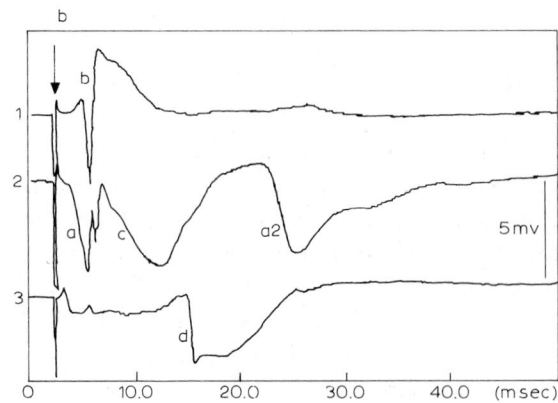

Fig. 1. Reverberation of neuronal impulses in the entorhinal cortex (EC) – hippocampus – EC circuitry. a: schematic diagram of the major excitatory connections in the hippocampal formation. b: evoked field potentials recorded simultaneously in 3 different layers of the CA1-dentate gyrus axis (heavy arrows in (a)) in response to a single volley delivered to the perforant path (double arrow in (a), single arrow in (b)). Letters indicate the anatomical substrates (a) of the successive potentials. a, depolarization of granule cells (gc) and feedforward inhibitory interneurons; b, summed action potentials of gc; c, disynaptic activation of hilar (hil) mossy cells and other interneurons by the mossy fibers (mf), and reactivation of gc by the associational (assoc) afferents; d, depolarization of CA1 pyramidal cells by the Schaffer collaterals of the CA3 pyramidal neurons. a2, reactivation of gc by the EC input. Such reverberation is only rarely observed in the intact animal.

Longitudinal organization of the physiological activity in the hippocampus

Evoked responses

To monitor the temporally coherent functional units along the long axis of the hippocampus, we developed a method for multisite recording of spontaneous and evoked field and cell responses by a multielectrode probe (Fig. 2) (Buzsáki et al., 1989a). By inserting 16 microelectrodes into the same cytoarchitectonic region along the

longitudinal axis in the hippocampus we are able to record electrophysiological patterns simultaneously and estimate the speed of propagation of population events during different behaviors.

Figure 3 illustrates the spatial distribution of evoked activity in the dentate gyrus and CA1 region. Stimulation of the angular bundle monosynaptically activates a substantial number of granule cells in the 3.0 mm strip of the recording area. This distance roughly corresponds to about one-third of the length of the rat hippocampus. The latency of response gradually increases with

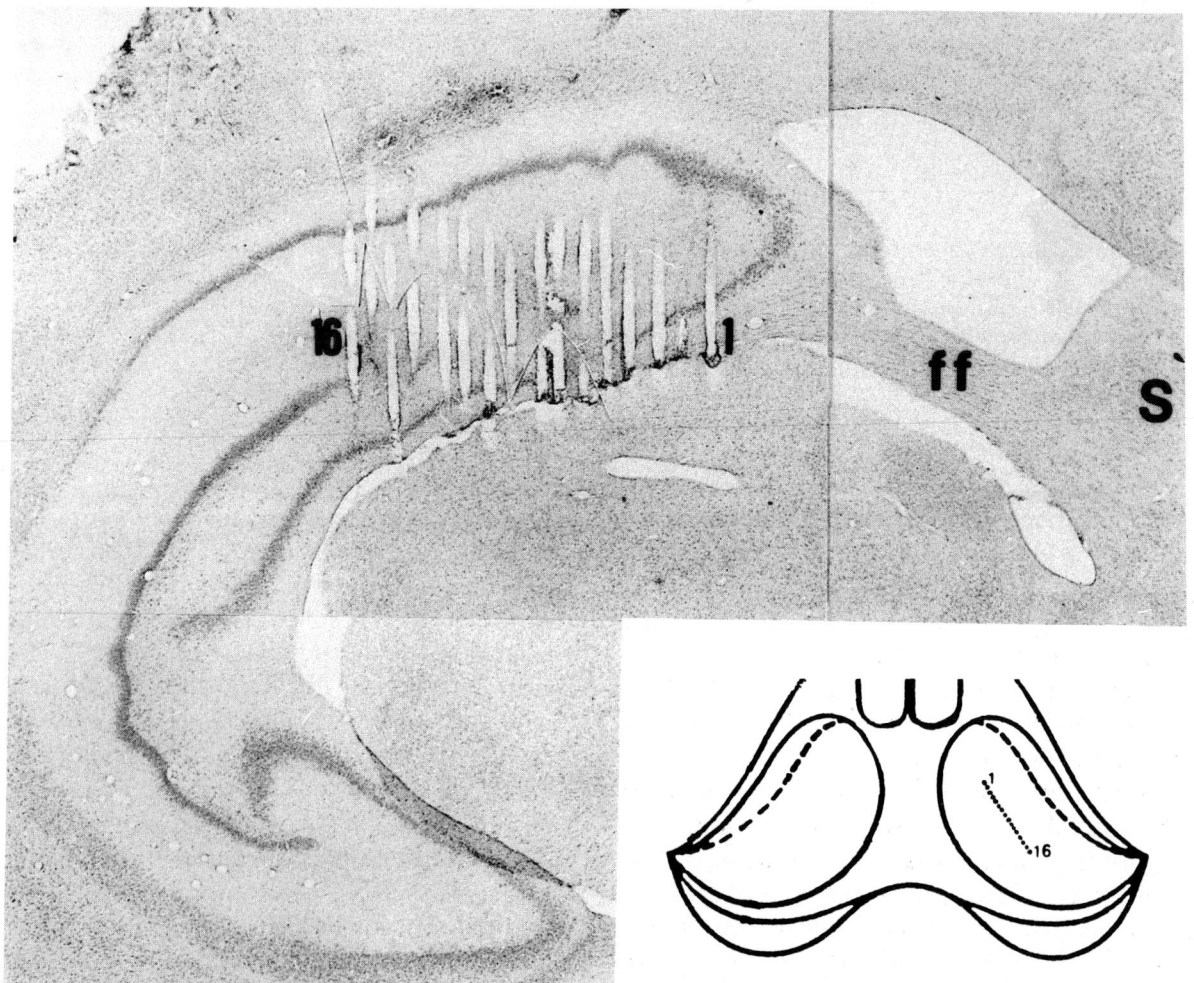

Fig. 2. Nissl-stained section along the long axis of the hippocampus. Photomontage of the tracks of recording microelectrodes (1–16). Inset illustrates the orientation of the electrode penetrations. ff, fimbria-fornix; s, septum.

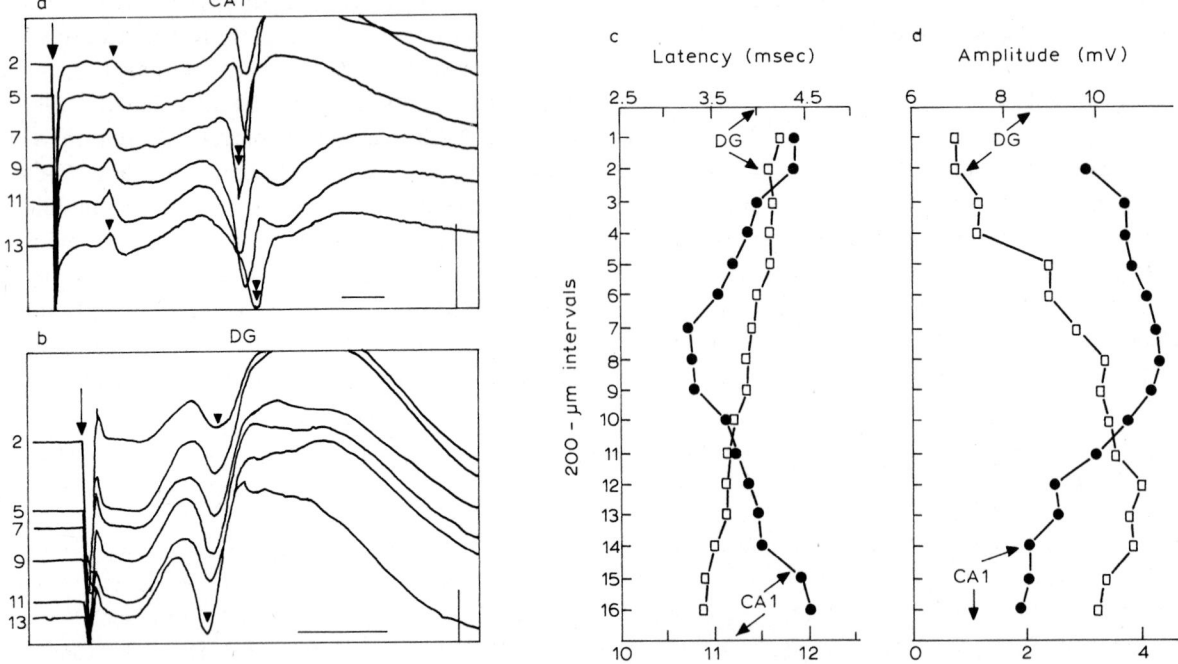

Fig. 3. Spatial distribution of evoked responses in CA1 and dentate gyrus (DG) along the long axis of the hippocampus. a and b: simultaneously recorded single evoked responses. The numbers indicate the position of the recording electrodes (see Fig. 2). Arrows: single pulse stimulation of the perforant path input. Arrowheads: dentate population spike. Double arrowheads: CA1 population spikes recorded simultaneously in the CA1 pyramidal layer. b: records were obtained from the hilus. Calibrations: 2.5 ms; 5 mV. c: distributions of peak latencies of the evoked population spikes in CA1 and DG. d: spatial distributions of the amplitude of the evoked population spikes. The electrodes were spaced at 200 μm intervals. Note gradual increase of response latency, and decrease of the population spike amplitude of the dentate potential but a V-shape curve of the CA1 responses, with latency minimum and amplitude maximum at electrodes 7 – 9.

distance from the stimulation site and the latency differences reflect an estimated 10 m/s conduction velocity of perforant path fibers. Extrapolating from our observation, it may be stated that simultaneous firing of neurons in the entorhinal cortex can induce discharges of granule cells within a time window of less than 1 ms, independent of the location of the cells.

Synchronous firing of the granule cells activates the CA3 pyramidal cells which, in turn, may discharge CA1 pyramidal neurons. This multisynaptic activation is very rare during exploratory (theta) behaviors, but may occur during sharp wave (SPW)-concurrent consummatory behaviors, immobility and slow wave sleep (Winson and Abzug, 1978; Buzsáki et al., 1983). Especially large amplitude responses can be evoked

at every level of the trisynaptic chain when the stimulus is delivered during a SPW-concurrent population burst (Buzsáki, 1986) or in a preparation with surgical removal of the subcortical hippocampal afferents (Buzsáki et al., 1989b). The spatial distributions of both the latency and amplitude of the CA1-evoked responses are substantially different from those of the dentate gyrus (Fig. 3). Even with large stimulus currents the latency difference of the CA1 population spikes in the recorded area (3.0 mm) is always larger than 1 ms (range: 1 to 5 ms). This implies that even under ideal conditions, simultaneous firing of entorhinal neurons will result in a delay of several ms in the trisynaptic activation of spatially distant CA1 pyramidal cells. Furthermore, in the CA1 region we always found a relatively short-latency and large-amplitude "beam" of population spikes, even though such patterns were not always observed in the dentate gyrus. This implies that an activated "focus" in CA1 emerges despite the relatively uniform activation of the granule cell population. Frequently, the largest amplitude and shortest latency population spikes in the CA1 region occurred in a plane approximately 1 – 1.5 mm more anterior to the activation maximum of the granule cells. This physiological finding is in line with the anatomical observation that CA3 cells send their Schaffer collaterals to more rostrally positioned CA1 pyramidal neurons (Tamamaki and Nojyo, 1988; Ishizuka et al., 1989).

This finding of context-dependent transmission of neuronal activity points to the importance of the distinction between anatomical and functional connectivity. While the *anatomical connectivity* (hardware) limits the operations of the network, it is the physiological principles of neuronal organization that determine the *state-dependent functional connections*.

Theta activity

Hippocampal rhythmic slow activity (RSA or theta) has been implicated in several functions, ranging from sensory processing to the voluntary control of movement (Grastyan et al., 1959; Bland, 1986; Vanderwolf, 1988). In the rat, hippocampal theta occurs during exploratory behaviors, such as sniffing, rearing, walking and the paradoxical phase of sleep (Vanderwolf, 1969). This rhythm is not intrinsic to the hippocampus, although the population organization of the structure endows the hippocampus to respond or "resonate" maximally at theta frequency (Bland et al., 1988; Traub et al., 1989). The external "pacemaker" for hippocampal rhythmicity resides in the septum (Petsche et al., 1962). Both cholinergic and GABAergic septal fibers project to the hippocampus and innervate both the principal cells and the GABAergic interneurons. Given the notoriously slow action of acetylcholine on hippocampal pyramidal neurons (Nicoll, 1985), it is

likely that the transfer of the septal pacemaker activity to the hippocampus is conveyed mainly via the septal GABA input – GABAergic interneuron – pyramidal cell circuitry (Buzsáki and Eidelberg, 1983; Buzsáki et al., 1983; Freund and Antal, 1988).

We examined the degree of synchrony of hippocampal theta in 3 dimensions of the structure. Theta waves were found highly coherent along the CA1-dentate gyrus and CA1-CA3 axes, despite the large phase-shifts that occurred at the level of the apical dendrites of the pyramidal cells and in the molecular layer of the dentate gyrus (Buzsáki et al., 1986). Similarly high coherence values were obtained when theta activity recorded from identical cytoarchitectonic regions of the two hemispheres were compared (Leung et al., 1982; Buzsáki et al., 1986). When microelectrodes were placed in the same fields along the long axis of the hippocampus, the theta waves occurred in phase (Fig. 4), and were highly coherent. It must be noted that the coherence values at other frequencies decreased abruptly within a few hundred microns (Buzsáki et al., 1986; Bullock et al., 1990). Furthermore, coherence values of irregular EEG in the theta band, recorded during immobility, also decreased rapidly with distance. The most parsimonious explanation of the highly synchronous

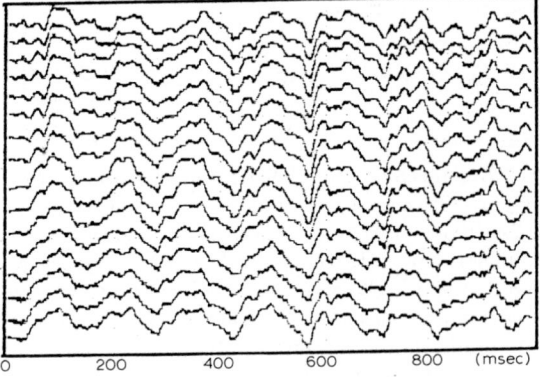

Fig. 4. Simultaneously derived theta waves from the stratum radiatum of CA1 along the long axis of the hippocampus (see Fig. 2) during running in a wheel. Electrode spacing: 200 μm. Note similar waveforms at all levels. Calibration: 1 mV. The uppermost trace is from the rostral pole of the hippocampus.

nature of hippocampal theta is that in the intact animal this rhythmicity is brought about by the command input from the septal pacemaker, as originally suggested by Petsche et al. (1962). The septal pacemaker – hippocampal resonator model is further supported by the observations that following septohippocampal disconnection, restoration of cholinergic reinnervation of the hippocampus by basal forebrain or brainstem

cholinergic grafts is not sufficient for the production of theta activity (Buzsáki et al., 1987).

Sharp wave-associated population bursts

In the absence of theta activity, irregular sharp waves (SPW) of 40 – 120 ms duration appear in the hippocampal record (Fig. 5). SPWs are observed, in order of incidence, during slow wave sleep, awake immobility, drinking, eating, face washing and body grooming (O'Keefe and Nadel, 1978; Buzsáki et al., 1983; Suzuki and Smith, 1988). The incidence of SPW ranges from 0.02 to 3/s during awake immobility. The importance of SPW is amplified by the fact that hippocampal SPWs have also been recorded from chimpanzees (Freemon et al., 1969) and humans (Freemon et al., 1970), whereas theta activity is present only in subprimate species (Vanderwolf, 1988).

The cellular correlates of theta and SPW are characteristically different. Although some "spatially sensitive" neurons (O'Keefe and Nadel, 1978) may show a sustained firing at 4 – 6/s when the rat walks through the "spatial field" of the cell, most pyramidal cells fire at a rate of 0.05/s or stop discharging altogether during theta-related behaviors. It is not known how many spatial cells determine a given location of the environment; therefore, we cannot estimate the percentage of pyramidal neurons whose firing rates are higher than those of the average population. Regarding the 0.05/s discharge frequency as typical, it follows that in a time window of 100 ms (about half theta cycle) about 0.005% of the pyramidal neurons will discharge. The firing pattern of pyramidal cells changes substantially during SPW-concurrent behaviors. Importantly, groups of pyramidal cells in CA1-3 and subiculum now fire in synchronous bursts associated with field SPW (Fig. 6). Examining the relationship of SPW and the probability of discharge of pyramidal neurons we found that the probability of coincidence of the two events is about 5% (range: 1 to 15%). Projecting this figure to the whole neuronal population, it is estimated that about 5% of all pyramidal

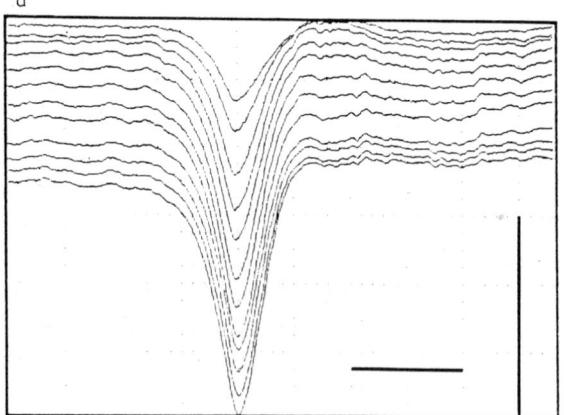

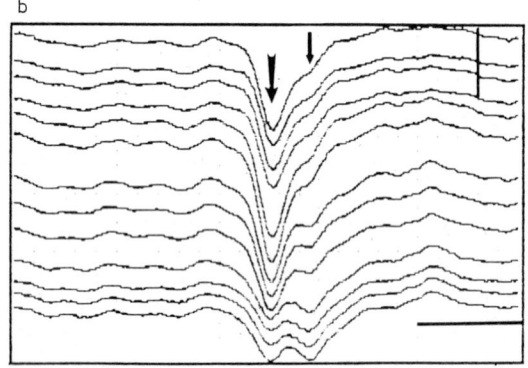

Fig. 5. Averaged SPWs ($n = 50$) recorded simultaneously from 12 (a) or 13 (b) microelectrodes along the longitudinal axis of the CA1 region of the hippocampus in two different animals. Recordings were made during alert immobility. Spacing between electrodes is 200 μm (see Fig. 2). All tips were positioned in the stratum radiatum. Note simultaneous occurrence of SPWs over a distance of 3.0 mm. The gradually increasing amplitude in (a) is due to an oblique positioning of the electrode array in the stratum radiatum. b: synchronous (large arrow) and delayed (small arrow) SPWs with different spatial amplitude maxima. The delayed SPW reflects slow (< 0.1 m/s) recruitment of neurons along the long axis of the hippocampus. Calibrations: 100 ms; 1 mV.

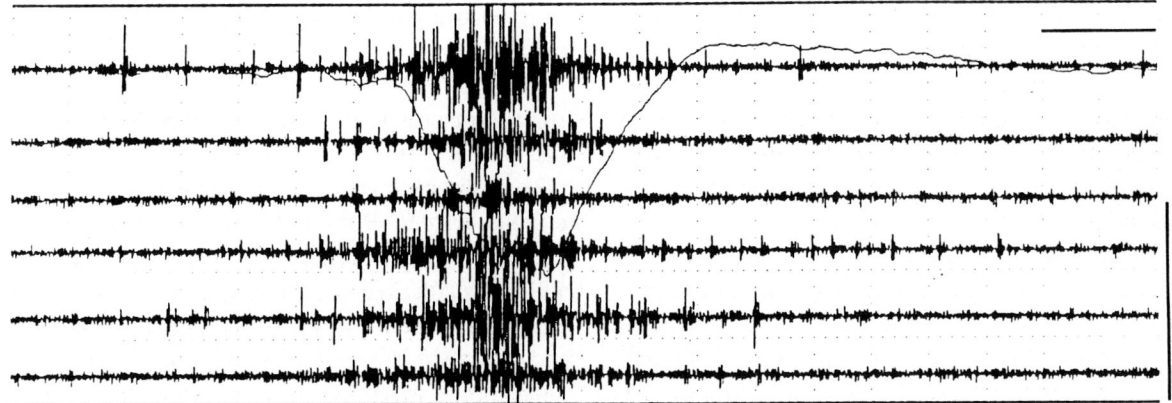

Fig. 6. SPW-concurrent population bursts recorded during awake immobility along the longitudinal axis of CA1 pyramidal layer. Distance between the first and last electrodes was 2.4 mm. Only 6 derivations with acceptable unit activity are shown. The filtered trace (1 – 70 Hz) was derived from an electrode in stratum radiatum. Note the synchronous nature of population bursts at all electrodes. Calibrations: 40 ms; 1 mV (field), 500 μV (units).

neurons discharge in the time window SPWs (40 – 120 ms). This figure corresponds to at least a 100-fold increase of population synchrony during hippocampal SPW relative to theta activity. Inhibitory interneurons also display a significant frequency increase during the SPW (Buzsáki et al., 1983), and there is very little neuronal activity of any kind between successive SPW. Despite the increased interneuronal activity during the SPW, the net excitability of the hippocampal network increases substantially, as demonstrated by the finding that stimuli delivered during the SPW-burst induced a several-fold increase of the evoked population spikes, relative to responses evoked in the absence of SPW (Buzsáki, 1986).

In contrast to theta, SPWs are intrinsically generated in the hippocampus, that is they are not induced actively by an extrahippocampal input. The trigger for the SPW is a synchronous population burst of CA3 pyramidal cells and hilar neurons. The population burst erupts virtually synchronously along the longitudinal extent of the hippocampus (Figs. 5 and 6). We suggested that subcortical afferents exert a tonic suppressive action on the synchronizing mechanisms of the CA3 and hilar regions (Buzsáki et al., 1983; Buzsáki, 1986). Indeed, surgical transection of the subcortical afferents to the hippocampus will convert

SPWs into very large amplitude (up to 12 mV) interictal spikes (Buzsáki et al., 1989). The high spatial coherence of the SPW-concurrent population burst of hippocampal neurons is explained by assuming that due to the time-locked release of subcortical tonic suppression neurons with the highest excitability (burst-initiator cells) begin recruiting their target cells virtually simultaneously along the long axis of the hippocampus (Buzsáki, 1986; Traub et al., 1989). The spatial synchrony is further facilitated by the extensive recurrent collateral system of the CA3 pyramidal neurons (Tamamaki, 1988). In addition to the fast synchronizing mechanisms, slow spread of population bursts via sequential recruitment of local circuitries (Miles et al., 1988) may also occur, resulting in delayed or double SPW-bursts (Fig. 5) (Buzsáki et al., 1989a, b).

Density of interneurons along the long axis of the hippocampus

The distribution of interneurons along the long axis of the dorsal hippocampus was investigated using parvalbumin immunocytochemistry. Coronal sections were taken at every 160 – 200 μm distance from the rostral end of the hippocampus to the curvature of the hippocampus (approx-

264

imately the same length as covered by our multielectrode). The cell density (number of parvalbumin-immunoreactive cells/mm²) was calculated in 4 subregions: stratum granulosum of the dentate gyrus, hilar region including hilar portion of the CA3 region (CA3c), stratum pyramidale of CA3a + b and CA1.

Immunoreactive neurons were not evenly distributed along the long axis of the hippocampus. The density of immunoreactive neurons was highest in the septal portion and decreased gradually towards the more posterior parts of the dorsal hippocampus. This pattern was most prominent in the hilar region (Fig. 7) and the stratum granulosum of the dentate gyrus, followed by the CA1 region. In the pyramidal layer of CA3a + b, the opposite, but statistically non-significant trend was observed. More importantly, a prominent periodicity of cell density with 200 μm distances was observed in the CA3a + b region.

The uneven distribution of the inhibitory interneurons may offer an anatomical basis for the emergence of distinct spatial distribution of physiological patterns, even when the principal cell populations are activated uniformly.

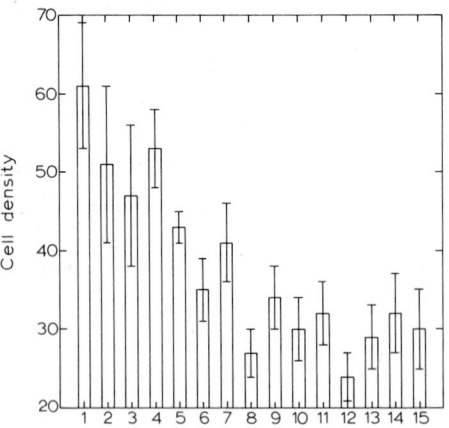

Fig. 7. Distribution of parvalbumin-immunoreactive neurons in the hilar area (hilus + CA3c) of the dorsal hippocampus. Coronal sections were taken at every 160–200 μm from the rostral pole (level 1) to the curvature (level 15). The cell density (immunoreactive cells/mm²) at each level reflects the mean and standard error calculated from sections of the same anatomical level in different rats (n = 9 hippocampi).

Long-term potentiation and hippocampal SPW-bursts

Long-term potentiation (LTP) of synaptic transmission is widely regarded as a candidate mechanism of memory formation in the central nervous system (Bliss and Lømo, 1973; see also Chapters by A.M. Lynch et al. and by G.S. Lynch et al., this volume). Basic requirements of LTP are (a) strong synaptic bombardment, preferably in bursts and (b) cooperative activity of a number of convergent afferent fibers (Douglas, 1977; McNaughton et al., 1978; Levy and Steward, 1979). Based on these and other requirements of LTP we suggested that the highly synchronous population bursts underlying the hippocampal SPWs are the most likely candidate pattern for the physiological induction of synaptic plasticity (Buzsáki, 1984, 1985). Briefly, it was hypothesized that during exploratory (theta) behaviors the acquired information is stored temporarily in the hippocampus and conversion to long-term storage occurs during SPW-associated behaviors (Buzsáki, 1989). At the cellular level we assumed that the entorhinal cortex – granule cells-mediated volleys produce a transient, short-lasting heterosynaptic potentiation in some of recurrent (associational) collaterals of the CA3 pyramidal neurons during exploratory activity. As a result, the interconnections among these information-carrying cells (e.g. spatial units) become more efficient and become the burst-initiator cells of the SPW-concurrent population events after the termination of the exploratory state. These "active" units are assumed to undergo potentiation during the theta state (a) because the convergence of granule cell inputs is maximum on these neurons (in addition to the direct perforant path activation), and (b) because the mossy fiber-mediated tetanizing inputs are co-active with the firing of only these cells.

The existence of heterosynaptic potentiation of the associational synapse in CA3 was recently demonstrated in the slice preparation. When single pulses delivered to the association fibers were coupled with strong trains of high-frequency bursts to the mossy fibers at theta frequency, a lasting potentiation of the associational terminals was observed. The potentiation effect, however, was absent or the synapses were even depressed when stimuli to the two afferent systems were delivered out-of-phase (Chattarji et al., 1989). It is important to emphasize in this context that in the freely behaving rat granule cells and CA3 pyramidal cells discharge on the same phase of theta waves (Buzsáki et al., 1983; Fox et al., 1986), and this conjunction is therefore the same as required for the potentiation effect in the slice.

The weakly potentiated cells therefore become the initiator cells of population bursts during subsequent SPW states due to the enhanced efficacy of their interconnections. The repeatedly occurring SPW-population bursts are hypothesized to produce sufficiently large depolarizations of the information-carrying burst-initiator cells in CA3 neurons and in their targets to induce plastic changes of the synapses of these neurons. In support of this hypothesis, we found that high-frequency stimulation of the entorhinal input modified the structure of the subsequently occurring spontaneous population bursts (Buzsáki, 1989).

The hypothesis of the two-stage process of LTP emphasizes the importance of behavioral states associated with neuronal population bursts (e.g. sleep states) in the formation of the memory trace and offers new insight into the information storing capacity of population events in anatomically-physiologically organized neuronal networks.

Reafferentation of information to the neocortex

Although the intact hippocampus is essential for depositing new memories, it is not the site for long-term storage of experience (Milner et al., 1968; Squire, 1986). Therefore, the question of how the hippocampus assists the formation of permanent memory trace in the neocortex must also be addressed (Teyler and DiScenna, 1986; Squire et al., 1989).

As we have discussed earlier, the major output of the hippocampus is the same structure as its dominant input: the entorhinal cortex. Although this structural-functional arrangement intuitively suggests that the hippocampus is an association-feedback device which potentiates neocortical representations, the physiological question – whether the hippocampal efferent pattern is able to re-access the same population of neurons that gave rise to the afferent pattern – remains a question for empirical analysis. The absence of a clear topographical relationship between the entorhinal cortex and the successive stages of the hippocampal formation would suggest a priori that the hippocampus would not retain information about the original source of the input in a simple way (Amaral and Witter, 1989; Squire et al., 1989).

When stimuli are delivered to the perforant path during a SPW-burst or when stimulation is done in animals with surgical removal of the subcortical hippocampal inputs, single volleys delivered to the perforant path occasionally evoke double or triple responses (Buzsáki et al., 1983; Buzsáki, 1986). These responses are due to the reverberation of neuronal impulses in the hippocampus – entorhinal cortex – hippocampus circuitry, each cycle requiring about 20–25 ms. We monitored the spatial distribution of the evoked responses along the long axis of the hippocampus testing the following hypothesis: the spatial pattern and the waveforms of the successive responses should be the same if the hippocampal efferent copy reactivates the same entorhinal neurons whose axons were stimulated by the electric shock, but substantially different if spatially segregated neurons are activated by the output volleys. The results of such an experiment are illustrated in Fig. 8. Stimuli, slightly above the threshold, were most effective in eliciting double responses. When second responses were present, their configuration and the spatial distribution of their amplitudes were quite similar to those of the first response. When individual neurons were isolated and responded to perforant path stimulation, they responded equally during the second cycle as well. These findings support the view that the output volley of the hippocampus selectively discharged the same or closely overlapping neurons in the entorhinal cortex whose axons had discharged the granule cells in the first place.

How can such a high-fidelity reafferent copy be retained with such extensive divergence of hippocampal axon collateral systems as described by

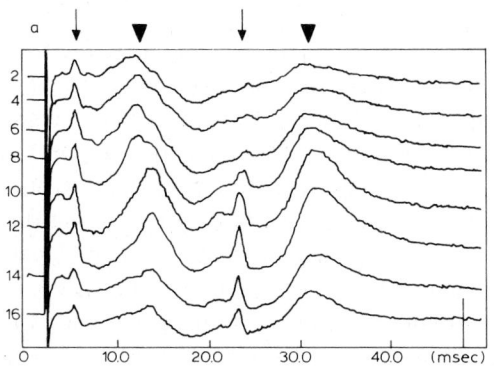

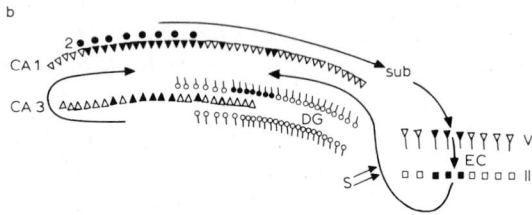

Fig. 8. Reverberation of neuronal impulses in the entorhinal cortex – hippocampus – entorhinal circuitry. a: simultaneously recorded field potentials from the stratum oriens of CA1 in response to single pulse stimulation of the perforant path. The distance between recording sites was 400 μm along the longitudinal axis of the hippocampus (see Fig. 2). Arrows: volume-conducted population spikes from the dentate gyrus. Large arrowheads: field responses generated in CA1. Note virtually identical spatial distribution of the early and late responses. Fimbria-fornix lesioned rat. b: circuit diagram of the neuronal events in a. Electrical stimulation (s) of the perforant path evoked neuronal firing of the granule cells of the dentate gyrus (DG), the CA3 and CA1 regions (filled cells). Dots in CA1 indicate the positions of recording electrodes 2 – 16. The population discharge of CA1 pyramidal neurons sequentially activated neurons in the subiculum (sub) and layer V of the entorhinal cortex (EC) which, in turn, reactivated the same population of layer II stellate cells (filled squares) whose axons were previously stimulated by the electrical pulse. These stellate neurons, in turn, reactivated the same or closely overlapping neuronal populations in the trisynaptic circuitry as during the first cycle. (Reproduced from Buzsáki, 1989.)

the anatomical analysis? A possible physiological explanation rests on the assumption that the active neurons in the CA3 region retained their excitability for at least 25 ms, perhaps coupled with surrounding lateral inhibition, and therefore even a relatively diffuse entorhinal volley preferentially reactivated the same subpopulation of CA3 cells. Such a physiological organization can selectively reinforce emerging patterns even in networks with relatively random connections (Edelman, 1987).

As discussed above, the same anatomical circuitry (hardware) can function in different modes of operations: the "open state" reflecting theta activity and the "closed state" corresponding to SPW-population bursts. Thus, the activity of the ascending subcortical inputs can reorganize the functional connectivity of the anatomical circuitry of the hippocampus into an entirely different mode of operation and thereby alter its output patterns (Buzsáki, 1989).

Combining the findings that activation of the entorhinal input determines the structure of the population burst (creation of initiator cells) with the high fidelity of reafferentation of the hippocampal input patterns, the following hypothesis may be put forward. A group of neurons in the entorhinal cortex is selectively active during explorative behavior and transiently activates a subset of CA3 pyramidal cells (e.g. spatial cells) directly and/or disynaptically via the granule cells. This activation results in heterosynaptic potentiation of these cells by the associational fibers terminating on the activated CA3 cells which neurons, in turn, become the burst-initiator cells of the subsequent SPW-associated population events at the termination of the exploratory activity. Given the substantially higher probability of the participation of the initiator cells in successive population bursts, it is likely that these cells will readdress the same population of neurons in the CA1, subiculum and the entorhinal cortex. These entorhinal cells, of course, are the same ones whose activity led to the creation of burst-initiator cells in the hippocampus. Because of the higher probability of convergence of population synchrony on the subset of neurons that carried information during the exploratory stage, the degree of depolarization of these neurons may reach the threshold of LTP during successive SPW-concurrent population bursts.

We briefly reviewed the three-dimensional organization of the physiological activity in the hippocampal formation. We conclude that the anatomical circuitry and the physiological patterns of the hippocampal formation are compatible with an active feedback device role of the hippocampus. We suggest that the afferent neuronal template originating in the neocortex may be consolidated by the population bursts of the hippocampus during consummatory states and sleep. Our findings also point to the necessity of studying physiological activity of the intact brain for assessing rules of network operations that cannot be revealed from anatomical or biophysical investigations.

Acknowledgements

The antibody against parvalbumin was a generous gift from Dr. K.G. Baimbridge. We thank Steve Forbes and Donna Chin for technical help. This research was supported by NINDS, the Whitehall Foundation, the Sandoz Foundation, ADRDA and the Office of Naval Research. L.S. Chen is an NRSA (NIH) Fellow.

References

Amaral, D.G. and Witter, M.P. (1989) A critique of the lamellar hypothesis of hippocampal organization in light of recent anatomical findings. *Neuroscience,* 31: 571–591.

Andersen, P., Bliss, T.V.P. and Skrede, K.K. (1971) Lamellar organization of hippocampal excitatory pathways. *Exp. Brain Res.,* 13: 222–238.

Bland, B.H. (1986) The physiology and pharmacology of hippocampal formation theta rhythms. *Prog. Neurobiol.,* 26: 1–54.

Bland, B.H., Colom, L.V., Konopacki, J. and Roth, S.H. (1988) Intracellular records of carbachol-induced theta rhythm in hippocampal slices. *Brain Res.,* 447: 364–368.

Bliss, T.V.P. and Lømo, T. (1973) Long-lasting potentiation of synaptic transmission in the dentate area of the anesthetized rabbit following stimulation of the perforant path. *J. Physiol. (Lond.),* 232: 331–356.

Bullock, T.H., McClune, M.C. and Buzsáki, G. (1990) Distribution of coherence of micro-EEG in the hippocampus of the rat asleep and awake. *Neuroscience,* in press.

Buzsáki, G. (1984) Feed-forward inhibition in the hippocampal formation. *Prog. Neurobiol.,* 22: 131–153.

Buzsáki, G. (1985) What does the "LTP model of memory" model? in B. Will, P. Schmitt and J.C. Dalrymple-Alford (Eds.), *Brain Plasticity, Learning and Memory,* Plenum, New York, pp. 157–166.

Buzsáki, G. (1986) Hippocampal sharp waves: their origin and significance. *Brain Res.,* 398: 242–252.

Buzsáki, G. (1989) Two-stage model of memory trace formation: a role for "noisy" brain states. *Neuroscience,* 31: 551–570.

Buzsáki, G. and Eidelberg, E. (1983) Phase relations of hippocampal projection cells and interneurons to theta activity in the urethane anesthetized rat. *Brain Res.,* 226: 334–338.

Buzsáki, G., Grastyan, E., Czopf, J., Kellenyi, L. and Prohaska, O. (1981) Changes in neuronal transmission in the rat hippocampus during behavior. *Brain Res.,* 225: 235–247.

Buzsáki, G., Leung, L.S. and Vanderwolf, C.H. (1983) Cellular bases of hippocampal EEG in the behaving rat. *Brain Res. Rev.,* 6: 139–171.

Buzsáki, G., Czopf, J., Kondakor, I. and Kellenyi, L. (1986) Laminar distribution of hippocampal rhythmic slow activity (RSA) in the behaving rat: current-source density analysis, effects of urethane and atropine. *Brain Res.,* 365: 125–137.

Buzsáki, G., Gage, F.H., Kellenyi, L. and Björklund, A. (1987) Restoration of rhythmic slow activity (theta) in the subcortically denervated hippocampus by embryonic CNS transplants. *Brain Res.,* 400: 321–333.

Buzsáki, G., Bickford, R.G., Ryan, L.J., Young, S., Prohaska, O., Mandel, R.J. and Gage, F.H. (1989a) Multisite recording of brain field potentials and unit activity in freely moving rats. *J. Neurosci. Methods,* 28: 209–217.

Buzsáki, G., Ponomareff, G.L., Bayardo, F., Ruiz, R. and Gage, F.H. (1989b) Neuronal activity in the subcortically denervated hippocampus: a chronic model for epilepsy. *Neuroscience,* 28: 527–538.

Chattarji, S., Stanton, P.K. and Sejnowski, T.J. (1990) Commissural synapses, but not mossy fiber synapses, in hippocampal field CA3 exhibit associative long-term potentiation and depression. *Brain Res.,* in press.

Douglas, R.M. (1977) Long-lasting synaptic potentiation in the rat dentate gyrus following brief high frequency stimulation. *Brain Res.,* 126: 361–365.

Edelman, G.M. (1987) *Neural Darwinism. The Theory of Neuronal Group Selection,* Basic Books, Inc., New York.

Fox, S.E., Wolfson, S. and Rank Jr., J.B. (1986) Hippocampal theta rhythm and the firing of neurons in walking and urethane anesthetized rats. *Exp. Brain Res.,* 62: 495–508.

Freemon, F.R. and Walter, R.D. (1970) Electrical activity of

268

human limbic system during sleep. *Comp. Psychiatry,* 11: 544 – 551.

Freemon, F.R., McNew, J.J. and Adey, W.R. (1969) Sleep of unrestrained chimpanzee: cortical and subcortical recordings. *Exp. Neurol.,* 25: 129 – 137.

Grastyan, E., Lissak, K., Madarasz, I. and Donhoffer, H. (1959) Hippocampal electrical activity during the development of conditioned reflexes. *Electroenceph. Clin. Neurophysiol.,* 11: 409 – 430.

Ishizuka, N., Weber, J. and Amaral, D.G. (1990) Organization of intrahippocampal projections originating from CA3 pyramidal cells in the rat. *J. Comp. Neurol.,* in press.

Leung, L.S., Lopes da Silva, F.H. and Wadman, W.J. (1982) Spectral characteristics of the hippocampal EEG in the freely moving rat. *Electroenceph. Clin. Neurophysiol.,* 54: 203 – 219.

Levy, W.B. and Steward, O. (1979) Synapses as associative memory elements in the hippocampal formation. *Brain Res.,* 175: 233 – 245.

McNaughton, B.L., Douglas, R.M. and Goddard, G.V. (1978) Synaptic enhancement in fascia dentata: cooperativity among coactive afferents. *Brain Res.,* 157: 277 – 293.

Miles, R., Traub, R.D. and Wong, R.K.S. (1988) Spread of synchronous firing in longitudinal slices from the CA3 region of the hippocampus. *J. Neurophysiol.,* 60: 1481 – 1496.

Milner, B., Corkin, S. and Teuber, H.L. (1968) Further analysis of the hippocampal amnesic syndrome: 14-year follow-up study of H.M. *Neuropsychology,* 6: 215 – 234.

Nicoll, R.A. (1985) The septo-hippocampal projection: a model of cholinergic pathways. *Trends Neurosci.,* 5: 533 – 536.

O'Keefe, J. and Nadel, L. (1978) *The Hippocampus as a Cognitive Map,* Clarendon, Oxford.

Petsche, H., Stumpf, C. and Gogolak, G. (1962) The significance of the rabbit's septum as a relay station between the midbrain and the hippocampus. The control of hippocampal arousal activity by septum cells. *Electroenceph. Clin. Neurophysiol.,* 14: 202 – 211.

Squire, L.R. (1986) Mechanisms of memory. *Science,* 232: 1612 – 1619.

Squire, L.R., Shimamura, A.P. and Amaral, D.G. (1989) Memory and the hippocampus. In J. Byrne and W. Berry (Eds.), *Neural Models of Plasticity,* Academic Press, New York.

Suzuki, S.S. and Smith, G.K. (1987) Spontaneous EEG spikes in the normal hippocampus. I. Behavioral correlates, laminar profiles and bilateral synchrony. *Electroenceph. Clin. Neurophysiol.,* 67: 348 – 359.

Suzuki, S.S. and Smith, G.K. (1988) Spontaneous EEG spikes in the normal hippocampus. II. Relations to synchronous burst discharges. *Electroencephal. Clin. Neurophysiol.,* 70: 84 – 95.

Tamamaki, N., Abe, K. and Nojyo, Y. (1988) Three-dimensional analysis of the whole axonal arbors originating from single CA2 pyramidal neurons in the rat hippocampus with the aid of a computer graphic technique. *Brain Res.,* 452: 255 – 272.

Teyler, T.J. and DiScenna, P. (1986) The hippocampal memory indexing theory. *Behav. Neurosci.,* 100: 147 – 154.

Traub, R.D., Miles, R. and Wong, R.K.S. (1989) Model of the origin of rhythmic population oscillations in the hippocampal slice. *Science,* 243: 1319 – 1325.

Vanderwolf, C.H. (1969) Hippocampal electrical activity and voluntary movement in the rat. *Electroenceph. Clin. Neurophysiol.,* 26: 407 – 418.

Vanderwolf, C.H. (1988) Cerebral activity and behavior: control by central cholinergic and serotonergic systems. *Int. Rev. Neurobiol.,* 30: 225 – 340.

Winson, J. and Abzug, C. (1978) Neuronal transmission through hippocampal pathways dependent on behavior. *J. Neurophysiol.,* 41: 716 – 732.

CHAPTER 20

Similarities in circuitry between Ammon's horn and dentate gyrus: local interactions and parallel processing

Philip A. Schwartzkroin[1,2], Helen E. Scharfman[1,*] and Robert S. Sloviter[3,4]

Departments of [1]Neurological Surgery, [2]Physiology and Biophysics, University of Washington, Seattle, WA 98195, U.S.A., [3]Neurology Research Center, Helen Hayes Hospital, New York State Department of Health, West Haverstraw, NY 10993, U.S.A. and [4]Departments of Pharmacology and Neurology, Columbia University, New York, NY 10032, U.S.A.

We present a "model" of hippocampal information processing based on a review of recent data regarding the local circuitry of Ammon's horn and the dentate gyrus. We have been struck by the parallels in cell type and connectivity in Ammon's horn and the dentate gyrus, and have focused on similarities between CA3 pyramidal cells and mossy cells. Important conclusions of our analysis include the following: (1) The idea of serial processing of afferent information, from one hippocampal subregion to the next, is inadequate and based on an over-simplification of circuitry; information processing undoubtedly occurs over parallel, as well as serial, pathways. (2) Local circuitry within a given hippocampal subregion gives rise predominantly to feedforward inhibition; recurrent inhibition is present, but less potent. (3) There are multiple populations of local circuit neurons, each of which has a specific function, characteristic interconnections, and special cell properties. It is misleading to categorize these cells into a single category of inhibitory interneuron.

Introduction

In this chapter, we will review our work on the local circuitry of the hippocampus – Ammon's horn as well as the dentate gyrus. In particular, we will consider the functional and structural properties of the various cell types found in both subregions. From these data, and data describing interactions among various cell types, we will try to derive some general principles of signal processing that may be applicable not only to the hippocampus, but to other cortical regions of the central nervous system.

Our work on hippocampus was guided initially by the traditional view of this structure as a tri-synaptic serial relay (Andersen, 1975). Figure 1A illustrates this view. This view of serial information transfer through the hippocampus has been explicitly or implicitly adopted by many laboratories involved in hippocampal research. The traditional view has also held that, within each subregion, local circuitry consists primarily of recurrent inhibition that is initiated by principal cell excitation and mediated by "basket cells" (Ramón y Cajal, 1911; Lorente de Nó, 1934; Andersen et al., 1964a, b). Figure 1B illustrates this local circuit interaction.

Our studies of hippocampal cell types and local circuitry have gradually convinced us that this view of the hippocampus is greatly over-simplified. Although initially of value in guiding research, these concepts may now impede efforts to elucidate hippocampal function. Clearly, the cir-

*Present address: Howard Hughes Medical Institute and Department of Neurobiology and Behavior, State University of New York at Stony Brook, Stony Brook, NY 11794, U.S.A.

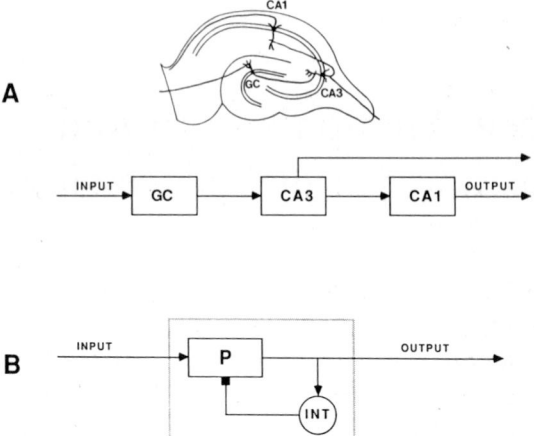

Fig. 1. Diagrammatic representations of hippocampal circuits, as traditionally presented. A: the tri-synaptic excitatory pathway through hippocampus. Input, in the form of perforant path activity, synaptically activates the granule cells (GC) of the dentate gyrus. Granule cell output, via the mossy fibers, excites CA3 pyramidal cells. The CA3 neurons project out of hippocampus (subicular, commissural, and subcortical projections), and also send collaterals that synapse on the dendrites of CA1-CA3 pyramidal cells. The CA1 cells project out of hippocampus to cortical and subcortical targets. B: local circuit interaction in the 3 major subregions indicated in A above. The excitatory input signal activates the principal cell (P) which in turn projects to the next major cell group. A collateral of the principal cell excites local interneurons (INT), which in turn inhibit the population of principal cells that excited them.

cuitry is more complex than suggested by ideas that were developed in the early days of hippocampal investigations. Recent data from many laboratories suggest that the general principles of hippocampal organization diverge significantly from the concepts of simple serial processing and recurrent inhibitory circuits. We propose that signal processing within the hippocampus is carried out via parallel systems that operate concomitantly with serial activity transfer. Further, our evidence indicates that the local circuitry within each hippocampal subregion consists of a rich variety of interneuron subtypes, each with somewhat different circuitry. Although recurrent inhibition certainly affects hippocampal function, feedforward inhibition plays a significant and perhaps dominant role.

Finally, we propose a functional model of the hippocampus based on its division into two cortical subregions, Cornu Ammonis (or Ammon's horn) and the dentate gyrus. We have been struck, in reviewing both electrophysiological and morphological data, with a set of intriguing parallels between Ammon's horn and the dentate gyrus, parallels that seem to organize the areas into basic processing units. These units involve two primary cell types within each subregion. Within the pyramidal cell region, the CA1 and CA3 pyramidal cells are output cells, with the CA1 cells providing the major efferent with respect to cortical interaction, and CA3 cells supplying the prominent contralateral connections (in addition to its subcortical output) (Blackstad, 1956; Gottlieb and Cowan, 1973; Swanson et al., 1981). In the dentate region, the granule cells constitute the "output" population; another cell type, the "mossy" cells, provide the major projection to contralateral dentate gyrus. Within each region, a variety of interneurons interact with these projection cells. The interneurons are characterized by different connectivities, different intrinsic cellular properties, and different neurotransmitters and other immunocytochemical markers.

In the following sections, we will illustrate the parallels between Ammon's horn and the dentate gyrus, comparing specific cell types and their roles within each region. It should be noted at the outset that, although we think the similarities and parallels are intriguing and potentially important for information processing in the hippocampus, we do not imply that these two regions parallel each other exactly. Clearly, there are important differences, and these will be identified.

Comparison between CA1 pyramidal cells and dentate gyrus granule cells

The properties of the CA1 pyramidal cells and granule cells have been explored at length in previous reports (see Schwartzkroin and Mueller, 1987, for review), and therefore will not be detailed here. For purposes of comparison, however, it is important to note that both cell populations receive input from the perforant path (Ramón y Cajal, 1911; Lorente de Nó, 1934; Steward and Scoville, 1976; Witter et al., 1988), and both populations serve as primary output cells for their respective regions (the CA1 cells for hippocampus in general, the granule cells for the dentate gyrus). Both are enmeshed in a complex interaction with a variety of interneurons, most of which appear to be inhibitory, but with each interneuron sub-population exhibiting distinctive properties (see below). The major cortical input to granule cells and CA1 pyramidal cells is from the perforant path, which is thought to use glutamate as the neurotransmitter (Cotman and Nadler, 1981). This excitatory amino acid apparently interacts with NMDA and non-NMDA-displaceable glutamate receptors (Watkins and Evans, 1981; Monaghan et al., 1983; Hablitz and Langmoen, 1986; Lambert and Jones, 1989). Although densely innervated by the perforant path, the "unitary" EPSP amplitude at the afferent-to-CA1 and afferent-to-GC synapse is modest ($100-150$ μV) (McNaughton et al., 1981; Sayer et al., 1988), and discharge of the postsynaptic neuron depends on summation of excitatory inputs. Both cell types receive modulatory influences from a variety of subcortical structures, including GABAergic and cholinergic inputs from the septum (Frotscher and Léránth, 1985; Freund and Antal, 1988), noradrenergic input from the locus coeruleus (Loy et al., 1980), and serotonergic input from raphe nuclei (Moore and Halaris, 1975). Finally, the pyramidal cells of CA1 and the granule cells are both apparently glutamatergic (Ottersen and Storm-Mathisen, 1984). Even apparent differences between CA1 and granule cells may, upon detailed analysis, give way to similarities. For example, CA1 receives input not only from the perforant path, but also from the collaterals of the CA3 pyramidal cells, whereas the primary excitatory input to granule cells is from the perforant path fibers. Recent morphological data, however, suggest that the dentate molecular layer, which contains dendrites of both granule cells and interneurons, also receives a dense,

presumably excitatory input from another source, the hilar mossy cells (Amaral, 1978; Ribak et al., 1985). Thus, in this input to granule cells, there is a parallel to the CA3 projection to CA1.

There are important differences between CA1 and granule cells which deserve comment. The CA1 cell population, at least under certain conditions, appears to be quite susceptible to damage; CA1 pyramidal cells are the hippocampal cells most sensitive to ischemic insults and some forms of hyperexcitability (Pulsinelli et al., 1982; Sloviter, 1983). Damage to the granule cells is much less common. Immunocytochemical analysis for calcium-binding proteins has shown that, although both the CA1 pyramidal cells and the dentate granule cells contain CaBP (calbindin-D_{28K}), the granule cell immunoreactivity is more intense than that in CA1 (Fig. 2A). The greater calcium-binding protein content of granule cells may help protect them from insults that trigger increases in intracellular calcium. At the single cell electrophysiological level, the relative insensitivity of granule cells is correlated with their extremely negative resting potential (as observed in intracellular recording) and their high threshold to excitatory input. At least in in vitro preparations, granule cells exhibit little spontaneous activity and fire synaptically-triggered action potentials only with relatively intense afferent input. Because of their negative resting potential, IPSPs in granule cells often appear to be depolarizing, whereas IPSPs in CA1 (recorded from pyramidal cell somata) are hyperpolarizing. However, when granule cells are appropriately depolarized, it is clear that they, like the CA1 pyramidal cells, exhibit both early and late component hyperpolarizing IPSPs. Thus, the pattern of synaptic activity in the two cell populations appears quite similar when the cells are driven by afferent input.

Comparison between CA3 pyramidal cells and mossy cells

The CA3 pyramidal cells of Ammon's horn have been studied extensively and are well characterized

(Wong et al., 1984), whereas relatively little information is available about mossy cells (see, however, Scharfman and Schwartzkroin, 1988). The focus of this section will therefore be on the mossy cells of the dentate hilus. However, it is worthwhile to point out some of the notable features of the CA3 pyramidal cells to facilitate comparison with mossy cells. The CA3 cells are the population of large pyramidal cells (Fig. 3B) in Ammon's horn, and receive afferent input from the perforant path on their distal apical dendrites (Hjorth-Simonsen and Jeune, 1972). In addition, they receive powerful synaptic input from the granule cells, the axons of which make up the mossy fiber pathway that terminates on CA3 proximal dendrites (Blackstad et al., 1970). The mossy

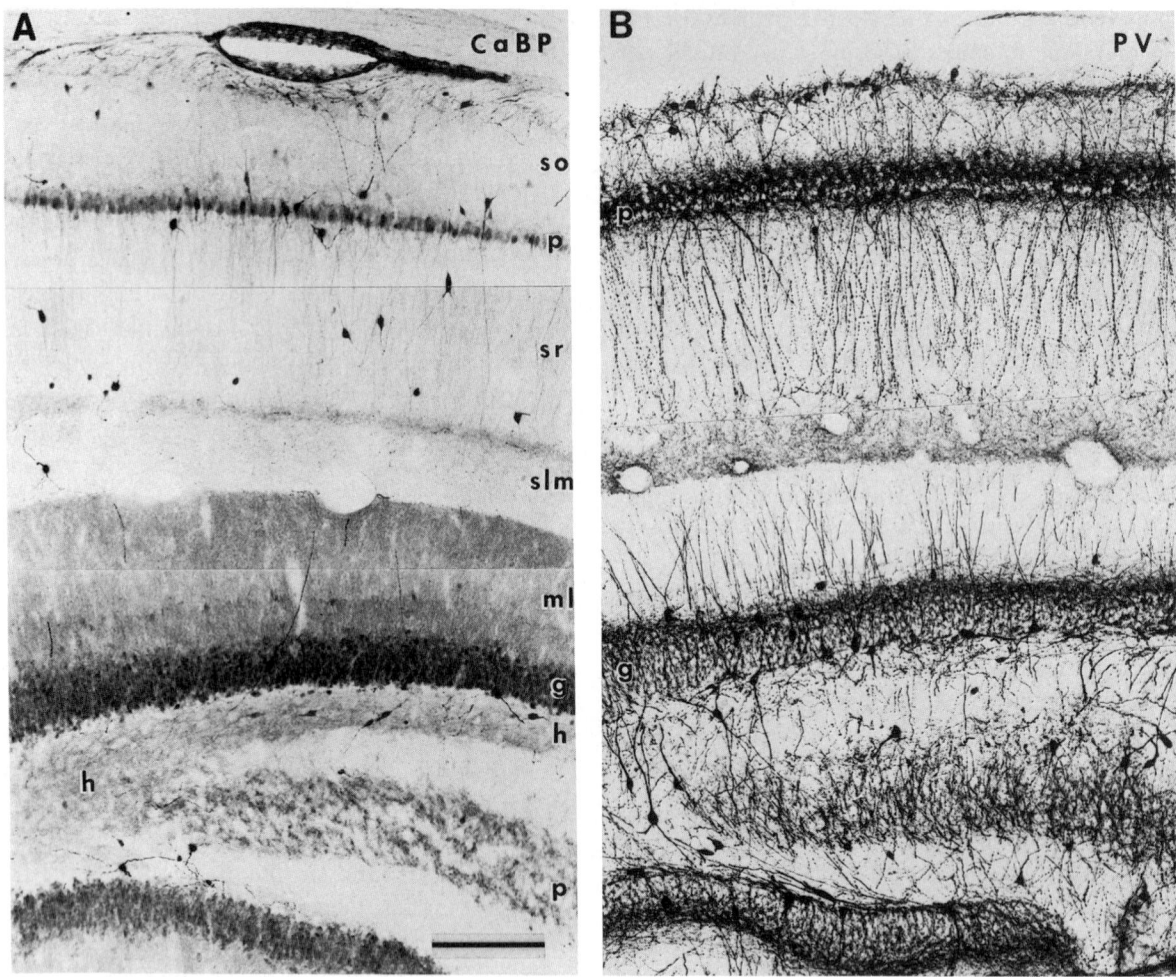

Fig. 2. Immunocytochemical demonstration of calcium-binding proteins in sections through the CA1 and dentate regions of hippocampus. A: Calbindin D_{28K} (CaBP)-like immunoreactivity. Note that CaBP staining is most dense in the dentate granule cell layer; the pyramidal cells of CA1 are less densely immunoreactive, and the CA3 pyramidal cells show no immunoreactivity. Scattered interneurons show dense CaBP immunoreactivity in all subregions. B: parvalbumin (PV)-like immunoreactivity. The dense staining around the pyramidal cell bodies in CA1 and granule cells in the dentate represents the axo-somatic plexuses formed by the basket cell subpopulation that is PV-immunoreactive. Abbreviations: so, stratum oriens; p, stratum pyramidale; sr, stratum radiatum; slm, stratum lacunosum-moleculare; ml, molecular layer of the dentate gyrus; g, granule cell layer; h, hilus. Calibration bar in A (for A and B) = 200 μm.

fiber input produces EPSPs when directly stimulated, and high amplitude spontaneous synaptic "noise" can be recorded in CA3 pyramidal cells, presumably due to synaptic release from mossy fiber terminals (Brown et al., 1979). Because the mossy fiber-to-CA3 "unitary" EPSPs are large, relatively little summation is needed to discharge CA3 neurons. Intrinsic properties of the CA3 pyramidal cells distinguished them from CA1, particularly the propensity of CA3 pyramidal cells to generate burst discharges when the cell is depolarized. Unlike the CA1 cell, which produces regular accommodating trains of action potentials when depolarizing current pulses are injected intracellularly, the CA3 pyramidal cell is likely to produce a burst arising from a large

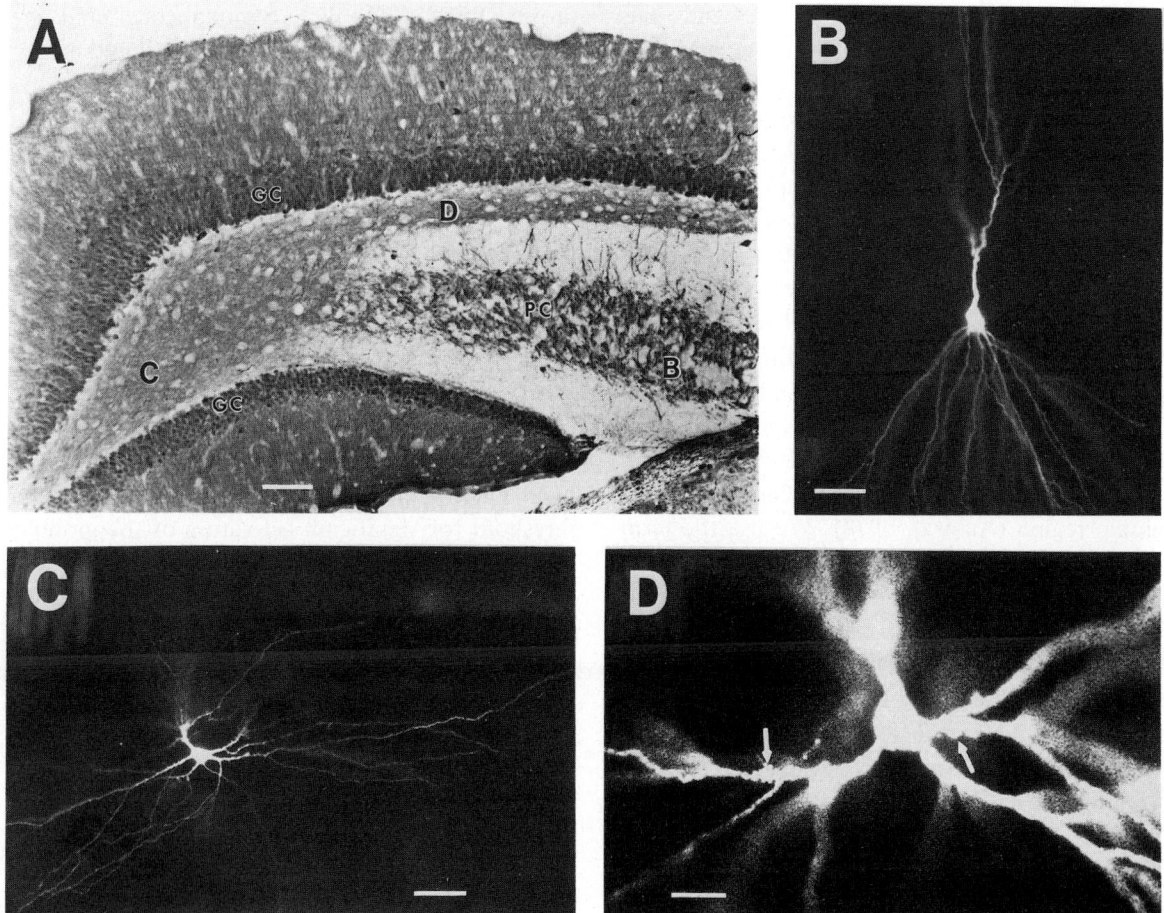

Fig. 3. A: overview of the dentate region (as seen with CaBP immunocytochemistry), showing the locations of the cells shown in B, C, and D. The hilus is the gray region just within the blades of the granule cell layers (GC). The pyramidal cell region of CA3c (PC) extends between the upper and lower blades of the granule cells, but ends as it approaches the hilus. Calibration bar = 95 μm. B: intracellularly stained (with Lucifer yellow) CA3c pyramidal cell, recorded at position B (as shown in part A of this figure). Calibration bar = 140 μm. C: a Lucifer yellow-stained mossy cell (located at position C on part A of this figure). The mossy cell is quite distinct from the CA3c pyramidal cell, with major dendrites that radiate out in a broad plane, extending across the hilus. Calibration bar = 100 μm. D: high-power micrograph of a different Lucifer yellow-stained mossy cell (located at position D in part A of this figure). Note the large swellings and elaborate spine-like processes on the proximal dendrites (arrows). Calibration bar = 20 μm. (C + D from Scharfman and Schwartzkroin (1988) *J. Neurosci.*, 8: 3812 – 3821. Reprinted with permission.)

depolarization. This latter event has been shown to be due primarily to a calcium current (Wong and Prince, 1978). The burst discharge propensity of these CA3 cells contributes to the role of the CA3 region as a "pacemaker" for interictal discharge in hippocampus (Wong and Schwartzkroin, 1982). The burst discharge propensity may also act as a "booster" mechanism, amplifying incoming excitatory signals from afferent pathways.

The CA3 region of Ammon's horn extends into the mouth of the dentate hilus (Fig. 3A), and ends where the CA3c cells (Lorente de Nó, 1934) become intermingled with hilar cells. The exact CA3c/hilar border is difficult to identify. Indeed, the distinction between dentate hilar neurons and CA3/CA4 pyramidal cells has been debated in the literature for a number of years. However, recent studies (Amaral, 1978) have clearly defined the boundaries of the dentate hilus, within which are found a variety of cell types including the mossy cells (Fig. 3C,D). The hilar cells have been referred to as "CA4 cells" (Lorente de Nó, 1934), a term that is inconsistent with the structural and functional association of this cell population with the dentate region (Amaral, 1978). We use the term "mossy cells" to refer to a specific subset of dentate hilar neurons. This descriptive name (Amaral, 1978) reflects the extremely dense coating of spines and "thorny excrescences" that covers their proximal dendrites, so that the cell appears to be covered with "moss" (Fig. 3D). These mossy cells constitute the most numerous of the hilar cell types (Amaral, 1978; Ribak et al., 1985), have large multi-polar cell bodies, and an extremely large dendritic tree that spans the hilus and can extend into the dentate molecular layer (Amaral, 1978). Like the CA3 pyramidal cells, axon collaterals of the mossy cells ramify ipsilaterally within the dendritic region of their target cells (i.e. the inner molecular layer of the dentate). Also like the CA3 pyramidal cell, mossy cells send axonal processes contralaterally. Whereas the contralateral projection of CA3 cells makes contact within the CA3 and CA1 regions, the mossy cell collateral projects to the homotopic inner molecular layer of the den-

tate gyrus (Laurberg and Sørensen, 1981).

Mossy cells are easily distinguishable electrophysiologically from surrounding interneurons and granule cells of the dentate region, but are similar to the CA3 pyramidal cells in many respects (Scharfman and Schwartzkroin, 1988) (Fig. 4). Mossy cells receive excitatory synaptic input from the axon collaterals of the granule cells which, like the mossy fiber terminals onto CA3 cells, produce large EPSPs (Fig. 4C). Simultaneous dual intracellular recordings from granule cells and mossy cells confirm that the mossy cells receive a significant direct excitatory input from the granule cells, and that this granule cell input produces very large unitary EPSPs on its postsynaptic target (Fig. 4D). The mossy cells display high input resistance and long time constants (Fig. 4A), again similar to the properties of CA3 pyramidal cells. Furthermore, the mossy cells, like the CA3 neurons, are burst-prone (Fig. 4B), and show high levels of baseline synaptic activity. Mossy cells respond to low-intensity perforant path stimulation with short-latency EPSPs, and are likely to discharge in a burst pattern in response to stimuli that are subthreshold for significant activation of the granule cell population.

The neurotransmitter system of the mossy cells, like the CA3 pyramidal cells, appears to be glutamatergic (Storm-Mathisen et al., 1983), although definitive evidence is still lacking. The CA3 pyramidal cells and mossy cells are also similar in their lack of calcium-binding proteins (Fig. 2). Immunocytochemical studies suggest that the mossy cells and CA3 pyramidal cells contain neither parvalbumin nor CaBP (Sloviter, 1989). The absence of calcium-binding proteins in these cells may be one explanation for their extreme vulnerability to damage in a number of animal models of tissue hyperexcitability.

Although the parallels between CA3 pyramidal cells and mossy cells are striking, they do differ importantly in a number of respects. Although there is a powerful excitatory afferent drive to CA3 pyramidal cells by the mossy fibers, these evoked EPSPs are abruptly and powerfully curtailed by

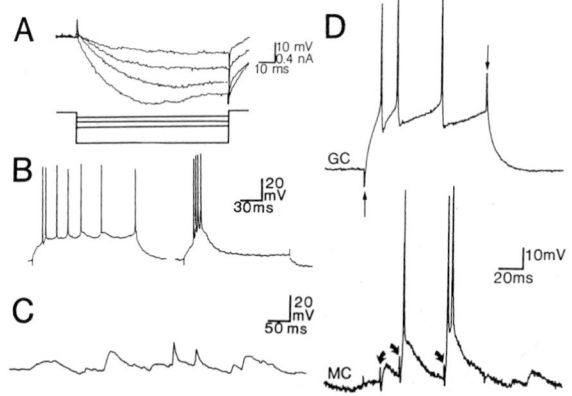

Fig. 4. Electrophysiology of mossy cells. A: response of the cell in Fig. 3D to hyperpolarizing current pulses (100 ms duration; 0.2, 0.3, and 0.6 nA). Resting membrane potential (RMP) of this cell was −60 mV. B: left: response of a mossy cell to a 0.3 nA, 300 ms depolarizing current pulse. RMP of this cell was −70 mV; right: the response of the cell in Fig. 3C to a 0.3 nA, 300 ms depolarizing pulse. Note that this cell discharged in a burst-like pattern in response to the depolarizing current. RMP = −65 mV. C: spontaneous activity recorded from a mossy cell that was hyperpolarized to a membrane potential of −74 mV from its RMP of −66 mV. Note the large amplitudes and varying waveforms of the spontaneous synaptic potentials. D: response of a granule cell (GC) to a 0.3 nA, 100 ms depolarizing current pulse (top), and of a simultaneously recorded mossy cell (MC) located approximately 300 μm away from the granule cell (bottom). Straight arrows in the top trace indicate the on and off artifacts of the current pulse. Curved arrows in the bottom trace indicate the coupling artifacts produced by granule cell action potentials. For each action potential discharge by the granule cell, there was a depolarizing synaptic potential (first spike) or spike discharge (second and third GC spike) evoked in the mossy cell. Granule cell RMP = −70 mV; mossy cell RMP = −60 mV. (A−C from Scharfman and Schwartzkroin (1988) *J. Neurosci.*, 8: 3812−3821. Reprinted with permission.)

IPSP activity (mediated via local circuitry) (Schwartzkroin and Kunkel, 1982). Little evidence of powerful inhibition onto mossy cells has been obtained in the electrophysiological studies on these cells, despite the fact that GABA-negative mossy cells exhibit GABA-LI terminals around their somata (Sloviter and Nilaver, 1987). Another apparent difference between CA3 and mossy cell circuitry is their association with glutamate receptor subtypes. There is a high density of kainate-displaceable glutamate receptors associated with

mossy fiber terminals on CA3 cells (Monaghan et al., 1985), and these cells are especially sensitive to intraventricularly injected kainate (Nadler et al., 1978). CA3 pyramidal cells do not appear to be affected by mossy fiber-mediated NMDA transmission (although the more distal input may have a significant NMDA component). In contrast, the NMDA subtype of glutamate receptor may play an important role in mossy cell activation. Preliminary data suggest that the vulnerability of mossy cells in some experimental paradigms can be blocked by treating the tissue with NMDA receptor blockers (Scharfman and Schwartzkroin, 1989a), although it is unclear whether this NMDA-related action is associated with perforant path or granule cell synapses onto mossy cells. Thus, both CA3 pyramidal cells and mossy cells are vulnerable to injury in specific experimental paradigms, but the mechanisms of their vulnerability appear to be somewhat different.

Interneuron populations of Ammon's horn and dentate gyrus

The classical Golgi studies of Ramón y Cajal (1911) and Lorente de Nó (1934) illustrated a large variety of interneuron cell types throughout the hippocampus. Despite the breadth of the anatomical data, physiological studies of the hippocampus compressed the interneuron population into one conceptual group, and attributed recurrent inhibition to these so-called "basket cells" (Andersen et al., 1964a, b). Recent studies − electrophysiological, morphological, and immunocytochemical − have reinforced the original observations of interneuron variety in both Ammon's horn and dentate gyrus (Amaral, 1978; Ribak and Seress, 1983; Kawaguchi and Hama, 1987; Lacaille et al., 1987; Sloviter and Nilaver, 1987; Lacaille and Schwartzkroin, 1988b). In our description of interneurons, we will try to convey some sense of the diversity of hippocampal interneuron cell types, describing what little we know about specific subpopulations and their connections. We will, however, inevitably over-simplify this subject area in an attempt at organization and clarity. We propose that there are significant parallels in the interneuron populations of Ammon's horn and dentate gyrus, and we will try to illustrate the similarities in interneuronal populations observed in these two major hippocampal regions. The initial basis for our categorization is electrophysiological observation made on the cell populations in the CA1 region (Lacaille et al., 1989). These data are supplemented with morphological and immunocytochemical findings in both Ammon's horn and dentate gyrus, as well as by recent electrophysiological studies in the dentate hilus.

The basket cells

One conspicuous population of interneurons in both the Ammon's horn and the dentate region are the so-called "basket cells". These are large neurons located within or adjacent to the pyramidale (Fig. 6A) or granulosum strata, with major dendritic trees that extend parallel to the dendrites of the principal cells into their respective dendritic regions (Amaral, 1978). The dendrites are aspinous, and receive a high density of synaptic contacts (Ribak and Anderson, 1980; Frotscher and Zimmer, 1983; Schwartzkroin and Kunkel, 1985). Clearly, these cells are in a position to receive powerful direct excitatory input not only via axon collaterals of the principal cell population – as would be required to mediate feedback inhibition – but also directly from major afferents. The basket cells are GABAergic (as shown with GABA and GAD immunocytochemistry) (Ribak et al., 1978; Gamrani et al., 1986) (Fig. 5A), and extend widely ramifying axonal processes that form terminal plexuses around pyramidal and granule cell bodies (Blackstad and Flood, 1963). A striking subpopulation of these GABAergic basket cells is immunopositive for the calcium-binding protein, parvalbumin (Fig. 2B) (Kosaka et al., 1987; Sloviter, 1989). In addition, another subpopulation of the basket cells contains cholecystokinin (CCK) (Kosaka et al., 1985; Sloviter and Nilaver,

1987); the function of CCK in these cells is presently unknown.

Electrophysiologically, the basket cells are identifiable by their short-duration action potentials, large hyperpolarizing after-potentials, and relatively high level of spontaneous activity (compared to the CA1 pyramidal cells and granule cells) (Schwartzkroin and Mathers, 1978; Kawaguchi and Hama, 1988) (Fig. 6A). They have relatively low activation thresholds; i.e., they can be activated with stimulus strengths below that required to discharge pyramidal cells (from stimulation in strata radiatum, oriens, or alveus) or granule cells (from perforant path stimulation). Dual intracellular recordings of basket cells and CA1 pyramidal cells have shown that the interneurons directly inhibit pyramidal cells, and also may receive direct excitatory PSPs from pyramidal cells. Thus, they are interposed in a circuitry that can mediate feedback inhibition as well as feedforward inhibition (Knowles and Schwartzkroin, 1981). Also striking in this interneuron population is the absence of spike firing accommodation (Fig. 6A). Unlike the pyramidal cells or granule cells, basket cells continue to fire action potentials at high rates when they are tonically depolarized.

Somatostatin- and neuropeptide Y-containing interneurons

In both the pyramidal cell and granule cell regions, there are populations of interneurons that show somatostatin-like immunoreactivity (SS-LI) (Köhler and Chan-Palay, 1982; Morrison et al., 1982; Sloviter and Nilaver, 1987) (Fig. 5B). Many of these cells also exhibit neuropeptide Y-like immunoreactivity (NPY-LI) (Köhler et al., 1987). In CA1, the SS interneuron population is localized primarily in the stratum oriens, and particularly at the border of oriens and alveus (Fig. 6B). Cell morphology is diverse, with most cells of medium size and somewhat spindle-shaped. They extend dendrites parallel to the axis of the alvear fibers, and also send long dendrites through strata oriens and pyramidale deep into strata radiatum and

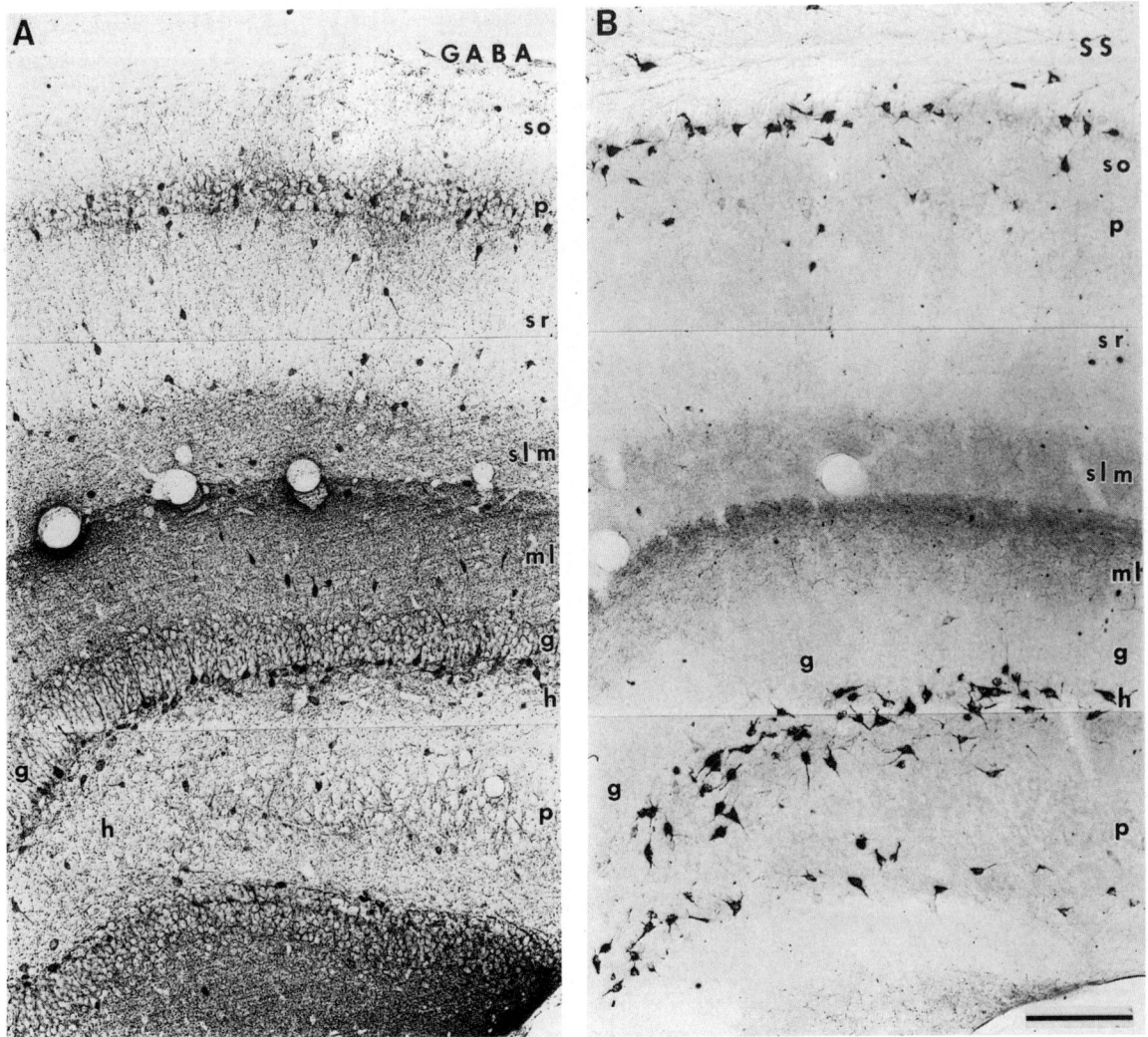

Fig. 5. Immunocytochemical demonstration of γ-aminobutyric acid (GABA) and somatostatin (SS) in sections through CA1 and the dentate gyrus of hippocampus. A: GABA-like immunoreactivity. Interneurons throughout CA1 and the dentate gyrus are immunoreactive. The densest concentrations of GABA-positive cells are the interneurons within the pyramidal layer of CA1, and those just basal to the granule cells in the dentate. Note that relatively few large cells in the hilus are GABA-immunoreactive. B: somatostatin immunoreactivity. Two major concentrations of SS-immunoreactive neurons are apparent in this profile. One group of cells lies at the border of stratum oriens and the alveus in CA1; the other group is composed of cells scattered within the dentate hilus. Abbreviations and calibration bar are as in Fig. 2.

lacunosum-moleculare of CA1. Axons of these neurons have been found to ramify around the cell bodies and apical dendrites of the CA1 pyramidal cells (Lacaille et al., 1987), but the major axonal ramification appears to be in stratum lacunosum-moleculare (Bakst et al., 1986; Haas et al., 1987; Naus et al., 1988), the region that receives the primary perforant path input. In the granule cell region, the SS-LI neurons are located throughout the dentate hilus. Here, too, the cells are often spindle-shaped and their major axonal projection forms a plexus in the dentate molecular layer where the perforant path terminals are found (Bakst et al., 1986). Data from a number of

278

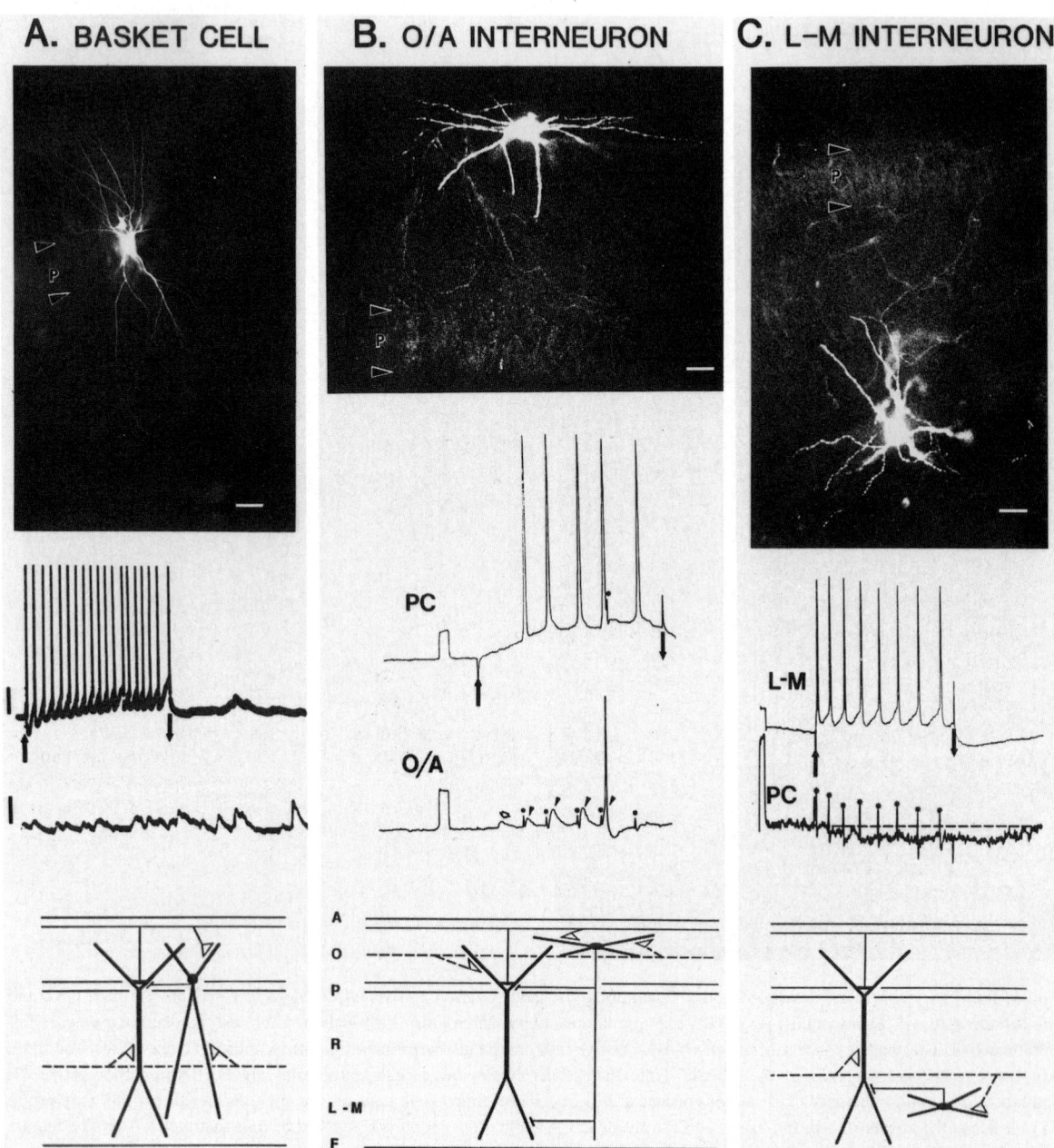

Fig. 6. Interneurons within the CA1 region of Ammon's horn. In each row, the top photo shows an example of an intracellularly stained (with Lucifer yellow) neuron; below each photo are electrophysiological traces illustrating salient features of the cell; finally, the diagram illustrates the interaction of that interneuron type with the CA1 pyramidal cell. A: basket cell. The soma is located within stratum pyramidale (P between arrowheads); aspinous apical and basal dendrites extend into stratum radiatum and stratum oriens (respectively), parallel to the apical and basal dendrites of the pyramidal cell. Calibration bar = 40 μm. Typical electrophysiological properties are illustrated in the two traces below. (From Schwartzkroin and Mathers (1978) *Brain Res.,* 157: 1–10. Reprinted with permission.) Upper: response to a 100 ms depolarizing current pulse (arrows show on and off of current). Note the high rate of firing, and the absence of spike firing adaptation. Spikes are clipped. Calibration bar at the start of the traces = 10 mV; time between arrows is 100 ms. Lower: recording of baseline activity in another such cell. Note the frequent spontaneously occurring synaptic

laboratories suggest that somatostatin (Gothert, 1980; Katayama and Kirai, 1989) and NPY (Colmers et al., 1987) may inhibit transmitter release from primary afferents. Preliminary results of electrophysiological studies in the hippocampus have shown that SS does depress perforant path EPSPs in granule cells when SS is ejected in the outer molecular layer. In CA1, SS ejected near the soma decreases IPSPs by a presynaptic mechanism (Scharfman and Schwartzkroin, 1989b). Thus, the role of SS as a presynaptic modulator of transmitter release has received support in both subregions of hippocampus. However, further studies are needed to elucidate the association of SS- and NPY-LI terminals with the perforant path terminal.

Immunocytochemically, many SS-containing neurons of CA1 and the dentate hilus co-localize GAD (Kosaka et al., 1988; Kunkel and Schwartzkroin, 1988). In the hilus, SS-containing cells contain neither parvalbumin nor CaBP (cf. Figs. 2,

5B), and like the mossy cells, are damaged by repetitive granule cell discharge (Sloviter, 1987). It has been hypothesized that the absence of calcium-binding protein in these cells is the reason for their vulnerability to activity-induced damage (Sloviter, 1989). In CA1, many interneurons of str. oriens exhibit either PV- or CaBP-LI, and do not display the extreme sensitivity of hilar SS cells (Fig. 2).

Electrophysiologically, both populations of SS-positive cells have been shown to receive monosynaptic short-latency inputs from primary afferents to hippocampus. The interneurons of CA1 are sensitive to stimulation in the alveus, strata oriens and radiatum, as well as in stratum lacunosum-moleculare (Lacaille et al., 1987); hilar SS cells are extremely sensitive to perforant path stimulation (Sloviter, 1987). Simultaneous intracellular recordings between CA1 pyramidal cells and oriens/alveus (O/A) interneurons have shown that the O/A cells receive direct excitatory input from the pyramidal cells (Fig. 6B), and also direct-

events. Calibration as in upper trace. Diagram: both pyramidal cell and basket cell are directly excited by afferents; the basket cell is also excited by the recurrent axon collateral of the pyramidal cell; the pyramidal cell is inhibited by the basket cell, primarily via axosomatic synapses. Excitatory synapses are shown by open triangles, inhibitory synapses by solid lines. Abbreviations for CA1 strata are: A, alveus; O, oriens; P, pyramidale; R, radiatum; L-M, lacunosum-moleculare; F, hippocampal fissure. B: oriens/alveus interneuron. The cell body is located at the border of stratum oriens and the alveus. Major dendritic processes radiate parallel to the alveus, but large processes also extend toward and through stratum pyramidale. The axonal arbor ramifies around pyramidal cells, and extends into the apical dendritic region of the CA1 pyramidal cell. Calibration bar = 40 μm. Electrophysiology of the interaction between an oriens/alveus interneuron and a CA1 pyramidal cell is illustrated in simultaneous intracellular impalements obtained from these cells. (From Lacaille et al. (1987) *J. Neurosci.*, 7: 1979–1983. Reprinted with permission.) Depolarizing current (100 ms between arrows) injected into the pyramidal cell (PC) (top trace) caused the cell to discharge a train of 5 action potentials. Spiking of the PC evoked excitatory postsynaptic potentials (first 3 pyramidal cell spikes) or spike discharge (clipped) (fourth pyramidal cell spike) in the O/A interneuron. Arrowheads in the bottom trace point to evoked EPSPs and spike. Asterisks show capacitative artifacts; open arrowhead in the bottom trace shows a PSP that is not associated with spike discharge in the recorded pyramidal cell. Calibration pulses at the beginning of each trace show 10 mV. Diagram: the O/A interneuron is directly activated by afferent input (as is the pyramidal cell). In addition, it receives recurrent excitatory input via the pyramidal cell axon (illustrated above). The O/A interneuron axonal plexus makes synaptic contacts on pyramidal cell body and dendrites, causing PC inhibition. C: lacunosum-moleculare interneuron. The cell body of the L-M interneuron is located at the border of strata radiatum and lacunosum-moleculare. This cell sends dendritic processes in all directions (primarily into strata radiatum and lacunosum-moleculare), extending as far as stratum pyramidale in CA1, and crossing the hippocampal fissure into the dentate gyrus. Axonal processes ramify for long distances. Calibration bar = 40 μm. Electrophysiological demonstration of interneuron inhibition of the pyramidal cell is seen in simultaneous intracellular recordings from an L-M interneuron (top trace) and a CA1 pyramidal cell (PC) (bottom trace). (From Lacaille and Schwartzkroin (1988) *J. Neurosci.*, 8: 1411–1424. Reprinted with permission.) A depolarizing current pulse (100 ms between arrows) injected into the L-M interneuron elicited spike firing in that cell; a resultant slow hyperpolarization was seen in the CA1 pyramidal cell. Asterisks in the bottom trace mark capacitative artifact from spike firing in the L-M interneuron. Calibration pulses at the beginning of each trace show 10 mV. Diagram: L-M interneurons and pyramidal cells both receive direct excitatory afferent input. The L-M interneuron inhibits the pyramidal cell, primarily via dendritically located synapses, but receives no excitatory axon collateral from the PC.

ly inhibit the pyramidal cells. Thus, like the basket cells, they are part of a circuit that can mediate both feedback and feedforward inhibition. Electrophysiological characterization of the SS-containing cells in the hilus, and their relationships to the other cell populations in the dentate gyrus, have not yet been addressed.

Other interneuron cell types

There are a variety of other interneuron cell types that deserve comment. In the CA1 region, an interneuron cell group located at the border of stratum radiatum and stratum lacunosum-moleculare (L-M interneurons) has been characterized electrophysiologically (Lacaille and Schwartzkroin, 1987a) (Fig. 6C). These cells differ from both the basket cells and O/A interneurons in their relatively low spontaneous activity, somewhat broader action potentials, and connectivity with the pyramidal cells. These cells do not receive excitatory input from pyramidal cell axon collaterals. Their afferent drive appears to come from pathways running through the strata radiatum and lacunosum-moleculare. They do, however, inhibit the pyramidal cells via a feedforward circuit (Lacaille and Schwartzkroin, 1987b) (Fig. 6C). Although their cell bodies are localized in a distinct layer of CA1, their dendrites extend throughout the dendritic region of the CA1 cells, and into the dendritic domain of the dentate gyrus. Similarly, their axonal ramifications make contact with both CA1 pyramidal cell and granule cell dendrites. This cell population spans the CA1-granule cell populations, perhaps providing a direct pathway for interaction between the two hippocampal regions. At the immunocytochemical level, the cell population is clearly GABAergic (Babb et al., 1988) (Fig. 5A), and many cells of this stratum exhibit CaBP-LI immunoreactivity (Sloviter, 1989). A subpopulation of these neurons exhibit vasoactive intestinal polypeptide-like immunoreactivity (VIP-LI) (Sloviter and Nilaver, 1987), although the role of this peptide is unknown. VIP cells have also been identified in the dentate hilus (Kosaka et al., 1985; Sloviter and Nilaver, 1987). It is noteworthy, for purposes of parallelism with CA1, that their cell bodies are often found in the dendritic domain of the dentate gyrus (the stratum moleculare) and their axons ramify in the granule cell layer and hilus.

Interneuron subpopulations in both pyramidal and granule cell regions are characterized by a number of other morphological, immunocytochemical, and electrophysiological features. As mentioned above, the peptide cholecystokinin is found in some GABAergic neurons in both regions. In addition, neuropeptide Y has been identified in a diverse population of interneurons (Köhler et al., 1986), some also immunoreactive for SS (Köhler et al., 1987), particularly within the dentate hilus. Electrophysiologically, interneurons within the dentate hilus can be categorized as particularly sensitive or not particularly sensitive to afferent stimulation. Since studies have suggested that the SS-containing interneuron population (which is also devoid of calcium-binding protein) is irreversibly damaged by repetitive granule cell discharge, it is tempting to associate the particularly sensitive interneurons (evaluated in in vitro studies) with these somatostatin-containing cells whose loss has been described in vivo (Sloviter, 1987). However, definitive demonstration of this association awaits further experiments.

It is important, at this point, to discuss briefly just what one means by the term "interneuron". Certainly, local circuit cells, such as the basket cells described above, are aptly described by the "interneuron" nomenclature in that their axons remain within the structure. What about mossy cells? Or even granule cells? These neurons are "projection" cells inasmuch as they send axons out of the local region of the cell body. However, their axons are confined to the hippocampus. Granule cells project no further than the CA3 pyramidal cell region, and mossy cell terminals are confined to the dentate molecular layer ipsilateral and contralateral to the cell body of origin. If the mossy cells were considered "interneurons", i.e. cells that modulate principal cell activity, they would be the first example of an excitatory interneuron identified in hippocampus. From a functional perspective, they seem to fit this definition. Our use of the term "interneuron" within this chapter refers to cells with axons that ramify within the region surrounding the cell body − that is, local circuit neurons. By this definition, neither the granule cells nor the mossy cells are truly "interneurons". This terminology, because it is solely descriptive of anatomical features, is rather limited. How does one describe a basket cell with a commissurally projecting axon that innervates the same principal cell population both ipsi- and contralaterally? Perhaps it is time to begin to describe cell types on the basis of their function as well as structure (e.g. excitatory projection cells, local circuit inhibitory neurons), and avoid generic labels when possible.

The striking features of local circuit neurons within the hippocampus, both Ammon's horn and dentate gyrus, can be summarized as follows:

(1) The variety of cell types, as characterized immunocytochemically, morphologically, and electrophysiologically, is overwhelming. It is unlikely that such a diverse set of cell types mediates a single or simple function.

(2) Although quite different in many respects from each other, the local circuit neurons share a number of electrophysiological and functional characteristics. Most, if not all, are inhibitory and are activated at very low afferent stimulation thresholds. Thus, they are in a position to mediate inhibition via feedforward mechanisms onto pyramidal cells and granule cells. Their sensitivity to input, lack of accommodation when depolarized, and tendency for high firing frequencies suggest that they can mediate powerful influences on the principal cells at input levels below those needed to excite the pyramidal or granule cells.

(3) Although some populations of local circuit neurons are sensitive to excitatory input, and may be destroyed by experimental manipulations or under pathological conditions, many are no more sensitive to trauma than the principal cells. In fact, some of the interneuron populations appear to be *more* resistant to damage than the principal cell. It is unclear what endows the specific cell types with sensitivity or resistance, but one intriguing possibility is the cell's content of calcium-binding proteins. Preliminary studies suggest that vulnerable cells that are low in calcium-binding proteins may be "protected" (from the lethal effects of calcium influx) if the cell is injected with a calcium chelator (Scharfman and Schwartzkroin, 1989a).

Discussion of the parallels between Ammon's horn and the dentate gyrus: principles of hippocampal organization

Given the above description of cell and synaptic organization for Ammon's horn and the dentate gyrus, there are several striking parallels that bear emphasis, and that are illustrated in the diagram of Fig. 7. Clearly, each of these hippocampal subregions has a set of "output neurons", as viewed within the context of cortical input and output. For Ammon's horn, that output population is the CA1 pyramidal cells, and, for the dentate gyrus, the granule cells. In each cell region, there is also a set of cells that have powerful excitatory internal collaterals. In Ammon's horn, these cells are the CA3 pyramidal cells; in the dentate gyrus, the mossy cells have a parallel role. Specifically, CA3 pyramidal cells project to the CA1 pyramidal and local circuit neuron populations, whereas the mossy cells appear to send a collateral system to the dentate molecular layer (although the precise target of these mossy cell collaterals, i.e. granule cell and/or local circuit neuron, has not yet been determined). Only mossy cells and CA3 pyramidal cells send major projections contralaterally to hippocampus. Strikingly, both mossy cells and CA3 pyramidal cells have a tendency toward burst discharge, and therefore appear to act as amplifiers of excitatory synaptic input. Finally, both cells types appear to be relatively sensitive to input from granule cell discharge.

Within the context of this circuitry, the CA3 pyramidal cells may be viewed as the activators of CA1 pyramidal cells and local circuit neurons.

282

Under some conditions, when the CA3 influence favors the activation of basket cells and other inhibitory interneurons, the net effect of CA3 input to CA1 may be primarily inhibitory. Similarly, in the dentate gyrus, the mossy cells may be viewed as the activators of their targets, the granule cells and local circuit neurons of the dentate gyrus. Here, too, the net effect of mossy cell output on its targets may be inhibitory if this output preferentially activates the inhibitory interneuron population. Such a scheme is consistent with experimental data which showed that commissural hilar stimulation (mediated primarily by mossy cells) excited presumed basket cells, and inhibited granule cell

population spikes (Buzsáki and Eidelberg, 1981; Douglas et al., 1983). This inhibitory commissural effect was blocked by bicuculline, leaving only weak excitatory effects on the granule cell population. According to this scenario, then, hilar mossy cells could be regarded as the "CA3" cells of the dentate gyrus. A major function of both CA3 pyramidal cells and dentate mossy cells would be to modulate the activity of the main output neurons by driving both inhibitory local circuit neurons and the output cells (the CA1 cells and granule cells). The balance of excitation and inhibition – and thus the net output – would depend on a complex integration of afferent signals

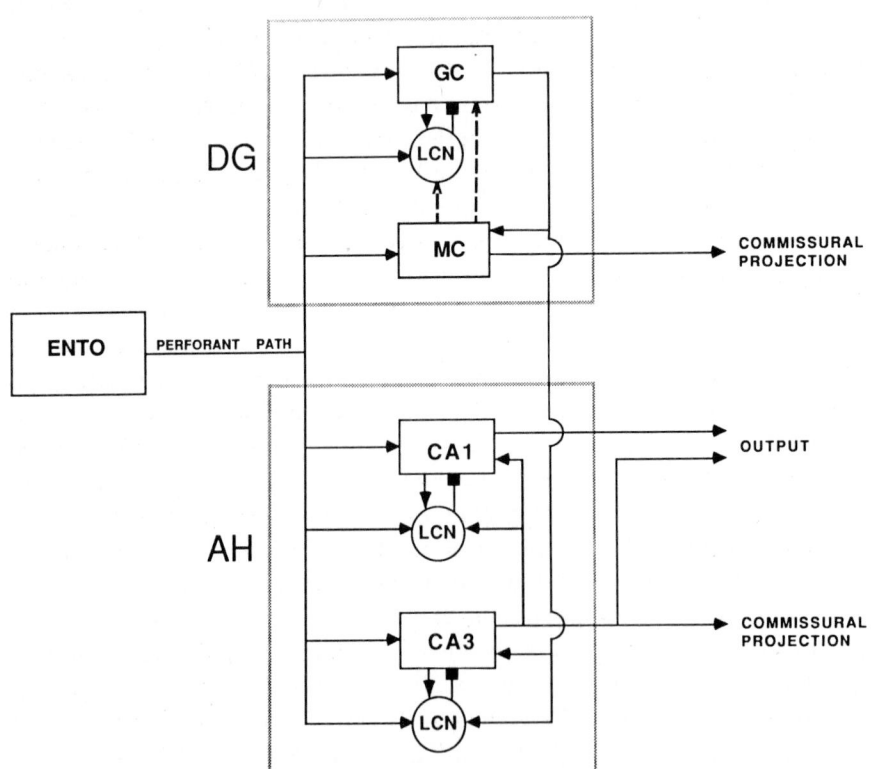

Fig. 7. Diagrammatic representation of local circuitry of the hippocampus, emphasizing: parallel inputs from the entorhinal cortex (ENTO) via the perforant path to each of the cell types in the dentate gyrus (DG) and Ammon's horn (AH); the somewhat analogous position of mossy cells (MC) in the dentate and CA3 pyramidal cells in Ammon's horn; the existence of both feedforward and feedback pathways for inhibition from local circuit neurons (LCN) onto granule cells (GC), CA1 pyramidal cells (CA1), and CA3 pyramidal cells (CA3). Interrupted lines emerging from the MC show proposed, but still to be experimentally verified, excitatory connections with GCs and LCNs.

that bias local circuit neuron and output cell thresholds relative to the input from CA3 and mossy cells.

In both Ammon's horn and the dentate gyrus, it is now clear that afferent input travels via parallel processing pathways, not only via the serial pathways traditionally used to describe hippocampus. Principal cells and local circuit neurons receive direct afferent input from the perforant path. Importantly, the direct afferent input to inhibitory interneurons in each subregion comprises part of a potent pathway for feedforward inhibition. Also striking within each subregion is the rich diversity of local circuit cell types, each of which may be involved in subtly different interactions with the principal cells and with each other. Distinct local circuit neuron subpopulations have already been identified, with specific circuitries, neurotransmitter content, metabolic levels, and calcium-binding protein capabilities. Despite this rich variety, Fig. 7 groups these local circuit neurons (LCNs) into a single category − in part to simplify the figure, but also to emphasize some important and distinctive properties shared by LCNs. As has long been suspected, most LCNs are GABAergic, and presumably mediate inhibition. Most of these interneuron populations also have low thresholds to afferent stimulation, a relative absence of accommodation, and a tendency for repetitive discharge. They are thus well equipped to inhibit, via feedforward circuitry, the output of the principal cell population.

Clearly, there are important differences between the Ammon's horn and dentate gyrus regions. For example, CA1 neurons project completely out of hippocampus, whereas the granule cell projection is exclusively within the hippocampus. Granule cells are relatively stable and insensitive to insult, whereas the CA1 projection cells are often vulnerable to damage. Granule cells project powerfully onto the mossy cell population, whereas CA1 cells send no such projection to the CA3 pyramidal cells. The purpose of this chapter is not to prove that the subregions are precisely parallel in their function and structure. Rather, our goal has been to present a more realistic way of thinking about hippocampal circuitry and information processing (e.g. Fig. 7), which may be summarized as follows: first, the idea of "serial" processing of afferent information, from one hippocampal subregion to another, is misleading, and based on an oversimplification of hippocampal anatomy. The routing of afferent information occurs over "parallel", as well as "serial" pathways, with afferent inputs synapsing directly onto virtually all principal cells and LCNs of both Ammon's horn and dentate gyrus. Second, the local circuitry within a given region most certainly involves not only feedback, but also feedforward actions of LCNs. In fact, the feedforward effect may be primary, given the finding of a low threshold of LCNs to direct afferent input. Third, there are multiple LCN populations, each with specific function, characteristic interconnections, and special cell properties. Some of these cell populations appear in both Ammon's horn and the dentate gyrus; many of them contain GABA and a colocalized peptide. Although we do not yet understand the specific roles of these LCN subpopulations, it would be a mistake to assume that they all play equivalent roles in hippocampal circuitry. We believe that these concepts may more closely approximate the manner in which hippocampal information is routed and integrated, and may also be applicable to analyses of cortical structures in other parts of the central nervous system.

Acknowledgements

The work reviewed in this chapter was supported by an equipment gift from the Helen Hayes Hospital Citizens Advisory Council and by NIH Grant NS 18201 to R.S.S.; by NIH Grants NS 18895, NS 15317, and NS 20482 to P.A.S.; and by NIH postdoctoral training Grant NS 01744 to H.E.S. P.A.S. is a research affiliate of the Child Development and Mental Retardation Center, University of Washington, Seattle, Washington.

284

References

Amaral, D.G. (1978) A Golgi study of cell type in the hilar region of the hippocampus in the rat. *J. Comp. Neurol.,* 132: 851 – 914.

Andersen, P. (1975) The organization of hippocampal neurons and their interconnections. in R.L. Isaacson and K.H. Pribram (Eds.), *The Hippocampus: Structure and Development, Vol. 1,* Plenum, New York, pp. 155 – 175.

Andersen, P., Eccles, J.C. and Løyning, Y. (1964a) Location of postsynaptic inhibitory synapses on hippocampal pyramids. *J. Neurophysiol.,* 27: 592 – 607.

Andersen, P., Eccles, J.C. and Løyning, Y. (1964b) Pathway of postsynaptic inhibition in the hippocampus. *J. Neurophysiol.,* 27: 608 – 619.

Babb, T.L., Pretorius, J.K., Kupfer, W.R. and Brown, W.J. (1988) Distribution of glutamate-decarboxylase immunoreactive neurons and synapses in the rat and monkey hippocampus: light and electron microscopy. *J. Comp. Neurol.,* 278: 121 – 138.

Bakst, I., Avendano, C., Morrison, J.H. and Amaral, D.G. (1986) An experimental analysis of the origins of somatostatin-like immunoreactivity in the dentate gyrus of the rat. *J. Neurosci.,* 6: 1452 – 1462.

Blackstad, T.W. (1956) Commissural connections of the hippocampal region in the rat, with special reference to their mode of termination. *J. Comp. Neurol.,* 105: 417 – 538.

Blackstad, T.W. and Flood, P.R. (1963) Ultrastructure of hippocampal axosomatic synapses. *Nature (Lond.),* 198: 542 – 543.

Blackstad, T.W., Brink, K., Hem, J. and Jeune, B. (1970) Distribution of hippocampal mossy fibers in the rat: an experimental study with silver impregnation methods. *J. Comp. Neurol.,* 138: 433 – 449.

Brown, T.H., Wong, R.K.S. and Prince, D.A. (1979) Spontaneous miniature synaptic potentials in hippocampal neurons. *Brain Res.,* 177: 194 – 199.

Buzsáki, G. and Eidelberg, E. (1981) Commissural projections to the dentate gyrus of the rat: evidence for feed-forward inhibition. *Brain Res.,* 230: 346 – 350.

Colmers, W.F., Lukowiak, K. and Pittman, Q.J. (1987) Presynaptic action of neuropeptide Y in area CA1 of rat hippocampal slice. *J. Physiol. (Lond.),* 383: 285 – 299.

Cotman, C.W. and Nadler, J.V. (1981) Glutamate and aspartate as hippocampal transmitters: biochemical and pharmacological evidence. In P.J. Roberts, J. Storm-Mathisen and G.A.R. Johnston (Eds.), *Glutamate: Transmitter in the Nervous System,* Wiley, New York, pp. 177 – 154.

Douglas, R.M., McNaughton, B.L. and Goddard, G. (1983) Commissural inhibition and facilitation of granule cell discharge in fascia dentata. *J. Comp. Neurol.,* 219: 285 – 294.

Freund, T.F. and Antal, M. (1988) GABA-containing neurons in the septum control inhibitory interneurons in the hippocampus. *Nature (Lond.),* 336: 170 – 173.

Frotscher, M. and Léránth, C. (1985) Cholinergic innervation of the rat hippocampus as revealed by choline acetyltransferase immunocytochemistry: a combined light and electron microscopic study. *J. Comp. Neurol.,* 239: 237 – 246.

Frotscher, M. and Zimmer, J. (1983) Commissural fibers terminate on non-pyramidal neurons in the guinea pig hippocampus – a combined Golgi/EM degeneration study. *Brain Res.,* 265: 289 – 293.

Gamrani, H., Onteniente, P., Seguela, P., Geffard, M. and Calas, A. (1986) Gamma-aminobutyric acid-immunoreactivity in the rat hippocampus. A light and electron microscopic study with anti-GABA antibodies. *Brain Res.,* 364: 30 – 38.

Gothert, M. (1980) Somatostatin selectivity inhibits noradrenaline release from hypothalamic neurones. *Nature (Lond.),* 288: 86 – 88.

Gottlieb, D.I. and Cowan, W.M. (1973) Autoradiographic studies of the commissural and associational connections of the hippocampus and dentate gyrus of the rat. I. The commissural connection. *J. Comp. Neurol.,* 149: 383 – 422.

Haas, H.L., Hermann, A., Greene, R.W. and Chan-Palay, V. (1987) Action and location of neuropeptide tyrosine (Y) on hippocampal neurons of the rat in slice preparation. *J. Comp. Neurol.,* 257: 208 – 215.

Hablitz, J.J. and Langmoen, I.A. (1986) *N*-methyl-D-aspartate receptor antagonists reduce synaptic excitation in the hippocampus. *J. Neurosci.,* 6: 102 – 110.

Hjorth-Simonsen, A. and Jeune, B. (1972) Origin and termination of the hippocampal perforant path in the rat studied by silver impregnation. *J. Comp. Neurol.,* 144: 215 – 232.

Katayama, Y. and Hirai, K. (1989) Somatostatin presynaptically inhibits transmitter release in feline parasympathetic ganglia. *Brain Res.,* 487: 62 – 68.

Kawaguchi, Y. and Hama, K. (1987) Two subtypes of non-pyramidal cells in rat hippocampal formation identified by intracellular recording and HRP injection. *Brain Res.,* 411: 190 – 195.

Kawaguchi, Y. and Hama, K. (1988) Physiological heterogeneity of nonpyramidal cells in rat hippocampal CA1 region. *Exp. Brain Res.,* 72: 494 – 502.

Knowles, W.D. and Schwartzkroin, P.A. (1981) Local circuit interactions in hippocampal brain slices. *J. Neurosci.,* 1: 318 – 322.

Köhler, C. and Chan-Palay, V. (1982) Somatostatin-like immunoreactive neurons in the hippocampus: an immunocytochemical study in the rat. *Neurosci. Lett.,* 34: 259 – 264.

Köhler, C., Eriksson, I., Davies, S. and Chan-Palay, V. (1986) Neuropeptide Y innervation of the hippocampal region in the rat and monkey brain. *J. Comp. Neurol.,* 244: 384 – 400.

Köhler, C., Eriksson, L.G., Davies, S. and Chan-Palay, V. (1987) Co-localization of neuropeptide tyrosine and somatostatin immunoreactivity in neurons of individual subfields of the rat hippocampal region. *Neurosci. Lett.,* 78: 1–6.

Kosaka, T., Kosaka, K., Tateishi, K., Hamaoka, Y., Yanaihara, N., Wu, J.-Y. and Hama, K. (1985) GABAergic neurons containing CCK-8-like and/or VIP-like immunoreactivities in the rat hippocampus and dentate gyrus. *J. Comp. Neurol.,* 239: 420–430.

Kosaka, T., Katsumaru, H., Hama, K., Wu, J.-Y. and Heizmann, C.W. (1987) GABAergic neurons containing the Ca^{2+}-binding protein parvalbumin in the rat hippocampus and dentate gyrus. *Brain Res.,* 419: 119–130.

Kosaka, T., Wu, J.-Y. and Benoit, R. (1988) GABAergic neurons containing somatostatin-like immunoreactivity in the rat hippocampus and dentate gyrus. *Exp. Brain Res.,* 71: 388–398.

Kunkel, D.D. and Schwartzkroin, P.A. (1988) Ultrastructural characterization and GAD co-localization of somatostatin-like immunoreactive neurons in CA1 of rabbit hippocampus. *Synapse,* 2: 371–381.

Lacaille, J.-C. and Schwartzkroin, P.A. (1988a) Stratum lacunosum-moleculare interneurons of hippocampal CA1 region. I. Intracellular response characteristics, synaptic responses, and morphology. *J. Neurosci.,* 8: 1400–1410.

Lacaille, J.-C. and Schwartzkroin, P.A. (1988b) Stratum lacunosum-moleculare interneurons of hippocampal CA1 region. II. Intrasomatic and intradendritic recording of local circuit interactions. *J. Neurosci.,* 8: 1411–1424.

Lacaille, J.-C., Mueller, A.L., Kunkel, D.D. and Schwartzkroin, P.A. (1987) Local circuit interactions between oriens/alveus interneurons and CA1 pyramidal cells in hippocampal slices: electrophysiology and morphology. *J. Neurosci.,* 7: 1979–1993.

Lacaille, J.-C., Kunkel, D.D. and Schwartzkroin, P.A. (1989) Electrophysiological and morphological characterization of hippocampal interneurons. In V. Chan-Palay and C. Köhler (Eds.), *The Hippocampus; New Vistas,* Alan R. Liss, New York, pp. 287–305.

Lambert, J.V.L. and Jones, R.S.G. (1989) Activation of N-methyl-D-aspartate receptors contributes to the EPSP at perforant path synapses in the rat dentate gyrus *in vitro*. *Neurosci. Lett.,* 97: 323–328.

Laurberg, S. and Sørensen, K.E. (1981) Associational and commissural collaterals of neurons in the hippocampal formation (hilus fasciae dentatae and subfield CA3). *Brain Res.,* 212: 287–300.

Lorente de Nó, R. (1934) Studies on the structure of the cerebral cortex. II. Continuation of the study of the ammonic system. *J. Psychol. Neurol.,* 46: 113–177.

Loy, R., Koziell, D.A., Lindsey, J.D. and Moore, R.Y. (1980) Noradrenergic innervation of the adult rat hippocampal formation. *J. Comp. Neurol.,* 189: 699–710.

McNaughton, B.L., Barnes, C.A. and Andersen, P. (1981) Synaptic efficacy and EPSP summation in granule cells of rat fascia dentata studied *in vitro*. *J. Neurophysiol.,* 46:

952–966.

Monaghan, D.T., Holets, V.R., Toy, D.W. and Cotman, C.W. (1983) Anatomical distributions of four pharmacologically distinct ^{3}H-L-glutamate binding sites. *Nature (Lond.),* 306: 176–179.

Monaghan, D.T., Yao, D. and Cotman, C.W. (1985) L-[^{3}H]-glutamate binds to kainate-, NMDA-, and AMPA-sensitive binding sites: an autoradiographic analysis. *Brain Res.,* 340: 378–383.

Moore, R.Y. and Halaris, A.E. (1975) Hippocampal innervation by serotonin neurons of the midbrain raphe in the rat. *J. Comp. Neurol.,* 164: 171–184.

Morrison, J.H., Benoit, R., Magistretti, P.J., Ling, N. and Bloom, F.E. (1982) Immunohistochemical distribution of pro-somatostatin-related peptides in hippocampus. *Neurosci. Lett.,* 34: 137–142.

Nadler, J.V., Perry, B. and Cotman, C.W. (1978) Intraventricular kainic acid preferentially destroys hippocampal pyramidal cells. *Nature (Lond.),* 271: 676–677.

Naus, C.C.G., Morrison, J.H. and Bloom, F.E. (1988) Development of somatostatin-containing neurons and fibers in the rat hippocampus. *Dev. Brain Res.,* 40: 113–121.

Ottersen, O.P. and Storm-Mathisen, J. (1984) Glutamate- and GABA-containing neurons in the mouse and rat brain, as demonstrated with a new immunocytochemical technique. *J. Comp. Neurol.,* 229: 374–392.

Pulsinelli, W., Brierly, J. and Plum, F. (1982) Temporal profile of neuronal damage in a model of transient forebrain ischemia. *Ann. Neurol.,* 11: 491–498.

Ramón y Cajal, S. (1911) *Histologie du Système Nerveux de l'Homme et des Vertebrés,* Maloine, Paris.

Ribak, C.E. and Anderson, L. (1980) Ultrastructure of the pyramidal basket cells in the dentate gyrus of the rat. *J. Comp. Neurol.,* 192: 903–916.

Ribak, C.E. and Seress, L. (1983) Five types of basket cells in the hippocampal dentate gyrus. A combined Golgi and electron microscopic study. *J. Neurocytol.,* 12: 577–597.

Ribak, C.E., Vaughn, J.E. and Saito, K. (1978) Immunocytochemical localization of glutamic acid decarboxylase in neuronal somata following colchicine inhibition of axonal transport. *Brain Res.,* 140: 315–332.

Ribak, C.E., Seress, L. and Amaral, D.G. (1985) The development, ultrastructure and synaptic connections of the mossy cells of the dentate gyrus. *J. Neurocytol.,* 14: 835–857.

Sayer, R.J., Redman, S.J. and Andersen, P. (1988) Amplitude fluctuations in small EPSPs recorded from CA1 pyramidal cells in the guinea pig hippocampal slice. *J. Neurosci.,* 9: 840–850.

Scharfman, H.E. and Schwartzkroin, P.A. (1988) Electrophysiology of morphologically identified mossy cells of the dentate hilus in guinea pig hippocampal slices. *J. Neurosci.,* 8: 3812–3821.

Scharfman, H.E. and Schwartzkroin, P.A. (1989a) Protection of dentate hilar cells from prolonged stimulation by intracellular calcium chelation. *Science,* 246: 257 – 260.

Scharfman, H.E. and Schwartzkroin, P.A. (1989b) Selective depression of GABA-mediated IPSPs by somatostatin in area CA1 of rabbit hippocampal slices. *Brain Res.,* 493: 205 – 211.

Schwartzkroin, P.A. and Kunkel, D.D. (1982) Electrophysiology and morphology of the developing hippocampus of fetal rabbits. *J. Neurosci.,* 2: 448 – 462.

Schwartzkroin, P.A. and Kunkel, D.D. (1985) Morphology of identified interneurons in the CA1 regions of guinea pig hippocampus. *J. Comp. Neurol.,* 232: 205 – 218.

Schwartzkroin, P.A. and Mathers, L.H. (1978) Physiological and morphological identification of a nonpyramidal hippocampal cell type. *Brain Res.,* 157: 1 – 10.

Schwartzkroin, P.A. and Mueller, A.L. (1987) Electrophysiology of hippocampal neurons. In E.G. Jones and A. Peters (Eds.), *Cerebral Cortex. Vol. 6. Further Aspects of Cortical Function, Including Hippocampus,* Plenum, New York, pp. 295 – 343.

Sloviter, R.S. (1983) "Epileptic" brain damage in rats induced by sustained electrical stimulation of the perforant path. I. Acute electrophysiological and light microscopic studies. *Brain Res. Bull.,* 10: 675 – 697.

Sloviter, R.S. (1987) Decreased hippocampal inhibition and a selective loss of interneurons in experimental epilepsy. *Science,* 235: 73 – 76.

Sloviter, R.S. (1989) Calcium binding protein (Calbindin-D_{28K}) and parvalbumin immunocytochemistry: location in the rat hippocampus with specific reference to the selective vulnerability of hippocampal neurons to seizure activity. *J. Comp. Neurol.,* 280: 183 – 196.

Sloviter, R.S. and Nilaver, G. (1987) Immunocytochemical localization of GABA-, cholecystokinin-, vasoactive intestinal polypeptide- and somatostatin-like immunoreactivity in the area dentata and hippocampus of the rat. *J. Comp. Neurol.,* 256: 42 – 60.

Steward, O. and Scoville, S.A. (1976) Cells of origin of entorhinal afferents to the hippocampus and fascia dentata of the rat. *J. Comp. Neurol.,* 169: 347 – 370.

Storm-Mathisen, J., Leknes, A.K., Bore, A.T., Vaaland, J.L., Edminson, P., Haug, F.-M.S. and Ottersen, O.P. (1983) First visualization of glutamate and GABA neurones by immunocytochemistry. *Nature (Lond.),* 301: 517 – 520.

Swanson, L.W., Sawchenko, P.E. and Cowan, W.M. (1981) Evidence for collateral projections by neurons in Ammon's horn, the dentate gyrus, and the subiculum: a multiple retrograde labeling study in the rat. *J. Neurosci.,* 1: 548 – 559.

Watkins, J.C. and Evans, R.H. (1981) Excitatory amino acid transmitters. *Annu. Rev. Pharmacol. Toxicol.,* 21: 165 – 204.

Witter, M.P., Griffioen, A.W., Jorritsma-Byham, B. and Krijnen, J.L.M. (1988) Entorhinal projections to the hippocampal CA1 region in the rat: an underestimated pathway. *Neurosci. Lett.,* 85: 193 – 198.

Wong, R.K.S. and Prince, D.A. (1978) Participation of calcium spikes during intrinsic burst firing in hippocampal neurons. *Brain Res.,* 159: 385 – 390.

Wong, R.K.S. and Schwartzkroin, P.A. (1982) Pacemaker neurons in the mammalian brain: mechanisms and function. In D.O. Carpenter (Ed.), *Cellular Pacemakers, Vol. 1. Mechanisms of Pacemaker Generation,* Wiley, New York, pp. 237 – 254.

Wong, R.K.S., Traub, R.D. and Miles, R. (1984) Epileptogenic mechanisms as revealed by studies of the hippocampal slice. In P.A. Schwartzkroin and H.V. Wheal (Eds.), *Electrophysiology of Epilepsy,* Academic, London, pp. 253 – 275.

Animals were individually housed in 53.5 × 29 cm plastic tub cages. Following acclimatization, the rats were placed on a food-restricted diet and maintained at roughly 80% of their free feeding weights. Over a period of several weeks, the animals were adapted to a radial 8-arm maze (see Fig. 2) and were trained to perform a standard spatial working memory task (Olton and Samuelson, 1976) in which they were required to obtain chocolate milk reward (0.1 ml) from the end of each arm. The majority of rats (80%) were next trained on a forced choice procedure in which each maze arm was presented in random sequence on a given trial (e.g. Barnes et al., 1983). Training was continued until the animals would perform 12 consecutive trials. The remainder of the rats were trained to perform multiple trials using the working memory procedure in which a short delay was imposed between the rat's fourth and fifth arm choices. Considerable experience with recording from hippocampal cells during both of these procedures has failed to reveal any obvious differences in firing characteristics between the two. The results are therefore considered together in the present report. The radial 8-arm maze (for details see Mizumori et al., 1989b) was located in a 12 × 12 ft room that was illuminated by a 40 W lamp located on the south wall. Numerous remote visual cues that could be used for spatial orientation were distributed around the room.

After the rats were well trained on the radial maze, surgery was performed for implantation of microdrives and electrodes for extracellular single unit recording. The recording technique involved the use of "stereotrodes" (McNaughton et al., 1983b) that were constructed in either of two ways. For roughly half of the animals two strands of lacquer-coated 20-μm tungsten wire were cemented together using Epoxylite. For the other half, 25-μm teflon-coated platinum-iridium wires were twisted together. The ends of the wires were cut with sharp scissors so that the exposed tips were approximately parallel and separated by roughly 10 – 15 μm of insulating material. Each stereotrode was cemented into a 30-gauge guide cannula leaving

1 – 2 mm of free electrode protruding. The guide cannulae were mounted on miniature micromanipulators (McNaughton et al., 1989) that were permanently attached via dental acrylic to the animal's head. Prior to implantation, the electrode tip impedances were reduced by electroplating with gold or platinum black. Final tip impedances ranged from 200 – 750 kΩ.

The series of experiments described here involved recording from 4 principal target sites (see Fig. 3, and Table I): the CA1 and CA3c pyramidal fields of the dorsal hippocampus, both dorsal and

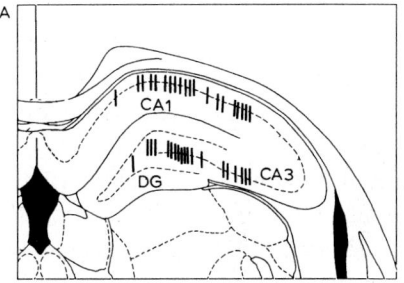

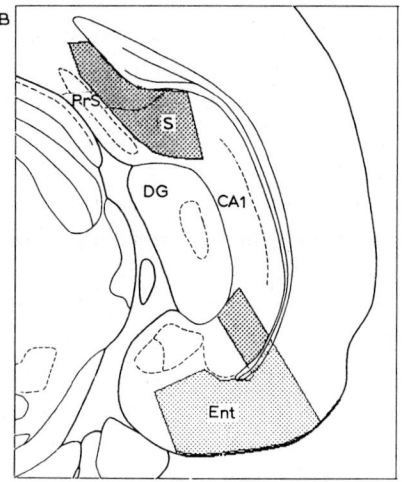

Fig. 3. Diagram of areas from which cells in CA1, CA3, entorhinal cortex and subiculum were recorded in this study. The bars in A show the extent over which CA1 and CA3c cell layers were sampled with our electrode penetrations. The dark stippled area in B shows the general dorsal and ventral regions from which cells in the subicular sample were recorded. The light stippled area in B shows the region of electrode penetrations through entorhinal cortex. The coronal sections shown here are adapted from Figs. 22 and 27 of Paxinos and Watson (1982).

TABLE I

Spike waveform parameters of cells recorded in the hippocampal formation in the present study

Cell type	Number of rats contributing cells	Total number of cells recorded	Spike height (μV)		Spike width (μs)	
			$\bar{x}$	S.E.M.	$\bar{x}$	S.E.M.
CA1 CS	9	120	108.0	5.2	359.7	19.0
CA1 θ	10	42	101.5	7.8	274.1	16.3
CA3 CS	16	220	102.3	3.8	266.6	6.7
CA3 θ	16	52	120.9	9.2	223.9	11.5
Subiculum	12	194	103.5	5.6	346.0	7.4
Entorhinal	5	45	81.7	2.4	405.1	14.0

ventral subiculum, and the entorhinal cortex. Within the CA3c sample, it is possible that some of the cells recorded were actually in the surrounding hilar region of the fascia dentata. The accuracy of the electrode localization methods would not have permitted us to make this precise distinction. The recording electrodes were oriented according to the selected target using the stereotaxic coordinate system of Paxinos and Watson (1982). Under deep anesthesia (33 mg/kg Nembutal), a small craniotomy was made over the appropriate target, the dura was slit with a sharp needle, and the electrode tips were inserted roughly 1 mm into cortex. The craniotomy was then filled either with medical grade silastic (Dow Corning) or low melting point bone wax up to a level at which the openings of the guide cannulae were covered. The entire assembly was then encased in dental acrylic that was firmly anchored to the skull by previously implanted stainless steel jeweler's screws. In addition to the stereotrodes, single reference wires were implanted in or near the corpus callosum within 2 – 3 mm of the stereotrode site. Following surgery, bicillin was injected (i.m.) into each hindleg, and rats were closely monitored until full recovery was apparent.

Approximately 2 weeks following surgery, rats were reintroduced to the maze task and adapted to wearing the 5-channel FET headstage for unit recording (Fig. 2). The stereotrodes were advanced in roughly 20-μm steps until cells in the appropriate target zone were encoutered. When the electrodes

were near the target zone, they were advanced by no more than about 100 μm per day, usually much less. This greatly facilitated long-term stability of the recording situation. The principle of the stereotrode recording technique is illustrated in Fig. 4 and described in detail elsewhere (McNaughton et al., 1983b; McNaughton et al., 1989; Mizumori, et al., 1989b). During recording sessions, the position of the animal was tracked by monitoring an infrared LED mounted on the headstage assembly. The position coordinates of the diode were sampled at 20 Hz, and stored on a PDP 11/23 computer. The spatial resolution was estimated to be 1.8 cm per pixel. Unit activity was amplified between 5000 and 10,000 times, filtered between 600 Hz and 6 kHz (50% attenuation frequencies), and acquired concurrently with the position data.

Spatial selectivity was the primary behavioral correlate of unit activity that was of interest in the present investigation. This was assessed by computing the average firing rate of each cell as a function of spatial location and radial orientation (i.e. inward vs outward motion) on the maze surface (see McNaughton et al., 1983a). These data were expressed in radial histogram form corresponding to the radial 8-arm maze. Examples of spatially selective and non-selective neurons recorded from the CA1 and CA3 cell regions are illustrated in Fig. 5. A "spatial selectivity score" was computed by dividing the aggregate rate for the arm/direction exhibiting the highest overall rate by the average of the rates for all other arms and radial directions. Note that this particular measure emphasizes spatial *selectivity* as opposed to spatial *consistency*. Cells with a single well-defined firing field would yield high specificity scores. On the other hand, a spatially consistent pattern of firing involving either one field covering several arms, or multiple fields distributed over the maze, would receive a low score. Moreover, for highly selective

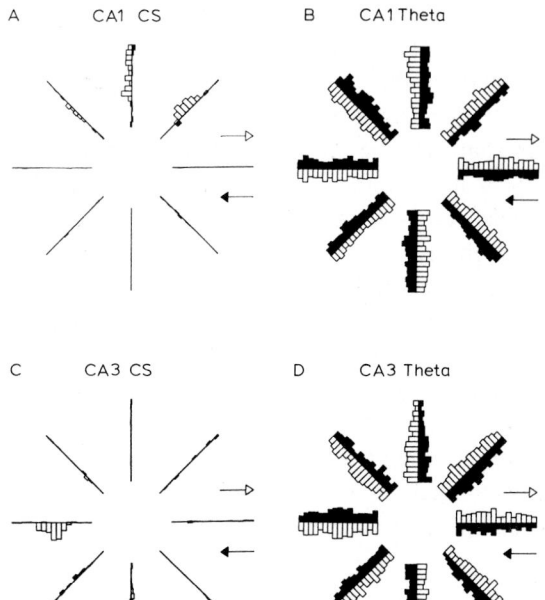

Fig. 5. Examples of the spatial firing rate distributions on the radial 8-arm maze for a CA1 complex spike cell (A), a CA1 theta cell (B), a CA3 complex spike cell (C), and a CA3 theta cell (D). Individual radial histograms correspond to each of the maze arms, with the open bars representing the average firing rates when the rat moved outward on an arm and the closed bars the rates while moving inward towards the center of the maze. These means represent the averages of 12 complete trials on the maze. Notice the greater spatial selectivity of the complex spike cells compared with the theta cells for each of these hippocampal subfields. Note also the directional selectivity of the complex spike cells, a characteristic feature of their activity on the radial maze.

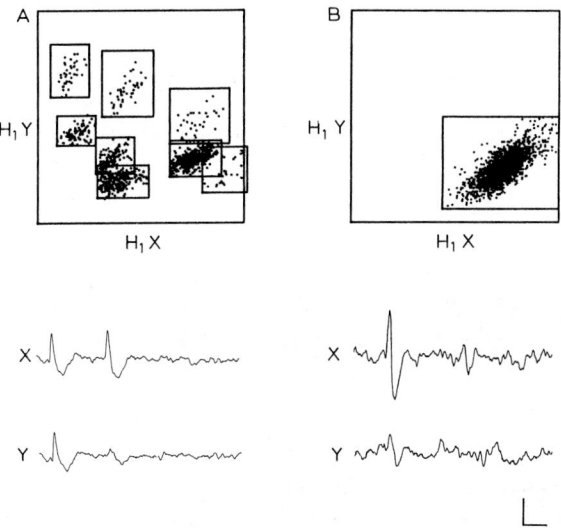

Fig. 4. The fundamental principle of the stereotrode is based on the fact that extracellularly recorded neuronal signals decline in amplitude approximately inversely with distance from the recording electrode. If two recording electrodes are located at different distances from a cell, they will record different spike amplitudes. In general, however, within a local cluster of cells different cells will have different ratios of distances from the two electrodes. Thus if one plots the amplitude of spikes on one channel vs their amplitude on the other (e.g. H_1Y vs H_1X), then different cells will produce different clusters in the X/Y plane. Using this tendency to cluster, plus additional information about spike waveshape (e.g. duration), the stereotrode thus provides a means of separating cells that would otherwise be virtually indistinguishable. A good example of this is shown in part A in which 8 CS cells from the CA3 region are simultaneously separated. The analog trace below the scatter plot illustrates a clear case where two units would have been confused if recorded on the X channel alone, but in conjunction with the Y channel record are clearly separable. Part B illustrates a case of single well-isolated theta cell in CA1. Calibration bar = 58 μV, 1 ms.

cells in which firing is restricted to only part of a single arm, this measure underestimates the true selectivity. As will be demonstrated in the results section, some clear cases of spatially consistent firing were found in the entorhinal cortex and subiculum in spite of rather low spatial selectivity scores.

In addition to spatial characteristics, the overall mean firing rates were measured, as well as estimates of maximum rates achieved by a given cell over any 100 ms period. For each cell, autocorrelation functions were also plotted for the com-

294

plete data set. These plots were used as a qualitative indication of whether the unit firing was rhythmically modulated and whether there was a tendency to fire in complex spike bursts. The latter characteristic was manifested as a sharp central peak in the autocorrelation function, examples of which are shown in Fig. 6. Measures of the waveform characteristics of the single units, including spike height and the width of the spike measured from its maximum to minimum value, were also recorded.

No data were included unless a minimum of 6 complete trials on the radial maze was completed. Statistical comparisons were carried out using a one-way analysis of variance and the Fischer posthoc test, with alpha set at the 0.05 level. For most cells, a complete set of measurements was available. However, in a few cases, one or another of the measures was not available. In most instances this resulted from computer magnetic storage media faults. This is reflected in slight variations in the degrees of freedom in the various tests described below.

Results

A total of 673 cells was recorded from 41 rats, and the mean number of trials completed per recording session for all cells and rats was 10.2. The numbers of cells recorded in each region can be found in Table I. The amplitude of the recorded spike signals did not differ greatly among areas or cell

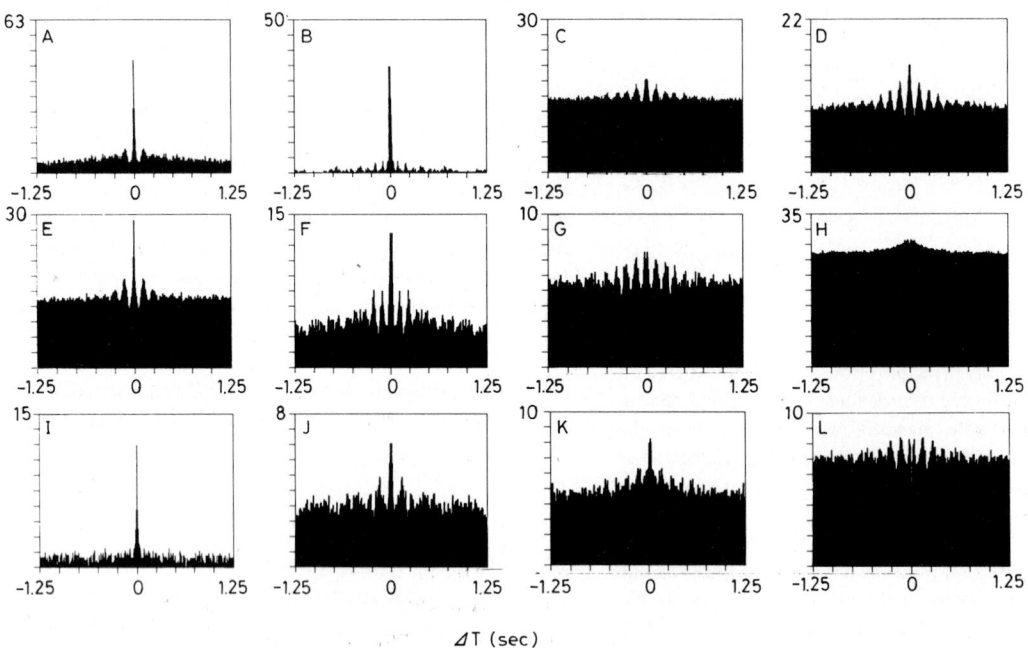

Fig. 6. Representative examples illustrating the range of autocorrelation functions observed in the CA fields (A – D), the subiculum (E – H), and the entorhinal cortex (I – L). The autocorrelation function is a measure of the expectation of firing at times $T \pm \Delta T$ given the occurrence of a spike at time T. The ordinates represent number of occurrences per time lag interval divided by the width of the interval. This has units of Hz. In the CA fields the discharge of complex spike cells (A,B) is characterized by the frequent occurrence of short bursts of spikes with short interspike intervals. This results in a sharp central peak in the autocorrelation function. By contrast the discharge of theta cells (C,D) is characterized by rhythmic firing with a fundamental frequency of about 7 Hz. This results in a series of peaks of declining amplitude on either side of zero delay. In subiculum and entorhinal cortex, such a clear separation on the basis of firing pattern was not possible. A few cells in entorhinal cortex exhibited complex spike bursting comparable to the complex spike cells in CA fields (e.g. I). However in most cases, in both the entorhinal cortex and subiculum, the patterns were intermediate between theta and the complex spike patterns of the CA fields.

types ($F_{5,621} = 1.83$, $P = 0.11$) although, as is shown in Table I, units recorded in the entorhinal cortex tended to have smaller signals, whereas theta cells recorded in CA3c tended to have the largest signals. More interesting were the differences in the spike width measures between cell types and areas ($F_{5,627} = 22.15$, $P = 0.0001$). In each of the two hippocampal subfields, CS cells exhibited significantly broader spikes than did theta cells. However, the overall spike widths for CS cells in CA3 were substantially less than for their counterparts in CA1. The populations of spikes recorded in subiculum and entorhinal cortex were also broader than either of the theta cell categories, with entorhinal cells forming the broadest waveform group.

Histograms showing the mean and maximum firing rates according to region and cell class are shown in Fig. 7. There were large differences between regions and cell types in mean ($F_{5,644} = 70.35$, $P = 0.0001$) and maximum ($F_{5,634} = 11.74$, $P = 0.001$) discharge rates. CA1 and CA3 CS cells exhibited comparable low average discharge rates, whereas the theta cells in the corresponding areas exhibited the highest average discharge rates. The mean rates for subicular cells were surprisingly high, falling roughly halfway between the CS and theta cell values. Entorhinal rates were significantly lower than subiculum rates. Although the mean entorhinal rates were roughly twice those of the CA3 and CA1 CS cell rates, this difference was only statistically significant for the CA3 comparison. The pattern for maximum rates was similar to the pattern for the mean rates, although the overall differences among areas and classes were much smaller.

Within each area and cell category the frequency distributions for observed mean rates were unimodal (see Fig. 8). For non-theta cells the CA3 CS cell mean rate distribution was the most skewed towards low rates, while that for the subiculum was the least skewed in this direction. Theta cells in both pyramidal fields exhibited the broadest spread of mean rates with modal values between 5 and 10 Hz. Complex spike cells in CA1 and CA3

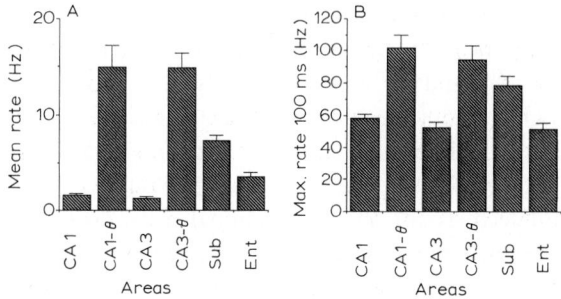

Fig. 7. Histograms illustrating the mean (A) and maximum (B) firing rates of neurons recorded in various subfields of the hippocampal formation of rats performing multiple trials on a radial 8-arm maze task. The maximum rates refer to the maximum observed over any 100 ms period. Abbreviations: CA1, complex spike cells in CA1; CA3, complex spike cells in CA3; CA1-θ, theta cells in CA1; CA3-θ, theta cells in CA3; Sub, subiculum cells; Ent, entorhinal cortex cells.

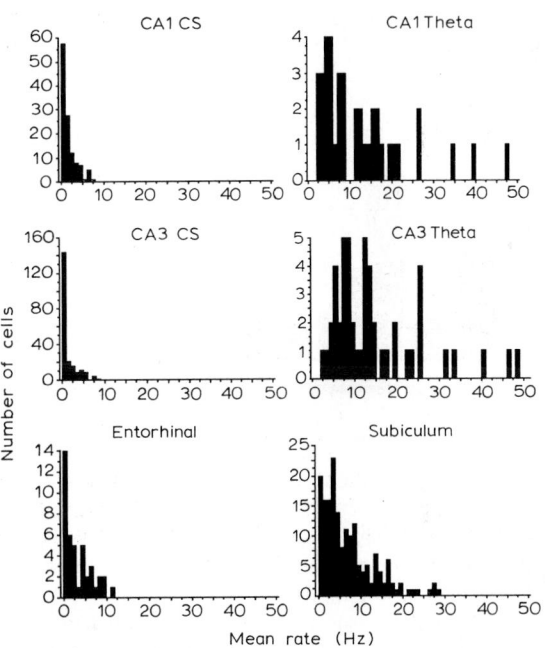

Fig. 8. Frequency distributions for mean firing rates of neurons recorded in the various subfields of the hippocampal formation of rats performing a radial 8-arm maze task. Although the overall mean rates were not significantly different between CA1 and CA3, the distribution for CA3 CS cells was the most skewed towards lower rates of any cell category. Of the non-theta cells subicular units showed the least proportion of low discharge rates. Entorhinal units were intermediate between CA1 CS cells and subiculum.

were generally characterized by the presence of a sharp peak in the autocorrelation function (see Fig. 6A and B) with some cells also showing a slight periodicity at about 7 Hz. Some entorhinal units exhibited similar burst discharge characteristics (see Fig. 6I), although this was rarely as pronounced as for the hippocampal cells. Autocorrelation functions dominated by burst discharge were even more rarely encountered among subicular cells. Many cells in both entorhinal cortex and subiculum exhibited rhythmic autocorrelation functions whether burst discharge was present or not. Most theta cells recorded in the hippocampus exhibited rhythmic autocorrelation functions (see Fig. 6C and D), often with a reduced probability of discharge at the very short interspike intervals at which CS cells show increased probability. Because of the overall higher discharge rates, the reduced tendency towards bursting and the frequent occurrence of rhythmic modulation, we were

unable except for a few cases to make clear distinctions between CS and theta modes of firing in either entorhinal cortex or subiculum. Thus, all cells in these areas are presented as a single class. The extent of possible distortion in the overall between-area comparisons that may have been introduced by this procedure is considered in the discussion.

Although there were large differences in spatial specificity scores among areas ($F_{5,618} = 10.49$, $P = 0.0001$), the pattern of scores observed was generally inconsistent with the "assembly-line" hypothesis outlined in the introduction (see Fig. 9). While specificity increased dramatically from entorhinal cortex to CA3 CS cells as expected by the hypothesis, the CS cells in CA1 were significantly *less* specific than those in CA3. Furthermore, cells in the subiculum exhibited practically no specificity according to this measure. As found in previous studies (McNaughton et al.,

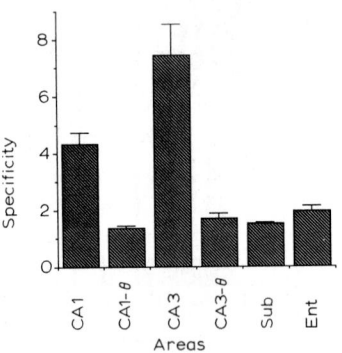

Fig. 9. Spatial specificity was defined on the basis of the distribution of firing rates over the 8-arm maze (see example in Fig. 5). The specificity index was computed by finding the arm and radial direction exhibiting the highest average firing rate, and dividing this rate by the average firing rate of the other arms and directions. This score provides a rough index of compactness of spatial tuning. It should be emphasized, however, that a low specificity score does not preclude the possibility of spatially consistent firing distributed among a number of locations on the maze. The surprising feature that emerges from this analysis is that spatial specificity declines rather than increases in the progression from CA3 to CA1 to the subiculum. As seen in Fig. 11 spatially consistent firing could be found in a significant number of subicular cells even though none showed highly restricted "place fields" frequently observed in hippocampal areas CA1 and CA3. Abbreviations as in Fig. 7.

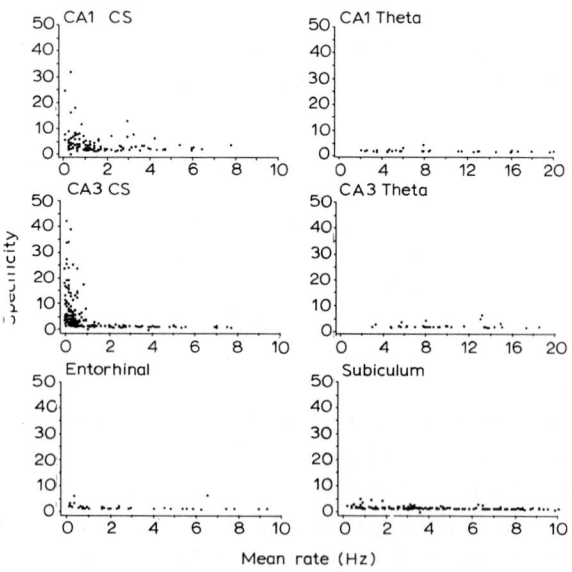

Fig. 10. Scatter plots of spatial specificity scores versus mean overall firing rates for cells in the various subfields on the hippocampal formation. These plots indicate that even if the differences in overall mean firing rate are taken into account, for a given mean rate, entorhinal and subicular cells are much less spatially selective than are CA1 and CA3 complex spike cells. Note difference in horizontal scale for theta cells, and the truncation of the rate axis at 10 Hz for the other cell categories.

1983a; Mizumori et al. 1989b), hippocampal theta cells also exhibited very little evidence of spatial selectivity. For the cell classes that exhibited significant specificity, there was a strong reciprocal relationship between the specificity score and the mean firing rate. Figure 10 illustrates that even when cells were equated for mean firing rate, entorhinal and subicular cell activity displayed little, if any, spatial specificity compared to hippocampal CS cells.

Although the spatial specificity indices in entorhinal cortex and subiculum were surprisingly low, there was, nevertheless, evidence for spatially *consistent* firing in both of these areas. A few entorhinal cells and a substantial proportion of subicular cells exhibited non-uniform distributions of mean rates over the maze surface. Examples of the most obviously selective cases for the two areas are shown in Figs. 11 and 12. Particularly in the subiculum, cases were found in which firing rates on several arms were substantially different from the others. Sometimes these included adjacent arms, but non-adjacent arms could also be includ-

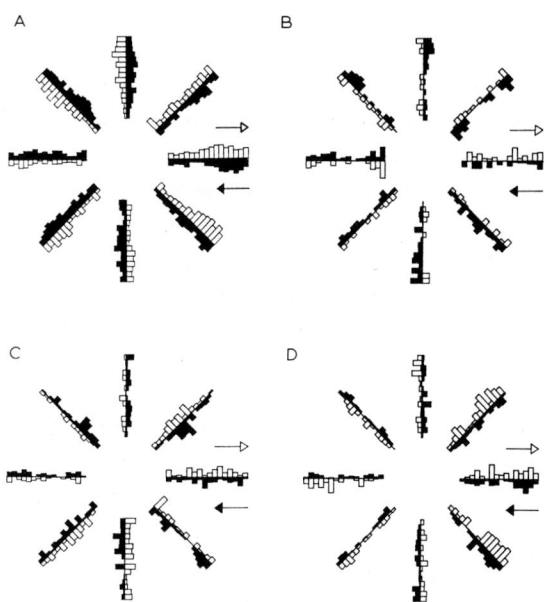

Fig. 12. Spatial firing rate distribution plots for 4 different entorhinal cells (see Fig. 5 for explanation). These examples illustrate the clearest cases of spatial consistency in firing that were observed in this sample of entorhinal cells.

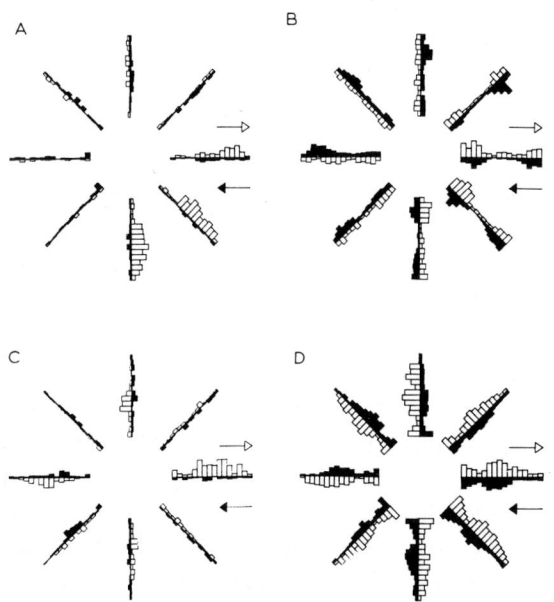

Fig. 11. Spatial firing rate distribution plots for 4 different subicular cells (see Fig. 5 for explanation). These cells were selected to illustrate the type of coarse, spatially consistent firing patterns found in some subicular cells.

ed. Again, these patterns were much more rarely encountered in entorhinal cortex.

Discussion

The simplest view of the role of the hippocampal formation in spatial information processing is that highly compact representations of local regions of the environment are somehow constructed within hippocampal circuitry through the conjunction of inputs conveying information about the various sensory features encountered in a particular place. For example, a given hippocampal cell might reflect the specific conjunction of features A, B, C and D, any one of which might occur in several locations in the environment with the complete set being unique to a single location. According to this view, one would expect to find less spatial selectivity towards the input side of the system, as for example was found in the present study for the entorhinal cortex, because cells would be firing in relation to the individual features rather than the overall collections. Given the results of McNaughton et al. (1989), that the granule cells of the dentate gyrus are not necessary for the expression of spatially selective discharge in CA3 pyramidal cells, it is reasonable to conclude that CA3 plays a pivotal role in generating a conjunctive code for spatial stimuli. What is at first surprising, however, is the progressive *loss* of spatial selectivity from CA3 to CA1 and again from CA1 to the subiculum.

A possible explanation for the latter pattern of results can be derived from considerations of the requirement of optimizing information storage capacity (see Marr, 1969, 1971). In order to maximize the number of different events that a distributed network can store, the relative overlap among events must be kept as low as possible. This requires that a given cell participates in relatively few events and thus has a low average discharge rate. Systems that transmit but do not store information can afford to employ a much more completely distributed representation in which the overall average firing rates are higher and in which each cell participates in a substantial proportion of the events experienced by the system. It is well-established that synapses within CA3 recurrent circuits as well as their Schaffer collateral projections to CA1 are highly modifiable (Schwartzkroin and Wester, 1975; Bliss et al., 1983), suggesting that these systems are involved in information storage. The foregoing considerations lead to the prediction that the output terminals of subicular cells should, in general, be only weakly or possibly slowly modifiable. We know of no available data that can address this prediction at present.

There are several technical caveats that need to be addressed in assessing and interpreting the results of the present investigation. Firstly, we were not able clearly to separate cells in subiculum and entorhinal cortex into the theta and CS categories that hippocampal cells fall into naturally. Although pooling these two classes (if they are present) would have reduced the overall specificity measures, this could not account for the lack of

specificity in cells with low-average discharge rates (see Fig. 10). Moreover, theta cells in the CA fields constituted only about 20% of the total sample. If the specificity data for CS and theta cells in the CA fields are pooled, the mean specificity is still significantly greater than that of either the subiculum or the entorhinal samples. Thus we are confident that the lack of precise spatial specificity in the latter two areas is not a result of our failure to make a clear distinction between these cell classes. Secondly, within entorhinal cortex, it was not possible to discriminate among the different cell layers of that region. In particular, we have no way of knowing how many, if any, of our sample included the cells of layers 2 and 3 that constitute the major sources of input from the entorhinal cortex to the hippocampal subfields. Moreover, the deeper layers of the entorhinal cortex receive a strong projection from the subiculum (Köhler, 1985), and this could to some extent account for the low spatial selectivity in the overall sample. Further studies will be required in which hippocampally projecting neurons in entorhinal cortex are identified by antidromic activation before this issue can be resolved.

A final caveat relates to the quality of single unit isolation. The stereotrode technique represents a substantial improvement in the ability reliably to isolate neurons, particularly smaller ones, compared to the single microwire techniques typically employed in chronic recording experiments in freely moving rats. However, even this method is subject to a variable error in regions where high overall levels of population activity lead to a substantial probability that spike signals from different cells will overlap in time. Such overlap degrades the quality of isolation of single units. Subicular cells have been notoriously difficult to isolate for this reason, and this difficulty may contribute to the low spatial selectivity scores in our sample of subicular recordings. However, the extremely low average selectivity, as well as the observation that spatial selectivity is already declining between CA3 and CA1, makes it unlikely that poor isolation is the entire explanation or even the principal one. Moreover, if subicular cells exhibited spatial specificity comparable to that observed in CA1 and CA3, then it should be easier rather than more difficult to isolate them, because their cell bodies are packed substantially less densely. Thus the very fact that the overall mean rates are higher, with frequently overlapping spike waveforms, is itself evidence for low spatial selectivity. More refined recording techniques, however, will be required for a completely accurate characterization of the discharge characteristics of these cells in relation to spatial behavior.

In conclusion, the analogy presented in the introduction might provide an accurate characterization of the sequential stages of hippocampal processing of spatial information if one assumes that the desired final product is a highly distributed representation of space rather than a highly discrete one. It appears that discrete spatial representations *are* constructed within early stages of the process for some purpose intrinsic to the hippocampus itself, possibly that of rapid information storage. These compact representations appear not to be passed back to the cortex via the subiculum. Rather, the information leaving the hippocampus through the subiculum seems to consist of much more highly distributed representations, constructed perhaps through the convergence and disjunction of a number of unrelated hippocampal place cells.

Acknowledgements

We thank C. Wood and K. Grewel for assistance with these experiments, G. Rao for help with figure preparation, and M. Mozer and J.L. McClelland for useful discussions. This research was supported by PHS Grants AG-03376 to C.A.B. and NS-20331 to B.L.M., and S.J.Y.M. was supported by NRSA fellowship AG-05475. C.A.B. and B.L.M. would also particularly like to thank Professor Theodor Blackstad for his enthusiasm and encouragement during the formative stages of our research careers and for sharing at least some of the available computer time at the University of Oslo Institutes of Anatomy and Neurophysiology on Saturday mornings.

References

Andersen P., Holmqvist, B. and Voorhoeve, P.E. (1966) Entorhinal activation of dentate granule cells. *Acta Physiol. Scand.*, 66: 448 – 460.

Andersen, P., Bliss, T.V.P. and Skrede, K.K. (1971) Lamellar organization of hippocampal excitatory pathways. *Exp Brain Res.*, 13: 222 – 238.

Barnes, C.A., McNaughton, B.L. and O'Keefe, J. (1983) Loss of place specificity in hippocampal complex-spike cells of senescent rat. *Neurobiol. Aging*, 4: 113 – 119.

Blackstad, T.W. (1958) On the termination of some afferents to the hippocampus and fascia dentata. *Acta Anat.*, 35: 203 – 214.

Bliss, T.V.P., Lancaster, B. and Wheal, H.V. (1983) Long-term potentiation in commissural and Schaffer projections to hippocampal CA1 cells: an *in vivo* study in the rat. *J. Physiol. (Lond.)*, 341: 617 – 626.

Cajal, S.R. (1911) *Histologie du Système Nerveux de l'Homme et des Vertébrés.* A. Maloine, Paris.

Christian, E.P. and Deadwyler, S.A. (1986) Behavioral functions and hippocampal cell types: evidence for two nonoverlapping populations in the rat. *J. Neurophysiol.*, 55: 331 – 348.

Fox, S.E. and Ranck Jr., J.B. (1975) Localization and anatomical identification of theta and complex spike cells in dorsal hippocampal formation of rats. *Exp. Neurol.*, 49: 299 – 313.

Fox, S.E., and Ranck Jr., J.B. (1981) Electrophysiological characteristics of hippocampal complex-spike and theta cells. *Exp. Brain Res.*, 41: 399 – 410.

Köhler, C. (1985) Intrinsic projections of the retrohippocampal region in the rat brain. I. The subicular complex. *J. Comp. Neurol.*, 236: 504 – 522.

Kubie, J.L. and Ranck Jr., J.B. (1983) Sensory-behavioral correlates in individual hippocampus neurons in three situations: space and context. In W. Seifert (Ed.), *Neurobiology of the Hippocampus*, Academic Press, New York, pp. 433 – 447.

Leonard, B.W. and McNaughton, B.L. (1990) Spatial representation in the rat: conceptual, behavioral, and neurophysiological perspectives. In R. Kesner and D.S. Olton (Eds.), *The Neurobiology of Comparative Cognition.* Lawrence Erlbaum Assoc., Hillsdale, NJ, pp. 363 – 422.

Marr, D.A. (1969) A theory of cerebellar cortex. *J. Physiol. (Lond.)*, 202: 437 – 470.

Marr, D.A. (1971) Simple memory: a theory for archicortex. *Phil. Trans. Roy. Soc. Ser. B,* 262: 23 – 81.

McNaughton, B.L., Barnes, C.A. and O'Keefe, J. (1983a) The contributions of position, direction, and velocity to single unit activity in the hippocampus of freely-moving rats. *Exp. Brain Res.*, 52: 41 – 49.

McNaughton, B.L., O'Keefe, J. and Barnes, C.A. (1983b) The stereotrode: a new technique for simultaneous isolation of several single units in the central nervous systeem from multiple unit records. *J. Neurosci. Methods*, 8: 391 – 397.

McNaughton, B.L., Barnes, C.A., Meltzer, J. and Sutherland, R.J. (1989) Hippocampal granule cells are necessary for spatial learning but not for spatially-selective pyramidal cell discharge. *Exp. Brain Res.*, 485 – 496.

Mitchell, S.J. and Ranck Jr., J.B. (1977) Firing patterns and behavioral correlates of neurons in entorhinal cortex of freely-moving rats. *Soc. Neurosci. Abstr.*, 3: 202.

Mizumori, S.J.Y., McNaughton, B.L. and Barnes, C.A. (1989a) A comparison of supramammillary and medial septal influences on hippocampal field potentials and single-unit activity. *J. Neurophysiol.*, 61: 15 – 31.

Mizumori, S.J.Y., McNaughton, B.L., Barnes, C.A. and Fox, K.B. (1989b) Preserved spatial coding in hippocampal CA1 pyramidal cells during reversible suppression of CA3 output: evidence for pattern completion in hippocampus. *J. Neurosci.*, 3915 – 3928.

Muller, R.U., Kubie, J.L. and Ranck Jr., J.B. (1987) Spatial firing pattern of hippocampal complex-spike cells in a fixed environment. *J. Neurosci.*, 7: 1935 – 1950.

O'Keefe, J. (1976) Place units in the hippocampus of the freely-moving rat. *Exp. Neurol.*, 51: 78 – 109.

O'Keefe, J. and Conway, D.H. (1978) Hippocampal place units in the freely moving rat: why they fire where they fire. *Exp. Brain Res.*, 31: 573 – 590.

O'Keefe, J. and Dostrovsky, J. (1971) The hippocampus as a spatial map. Preliminary evidence from unit activity in the freely-moving rat. *Brain Res.*, 34: 171 – 175.

O'Keefe, J. and Nadel, L. (1978) *The Hippocampus as a Cognitive Map.* Clarendon Press, Oxford.

O'Keefe, J. and Speakman, A. (1987) Single unit activity in the rat hippocampus during a spatial memory task. *Exp. Brain Res.*, 68: 1 – 27.

Olton, D.S. and Samuelson, R.J. (1976) Remembrance of places passed: spatial memory in rats. *J. Exp. Psychol.: Ani. Behav. Proc.*, 2: 97 – 116.

Olton, D.S., Branch, M. and Best, P.J. (1978) Spatial correlates of hippocampal unit activity. *Exp. Neurol.*, 58: 387 – 409.

Paxinos, G. and Watson, C. (1982) *The Rat Brain in Stereotaxic Coordinates*, Academic Press, Sydney.

Quirk, G.J. and Ranck Jr., J.B. (1986) Firing of single cells in entorhinal cortex is location specific and phase locked to hippocampal theta rhythm. *Soc. Neurosci. Abstr.*, 12: 1524.

Ranck Jr., J.B. (1973) Studies on single neurons in dorsal hippocampal formation and septum in unrestrained rats. I. Behavioral correlates and firing repertoires. *Exp. Neurol.*, 41: 461 – 535.

Rose, G. (1983) Physiological and behavioral characteristics of dentate granule cells. In W. Seifert (Ed.), *The Neurobiology of the Hippocampus*, Academic Press, New York, pp. 449 – 472.

Schwartzkroin, P.A. and Wester, K. (1975) Long-lasting facilitation of a synaptic potential following tetanization in the *in vitro* hippocampal slice. *Brain Res.*, 89: 107 – 119.

Steward, O. and Scoville, S.A. (1976) Cells of origin of entorhinal cortical afferents to the hippocampus and fascia dentata of the rat. *J. Comp. Neurol.*, 169: 347 – 370.

Witter, M.P., Griffioen, A.W., Jorritsma-Byham, B. and Krinjinen, J.L.M. (1988) Entorhinal projections to the hippocampal CA1 region in the rat: an underestimated pathway. *Neurosci. Lett.*, 85: 193 – 198.

J. Storm-Mathisen, J. Zimmer and O.P. Ottersen (Eds.)
Progress in Brain Research, Vol. 83
© 1990 Elsevier Science Publishers B.V. (Biomedical Division)

CHAPTER 22

A computational theory of the hippocampal cognitive map

John O'Keefe

Department of Anatomy and Developmental Biology, University College London, Gower Street, London WC1E 6BT, U.K.

Evidence from single unit and lesion studies suggests that the hippocampal formation acts as a spatial or cognitive map (O'Keefe and Nadel, 1978). In this chapter, I summarise some of the unit recording data and then outline the most recent computational version of the cognitive map theory. The novel aspects of the present version of the theory are that it identifies two allocentric parameters, the centroid and the eccentricity, which can be calculated from the array of cues in an environment and which can serve as the bases for an allocentric polar co-ordinate system. Computations within this framework enable the animal to identify its location within an environment, to predict the location which will be reached as a result of any specific movement from that location, and conversely, to calculate the spatial transformation necessary to go from the current location to a desired location. Aspects of the model are identified with the information provided by cells in the hippocampus and dorsal presubiculum. The hippocampal place cells are involved in the calculation of the centroid and the presubicular direction cells in the calculation of the eccentricity.

Introduction

Based on a summary of the single-unit and lesion data available at the time, O'Keefe and Nadel (1978) suggested that the hippocampus acted as a cognitive map. In infra-human species such as the rat, the cognitive map was confined to the analysis and manipulation of spatial information; but for the human the concept was broadened to include the notion of a semantic map in the left hippocampus. This map acted to organize abstract linguistic material into a map-like narrative. The right human hippocampus was held to function as a purely spatial system.

Subsequent experimental work has provided strong evidence for the spatial role of the hippocampus in infra-human species: single unit recordings in the hippocampus of the freely moving rat have confirmed the existence of the place cells and substantiated many of the properties at-tributed to them (O'Keefe and Dostrovsky, 1971; Ranck, 1973; O'Keefe, 1976, 1979; Hill, 1978; O'Keefe and Conway, 1978; Olton et al., 1978; Muller and Best, 1980; Hill and Best, 1981; Kubie and Ranck, 1983; Christian et al., 1986; Breese et al., 1987; Eichenbaum et al., 1987; Muller and Kubie, 1987; Muller et al., 1987). In brief these papers show that the place cells account for a large percentage of the hippocampal complex-spike cells recorded ($> 50\%$) and have the following properties:

(1) The firing of each place cell is restricted to a contiguous patch of an environment or, in some cases, to two such patches. The same cell often has a field in more than one environment (Kubie and Ranck, 1983).

(2) Neighbouring cells in the hippocampus have place fields distributed around an environment and do not show the type of clustering of receptive fields found in the neocortex (O'Keefe, 1976;

Muller et al., 1987; O'Keefe and Speakman, 1987). It should be noted however that there is a problem with the use of extracellular recording here since small groups of neighbouring cells may have nearly identical waveforms and this might be counted as a single unit. The development of the bipolar "stereotrode" (McNaughton et al., 1983b) and more recently a 4 electrode "tetrode" version (Recce and O'Keefe, 1989) may allow a definitive resolution of this question. These techniques permit better separation of closely spaced cells on the basis of their differing extracellular potentials on the different electrodes.

(3) The firing of a complex spike cell within its place field may or not be dependent on the direction in which the animal is facing. In the original account (O'Keefe, 1976) it was noted that some cells were directional while others were not. Subsequently McNaughton et al. (1983a) found that a large majority of cells recorded in the radial arm maze were dependent on the direction in which the animal was running (inward or outward on the arm). More recently Bostock et al. (1988) have reported that none of the 14 place cells recorded in a cylinder had directional fields. It appears that the place cells can be directional or non-directional depending on some as yet unknown aspect of the testing situation.

(4) The place cells can identify their firing field on the basis of a limited, redundant set of environmental cues. Experiments in which the rat was forced to use a limited number of spatial cues to locate places in an environment (cue-controlled environment) showed that any two of the 4 original cues could be used to do so (O'Keefe and Conway, 1978). This finding suggests that the representation of an environment within the hippocampus is not directly driven by particular sensory cues but that these cues can be used to locate the orientation of the representation relative to the environment.

(5) The hippocampus acts as a memory store for spatial information or is downstream from such a store. Place cells in the hippocampus act as memory cells. In a cue-controlled environment, once the correct pattern of firing has been set up

in a group of place cells this pattern is maintained even after the spatial cues have been removed (O'Keefe and Speakman, 1987). Not only is the pattern maintained for the parts of the maze where the rat has perceived the spatial cues during the beginning of that trial but also for the rest of the maze as well. There are several possible explanations for this latter finding, all of which would suggest that the hippocampus or some related structure is capable of manipulating or transforming the representation of an environment or places in it, in addition to storing these representations.

Models of the hippocampus

The simplest model which attempts to explain these results is the matrix associator model of McNaughton (1988). He proposes that the place cell firing represents the local view which the animal has when it faces in a particular direction in a place and that the hippocampus is part of a system which calculates the expected view which will result when the animal makes a movement from this position. The computation consists of the association of the matrix representing the current local view with a transition matrix representing the actual movement to be made (turn left, go straight etc.) in order to produce the subsequent local view matrix. The model emphasises the finding that the place cells can be directionally sensitive and interprets this to mean that the inputs to these cells are essentially egocentric. The theory bears strong resemblance to the stimulus-response behaviourist theories of Hull and Spence (see also the taxon systems of O'Keefe and Nadel, 1978) and shares many of their strengths and weaknesses. The strengths lie in the simplicity of representation of both the environment and the movement as matrices and the limiting of the computation to matrix association by addition. The weaknesses are (a) the great burden placed on the memory storage capacities of the system since each view and each movement must be stored separately and (b) the apparently limited creativity of the system. This latter depends entirely on generalization from the view at one environmental location to that at a neighbouring location and on the ability of a system external to the hippocampus to compute turn equivalents such as the fact that 3 left turns of 90° are equal to 1 right turn of 90°. Similarly, it remains to be seen whether the model has enough power to explain the ability of a rat to extrapolate from known to unknown parts of an environment, to generate detours when the usual path is blocked, or to provide the cohesiveness between a set of place representations which identifies one environment as opposed to another.

It should be noted that much of the power of this system is located in the postulated motor equivalences and it is these that we should examine carefully. In the absence of an underlying *spatial* system it would appear that all of the possible combinations would need to be stored. Thus not only would the system need to know that 3 left turns = 1 right but that 2 lefts = 2 rights = 1 aboutface ≠ 2 aboutfaces. In contrast 2 straight turns = 1 straight. Since there are a large number of such equivalents these would all need to be stored and there would need to be a computational device for calculating the results of combining them. A perhaps more problematic concern is that, except under the limited circumstances of a pure rotational movement of the sort encouraged by testing apparatuses like the radial maze, the above equivalences do *not* obtain. For example, 3 left turns with straight movements between them can be equivalent to a single right turn or a left turn or an aboutface depending on the relative distances of the intervening straight movements. Unless the distances are incorporated into the computations within the framework of a spatial system these alternatives cannot be distinguished.

Alternative models are based on the idea that the hippocampus generates a spatial framework within which the above equivalences would be valid and that the computations are performed on the representations within this framework. I have recently published a description of one such model which is a compromise between an egocentric system and a fully non-egocentric one (O'Keefe,

1988). Following a brief description of that model, I will present a more recent model which is a fully allocentric, non-egocentric one.

In the first model (O'Keefe, 1988), the spatial framework is centred on the animal's head and moves with it as it moves around an environment. Cues are identified within this framework by their sensory features, their angle and their distance from the origin. The angle which each observed cue makes with this ego-centric framework is given directly by the sensory systems but the distance must be calculated. This latter is based on a motion parallax system whereby the difference between the expected and actual locations of an environmental cue as the animal explores an environment is used to calculate an estimate of the distance of that cue. Movements of the animal are represented as transforms (translations plus rotations) of the rat-centred spatial framework. Predictions of the consequence of a movement are generated by the system by the matrix multiplication of the matrix of place cell firing representing the current location by the transform matrix which represents the movement in terms of a translation and rotation of the reference framework. The system also calculates the inverse matrix of the present location. When this is multiplied by a matrix representing a desired location (e.g. a goal), the result is the transform matrix (spatial translation + rotation) necessary to move to that desired location. In this way the system can direct the motor system to move the animal to any part of a known environment. In this model, the representation of the current location is identified with the firing of cells in the CA3 field, the inverse matrix of the current location with the firing pattern across the cells of the CA1 field, and the transform matrix with the theta mechanism which is partly located in the medial septum and partly in the inhibitory interneuron – basket cell network of the hippocampus itself.

Although this model is compatible with some of the features of hippocampal anatomy and physiology and is capable of generating novel behaviours and of guiding the animal's behaviour from one place to another, it has several properties which may limit its application to the hippocampus. First, although it is a spatial system and derives much of its properties from this fact, it is still an egocentric spatial system and thus does not fulfill all of the conditions associated with an allocentric cognitive map. It cannot, for example, account for the fact that the place cells are non-directional under some circumstances. Furthermore, the cues represented within this system remain independent of each other and do not exhibit the cohesion attributed to such maps. It is not clear, for example, why the removal of a cue from such a system would have an effect on the representation of an environment but would not completely alter that representation.

An allocentric cognitive map theory

In an attempt to overcome some of these difficulties I have been working on an allocentric model for the cognitive map. The distinguishing properties of this model are that it references places in an environment not to a framework centred on the animal's body but to a framework fixed to the environment. This relies on the results of two independent computations performed on the cue representations in egocentric framework to yield two measures which are independent of the animal's current location and which can form the basis of a non-egocentric spatial framework. The first of these calculations is the geometric centroid of the set of cues which make up the environment and the second is a polarizing direction derived from the average slope of the lines drawn between each pair of cues. The former serves as the origin of the allocentric framework and the latter provides a reference direction from which polar angles can be measured. Together they specify the core of the cognitive mapping system. Both depend on a previous calculation of the distance of each cue from the rat within egocentric space. In the next sections, I will outline these processes in more detail.

The present model uses some of the ideas con-

tained in the previous model but in general attempts to overcome the aforementioned weaknesses. It does so by postulating a set of computational processes which enable the mapping system to calculate several aspects of a set of cues which uniquely identify that environment and which serve as the foundation on which to build an allocentric framework. Following the previous model, I assume that cues in the environment are represented within the neocortical sensoria as a bundle of qualities (proximal size, modality, intensity etc.) and are set within an egocentric framework centred on the rat's head (or body). Each cue is represented independently of all the others and there is no interaction (except where one occludes the other).

Before these data arrive at the mapping system, they need to be supplemented by a calculation

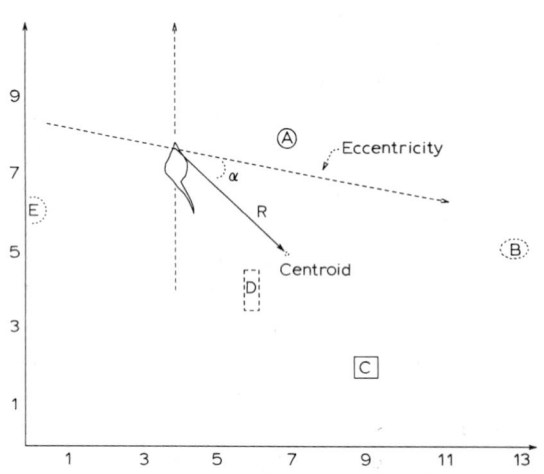

Fig. 1. A rat finds itself within an environment consisting of 5 cues A – E. A Cartesian framework with arbitrary metric has been superimposed upon the environment for identification of cue locations and for calculations. The dotted line through the animal's head represents the axis of an ego-centric polar coordinate framework centred on the head (E-space). This moves with the animal as it moves through the environment. The centroid is a location in the environment which does not change with the animal's movements and is estimated by the vector summation of the cue vectors. The second parameter, the eccentricity, is also derived from the cues, representing the average slopes of all the cue-pairs in E-space. α is the angle between the centroid vector and the eccentricity axis. R is the distance to the centroid.

which uses the movement parallax generated by each cue as the animal moves around an environment as a clue to its veridical distance in egocentric space (henceforth called E-space in contrast to the allocentric space generated in the cognitive mapping system: A-space). The data presented to the mapping system, then, consists of a set of cues each located in E-space by a distance and angle. The mapping system computes two pieces of information from these data: the geometrical centroid of the set of cues and the eccentricity of the distribution of the same cues. The first is used as the centre of a polar A-space framework while the second provides a direction which can be used as a reference from which angles in A-space can be measured. An example of these two parameters is shown in Fig. 1. In the next section I will set out a concrete proposal about the method by which these parameters are calculated.

Figures 1 – 3 show the mean vectors for the set of cues A – E from two orientations and two locations in the environment. Note that the length of vector **R** does not change as the animal rotates in a fixed location (Figs. 1 and 2) but that both the length R and the angle α of the centroid vary with translation movements regardless of whether or

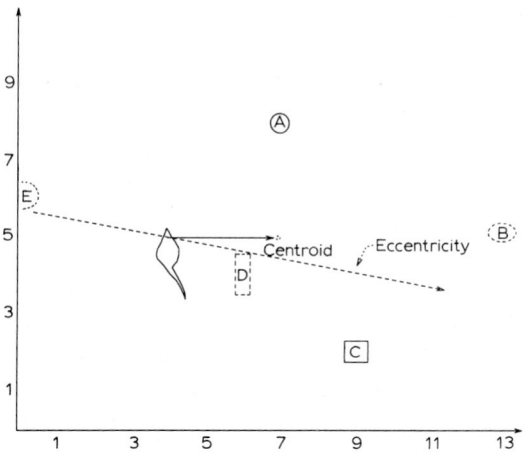

Fig. 3. The magnitude of the centroid vector changes with pure translation movements but unless there is an associated rotation the angle of eccentricity remains the same everywhere in the environment.

not these are associated with rotations (Figs. 1 and 3).

Computation of the eccentricity and centroid of an environment

The first measure derived from the distribution of cues in an environment is the eccentricity. This is defined as the deviation from symmetry or isotropism of the cue configuration in different directions. It can be measured as follows: at any given location in an environment a line drawn between two cues has a slope in E-space defined as

$$\text{Slope EC} = \frac{\Delta X}{\Delta Y} = \frac{AX - BX}{AY - BY} = \frac{A \sin \beta - B \sin \delta}{A \cos \beta - B \cos \delta}$$

where β and δ are the angles which the A and B cues make with the E-space polar axis. Notice that this measure depends on having previously assigned a veridical distance to the cues A and B. Now the interesting property of this slope measure is that although it varies as a function of rotational movements it is invariant with translation movements, i.e. it is identical at all locations in the environment for identical headings or directions of

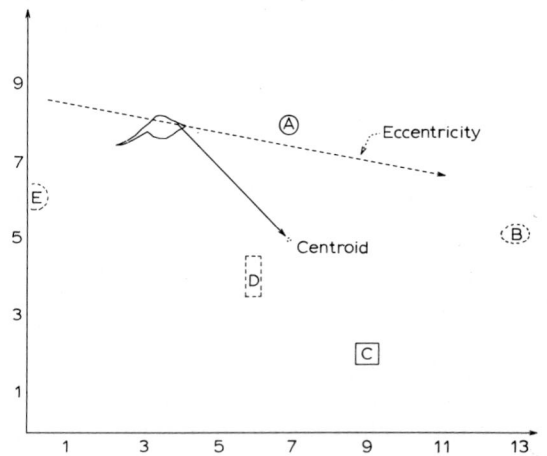

Fig. 2. The magnitude or distance measure of the centroid does not change with an inplace pure rotational movement. Here is shown such a rotation at the location of Fig. 1. In contrast, the animal's orientation with respect to the eccentricity axis does vary with rotations.

pointing. It follows that it can be used as a measure of direction: averaging across the slopes for all of the cue pairs in an environment gives the overall slope which can serve as a measure of the eccentricity of the cue distribution in a particular environment. The overall slope for the set of cues A − E is drawn on the diagram of Fig. 1. The overall eccentricity calculation could be carried out in several stages. Instead of taking all of the cue pairs at once, small subsets could be used to produce different estimates of the eccentricity and these in turn could be averaged to get the overall eccentricity. Figure 4 shows the result of estimates of the eccentricity based on the slopes of two pairs of cues each.

The centroid of the environment is defined as the geometric centre or centre of mass of the cues in the environment. This is calculated by taking the grand mean vector of the cue vectors in either A-space or E-space. In E-space each cue angle would be calculated from the egocentric head direction; in A-space the angle would be taken relative to the allocentric direction of eccentricity.

$$\boldsymbol{R} = \frac{1}{N} \sum_{i=1}^{N} \boldsymbol{V}$$

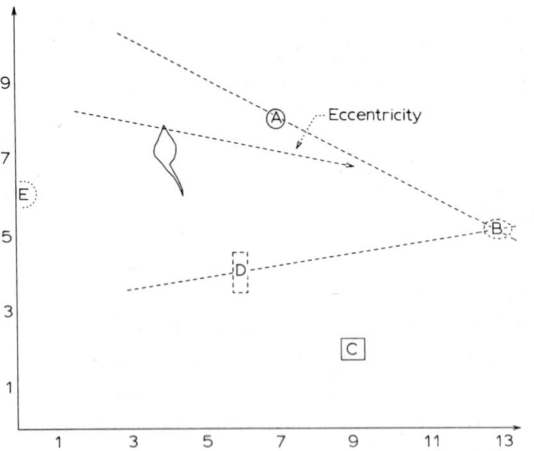

Fig. 4. The eccentricity direction is calculated by averaging across all of the slopes of the pairs of cues in the environment. In addition to the overall eccentricity, the slopes of cue pairs AB and BD are shown.

In order to take the vector average, it is convenient to separate each cue vector $\boldsymbol{R}$ into X and Y components

$$X = \boldsymbol{R} \sin \alpha$$
$$Y = \boldsymbol{R} \cos \alpha$$

The X's and Y's are summed independently and recombined to give the grand mean distance to the centroid R and the angle of vector α.

$$R^2 = \left(\frac{1}{N} \sum X\right)^2 + \left(\frac{1}{N} \sum Y\right)^2$$

$$\tan^{-1} \alpha = \frac{\sum X}{\sum Y}$$

Note that the length of the grand mean vector is a measure of the variance of the individual cue vectors or more exactly, a measure of the concentration of these vectors around the mean direction.

In a manner similar to the sequential computation of the eccentricity, the centroid vector $\boldsymbol{R}$, α can also be calculated in several stages. Small subsets of the cue vectors can be averaged to produce partial estimates of the grand average centroid and these in turn may be averaged to get the overall result. Figure 5 shows several intermediate vectors derived from the group of cues shown in Fig. 1 when the animal is at location I. In a subsequent section, I will suggest that one aspect of these intermediate centroid vectors might be encoded in place cell firing.

The two parameters, the centroid and the eccentricity, jointly define an allocentric space which is independent of the animal's movements but which can be used to locate the animal's current position and that of other places in the environment, for example, the location of food, water or dangerous objects. They can also provide a mechanism for assessing the coherence of the environmental representation and for detecting changes in the cue configuration: the absence or movements of existing cues or the appearance of new cues. In the next sections I will outline how the system predicts the results of movements and conversely, how it

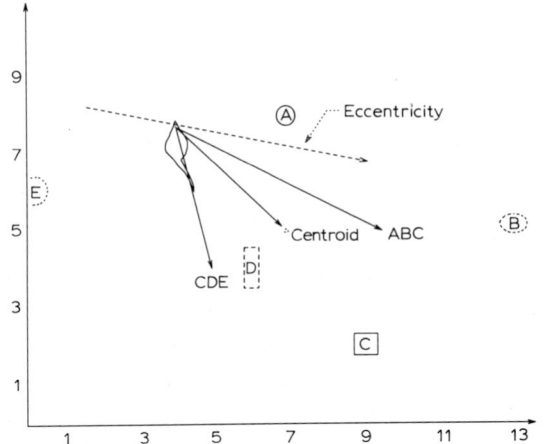

Fig. 5. The centroid is calculated by taking the vector average of all of the cues. Partial estimates of the centroid are given by the vector averages of subsets of cues. The centroid estimates based on cue subsets ABC and CDE are shown in addition to the centroid. Note that these vectors are different from the centroid and from each other.

allows for the calculation of the movements required to go from the current location to a goal.

Prediction of the centroid vector from the next location following a movement

As the animal moves around a familiar environment, the mapping system is continually predicting the changes in the centroid co-ordinates as a result of each movement. Each movement has a distance (M) and a direction component (γ) relative to the A-space defined by the centroid and the eccentricity. This vector, when combined with the vector representing the current location in A-space yields the new location vector. This process is shown in Figs. 6 and 7 for a movement within the space shown in Fig. 1 (cues A – E have been omitted from the figure for clarity). The rat begins its movement at location I ($X = 4$, $Y = 8$) and moves to location II ($X = 10$, $Y = 6$). The start location is represented as a vector with length $R_1 = 4.24$ and direction angle relative to the axis of eccentricity $\alpha_1 = 37.15°$ while the movement is represented as a vector of length $M = 6.32$ and

angle $\gamma = 10.58°$. The new centroid vector can be obtained by vector subtraction. In the example given

$$R_2X = R_1X - MX$$

$$R_1X = 4.24 \sin 37.15° = 2.56$$

$$MX = 6.32 \sin 10.58° = 1.16$$

$$R_2X = 2.56 - 1.16 = 1.40$$

and

$$R_2Y = R_1Y - MY$$

$$R_1Y = 4.24 \cos 37.15° = 3.38$$

$$MY = 6.32 \cos 10.58° = 6.21$$

$$R_2Y = 3.38 - 6.21 = -2.83$$

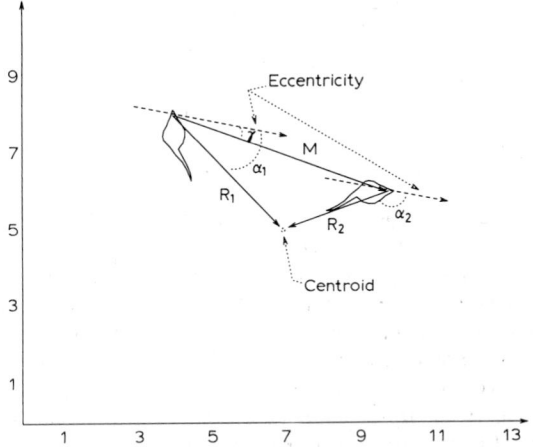

Fig. 6. Schema showing the movement from one location (on the left) to another (on the right) as a vector M with amplitude M and angle relative to the axis of eccentricity γ. The centroid vectors R_1 and R_2 from the start and finish location are also shown. Their angles relative to the axis of eccentricity are labelled α_1 and α_2 respectively.

Therefore the new location centroid vector is

$$\boldsymbol{R}_2 = (\boldsymbol{R}_2 X^2 + \boldsymbol{R}_2 Y^2)^{0.5} = 3.16$$

$$\alpha_2 = \tan^{-1} \frac{\boldsymbol{R}_2 Y}{\boldsymbol{R}_2 X} = 153.68°$$

This vector calculation is true for any set of vectors which add up to $\boldsymbol{R}$ and the system therefore will predict the final location on the basis of any set of equivalent movements.

This system has several uses. First, it can be used to define co-ordinates for regions of an environment in which there are few or even no sensory cues available. Second, it can allow two environments with no overlap of cues to be integrated. Third, it can be used to choose between the representations of two different environments

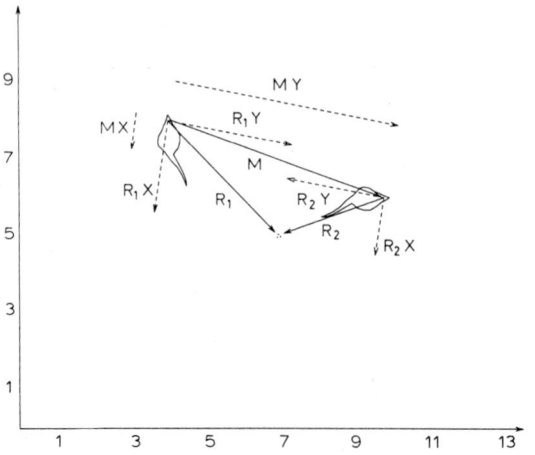

Fig. 7. Schema showing how the A-space formed from the centroid and eccentricity is used to calculate the new location after a movement. The movement vector $\boldsymbol{M}$ is decomposed into orthogonal components $\boldsymbol{M}X$ and $\boldsymbol{M}Y$ along and at right angles to the axis of eccentricity. $\boldsymbol{R}_1$ and $\boldsymbol{R}_2$ are the centroid vectors from the two locations and these are also decomposed into their X and Y components. α_1 and α_2 are the angles which the centroid vectors $\boldsymbol{R}_1$ and $\boldsymbol{R}_2$ make with the axis of eccentricity. Subtraction of these orthogonal components of the start location and the movement vectors and their recombination yields the new location vector. The inverse process is used to calculate the movement transform required to go from one location to the other. Here the centroid vectors of the two locations are decomposed in the A-space framework and their respective components subtracted in order to yield the movement vector $\boldsymbol{M}$.

where the calculations of the co-ordinates of the centroid from the initial arrays of sensory inputs do not allow this.

Generation of the movement transform

Part of the function of the mapping system is to enable the animal to navigate from its current location in an environment to a desirable location or goal. I have previously suggested (O'Keefe, 1988) that this computation involves the generation of the inverse matrix of the current location and its combination with the matrix representing the desired location, this latter having been stored during previous experience with the environment. A similar model is proposed for the present theory. In this case the goal of the computation is to calculate the movement vector $\boldsymbol{M}$, given a start location I and a goal location II. The calculation proceeds in a fashion similar to that of the previous section except that the amplitude and direction of the $\boldsymbol{M}$ vector have to be calculated from the component $\boldsymbol{R}_1$ and $\boldsymbol{R}_2$ centroid vectors (see Fig. 7). The movement translation required to go from the current location to a desired location is given by the equations:

$$\boldsymbol{M}^2 = \boldsymbol{M}X^2 + \boldsymbol{M}Y^2$$

$$\gamma = \tan^{-1} \frac{\boldsymbol{M}X}{\boldsymbol{M}Y}$$

where

$$\boldsymbol{M}X = \boldsymbol{R}_1 X - \boldsymbol{R}_2 X$$

$$\boldsymbol{M}Y = \boldsymbol{R}_1 Y - \boldsymbol{R}_2 Y$$

$\boldsymbol{M}X$ and $\boldsymbol{M}Y$ represent the respective differences of the X and Y components of the distances to the centroid from each of the locations. Behaviourally these measures could be translated into action by motor system commands which rotated the animal at the first location through an angle of γ to bring it into line with the goal and then moved it in a straight line a distance of M. Notice that this transform vector is continuously modified during the movement so that if it is not possible for the animal to take the straight line course to the goal, detours can be calculated. For example, if the straight line path is blocked and the animal is faced with several alternative routes, it can test the "efficiency" of these alterations by calculating which offers the minimum deviation from the optimal choice. Generally this will be equivalent to the minimum angular deviation at the choice point. One form of learning might involve the storage of optimal choices where experience has shown that the minimum overall detour vector differs from the minimum angle at the choice (because the detour length in that direction was longer).

Relationship of the model to the hippocampal system

The model suggests that the hippocampus proper and the subicular region together constitute the neural basis of the cognitive map. Further it suggests that different aspects of the spatial computations are carried out in different regions. The similarity of the fields of the place fields found in CA3 and CA1 of the hippocampus to the elements which compute the distance parameter of the centroid suggest that the hippocampus proper is involved in the calculations of the centroid of the environment from cue vectors presented to it via the entorhinal cortex. Similarly, the similarity of the direction-computing elements to the direction cells of dorsal presubiculum suggests that this is the area where the environmental eccentricity measure is computed.

How the centroid computations might be mapped onto the hippocampal area

In my previous model (O'Keefe, 1988) I suggested that the distances of the cue vectors in E-space were computed in the hippocampus proper and fed back to the entorhinal cortex where they were stored. According to the present model, this com-

putation takes place either in the entorhinal cortex itself or in its neocortical afferents (including the parietal cortex). The resulting R's are decomposed into their X and Y components so that they can be vector-summed rather than linearly summed. One of the major computational functions attributed to the hippocampal and subicular areas on this model is that of trigonometric decomposition of a vector into its orthogonal components or projection of the vector onto the X and Y axes either of E-space or A-space. While it is possible to accomplish this by the use of parallel or iterative computations which employ simple elements, a more intriguing possibility is that the trigonometric conversions are carried out by the theta system. On this model the primary function of the theta system is to cause the granule and pyramidal cells to oscillate with a sinusoid wave. Control of the amplitude and phase relations amongst the oscillators enables these cells to calculate the quantity $R \sin \alpha$ where R is the strength of the input or the amplitude of the sinusoid and α is the phase angle of the input relative to other oscillators or to the septal clock. Although the idea will not be explored further here this mechanism might involve NMDA receptors as well as the cholinergic system. NMDA has been shown to set up membrane oscillations in neocortical cells after synaptic activity had been blocked by tetrodotoxin (Flatman et al., 1983).

At this stage of our understanding it is only possible to speculate about the loci of such computations. Place-coded cells have been reported in layers II and III of the entorhinal cortex as well as in the hippocampus proper (Quirk and Ranck, 1987). These cells give rise to the perforant path which appears to be the main conduit for neocortical input to the hippocampal region. Anatomical studies suggest that the primary connection between the presubicular direction system and the hippocampal place system is via a projection of the former to layer III of the entorhinal cortex (Köhler, 1985). Connections from the hippocampus proper to the presubiculum are sparse but there is one from the subiculum (Köhler, 1985). On the present scheme, this would imply that the entorhinal cells are influenced by the eccentricity parameter and suggests that the egocentric cue vectors arriving from the neocortex are mapped into allocentric co-ordinates at this stage. This is accomplished by rotating each vector by the angle of the eccentricity direction in head-centred space. Vector rotation could be accomplished by phase-shifting of the sinusoid which could in turn be done by simple addition.

According to this theory the next computation requires the cue vectors to be decomposed into orthogonal vectors to permit vector addition. If the computation is performed by sinusoids then the calculation of the cos component could be carried out by a 90° phase shift of the sin value. This phase shift might be one of the operations performed by the dentate granule cells on the entorhinal input. The X and Y components for a set of cues would then be recombined in the CA3 field, one component carried in on the direct entorhinal input and the other via the dentate phase-shifted input. Here the place field firing of each pyramidal cell would represent the vector average of a small subset of cues in A-space or what is equivalent, the estimate of the distance (actually inverse distance) to the centroid based on that cue subset. This centroid measure would be encoded in the CA3 place cell firing pattern. Averaging over all such subsets would give the best estimate of the grand centroid distance. I have previously suggested that this averaging could take place via the CA3 collateral network and that one of the roles of the inhibitory network is to normalize the computations (O'Keefe, 1988).

The differences between the place cells of the CA3 and CA1 fields of the hippocampus are not marked and the present theory does not provide any well-motivated, distinctive role for the CA1 field. Perhaps the CA1 field is the place where the location which is predicted to result from the current movement is computed. The need for a separate brain region might arise from the fact that the calculation involves a subtraction rather than an addition of vectors. On this view the CA1 pyramids combine information about the current location arriving along the Schaffer collateral pathway from CA3 with information about the direction and distance of the movement generated by the medial septal/diagonal band region or from some other as yet unidentified brain region.

The inverse calculation for deriving the distance and direction of a desired goal from the present location would be carried out in the next stage of the circuit, in the subicular area. Information about the locations of desirable objects such as food and water would be located and combined with information about the current location coming from the hippocampus proper.

Relation to the place cell data

According to the present model the firing rate of the place cells codes an estimate of the inverse distance to the centroid of the sensory array. Each cell uses a different subset of the overall cue array and therefore each place field is different. Neighbouring place cells code for different sets of cues: depending on the spatial arrangement of those cues within the environment there may be greater or lesser topographic organization amongst the place fields of a group of neighbouring cells. The grand vector sum of a large group of place cell fields should yield a good value for the centroid — another way of saying this is that they should be spread homogeneously around the environment. This appears to be the case (O'Keefe 1979; Muller et al., 1987). Furthermore, many of the fields away from the edges of symmetrical environments should approximate to gaussians and inspection of the Muller et al. data suggests that this is also the case. The place fields in CA3 and CA1 do not appear to differ from each other in any marked way. This may mean that the present methods of recording and representing the place fields are missing an important aspect of their information content or that the difference is a subtle one of the type suggested above. Muller and Kubie (1986) have suggested that the place cell firing may be better correlated with the rat's future location than with its present location.

In the O'Keefe and Speakman (1987) experiment it was found possible to rotate the place fields around the centre of a + maze by rotating a set of controlled spatial cues by steps of 90°, 180° or 270°. For example, a field in the North arm on trial 1 would appear on the East arm on trial 2 when the spatial cues had been rotated by 90° clockwise in the interval. Furthermore, the fields remained in the correct location if the spatial cues were removed after a 30-s exposure. Within the present model, these data might suggest that the controlled spatial cues are responsible primarily for setting the eccentricity parameter but not the centroid. This latter would be set by the maze cues themselves as well as by the stationary background cues which were not moved from trial-to-trial. As the controlled cues were rotated by multiples of 90° the field shape which was given by the background cues and coded for the distance to the centroid would remain unchanged but its location relative to the room would rotate with the eccentricity. Memory on each trial would consist of a temporary fixation of the axis of eccentricity relative to the stable centroid cues. At the end of each trial the eccentricity would reset to a default value ready to be altered at the beginning of the next.

Acknowledgements

I would like to dedicate this chapter to Professor Theodor Blackstad in recognition of his pioneering contributions to the anatomy of the hippocampus. His humility and patient attention to detail have been a life-long source of admiration and inspiration. The work reported here has been supported by the Medical Research Council of Britain and by a grant from the Sloan Foundation.

References

Bostock, E., Taube, J. and Muller, R.U. (1988) The effects of head orientation on the firing of hippocampal place cells. *Soc. Neurosci. Abstr.*, 13 (no. 51.7): 127.

Breese, C.R., Hampson, R.E. and Deadwyler, S.A. (1989) Hippocampal place cells: stereotypy and plasticity. *J. Neurosci.*, 9: 1097 – 1111.

Christian, E.P. and Deadwyler, S.A. (1986) Behavioral functions and hippocampal cell types: evidence for two nonoverlapping populations in the rat. *J. Neurophysiol.*, 55: 331 – 348.

Eichenbaum, H., Kuperstein, M., Fagan, A. and Nagode, J. (1987) Cue-sampling and goal-approach correlates of hippocampal unit activity in rats performing an odor discrimination task. *J. Neurosci.*, 7: 716 – 732.

Flatman, J.A., Schwindt, P.C., Crill, W.E. and Stafstrom, C.E. (1983) Multiple actions of N-methyl-D-aspartate on cat neocortical neurons in vitro. *Brain Res.*, 266: 169 – 173.

Hill, A.J. (1978) First occurrence of hippocampal spatial firing in a new environment. *Exp. Neurol.*, 62: 282 – 297.

Hill, A.J. and Best, P.J. (1981) Effects of deafness and blindness on the spatial correlates of hippocampal unit activity in the rat. *Exp. Neurol.*, 73: 204 – 217.

Köhler, C. (1985) Intrinsic projections of the retrohippocampal region in the rat brain. I. The subicular complex. *J. Comp. Neurol.*, 236: 504 – 522.

Kubie, J.L. and Ranck, J.B. (1983) Sensory-behavioral correlates in individual hippocampus neurons in three situations: space and context. In W. Seifert (Ed.) *Neurobiology of the Hippocampus*, Academic Press, London, pp. 433 – 447.

McNaughton, B.L. (1988) Neural mechanisms for spatial computation and information storage. In L. Nadel, L.A.Cooper, P. Culicover and R.M. Harnish (Eds.), *Neural Connections and Mental Computations*, MIT Press, Cambridge, MA, pp. 285 – 350.

McNaughton, B.L., Barnes, C.A. and O'Keefe, J. (1983a) The contributions of position, direction and velocity to single unit activity in the hippocampus of freely-moving rats. *Exp. Brain Res.*, 52: 41 – 49.

McNaughton, B.L., O'Keefe, J. and Barnes, C.A. (1983b) The stereotrode: a new technique for simultaneous isolation of several single units in the central nervous system from multiple unit records. *J. Neurosci. Methods*, 8: 391 – 397.

Miller, V.M. and Best, P.J. (1980) Spatial correlates of hippocampal unit activity are altered by lesions of the fornix and entorhinal cortex. *Brain Res.*, 194: 311 – 323.

Muller, R.U. and Kubie, J.L. (1986) Introduction of time into the study of place cells. *Soc. Neurosci. Abstr.*, 12 (No. 141.8): 521.

Muller, R.U. and Kubie, J.L. (1987) The effects of changes in the environment on the spatial firing of hippocampal complex-spike cells. *J. Neurosci.*, 7: 1951 – 1968.

Muller, R.U., Kubie, J.L. and Ranck, J.B. (1987) Spatial firing patterns of hippocampal complex-spike cells in a fixed environment. *J. Neurosci.*, 7: 1935 – 1950.

O'Keefe, J. (1976) Place units in the hippocampus of the freely moving rat. *Exp. Neurol.*, 51: 78 – 109.

O'Keefe, J. (1979) A review of the hippocampal place cells. *Prog. Neurobiol.*, 13: 419 – 439.

312

O'Keefe, J. (1988) Computations the hippocampus might perform. In L. Nadel, L.A. Cooper, P. Culicover and R.M. Harnish (Eds.), *Neural Connections and Mental Computations*, MIT Press, Cambridge, MA, pp. 225–284.

O'Keefe, J. and Conway, D.H. (1978) Hippocampal place units in the freely moving rat: why they fire where they fire. *Exp. Brain Res.*, 31: 573–590.

O'Keefe, J. and Dostrovsky, J. (1971) The hippocampus as a spatial map. Preliminary evidence from unit activity in freely moving rats. *Brain Res.*, 34: 171–175.

O'Keefe, J. and Nadel, L. (1978) *The Hippocampus as a Cognitive Map,* Clarendon Press, Oxford.

O'Keefe, J. and Speakman, A. (1987) Single unit activity in the rat hippocampus during a spatial memory task. *Exp. Brain Res.*, 68: 1–27.

Olton, D.S., Branch, M. and Best, P.J. (1978) Spatial correlates of hippocampal unit activity. *Exp. Neurol.*, 58: 387–409.

Quirk, G.J. and Ranck, J.B. (1986) Firing of single cells in entorhinal cortex is location specific and phase locked to hippocampal theta rhythm. *Soc. Neurosci. Abstr.*, 13 (no. 413.2): 1524.

Recce, M. and O'Keefe (1989) The tetrode: an improved technique for multi-unit extracellular recording. *Soc. Neurosci. Abstr.*, 15 (no. 490.3): 1250.

J. Storm-Mathisen, J. Zimmer and O.P. Ottersen (Eds.)
Progress in Brain Research, Vol. 83
© 1990 Elsevier Science Publishers B.V. (Biomedical Division)

CHAPTER 23

GABAergic mechanisms in the CA3 hippocampal region during early postnatal life

Y. Ben-Ari, C. Rovira, J.L. Gaiarsa, R. Corradetti*, O. Robain and E. Cherubini

INSERM U – 29, 123 Bd. de Port-Royal, 75014 Paris, France

The developmental pattern of GABAergic neurons in the rat hippocampus during the first week of postnatal life shows several particularities both from a morphological and physiological point of view: (1) GABA immunoreactive neurons which are initially localized in a deep and superficial layer, progressively disappear from these two layers. From the end of the first postnatal week, GABAergic neuronal somata appear throughout the whole hippocampus, but GABA immunoreactive terminal structures are not frequent until the second postnatal week. (2) Intracellular observations in slices reveal the presence in CA3 pyramidal neurons between P0 and P6 (postnatal days) of spontaneous giant depolarizing potentials (GDPs); these are mediated by GABA acting on $GABA_A$ receptors and modulated presynaptically by NMDA receptors. During this period of development, GABA and $GABA_A$ analogues have a depolarizing action at resting membrane potential. Bicuculline at this developmental stage blocks completely spontaneous and evoked synaptic potentials. During the second postnatal week, when GABA responses shift from depolarizing to hyperpolarizing, bicuculline induces spontaneous interictal discharges. It is suggested that the positive feedback of the GABAergic interneuron on the pyramidal neuron during the first week of life may account for the generation of GDPS which may play an important role in synaptogenesis.

Introduction

In the adult hippocampus – as in many other brain structures – excitatory and inhibitory events are primarily mediated by glutamate and GABA respectively. In CA3 pyramidal neurons, the excitatory postsynaptic potentials (EPSPs) evoked by mossy fibre stimulation are mediated through the activation of non-*N*-methyl-D-aspartate (non-NMDA) type of receptors since they are blocked by the relatively specific non-NMDA receptor antagonist – CNQX (Drejer and Honoré, 1988; Neuman et al., 1988) but not by the specific NMDA receptor antagonist D-2-amino-5-phosphonovalerate (APV). In the CA3 region hip-

pocampal EPSPs include also an NMDA-mediated component, which at resting membrane potential is blocked by Mg^{2+}. This component is readily revealed when Mg^{2+} is removed from the perfusing solution (Neuman et al., 1988b). It is therefore reminiscent of that which plays an important role in a long-term potentiation of synaptic transmission in CA1 (Collingridge et al., 1988). This and other observations (see Collingridge and Bliss, 1987) reflect the important role of NMDA-mediated events on synaptic plasticity.

In the adult hippocampus inhibitory activity is primarily mediated by GABA. Thus, stimulation of the mossy fibres evokes a fast and a slow inhibitory postsynaptic potential (IPSP). The fast IPSP is mediated by GABA acting on bicuculline-sensitive $GABA_A$ receptors coupled to Cl^- channels (Ben Ari et al., 1981), whereas the slow IPSP is mediated by GABA acting on bicuculline insensitive $GABA_B$ receptors coupled to K^+ channels

---

* Present address: Department of Preclinical and Clinical Pharmacology, University of Florence, Viale G.B. Morgagni 65, 50134 Firenze, Italy.

(Alger, 1984). The early postnatal period is characterized by important and abrupt changes notably in brain transmitter markers (Dupont et al., 1987; Garthwaite et al., 1987). There are several examples of transient expression of receptors (Parnavelas and Cavanagh, 1988) uncluding in the hippocampal formation (Tremblay et al., 1988; Represa et al., 1989). In vitro studies suggest that these changes may reflect the contribution of transmitters to growth, synapse formation and stabilization or regression of connections (Mattson, 1988). In vivo experiments reflect the important role of NMDA-mediated events in developmental plasticity (Kleinschmidt et al., 1987; Tsumoto et al., 1987).

In this report we have examined by immunocytochemistry the early ontogenesis of GABAergic neurons in the rat hippocampus and analyzed in slices the changes in GABA receptors and excitatory amino acid mediated synaptic transmission which occur during this developmental period. We report during the first postnatal week the presence in CA3 pyramidal neurons of spontaneous giant depolarizing potentials (GDPs), which are mediated by GABA acting on $GABA_A$ receptors and modulated presynaptically by NMDA receptors.

Results

GABA immunocytochemistry in early postnatal life

GABAergic neurons have an early neurogenesis. Using tritiated thymidine and immunocytochemistry several studies indicate that GABAergic neurons are generated between E13 and E15 embryonic age (Amaral and Kurz, 1985; Lubbers et al., 1985; Soriano et al., 1986, 1989a), 2 days before pyramidal neurons (Bayer, 1980). In the fascia dentata GABAergic neurons are also generated before birth (Soriano et al., 1989b).

Using an immunocytochemical approach with GABA antibody in semi-thin sections (10 μm) we have recently studied the developmental changes in GABA distribution in early postnatal life (Rozenberg et al., 1989). Our observations can be summarized as follows:

(1) GABA immunolabelling is observed 2 – 4 days after the last mitosis (i.e. E18). GABA-immunoreactive neurons are initially located primarily in two layers: a deep layer in the intermediate zone and a superficial layer in the marginal zone just above the hippocampal fissure. A similar pattern of distribution has been observed in the visual cortex (Chronwall and Wolff, 1980; Lauder et al., 1986). Both layers are largely transient since they disappear postnatally; the underlying mechanisms have not been clarified (cellular death, migration, or transient expression of GABA in some neurons). An adult pattern of GABA distribution is observed starting from P10.

(2) Although GABA-immunoreactive neurons are visible as early as E18, GABAergic boutons around the cell bodies of pyramidal neurons are observed only starting from P6 (Fig. 1B). At this stage, there are only few GABA-positive puncta around some pyramidal cells (Fig. 1B), and an adult pattern of 15 – 20 GABA-positive puncta around cell pyramidal neuron (e.g. Woodson et al., 1988) is conspicuous at P18 (Fig. 1C). A similar delay between the presence of GABAergic neuron somata and terminals is also visible in the fascia dentata (Rozenberg et al., 1989).

GABA is the principal "excitatory" transmitter in early postnatal life

Intracellular recordings from over 300 CA3 neurons from immature hippocampal slices revealed the presence of spontaneous giant depolarizing potentials (GDPs) in over 85% of the neurons between P0 – P8, but not after (Fig. 2A,B). GDPs consisted of a 300 – 500 ms large depolarization (25 – 50 mV) with superimposed fast action potentials. GDPs were network-driven synaptic potentials (and not endogenous potentials) since: (1) they were synchronous with field potentials recorded with extracellular electrodes positioned in the stratum radiatum (Fig. 2C); (2) they were syn-

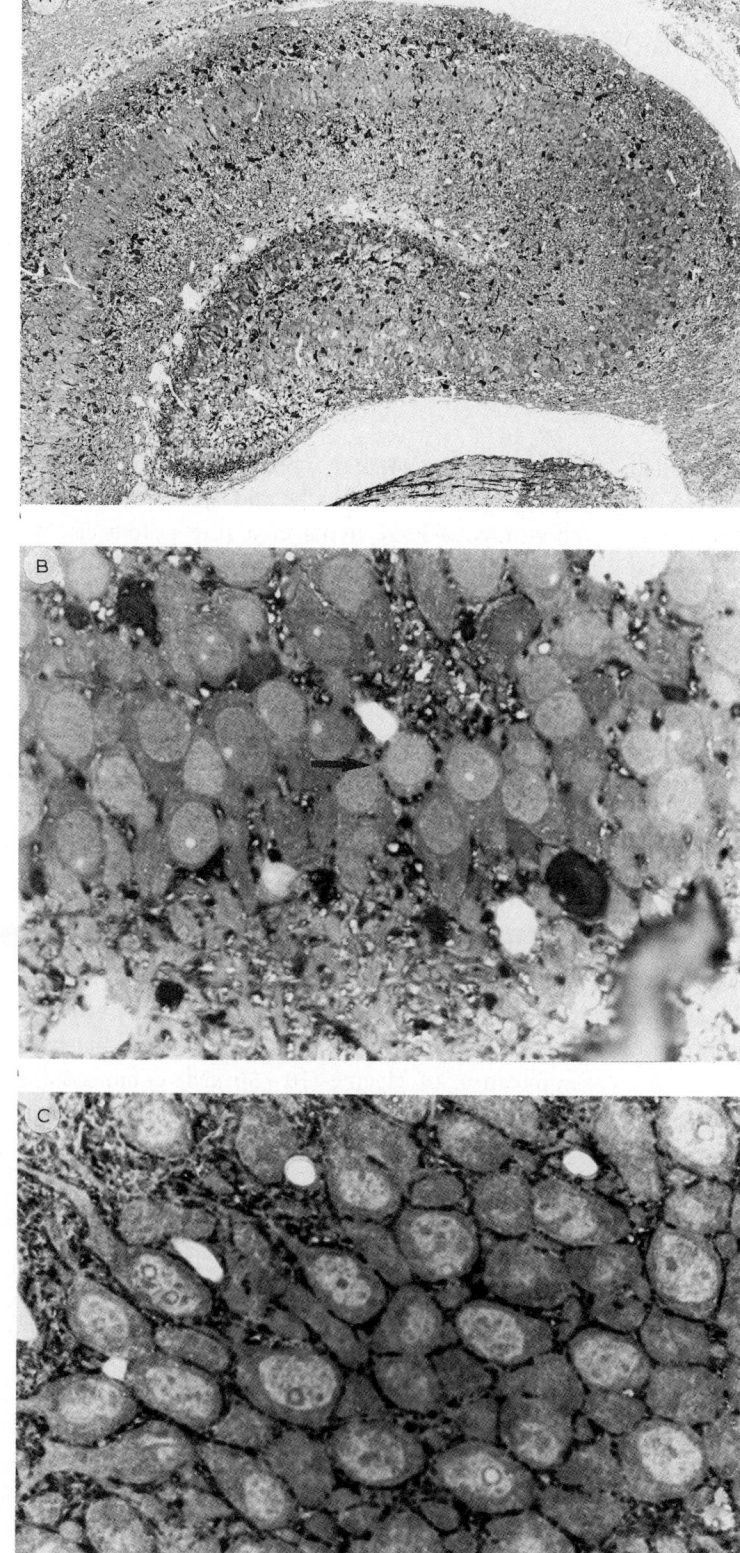

Fig. 1. Distribution of GABA immunoreactivity at P3 (A), P6 (B), and P18 (C). Semithin sections (10 μm), ×60 (A), ×360 (B,C). Note that already at P3 numerous GABA neurons are conspicuous in stratum oriens and stratum radiatum; GABA-positive puncta are not obeserved at P3, a few puncta are observed at P6, and the adult patern is found at P18.

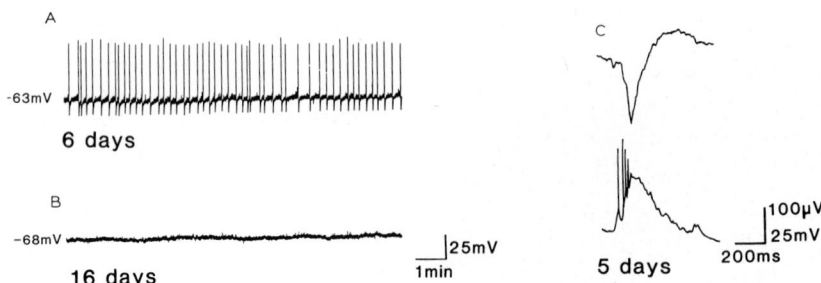

Fig. 2. Spontaneous GDPs in CA3 are generated by a network. A: spontaneously occurring GDPs in a 6-day-old rat. B: GDPs are not present at the end of the second postnatal week. C: concomitant extracellular (upper trace) and intracellular (lower trace) recordings of a GDP in a 5-day-old rat.

chronous in pairs of CA3 neurones recorded simultaneously. GDPs were mediated by GABA acting on GABA$_A$ receptors since they were blocked by bicuculline (1 – 10 μM); in this period of development bicuculline induced a small membrane hyperpolarization (4 ± 2 mV) and blocked spontaneous synaptic noise. It is worth noting that from the end of the second postnatal week, when GDPs are no longer present, bicuculline induced interictal discharges, as in adult neurons. Furthermore, GDPs reversed polarity at the same potential as exogenously applied GABA or isoguvacine (a GABA$_A$ agonist) (i.e. – 20 mV and – 50 mV with KCl- and K-methylsulfate-filled electrodes respectively). Electrical stimulation of the hilar region also induced GDPs. Like spontaneous GDPs they were blocked by bicuculline (1 – 10 μM) and reversed polarity at the same potential as GABA and/or isoguvacine.

It is likely that the depolarizing action of GABA is due to a reversed Cl gradient (in comparison to adult); the underlying mechanisms have not yet been clarified. However, regardless of the mechanisms underlying the depolarizing action of GABA, it is clear that GDPs are excitatory events since they reached the threshold for spike generation in spite of the fall in input resistance. Therefore at this period of development GABA-mediated GDPs and synaptic noise constitute the principal excitatory drive of CA3 pyramidal neurons. There is a transitional period at the end of the first postnatal week during which GDPs disappeared progressively and were replaced by spontaneous large hyperpolarizing potentials. As GDPs, these were mediated by GABA acting on GABA$_A$ receptors. Interestingly, bicuculline blocked these large hyperpolarizing potentials and generated interictal discharges as in adult neurons.

NMDA receptors modulate GABA-mediated GDPs in early postnatal life

Bath application of NMDA receptor antagonists (APV 10 – 50 μM, Fig. 3), APH (10 – 50 μM), CPP (10 – 50 μM) or NMDA channel blockers (phencyclidine 1 μM or ketamine 20 μM) reduced or blocked spontaneous (or evoked) GDPs. In contrast to bicuculline they did not block the synaptic noise. More recently we have also found that bath application of glycine (10 – 30 μM) enhanced the frequency of GDPs without modifying their amplitude or duration (Fig. 4). These effects were mediated by the glycine allosteric site of NMDA receptors (Johnston and Ascher, 1987) since they were insensitive to strychnine (1 μM) and they were mimicked by D-serine. The enhancement of GDP frequency by glycine was blocked by APV, APH (50 μM) or by bicuculline (10 μM). From the end of the second postnatal week, when GDPs were absent, higher concentrations of glycine (200 μM, Fig. 4) did not produce any effect on spontaneous synaptic noise, membrane potential and

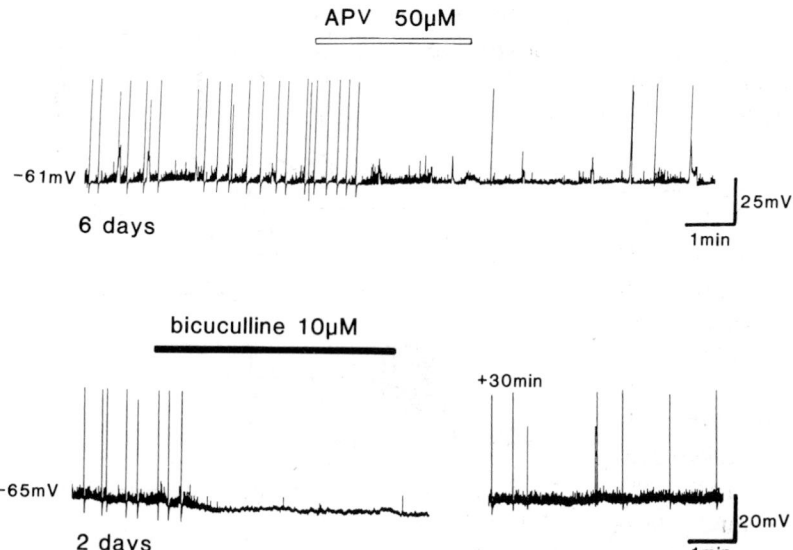

Fig. 3. GDPs are blocked by the NMDA receptor antagonist APV (upper trace) and by the GABA$_A$ antagonist bicuculline (lower trace); the two recordings are from two different neurons.

input resistance. Furthermore, the effects of sub-threshold concentrations of NMDA (0.1 μM) were considerably potentiated by concomitant application of glycine or D-serine (10 – 20 μM) which by themselves were inactive on these neurons. Interestingly, in the presence of TTX (1 μM) which blocks propagated activity, glycine (up to 50 μM) or D-serine (20 – 50 μM) had no effect on membrane potential, input resistance or NMDA induced membrane depolarization. In voltage-clamped neurones glycine or D-serine had no effect on the APV-sensitive inward current generated by bath application of NMDA. Therefore, the effects of glycine were not mediated by a direct action on pyramidal neurons.

GABA responses in early postnatal life do not desensitize

Immature cells were very sensitive to GABA and GABA$_A$ agonists (isoguvacine or THIP). The GABA$_A$ responses were blocked by bicuculline with an apparent PA_2 of 6.8. A particular feature of GABA response in immature neurons was the

absence of receptor desensitization. Bath applications of GABA (100 – 300 μM), isoguvacine or THIP (10 – 30 μM, Fig. 5), which are poor substrates for uptake system, induced a peak inward current which after a few seconds declined to a plateau level. The decline was not associated to changes in leak conductance, ruling out the possibility of a receptor desensitization; it is likely due to a change in the driving force to chloride which occurs during long applications of GABA.

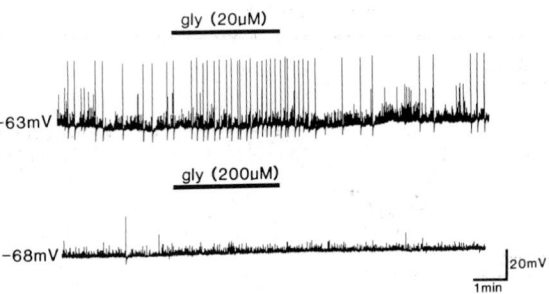

Fig. 4. Glycine increases the frequency of GDPs during the first postnatal week (upper trace: 5-day-old rat) and in the adult rat (lower trace). Higher concentration of glycine has no effects on membrane potential or synaptic noise.

318

Discussion

Interaction between GABA and excitatory amino acid mediated events in early postnatal life

Figure 6 illustrates the proposed wiring diagram underlying the generation of GDPs. The GABAergic interneuron oscillates in response to the activation of NMDA receptors by glutamate released by axon collaterals of pyramidal cells. The Ca^{2+} influx, induced by the activation of the NMDA channel will activate a Ca^{2+} dependent K^+ conductance which will repolarize the cell. (e.g. the well-documented case of the cells in the Lamprey spinal cord, Grillner et al., 1987). The oscillating GABAergic interneuron would release GABA. The depolarization induced by GABA will promote a positive feedback loop through which the synchronous discharge of a population of pyramidal cells might be produced. Interestingly, Dun and Mo (1989) have recently shown that in immature sympathetic ganglion cells, NMDA modulates the glycinergic IPSP suggesting that the presynaptic control of inhibitory amino acid release by NMDA may be a general feature of the immature circuit. There are in fact several indications that NMDA receptors may play a particularly important role in developmental plasticity: (1) In the visual system, NMDA antagonists block the processing of visual information in the immature but not adult rat (Tsumoto et al., 1987). (2) In the

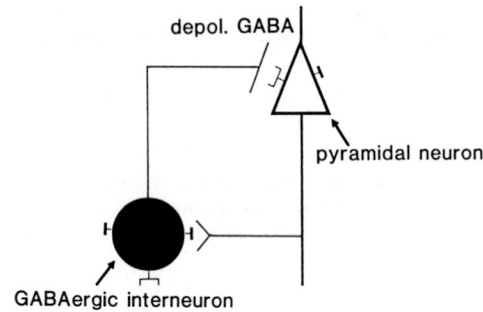

Fig. 6. Model of oscillatory behaviour of immature CA3 hippocampal neurons (see text).

hippocampus, there is a transient enhanced density of NMDA binding sites during early postnatal life; the density of specific glutamate binding sites in the Ammon's horn increases significantly from P4 (postnatal day) to P8 and then there is a highly significant decrease (Tremblay et al., 1988); these changes are due to a transient increase (at P8) in the density of NMDA sites and not to a change in affinity (ibid). A study in the human hippocampus shows a similar development curve with a peak at foetal week 23 – 27 (Represa et al., 1989). (3) The inward currents generated by NMDA are often less voltage-dependent during this period than in adult neurons (Ben-Ari et al., 1988). This will facilitate

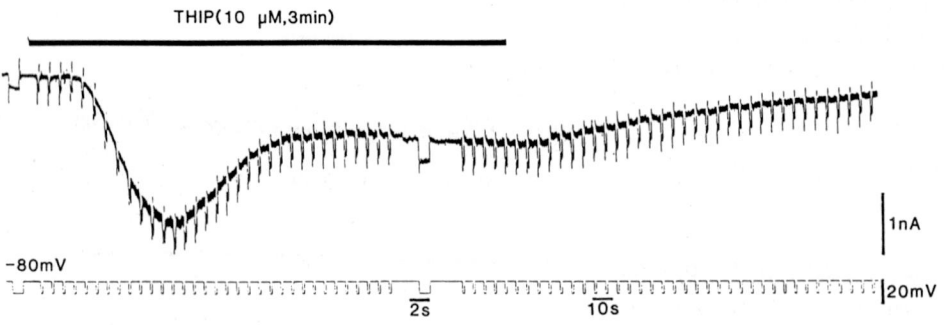

Fig. 5. Lack of desensitization of the response to THIP in early postnatal life. Inward current produced by bath application of THIP (10 μM). The cell was held at -80 mV and 10 mV (1 s duration), hyperpolarizing voltage steps were applied to the cell. Note that the increase in leak conductance was constant in spite of the decline in the inward current.

the contribution of NMDA-mediated events at resting membrane potential. (4) The contribution of NMDA reeptors in early postnatal life is also suggested by the observations that glycine potentiates spontaneous activity only during this period. We suggest the existence of a heterogeneous population of strychnine-insensitive glycine sites. The high-affinity sites (submicromolar K_d see Johnston and Ascher, 1987; Kemp et al., 1988; Kleckner and Dingledine, 1988; Kessler et al., 1989) present in adult or immature hippocampus would be saturated in slices (or in situ) by the endogenous concentrations of glycine (McGale et al., 1977). We postulate the existence of an additional lower affinity glycine site which would be located on the somata or terminals of GABAergic interneurons. Changes in the local concentrations of glycine could modulate GDPs and synaptic noise by altering the sensitivity of the interneurons to glutamate. This site would disappear by the end of the first postnatal week.

Mechanisms of action and possible physiological relevance of depolarizing action of GABA in early postnatal life

The mechanisms underlying the depolarizing action of GABA are presently unknown but it is possible that in immature cells − like following dendritic application of GABA on adult hippocampal neurons (Andersen et al., 1980) − there is a modified chloride gradient resulting from a unidirectional chloride pump (Misgeld et al., 1986). Alterations in intracellular pH at this developmental stage − due to different metabolic patterns − may also contribute to the reversed Cl^- gradient because of the permeability of the channel to bicarbonate (Kaila and Viopo, 1987). It will be important to determine the relation between the alterations in properties of GABA responses at this early stage and the developmental modifications as determined in molecular biology in the subunits of the $GABA_A$ receptor channel complex (William et al., 1988).

Interestingly, there are now several indications that GABA has a trophic role in immature neurons. At birth GABAergic interneurons are present but GABAergic terminals are seldom observed and electronmicroscopic studies in fact suggest that at this early developmental stage the synapses are primarily asymmetric and have several immature features, notably lack of postsynaptic thickenings, few synaptic vesicles etc. (McLaughlin et al., 1975; Blue and Parnavelas, 1983; Bahr and Wolf, 1985). Other observations suggest that a non-synaptic release of GABA may precede GABAergic synaptogenesis (Hicks and al., 1986.) This release may originate from growth cones (Gordon-Weeks et al., 1984). Since GABA provides most of the ongoing excitatory drive at this stage, it is possible that GABA-mediated GDPs represent a significant signal in the growth and differentiation of CA3 pyramidal neurons. The delayed maturation of excitatory amino acid mediated connections − in particular the mossy fibre system which has been elegantly studied by Blackstad and Kjaerheim (1961), may well provide a signal promoting the stabilization of one type of GABAergic synapses and the regression of another. Using selective lesions or deafferentations or roller cultures it is possible to test the sequence of events and the mechanisms governing the interactions between GABA and excitatory amino acids in early development. This provides a particularly adequate model of the regulation by transmitters and synaptic activity of synaptogenesis and the shape and extent of arborizations of target neurons.

References

Alger, B.E. (1984) Characteristics of a slow hyperpolarizing synaptic potential in rat hippocampal pyramidal cells in vitro. *J. Neurophysiol.,* 52: 892 – 910.

Amaral, D.G. and Kurz, J. (1985) The time of origin of cells demonstrating glutamic acid decarboxylase like immunoreactivity in the hippocampal formation of the rat. *Neurosci. Lett.,* 59: 33 – 39.

Andersen, P., Dingledine, R., Gjerstad, L., Langmoen, I.A. and Mosfeldt Laursen, A. (1980) Two different responses of hippocampal pyramidal cells to application of gamma-

320

aminobutyric acid. *J. Physiol. (Lond.)*, 305: 279–296.

Bahr, S. and Wolff, J.R. (1985) Postnatal development of axosomatic synapses in the rat visual cortex: morphogenesis and quantitative evaluation. *J. Comp. Neurol.*, 233: 405–420.

Bayer, S. (1980) Development of the hippocampal region in the rat. I. Neurogenesis examined with (3H) thymidine autoradiography. *J. Comp. Neurol.*, 190: 87–114.

Ben-Ari, Y., Krnjević, K., Reiffenstein, R.J. and Reinhardt, W. (1981) Inhibitory conductance changes and action of γ-aminobutyrate in rat hippocampus. *Neuroscience*, 6: 2445–2463.

Ben-Ari, Y., Cherubini, E. and Krnjevic, K. (1988) Changes in voltage dependence of NMDA currents during development. *Neurosci. Lett.*, 94: 88–92.

Ben-Ari, Y., Cherubini, E., Corradetti, R. and Gaiarsa, J.L. (1989) Giant synaptic potentials in immature rat CA3 hippocampal neurones. *J. Physiol. (Lond.)* 416: 303–325.

Blackstad, T.W. and Kjaerheim, A. (1961) Special axondendritic synapses in the hippocampal cortex: electron and light microscopic studies on the layer of mossy fiber. *J. Comp. Neurol.*, 117: 133–146.

Blue, M. and Parnavelas, J.G. (1983) The formation and maturation of synapses in the visual cortex of the rat. Quantitative analysis. *J. Neurocytol.*, 12: 697–712.

Chronwall, B. and Wolff, J.R. (1980) Prenatal and postnatal development of GABA-accumulating cells in the occipital neocortex of rat. *J. Comp. Neurol.*, 190: 187–208.

Collingridge, G.L. and Bliss, T.V.P. (1987) NMDA receptors in long term potentiation. *Trends Neurosci.*, 10: 289–293.

Collingridge, G.L., Herron, C.E. and Lester, R.A.J. (1988) Synaptic activation of N-methyl-D-aspartate receptors in the Schaffer collateral-commissural pathway of rat hippocampus. *J. Physiol. (Lond.)*, 399: 283–300.

Drejer, J. and Honoré, T. (1988) New quinoxalinediones show potent antagonism of quisqualate responses in cultured mouse cortical neurons. *Neurosci. Lett.*, 87: 104–108.

Dun, N.J. and Mo, N. (1989) Inhibitory postsynaptic potentials in neonatal rat sympathetic preganglionic neurones in vitro. *J. Physiol. (Lond.)*, 410: 267–281.

Dupont, J.L., Gardette, R. and Crepel, F. (1987) Postnatal development of the chemosensitivity of rat cerebellar Purkinje cells to excitatory amino acids: an in vitro study, *Dev. Brain Res.*, 34: 59–68.

Garthwaite, G., Yamini, B. and Garthwaite, J. (1987) Selective loss of Purkinje and granule cell responsiveness to N-methyl-D-aspartate in rat cerebellum during development. *Dev. Brain Res.*, 36: 288–292.

Gordon-Weeks, P.R., Lockerbie, R.O. and Pearce, B.R. (1984) Uptake and release of 3H GABA by growth cones isolated from neonatal rat brain. *Neurosci. Lett.*, 52: 205–212.

Grillner, S., Wallen, P., Dale, N., Brodin, L., Buchanan, J. and Hill, R. (1987) Transmitters, membrane properties and network circuity in the control of locomotion in lamprey.

Trends Neurosci., 10: 34–41.

Hicks, T.P., Ruwe, W.D. and Veale, W.L. (1986) Release of gamma-aminobutyric acid from the visual cortex of young kittens. *Dev. Brain Res.*, 24: 299–304.

Johnson, J.W. and Ascher, P. (1987) Glycine potentiates the NMDA response in cultured mouse brain neurons. *Nature (Lond.)*, 325: 529–531.

Kaila, K. and Viopo, J. (1987) Postsynaptic fall in intracellular pH induced by GABA-activated bicarbonate conductance. *Nature (Lond.)*, 330: 163–165.

Kleckner, N.W. and Dingledine, R. (1988) Requirement for glycine in activation of NMDA-receptors expressed in *Xenopus* oocytes. *Science*, 24: 835–837.

Kleinschmidt, A., Bear, M.F. and Singer, W. (1987) Blockade of NMDA receptors disrupts experience dependent plasticity of kitten striate cortex, *Science*, 238: 355–358.

Kemp, J.A., Foster, A.G., Leesor, P.D., Priestley, T., Tridgitt, R., Iversen, L.L. and Woodruff, O.N. (1988) 7-chlorotynurenic acid is a selective antagonist at the glycine modulatory site of the N-methyl-D-aspartate receptor complex. *Proc. Natl. Acad. Sci. U.S.A.*, 85: 6547–6550.

Kessler, M., Terramani, T., Lynch, G. and Baudry, M. (1989) A glycine site associated with N-methyl-D-aspartic acid receptors. characterization and identification of a new class of antagonists. *J. Neurochem.*, 52: 1319–1328.

Lauder, J.M., Han, V.K.M., Henderson, P., Verdoorn, T. and Towle, A.C. (1986) Prenatal ontogeny of the GABAergic system in the rat brain: an immunocytochemical study. *Neuroscience*. 19: 465–483.

Lübbers, K., Wolff, J.R. and Frotscher, M. (1985) Neurogenesis of GABAergic neurons in the rat dentate gyrus: a combined autoradiographic and immunocytochemical study. *Neurosci. Lett.*, 62: 317–322.

Matson, M.P. (1988) Neurotransmitters in the regulation of neuronal cytoarchitecture. *Brain Res. Rev.*, 13: 179–212.

Mac Gale, E.H.F., Pye, I.F. and Stonier, C. (1977) Studies of the interrelationship between cerebrospinal fluid and plasma amino acid concentration in normal individuals. *J. Neurochem.*, 29: 291–298.

Mc Laughlin, B.J., Wood, J.G., Saito, K., Roberts, E. and Wu, J.Y. (1975) The fine structural localization of glutamic acid decarboxylase in developing axonal processes and presynaptic terminals of rodent cerebellum. *Brain Res.*, 85: 355–371.

Misgeld, U., Deisz. R.A., Dodt, H.U. and Lux, W.D. (1986) The role of chloride transport in postsynaptic inhibition of hippocampal neurons. *Science*, 232: 1413–1415.

Neuman, R., Cherubini, E. and Ben-Ari, Y. (1988a) Endogenous and network burst induced by N-methyl-D-aspartate and Mg^{++} free medium on the CA3 region of the hippocampal slice. *Neuroscience*, 28: 393–399.

Neuman, R.S., Ben-Ari, Y., Gho, M. and Cherubini, E. (1988b) Blockade of excitatory synaptic transmission by 6-cyano-7-nitroquinoxaline-2,3-dione (CNQX) in the hippocampus in vitro. *Neurosci., Lett.,* 92: 64 – 68.

Parnavelas, J.G. and Cavanagh, M. (1988) Transient expression of neurotransmitters in the developing neocortex. *Trends Neurosci.* 11: 92 – 93.

Represa, A., Tremblay, E. and Ben-Ari, Y. (1989) Transient increase of NMDA binding sites in human hippocampus during development. *Neurosci. Lett.,* 99: 61 – 66.

Rozenberg, F., Robain, O., Jardin, L. and Ben-Ari, Y. (1989) Distribution of GABAergic neurons in rate fetal and early postnatal rat hippocampus. *Dev. Brain Res.,* 50: 177 – 187.

Soriano, E., Cobas, A. and Fairen, A. (1986) A synchronism in the neurogenesis of GABAergic and non GABAergic neurons in the mouse hippocampus. *Dev. Brain Res.,* 30: 88 – 92.

Soriano, E., Cobas, A. and Fairen, A. (1989a) Neurogenesis of glutamic acid decarboxylase immunoreactive cells in the hippocampus of the mouse. I: Regio Superior and Regio Inferior. *J. Comp. Neurol.,* 281: 568 – 602.

Soriano, E., Cobas, A. and Fairen, A. (1989b) Decarboxylase immunoreactive cells in the hippocampus of the mouse. II: Area dentata. *J. Comp. Neurol.,* 281: 603 – 611.

Tremblay, E., Roisin, M.P., Represa, A., Charriaut-Marlangue, C. and Ben-Ari, Y. (1988) Transient increased density of NMDA binding sites in the developing rat hippocampus, *Brain Res.,* 461: 393 – 396.

Tsumoto, T., Hagihara, K., Sato, H. and Hata, Y. (1987) NMDA receptors in the visual cortex of young kittens are more effective than those of adult cats, *Nature (Lond.),* 327: 513 – 514.

William, W., Morris, B.J., Darlison, M.G., Hunt, S.P. and Barnard, E.A. (1988) Distinct GABA A receptor and subunit mRNAs show differential patterns of expression in bovine brain. *Neuron,* 1: 937 – 947.

Woodson, W., Nitecka, L. and Ben-Ari, Y. (1988) Organisation of the GABAergic system in the rat hippocampus. *J. Comp. Neurol.,* 280: 254 – 271.

J. Storm-Mathisen, J. zimmer and O.P. Ottersen (Eds.)
Progress in Brain Research, Vol. 83
© 1990 Elsevier Science Publishers B.V. (Biomedical Division)

CHAPTER 24

Plasticity of identified neurons in slice cultures of hippocampus: a combined Golgi/electron microscopic and immunocytochemical study

Michael Frotscher, Bernd Heimrich and Herbert Schwegler

Institute of Anatomy, University of Freiburg, Albertstr. 17, D-7800 Freiburg, F.R.G.

The combined Golgi/electron microscope (EM) technique and immunocytochemistry for glutamate decarboxylase (GAD) were used to study the differentiation of pyramidal neurons and GABAergic inhibitory non-pyramidal cells in slice cultures of rat and mouse hippocampus. Golgi-impregnated and gold-toned cultures showed the characteristic curved structure of the Ammon's horn. Hippocampal regions CA1, CA3 and fascia dentata could easily be recognized. Pyramidal neurons in CA1 displayed all characteristics of this cell type known from Golgi studies in situ. A triangular cell body gives rise to a main apical dendritic shaft which gives off several side branches. Basal dendrites and the axon originate at the basal pole of the cell body. Apical and basal dendrites are densely covered with spines. As a characteristic feature of the cultured pyramidal cells, numerous spines were observed on the cell body. Most likely due to flattening of the slice during incubation, the pyramidal neurons in CA1 are no longer arranged in a densely packed layer. This results in more space between cell bodies which is filled in by numerous horizontal and basal dendrites originating from the pyramidal cell perikaryon. CA1 pyramidal neurons in slice cultures of the rat or mouse thus resemble the pyramidal neurons in the CA1 region of the primate hippocampus where a similar loose distribution of cell bodies is found. In the electron microscope, cell bodies and dendritic shafts of the gold-toned pyramidal cells formed symmetric synaptic contacts with presynaptic terminals. Numerous boutons were observed that established asymmetric synaptic contacts on gold-toned spines of peripheral pyramidal cell dendrites. This suggests that considerable synaptic reorganization takes place because in situ spines on peripheral dendritic segments are contacted mainly by extrinsic afferents. Like in situ, at least some of the terminals that establish symmetric synaptic contacts are GABAergic. In our immunocytochemical study we observed numerous GAD-positive terminals that formed a dense pericellular plexus around immunonegative cell bodies of pyramidal neurons. In the electron microscope these structures were identified as presynaptic boutons which formed symmetric synaptic contacts on cell bodies and dendritic shafts. They most likely originated from the GAD-positive neurons scattered in all layers of the slice culture. Our results have shown that the main cell types in the hippocampus, pyramidal neurons and GABAergic inhibitory non-pyramidal cells, survive and differentiate under the present culture conditions. Specific extrinsic afferents do not seem to be necessary for the induction and maintenance of the main structural characteristics of these cells. Our data also show that slice cultures of hippocampus provide a useful model for studies of dendritic and axonal plasticity.

Introduction

There are several reasons why the hippocampus has become a model for studies of neuronal plasticity. First, it is known from many studies that the hippocampus plays a major role in learning and memory processes and thus in neuronal plasticity (for review see Seifert, 1983; Köhler and Chan-Palay, 1989). Second, the hippocampus is a relatively simple cortical structure which can easily be isolated from the rest of the brain. The principal cells, pyramidal neurons in the hippocampus proper and the granule cells in the fascia dentata, are densely packed in single cell layers. Afferent fibers to them have been described as terminating in the surrounding dendritic zones in a laminated, nearly non-overlapping fashion. Most afferents run perpendicular to the longitudinal axis of the hippocampus thereby creating the lamellar organization of the hippocampus (Andersen et al., 1971). These anatomical peculiarities have led to the development of the transverse hippocampal slice preparation which is currently used in many laboratories. Hippocampal slices have become a useful tool for many kinds of neurophysiological studies, in particular for studies of neuronal plasticity. We are currently facing an exponentially growing number of studies on plastic phenomena of hippocampal neurons such as posttetanic potentiation and long-term potentiation, all performed on transverse slices of hippocampus and fascia dentata.

Major changes with regard to the structural plasticity of neurons take place during ontogenetic development when the cells differentiate their processes and form their synaptic connections. A fundamental question is to what extent the final structure and functional properties of a neuron are determined by the genetic capacity of the cell itself or by specific afferent fibers that establish synaptic contacts with it. This question may be addressed when considering tissue cultures of central neurons which lack all extrinsic afferents. Again, the hippocampus provides a useful model because it is now possible to culture transverse slices of hippocampal tissue (Gähwiler, 1981). In these slice cultures the organotypic organization of hippocampal neurons is preserved to a large extent.

In the present study we have used the combined Golgi/electron microscopic (EM) procedure (Blackstad, 1965; Fairén et al., 1977) to study morphological characteristics of single identified pyramidal neurons in slice cultures of hippocampus. Light and electron microscopic immunocytochemical studies employing an antibody against glutamate decarboxylase (GAD), the GABA-synthesizing enzyme, were performed to study inhibitory non-pyramidal neurons in the cultures. We have raised the following questions:
(1) Do the main types of hippocampal neurons, pyramidal neurons and GABAergic non-pyramidal cells survive and differentiate their

cell-specific morphological characteristics?
(2) To what extent are the differentiation and maintenance of structural characteristics of hippocampal neurons influenced by extrinsic afferents which are absent under culture conditions?
(3) To what extent is the lack of extrinsic afferents compensated for by neuronal plasticity (sprouting) of the cultured neurons?
Our observations of developing neurons in slice cultures were compared with previous and current Golgi/EM and immunocytochemical studies on the hippocampus in situ in adult and developing animals (e.g. Frotscher, 1983; Frotscher et al., 1984, 1988; Frotscher, 1988; Lübbers and Frotscher, 1988).

Material and methods

Preparation of slice cultures

For the preparation of slice cultures we adopted the method described by Gähwiler (1981; 1984a, b). Briefly, 1- to 6-day-old rats or mice were decapitated and the brain was aseptically removed from the skull. The hippocampi were prepared and cut perpendicular to the longitudinal axis into approximately 300 to 400-μm-thick slices by means of a McIlwain tissue chopper. Slices were collected in a petri dish in a buffer solution (Gähwiler, 1981, 1984a, b) and complete and well-preserved slices were selected. The slices were then placed on carefully cleaned coverslips and embedded in a clot of chicken plasma (Sigma, P3266) which was coagulated by the addition of a drop of thrombin. The coverslips with the slices were then put into plastic planar tubes and were cultured by means of the roller tube technique at 36°C in dry air. The roller drum was tilted 5° in order to ensure that the cultures were kept moist and oxygenated. The medium was prepared exactly as described by Gähwiler (1984a, b). The cultures were incubated for 3 weeks and were fed every third day (0.5 ml).

Golgi impregnation and gold-toning of slice cultures

For our combined Golgi/EM study the slice cultures were fixed using a solution of 1% glutaraldehyde and 1% paraformaldehyde in 0.12 M phoshate buffer (pH 7.3). After at least 15 min of fixation the slice cultures were removed from the coverslips with a brush and were Golgi-impregnated employing a modification of the section Golgi impregnation procedure (Freund and Somogyi, 1983) described in detail elsewhere (Frotscher and Leranth, 1986; Frotscher and Zimmer, 1986). In brief, the slice cultures were placed onto pieces of Parafilm slightly larger than the cultures and kept moist with phosphate buffer. Then, 5 – 10 cultures, with intervening Parafilm, were piled on top of each other so that each culture was sandwiched between two layers of Parafilm. The phosphate buffer was blotted with filter paper and the pile was covered with 5% agar to form a single "tissue block". These blocks were immersed in a freshly prepared osmium dichromate solution which in most cases contained 1 g of osmium tetroxide and 12 g of potassium dichromate in 500 ml distilled water for 4 – 7 days. In order to standardize the results the tissue blocks were incubated in the dichromate solution at a constant temperature (10 – 12°C). Thereafter, the tissue blocks were incubated in 0.75% silver nitrate for 24 – 48 h at room temperature. The cultures were then separated by cutting away the covering agar, and examined in the light microscope while immersed in a drop of 60% glycerol on the translucent Parafilm. Cultures containing well-impregnated neurons were removed from the Parafilm pieces and further processed according to the gold-toning procedure (Fairén et al., 1977). Non-impregnated cultures were again piled, covered with agar and subjected to another Golgi impregnation. In order to gold-tone fine axonal processes, the cultures wer put into petri dishes containing absolute glycerol and illuminated with cold white light for 2 h at room temperature (Blackstad, 1981; Fairén et al., 1981). Then, the cultures were rehydrated in a graded series of glycerol solutions (about 2 min each) and washed in 2 rinses of 20% glycerol.

In recent experiments we added potassium dichromate to the glycerol solutions which was found to prevent a de-impregnation of the cultures (Soriano et al., 1990). Gold-toning was performed by incubating the cultures in 0.05% gold tetrachloride in distilled water containing 20% glycerol. The addition of glycerol made it necessary to prolong the gold-toning up to 1 – 2 h. The cultures were then rinsed in distilled water. Reduction to metallic gold was accomplished by incubating the material in 0.05% oxalic acid for 4 min. After de-impregnation in 1% sodium thiosulphate for up to 1 h the sections were postfixed in 2% phosphate-buffered osmium tetroxide. The de-impregnation in sodium thiosulphate was controlled by light microscopic inspection of the cultures while they were immersed in the solution. The cultures were dehydrated (block-stained with uranyl acetate in 70% ethanol), and flat-embedded in Araldite between an aluminum foil and a transparent plastic foil. After hardening, the aluminum foil was removed and the gold-toned neurons were again examined under the light microscope, photographed and drawn using a Zeiss microscope equipped with a drawing tube. For electron microscopy, cultures containing selected samples of CA1 pyramidal neurons were re-embedded in plastic capsules. The neurons were closely trimmed and ultrathin serial sections were cut on a LKB Ultrotome 3, mounted on single-slot grids coated with Formvar film, stained with lead nitrate, and studied in a Siemens Elmiskop 101. To facilitate the identification of single processes in the electron microscope, the blocks were repeatedly taken out of the ultrotome and drawings of the remaining parts of the cells were made.

GAD immunostaining of slice cultures

For immunostaining, the cultures were fixed with a solution containing 4% paraformaldehyde, 0.08% glutaraldehyde and 15% saturated picric acid in 0.1 M phosphate buffer (Somogyi and Takagi, 1982). After fixation the cultures were carefully washed for 24 h in several changes of phosphate buffer. Prior to immunostaining the vials containing the cultures in 10% sucrose in phosphate buffer were briefly frozen in liquid nitrogen, thawed to room temperature, and carefully washed in phosphate buffer. In some experiments the cultures were frozen up to 3 times in order to improve the penetration of the antibodies through a layer of glia cells on top of the cultures. Following preincubation for 30 min in 10% normal rabbit serum in phosphate buffer, the cultures were incubated for 48 h at 4°C in sheep antiserum S3 against GAD (Oertel et al., 1982). The GAD antibody was diluted 1 : 2000 in 0.1 M phosphate buffer containing 1% normal rabbit serum and 0.1% NaN_3. Immunostaining was performed according to the peroxidase-antiperoxidase (PAP) technique of Sternberger et al. (1970), which included incubation of the cultures in rabbit antisheep immunogammaglobulin (Miles Yeda Ltd., 1 : 40 dilution, 20°C, 1.5 h) followed by goat PAP complex (Sternberger-Meyer Immunocytochemicals Inc., Jarrettsville, MD, 1 : 40 dilution, 20°C, 2 h) with washing in several changes of phosphate buffer between each two incubation steps. The tissue-bound peroxidase was finally visualized by incubating the cultures with 3,3-diaminobenzidine (0.07%) and H_2O_2 in Tris buffer (0.1 M, pH 7.6) for 5 – 10 min. In parallel control experiments the cultures were incubated with all but the primary antiserum. No immunostaining was observed in the control cultures. After again washing in phosphate buffer the cultures were osmicated in 1% osmium tetroxide in 0.1 M phosphate buffer for 30 min, dehydrated and block-stained with uranyl acetate in 70% ethanol. The cultures were then flat-embedded in Araldite as described above.

Additional material

Golgi-impregnated or immunostained neurons in the slice cultures were compared to similarly treated cells in the hippocampus fixed by transcardial perfusion in situ. For this, a large amount of material from previous and current studies on the adult and developing rat hippocampus was available (see Introduction).

Results

Golgi/EM studies on pyramidal neurons in culture

The general histological organization of hippocampal slice cultures has been described in the first studies using this technique (Gähwiler, 1981; 1984a, b; Zimmer and Gähwiler, 1984). It is evident from these studies that the organotypic organization of hippocampus and fascia dentata is preserved in this preparation. This is also seen in the present Golgi-impregnated cultures (Fig. 1). The characteristic layers of principal cells, pyramidal neurons in the Ammon's horn and granule cells in the fascia dentata, are retained and the hippocampal fields CA1, CA3 and fascia dentata and hilus can be differentiated. Also, the orientation of the cells resembles very much the well-known arrangement seen in perfusion-fixed hippocampi. The pyramidal cells extend a main apical dendrite in the stratum radiatum and basal dendrites in the stratum oriens; granule cells form an extensive dendritic arbor in the molecular layer of the fascia dentata (Fig. 1). However, it is obvious both in thionin-stained (cf. Zimmer and Gähwiler, 1984) and Golgi-impregnated slice cultures (Figs. 1, 3) that the pyramidal neurons, particularly in CA1, are no longer arranged in a densely packed cell layer but are more loosely distributed than known from the hippocampus of perfusion-fixed rodents. The CA1 region in slice cultures of rats and mice thus resembles very much the CA1 region in the primate hippocampus in situ (Stephan, 1975, 1983; Frotscher et al., 1988).

In the present study we have used the Golgi technique to compare the differentiation of hippocampal neurons in slice cultures with that of the same cells in the rodent hippocampus fixed in situ by transcardial perfusion. The morphology of hippocampal neurons as seen after Golgi impregnation is well known from the early work by Golgi (1886), Sala (1891), Schaffer (1892), Koelliker (1896), Ramón y Cajal (1911), Lorente de Nó (1934) and the reader is referred to these studies and more recent reviews (e.g. Blackstad, 1963; 1967; Amaral, 1978; Frotscher, 1988) for detailed descriptions. Accordingly, we have concentrated here on the morphological characteristics of hip-

pocampal neurons in slice cultures. We have focused on pyramidal cells in CA1 in our correlated light and electron microscopic analysis because the fine structural characteristics of identified CA3 pyramidal neurons have recently been described by using intracellular injection of horseradish peroxidase (HRP) and light and electron microsopic techniques (Frotscher and Gähwiler, 1988).

Fig. 2a shows a typical CA1 pyramidal neuron in

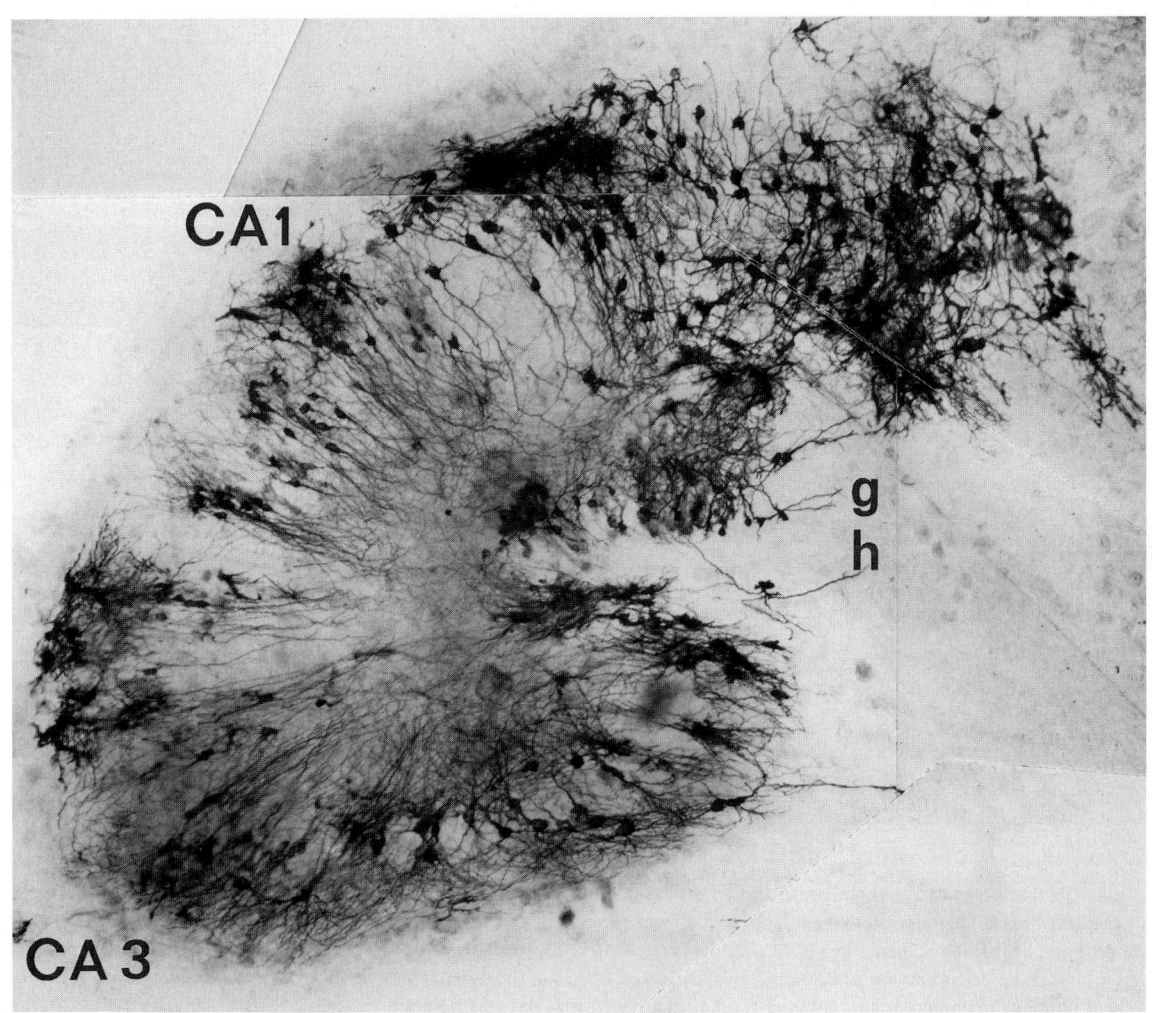

Fig. 1. Golgi-impregnated and gold-toned slice culture of mouse hippocampus cultured for 3 weeks. The characteristic curvature of the Ammon's horn is retained and hippocampal regions CA1 and CA3 and the granular layer (g) and hilus (h) of the fascia dentata can be identified. Most likely due to flattening of the culture, the cell bodies of pyramidal neurons, particularly in CA1, are no longer arranged in a densely packed cell layer. Note that the orientation of the main dendrites of pyramidal neurons and granule cells is preserved. ×120.

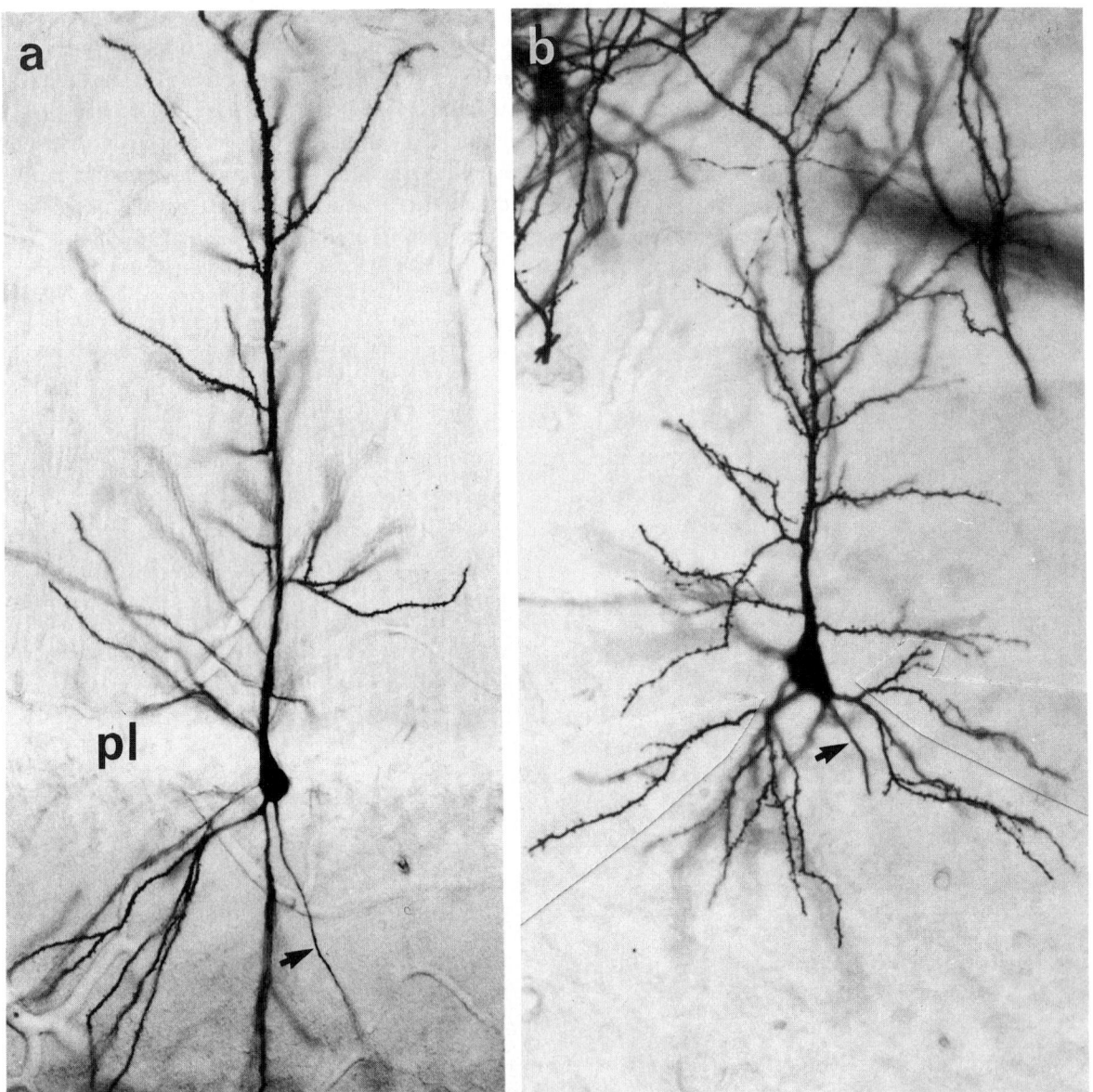

Fig. 2. a: Golgi-impregnated pyramidal cell in the adult rat hippocampus fixed in situ by transcardial perfusion. The cell was photographed after Golgi impregnation while the section was floating in a drop of glycerol. The cell displays the characteristic main apical dendrite, apical side branches and basal dendrites extending in stratum oriens. Arrow pointing to the axon which runs towards the alveus. Note the dense packing of unstained pyramidal cell bodies in the pyramidal layer (pl). ×300. b: CA1 pyramidal neuron in a slice culture of rat hippocampus cultured for 3 weeks. Photographed after Golgi impregnation while the culture was floating in a drop of glycerol. The cell exhibits all major structural characteristics of a normal CA1 pyramidal neuron, i.e., a triangular cell body which gives rise to the main apical dendrite, basal dendrites and apical side branches. All dendrites are densely covered with spines. As in situ, the axon (arrow) runs through stratum oriens. Note that the cell body is not located in a demarcated cell layer. As a result, there is space for horizontal dendrites originating from the cell body and extending laterally. ×430.

the hippocampus of an adult rat fixed in situ by transcardial perfusion. A single cell is impregnated in the densely packed, clearly demarcated pyramidal layer. The cell body has a triangular or ovoid shape giving rise to the main apical dendritic shaft which branches in stratum lacunosum-moleculare. On its way through the stratum radiatum the apical dendrite gives off several side branches. The axon and basal dendrites emerge from the basal pole of the cell body. With this dendritic arrangement, the cell has a bipolar appearance characteristic for the cells in this hippocampal field. After an initial spine-free segment the main apical dendrite as well as apical side branches and basal dendrites are densely covered with

spines. The axon traverses the stratum oriens and joins the alveus, the white matter of the hippocampus.

A very similar dendritic organization is seen in the Golgi-impregnated pyramidal cell in a slice culture cultivated for 3 weeks (Fig. 2b). Again, a main apical dendritic shaft arises from a triangular cell body and, after traversing stratum radiatum, it branches in stratum lacunosum-moleculare. As in Fig. 2a, only one cell is completely stained. However, due to the loose distribution of cell bodies no distinct layer of unstained pyramidal cells can be recognized. Numerous side branches originate at right angles from the main apical shaft. Several basal dendrites emerge directly from

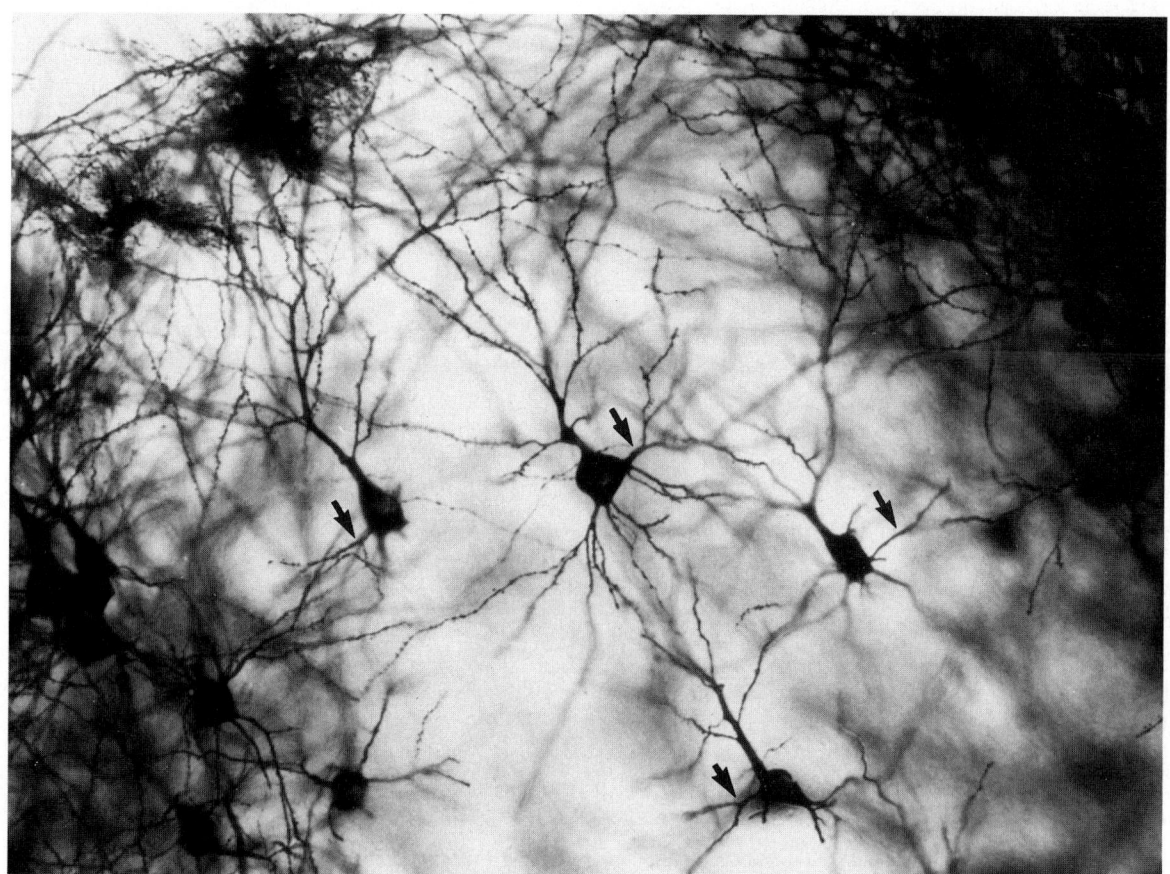

Fig. 3. Slice culture of rat hippocampus cultured for 3 weeks. Photographed after Golgi impregnation while the culture was floating in a drop of glycerol. A loose distribution of CA1 pyramidal cells provides space for abundant basal and horizontal dendrites originating from the cell body. Some horizontal dendrites labeled by arrows. ×470.

the basal pole of the cell body. As in the neuron fixed in situ, the axon is directed towards stratum oriens in the culture. Numerous spines can be seen on apical and basal dendrites although their number seems to be slightly reduced when compared with the cell shown in Fig. 2a. In contrast to normal pyramidal neurons, we have regularly observed somatic spines on the cell bodies of the cultured cells (Fig. 4a).

Probably due to more space between neighboring cell bodies in the CA1 region of the culture, horizontal dendrites extending laterally from the

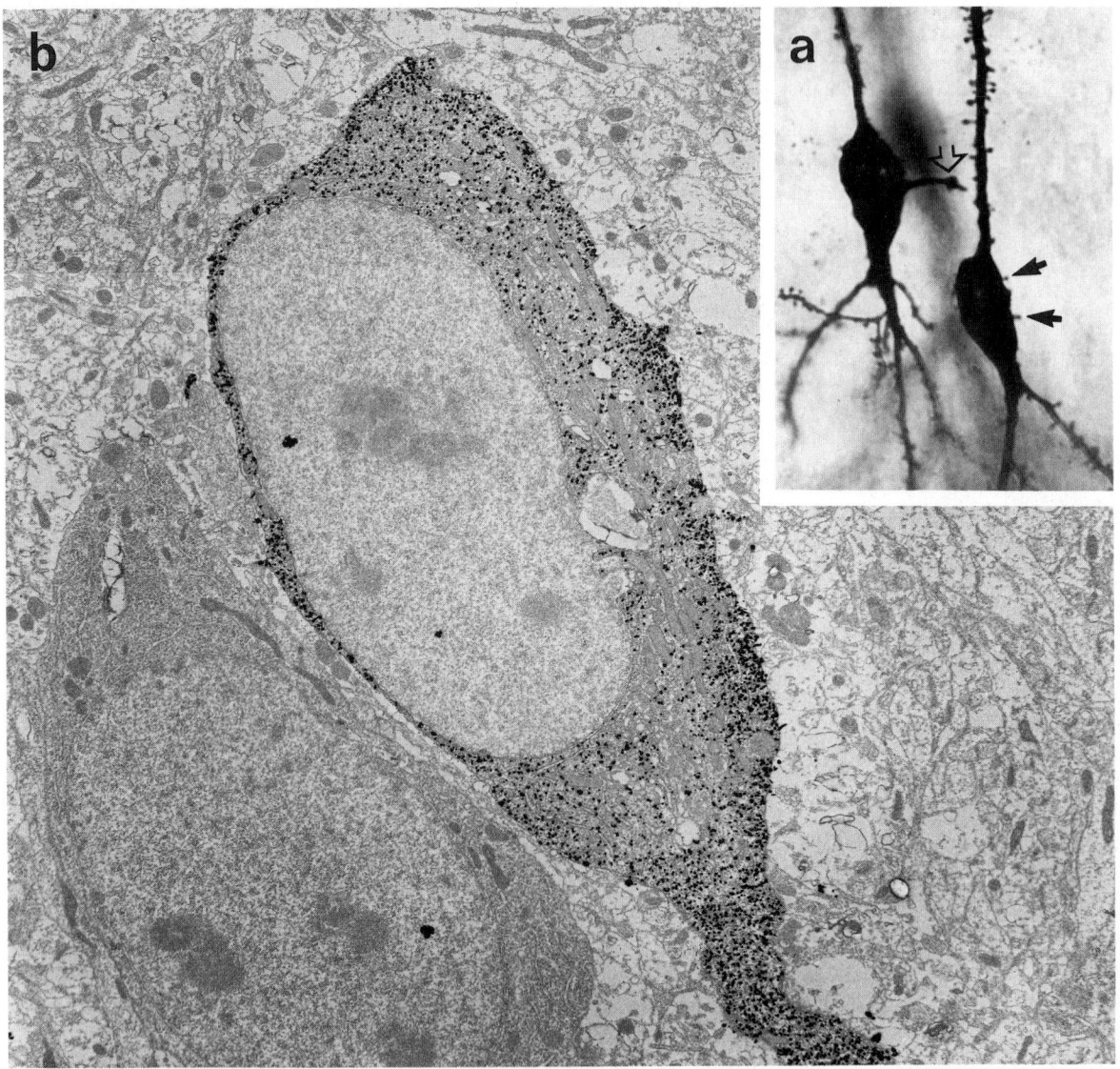

Fig. 4. a: two Golgi-impregnated and gold-toned CA1 pyramidal neurons in a slice culture of mouse hippocampus. The cell on the right is shown in b. Open arrow labels an outgrowing horizontal dendrite. Note density of spines on apical and basal dendrites. Small arrows point to somatic spines. ×720. b: electron micrograph of the cell body region of the neuron shown on the right in a. The nucleus which does not display indentations is surrounded by varying amounts of cytoplasm containing numerous mitochondria. ×8800.

cell body are apparent. This latter observation is better demonstrated in Fig. 3 which shows several loosely distributed Golgi-impregnated and gold-toned pyramidal cells. By their numerous horizontal and basal dendrites and by the varying length of the main apical shaft these cells resemble neocortical cells. A similar dendritic pattern has recently been described for pyramidal cells in the CA1 region of the primate hippocampus (Frotscher et al., 1988). Comparable to the situation in the slice culture, CA1 pyramidal cells in the primate brain are not arranged in a densely packed cell layer. The abundance of horizontal dendrites and somatic spines are the only clear-cut differences when CA1 pyramidal cells in slice cultures and in perfusion-fixed rats and mice were compared.

A total of 11 well-impregnated and gold-toned CA1 pyramidal cells in slice cultures of rats and mice were subjected to fine structural analysis. Fig. 4a and b show light and electron micrographs of an identified CA1 pyramidal neuron. The bipolar cell body contains an ovoid nucleus surrounded by varying amounts of cytoplasm in which a relatively high number of mitochondria were seen. Characteristic of pyramidal neurons the contour of the nuclear membrane was smooth and lacked deep infoldings. Deeply indented nuclei, nuclear rods and sheets as well as large amounts of perinuclear cytoplasm are characteristic features of non-pyramidal neurons in the hippocampus and fascia dentata (Ribak and Anderson, 1980; Seress and Ribak, 1985; Schlander and Frotscher, 1986). As in the hippocampus in situ presynaptic terminals form symmetric synaptic contacts on the cell bodies of pyramidal cells (Fig. 5a). It has already been mentioned that pyramidal neurons in slice cultures, in contrast to the hippocampus in situ, often exhibit somatic spines. Synaptic contacts on soma spines were exclusively asymmetric (Figs. 5b, 6a).

We were unable to find obvious differences in the fine structure of dendrites between identified pyramidal cells in slice cultures and in the hippocampus in situ. It should be mentioned, however, that accumulations of gold grains within the cytoplasm of the identified pyramidal cells often masked fine structural details (Fig. 5c,d). This was also true for the synaptic contacts formed on the gold-toned neurons in culture. To our surprise we have observed numerous synaptic contacts on dendritic shafts and spines of the cultured neurons although all extrinsic afferents were absent under the culture conditions (Figs. 5c,d, 6). Abundant synaptic contacts on shafts and spines of the identified pyramidal cells were seen on proximal as well as distal dendritic segments. In the hippocampus in situ cell bodies and proximal dendritic segments are mainly contacted by terminals of intrinsic origin whereas more distal dendritic segments in stratum radiatum and stratum oriens establish contacts with commissural fibers from the contralateral hippocampus (Blackstad, 1956). Most distal segments of apical dendrites which branch in the stratum lacunosum-moleculare are normally contacted by entorhinal afferents. The presence of synaptic contacts on all these dendritic segments of the cultured neurons suggests a considerable reorganization (sprouting) under the present culture conditions.

GAD-immunocytochemical studies on non-pyramidal neurons in culture

In our Golgi-impregnated cultures we have already seen a number of neurons that by the shape of their cell body and the orientation of their varicose dendrites resembled very much the GABAergic non-pyramidal neurons in the hippocampus and fascia dentata (Frotscher and Zimmer, 1983; Ribak and Seress, 1983; Seress and Ribak, 1985; Schlander and Frotscher, 1986; Lübbers and Frotscher, 1987). However, we could not exclude that these cells represented pyramidal neurons that have abnormally developed under the present culture conditions. Immunostaining for GAD, the GABA-synthesizing enzyme, seemed to be a more adequate method for a study of GABAergic non-pyramidal cells.

Initial attempts to stain the cultures for GAD were not very successful. Immunostained cultures

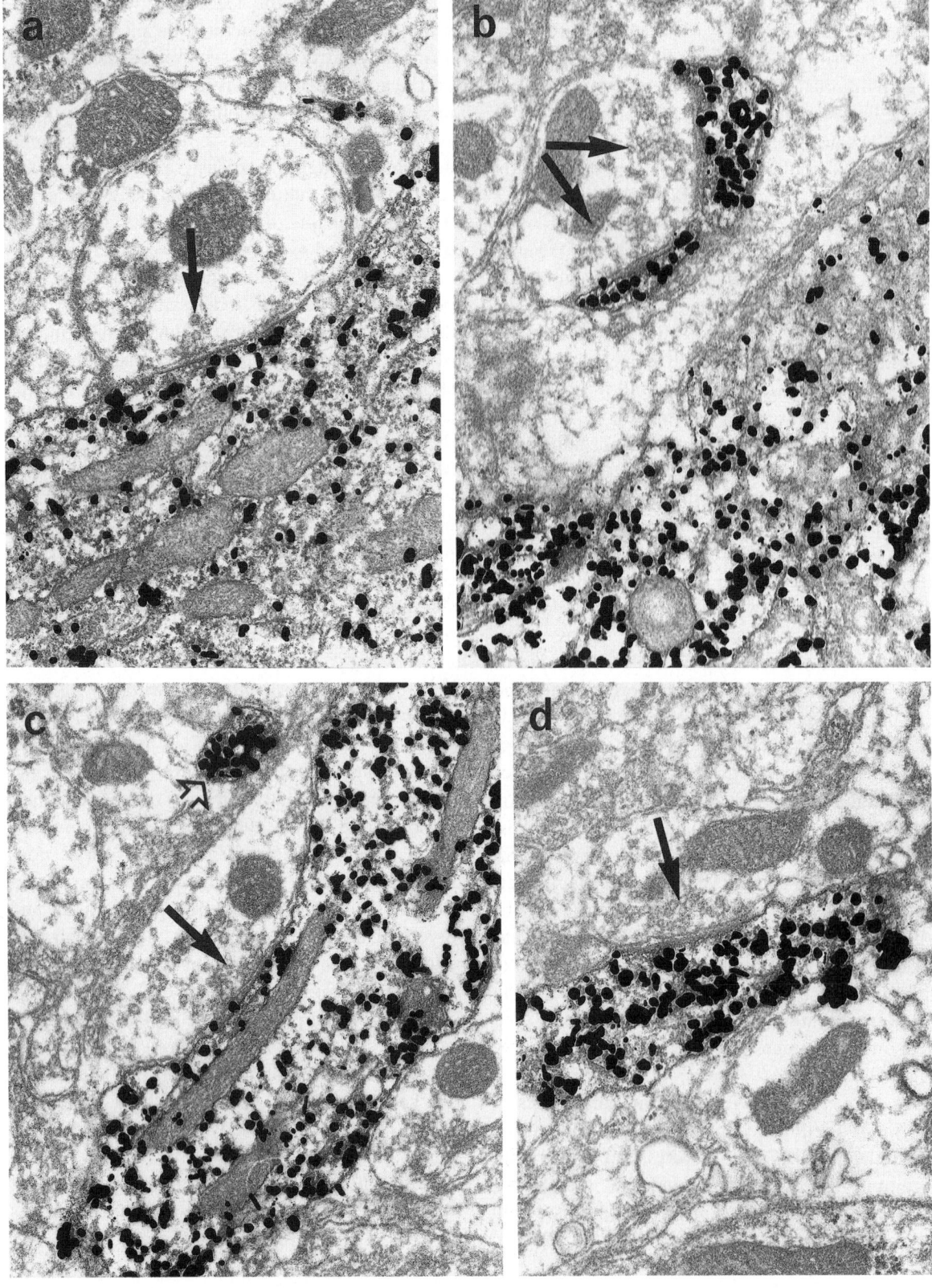

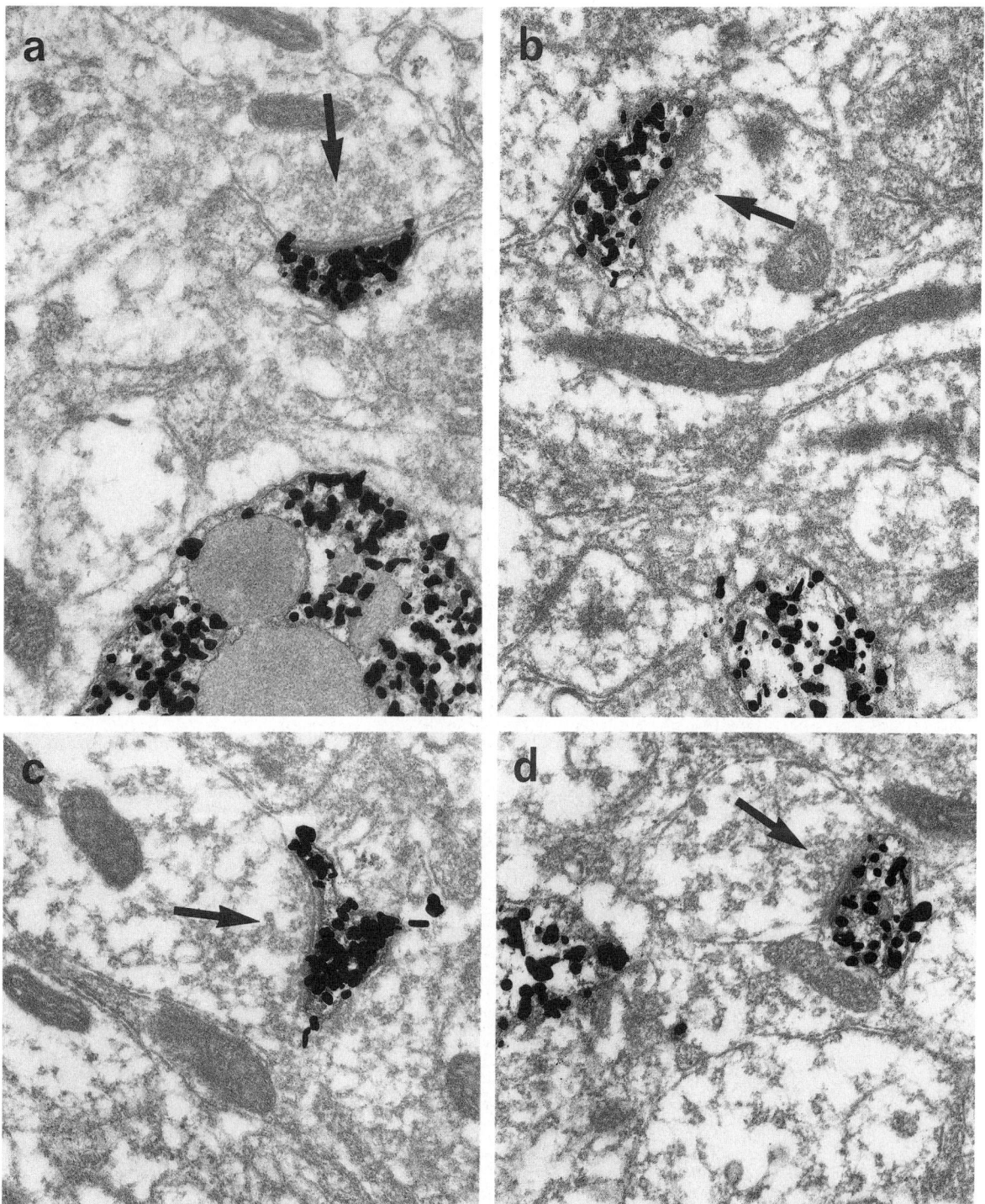

Fig. 6. Input synapses on spines of identified pyramidal cells in culture. Arrows pointing to synaptic contacts. a: somatic spine. b – d: spines on peripheral dendrites. ×36,000.

Fig. 5. Electron micrographs of Golgi-impregnated and gold-toned CA1 pyramidal neurons in culture. Input synapses of the identified cells. a: terminal forming symmetric synaptic contact (arrow) on cell body. b: bouton establishing asymmetric synaptic contact (arrows) on a soma spine. c,d: terminals in symmetric (c) and asymmetric (d) synaptic contact with dendritic shafts. Open arrow in c pointing to a dendritic spine. ×36,000.

334

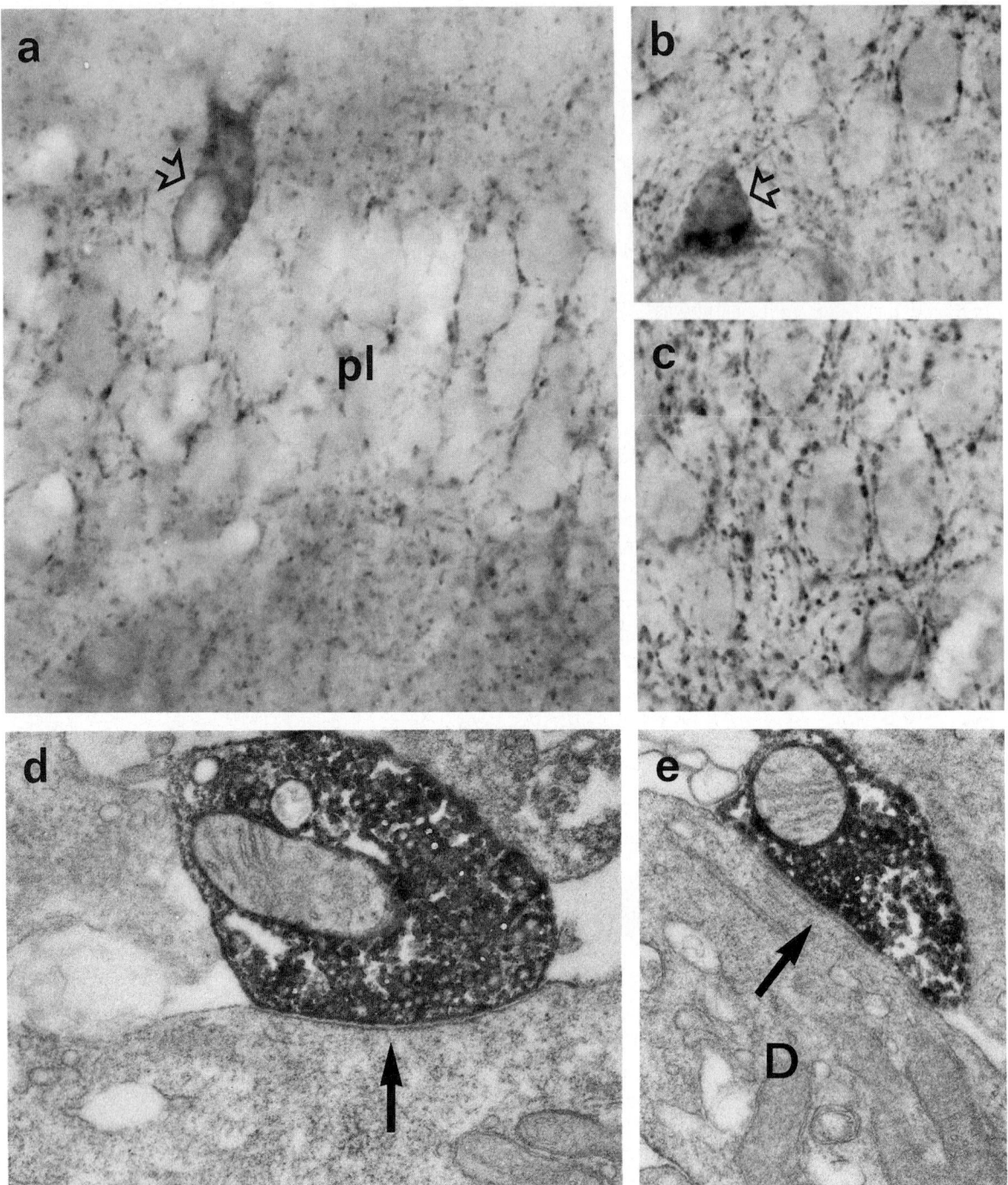

Fig. 7. a: Vibratome section of the CA1 region of an adult rat immunostained for GAD. Open arrow pointing to GAD-positive cell. Note terminal-like puncta surrounding densely packed immunonegative cell bodies in the pyramidal layer (pl). ×720. b,c: GAD immunoreactivity in a slice culture of rat hippocampus. Open arrow in b pointing to GAD-positive cell. Immunopositive terminal-like puncta form a dense plexus around immunonegative cell bodies in CA1. ×720. d,e: electron micrographs of GAD-positive boutons in a slice culture of rat hippocampus. The terminals establish symmetric synaptic contacts on cell body (d) and dendritic shaft (e). Arrows pointing to contact zones. D, dendrite. ×36,000.

and controls which were incubated with all but primary antiserum did not differ very much. We did not observe non-specific staining but were unsuccessful in labeling the typical pericellular baskets of GABAergic terminals as well as GABAergic neurons. In order to define the preparation better we recently cut some cultures transversally and found the whole slice culture covered by a layer of glia cells after an incubation period of 3 weeks. Obviously, the layer of glia cells prevented penetration of antibodies when we applied our standard immunocytochemical technique. This procedure does not include pretreatment with Triton X-100, the application of which damages the fine structure. In subsequent experiments we have thus repeated our freeze – thaw procedure, sometimes up to 3 times, in order to allow for a better penetration of the antibodies. This procedure in fact labeled GABAergic neurons and terminals but definitely affected the fine structural preservation of the tissue.

Fig. 7a shows a GAD-immunostained Vibratome section from a perfusion-fixed rat hippocampus. A GAD-positive cell body with its proximal dendrites is seen. Numerous terminal-like puncta surround the immunonegative cell bodies of CA1 pyramidal neurons.

A very similar staining pattern was observed in the slice cultures (Fig. 7b,c). Numerous GAD-positive fibers displayed a large number of varicose swellings in their course suggesting the existence of numerous en-passant contacts. In this manner a dense pericellular plexus was formed around immunonegative cell bodies of pyramidal neurons. GAD-immunoreactive cell bodies were observed (Fig. 7b). However, they did not show much staining of their dendrites which was most likely due to the lack of colchicine pretreatment that enhances GAD immunostaining of dendritic processes in vivo (Ribak et al., 1978).

Some cultures were thin-sectioned in order to study the fine structure of GAD-immunoreactive terminals. As could be expected after repeating the freeze – thaw treatment for at least 2 times, the fine structure of the tissue was not as well pre-served as in the case of the Golgi/EM material. This mainly included membrane disruptions and at some places a widening of the extracellular space. Numerous GAD-immunoreactive terminals densely filled with synaptic vesicles were observed which established symmetric synaptic contacts on immunonegative cell bodies and dendritic shafts of pyramidal cells. Examples are demonstrated in Fig. 7d and e.

Discussion

The present study has shown that the main cell types in the CA1 region of the hippocampus survive the preparation of slices at early postnatal stages and the subsequent cultivation for several weeks. Moreover, they differentiate and form their cell-specific characteristics under these conditions. This is remarkable because specific extrinsic afferents which normally provide the functional integration of these cells are absent. Here we will discuss our results by (1) referring to Golgi-impregnated and immunostained CA1 neurons fixed in situ by perfusion and (2) to experimental models of partially denervated or isolated hippocampal tissue.

It is well known that partial denervation of hippocampus and fascia dentata induces sprouting of the remaining intact afferents (cf. Cotman and Nadler, 1978). Similarly, hippocampal transplants lack their specific afferent innervation but are innervated by host fibers and sprouting intrinsic elements. Partial denervation and transplantation create conditions that, at least to a certain extent, are comparable with those in the present culture preparation. The slice culture is partially denervated hippocampal tissue and there is evidence from the present and recent studies that a considerable reorganization and sprouting of the surviving neurons in culture takes place (Zimmer and Gähwiler, 1984; Frotscher and Gähwiler, 1988).

As a starting point, it might be useful to compare identified hippocampal neurons in the presently described slice cultures and in acute slices. Acute slices are prepared in the very same way except that the tissue is usually taken from adult animals and the slices are used for experiments to be performed on the day of preparation. The neurons in acute slices have differentiated in situ and have established all their normal synaptic connections. Intracellularly stained neurons in hippocampal slices display in fact the same structural features as hippocampal neurons fixed in situ by transcardial perfusion (Claiborne et al., 1986; Frotscher and Misgeld, 1989). However, well-preserved neurons and neuropil were only observed in the central portion of the slice. Neurons and fibers closer to the cut surfaces of the slice always showed signs of degeneration due to damage during preparation (Frotscher et al., 1981; Misgeld and Frotscher, 1982). In an electron microscopic study of input synapses of intracellularly (HRP) stained neurons in acute hippocampal slices we were surprised to find a large number of well-preserved presynaptic terminals in the central portion of the slice although all extrinsic afferents were cut when the slice was prepared (Frotscher and Misgeld, 1989). Sealing of membranes obviously guarantees the survival of transected fibers for several hours before they eventually undergo degeneration. In fact, a large number of physiological studies have shown that the various afferent fibers to hippocampal neurons terminating in a laminated fashion in the different hippocampal layers can be activated in the acute slice (e.g. Misgeld, 1988).

The differences between acute slices and slice cultures are obvious. For slice cultures 1- to 6-day-old animals were used. At this postnatal stage both pyramidal and GABAergic non-pyramidal neurons had already formed (Bayer, 1980; Amaral and Kurz, 1985; Lübbers et al., 1985; Soriano et al., 1989) but were still very immature. Their differentiation takes place under culture conditions in the absence of all extrinsic afferents. All synaptic contacts formed are of intrinsic origin. After a cultivation period of 3 weeks, which was mainly used in the present experiments, all elements degenerating following slice preparation (i.e. the damaged outer zones) were eliminated from the tissue. This results in flattening of the culture which may also cause a widening of the pyramidal layer in CA1. We have regarded it as a main result of the present study that hippocampal neurons, pyramidal cells and GABAergic non-pyramidal neurons develop very similar morphological features in slice cultures when compared with the same cell types in acute slices and in perfusion-fixed hippocampi. This suggests that the differentiation and maintenance of a characteristic morphology of the dendritic arbor is not determined by specific extrinsic afferents. We have arrived at a very similar conclusion when we recently studied neuronal differentiation in embryonic hippocampal transplants (Frotscher and Zimmer, 1986, 1987). Again by using GAD immunocytochemistry and Golgi impregnation, which provides a unique staining of the entire dendritic arbor, we found that the transplanted neurons differentiated very similar structural characteristics as they do in situ. Also, the differentiation of characteristic postsynaptic elements, i.e. dendritic spines, said to be induced by specific afferent fibers (Hámori, 1973), takes place under the isolated conditions of transplants and slice cultures.

Our electron microscopic studies of identified cells in transplants and slice cultures have revealed asymmetric (Gray type I) synaptic contacts on dendritic spines and symmetric (Gray type II) contacts on cell bodies and dendritic shafts. Part of the symmetric synapses on cell bodies and dendritic shafts of pyramidal neurons are likely to be formed by boutons of GABAergic inhibitory terminals. In both hippocampal transplants (Frotscher and Zimmer, 1987) and slice cultures (Streit et al., 1989) GABAergic neurons survive and form their normal symmetric synaptic contacts on cell bodies and dendritic shafts (present study). In the slice cultures all terminals that form asymmetric synaptic contacts on spines of proximal and distal dendritic segments are of intrinsic origin. In situ asymmetric contacts on spines are largely formed by extrinsic fibers for instance from the entorhinal cortex (Nafstad, 1967), the medial septum (Frotscher and Leranth, 1985) and the contralateral hippocampus (Blackstad, 1970; Frotscher, 1983). In a recent electron microscopic study of intracellularly stained CA3 pyramidal cells in slice cultures (Frotscher and Gähwiler, 1988) we were able to demonstrate that the axons of the labeled cells formed an enormous number of collaterals including aberrant ones that have not been described in situ. This clearly demonstrates the capacity of the cultivated neurons to sprout in response to the loss of extrinsic afferent fibers. The cultures thus behave like transplanted hippocampal neurons (Zimmer and Gähwiler, 1984) and hippocampi partially denervated in situ (cf. Cotman and Nadler, 1978). The sprouting collaterals of the cultured pyramidal neurons are likely to establish the asymmetric synaptic contacts on spines. We have in fact found numerous intracellularly stained collaterals of pyramidal cells in slice cultures that formed asymmetric contacts on spines (Frotscher and Gähwiler, 1988). It cannot be ascertained whether these collaterals induce and maintain the formation of spines. However, we can conclude that specific extrinsic inputs are not required. Alternatively, pyramidal neurons form spines irrespective of potential inputs. As far as symmetric synaptic contacts are concerned, we have provided evidence that they are formed by inhibitory GABAergic neurons.

When regarding the dendritic organization of Golgi-impregnated CA1 pyramidal cells in culture, some abnormal traits were observed in the present study. A major finding was an increase in the number of horizontal and basal dendrites. The abundance of horizontal and basal dendrites is generally regarded as a late event in the phylogenetic development of pyramidal cells (Fig. 23 in Ramón y Cajal, 1911). A comparison of CA1 pyramidal cells in primates and small laboratory animals revealed in fact a considerable increase in the number of horizontal and basal dendrites in primates (Frotscher et al., 1988). CA1 pyramidal cells in the monkey hippocampus thus resembled very much neocortical pyramidal cells. Comparable to CA1 pyramidal cells in rat slice cultures, CA1 pyramidal neurons in the primate hippocam-

pus are not arranged in a densely packed cell layer (Stephan, 1975, 1983; Frotscher et al., 1988). In both cases the result seems to be a larger variability of the dendritic arbor. We conclude that pyramidal cells in the rodent hippocampus do already have the capacity to form abundant horizontal and basal dendrites as observed in the primate hippocampus. The development of these processes is, however, suppressed in situ due to the dense packing of pyramidal cell bodies. It is thus a larger amount of space between individual neurons that characterizes phylogenetic development of the CA1 region and not changes in the pyramidal cell's capacity to form more frequent dendritic branches.

In conclusion, the present study has shown that slice cultures of the rodent hippocampus provide a useful model to study dendritic and axonal plasticity. Our results also demonstrate that the hippocampal slice culture is a self-organizing system that is clearly different from the acute brain slice currently used in many neurophysiological laboratories. These differences have to be considered when data obtained in acute slices and slice cultures are compared.

Acknowledgements

The authors wish to thank G. Mueller for reading the manuscript and E. Thielen and B. Krebs for excellent technical assistance. This work was supported by the Deutsche Forschungsgemeinschaft (Fr 620/2 – 3).

References

Amaral, D.G. (1978) A Golgi study of cell types in the hilar region of the hippocampus in the rat. *J. Comp. Neurol.,* 182: 851 – 914.

Amaral, D.G. and Kurz, J. (1985) The time of origin of cells demonstrating glutamic acid decarboxylase-like immunoreactivity in the hippocampal formation of the rat. *Neurosci. Lett.,* 58: 33 – 40.

Andersen, P., Bliss T.V.P. and Skrede, K.K. (1971) Lamellar organization of hippocampal excitatory pathways. *Exp. Brain Res.,* 13: 222 – 238.

338

Bayer, S.A. (1980) Development of the hippocampal region in the rat. I. Neurogenesis examined with (^{3}H)thymidine autoradiography. *J. Comp. Neurol.,* 190: 87 – 114.

Blackstad, T.W. (1956) Commissural connections of the hippocampal region in the rat, with special reference to their mode of termination. *J. Comp. Neurol.,* 105: 417 – 537.

Blackstad, T.W. (1963) Ultrastructural studies on the hippocampal region. *Prog. Brain Res.,* 3: 122 – 148.

Blackstad, T.W. (1965) Mapping of experimental axon degeneration by electron microscopy of Golgi preparations. *Z. Zellforsch.,* 67: 819 – 834.

Blackstad, T.W. (1967) Cortical grey matter. A correlation of light and electron microscopic data. In H. Hydén (Ed.), *The Neuron,* Elsevier, Amsterdam, pp. 49 – 118.

Blackstad, T.W. (1970) Electron microscopy of Golgi preparations for the study of neuronal relations. In W.J.H. Nauta and S.O.E. Ebbesson (Eds.), *Contemporary Research Methods in Neuroanatomy,* Springer, Berlin, pp. 186 – 216.

Blackstad, T.W. (1981) Tract tracing by electron microscopy of Golgi preparations. In L. Heimer and M.J. RoBards (Eds.), *Neuroanatomical Tract-Tracing Methods,* Plenum Press, New York, pp. 407 – 440.

Claiborne, B.J., Amaral, D.G. and Cowan, W.M. (1986) A light and electron microscopic analysis of the mossy fibers of the rat dentate gyrus. *J. Comp. Neurol.,* 246: 435 – 458.

Cotman, C.W. and Nadler, J.V. (1978) Reactive synaptogenesis in the hippocampus. In C.W. Cotman (Ed.), *Neuronal Plasticity,* Raven, New York, pp. 227 – 271.

Fairén, A., Peters, A. and Saldanha, J. (1977) A new procedure for examining Golgi impregnated neurons by light and electron microscopy. *J. Neurocytol.,* 6: 311 – 337.

Fairén, A., DeFelipe, J. and Martinez-Ruiz (1981) The Golgi-EM procedure: a tool to study neocortical interneurons. In *Eleventh International Congress of Anatomy: Glial and Neuronal Cell Biology,* Alan R. Liss, New York, pp. 291 – 301.

Freund, T. and Somogyi, P. (1983) The section-Golgi impregnation procedure. I. Description of the method and its combination with histochemistry after intracellular iontophoresis or retrograde transport of horseradish peroxidase. *Neuroscience,* 9: 463 – 474.

Frotscher, M. (1983) Dendritic plasticity in response to partial deafferentation. In W. Seifert (Ed.), *Neurobiology of the Hippocampus.* Academic Press, London, pp. 65 – 80.

Frotscher, M. (1988) Neuronal elements in the hippocampus and their synaptic connections. In M. Frotscher, P. Kugler, U. Misgeld and K. Zilles (Eds.), *Neurotransmission in the Hippocampus, Adv. Anat. Embryol. Cell Biol. Vol. 111,* Springer-Verlag, Berlin, pp. 2 – 19.

Frotscher, M. and Gähwiler, B.H. (1988) Synaptic organization of intracellularly stained CA3 pyramidal neurons in slice cultures of rat hippocampus. *Neuroscience,* 24: 541 – 551.

Frotscher, M. and Leranth, C. (1985) Cholinergic innervation of the rat hippocampus as revealed by choline acetyltransferase immunocytochemistry: a combined light and electron microscopic study. *J. Comp. Neurol.,* 239: 237 – 246.

Frotscher, M. and Leranth, C. (1986) The cholinergic innervation of the rat fascia dentata: identification of target structures on granule cells by combining choline acetyltransferase immunocytochemistry and Golgi impregnation. *J. Comp. Neurol.,* 243: 58 – 70.

Frotscher, M. and Misgeld, U. (1989) Characterization of input synapses on intracellularly stained neurons in hippocampal slices: an HRP/EM study. *Exp. Brain Res.,* 75: 327 – 334.

Frotscher, M. and Zimmer, J. (1983) Commissural fibers terminate on non-pyramidal neurons in the guinea pig hippocampus – a combined Golgi/EM degeneration study. *Brain Res.,* 265: 289 – 293.

Frotscher, M. and Zimmer, J. (1986) Interacerebral transplants of the rat fascia dentata: a Golgi/electron microscope study of dentate granule cells. *J. Comp. Neurol.,* 246: 181 – 190.

Frotscher, M. and Zimmer, J. (1987) GABAergic non-pyramidal neurons in intracerebral transplants of the rat hippocampus and fascia dentata: a combined light and electron microscopic immunocytochemical study. *J. Comp. Neurol.,* 259: 266 – 276.

Frotscher, M., Misgeld, U. and Nitsch, C. (1981) Ultrastructure of mossy fiber endings in in vitro hippocampal slices. *Exp. Brain Res.,* 41: 247 – 255.

Frotscher, M., Leranth, C., Lübbers, K. and Oertel, W.H. (1984) Commissural afferents innervate glutamate decarboxylase immunoreactive non-pyramidal neurons in the guinea pig hippocampus. *Neurosci. Lett.,* 46: 137 – 143.

Frotscher, M., Kraft, J. and Zorn, U. (1988) Fine structure of identified neurons in the primate hippocampus: a combined Golgi/EM study in the baboon. *J. Comp. Neurol.,* 275: 254 – 270.

Gähwiler, B.H. (1981) Organotypic monolayer cultures of nervous tissue. *J. Neurosci. Methods,* 4: 329 – 342.

Gähwiler, B.H. (1984a) Development of the hippocampus in vitro: cell types, synapses and receptors. *Neuroscience,* 11: 751 – 760.

Gähwiler, B.H. (1984b) Slice cultures of cerebellar, hippocampal and hypothalamic tissue. *Experientia,* 40: 235 – 244.

Golgi, C. (1886) *Sulla Fina Anatomia degli Organi Centrali del Sistema Nervoso,* Hoepli, Milan.

Hámori, J. (1973) The inductive role of presynaptic axons in the development of postsynaptic spines. *Brain Res.,* 62: 337 – 344.

Köhler, C. and Chan-Palay, V. (Eds.) (1989) *The Hippocampus – New Vistas.* Alan R. Liss, New York.

Koelliker, A. v. (1896) *Handbuch der Gewebelehre des Menschen. Nervensystem des Menschen und der Thiere,* 6th edn., Engelmann, Leipzig.

Lorente de Nó, R. (1934) Studies on the structure of the cerebral cortex. II. Continuation of the study of the ammonic system. *J. Psychol. Neurol.,* 46: 113 – 177.

Lübbers, K. and Frotscher, M. (1987) Fine structure and synaptic connections of identified neurons in the rat fascia dentata. *Anat. Embryol.*, 177: 1–14.

Lübbers, K. and Frotscher, M. (1988) Differentiation of granule cells in relation to GABAergic neurons in the rat fascia dentata. Combined Golgi/EM and immunocytochemical studies. *Anat. Embryol.*, 178: 119–127.

Lübbers, K., Wolff, J.R. and Frotscher, M. (1985) Neurogenesis of GABAergic neurons in the rat dentate gyrus: a combined autoradiographic and immunocytochemical study. *Neurosci. Lett.*, 62: 317–322.

Lugaro, E. (1893) Contributo alla Fina Anatomia del Grande Piede del Hippocampo. *Arch. Sci. Med.*, 18: 113–142.

Misgeld, U. (1988) Membrane properties and postsynaptic responses of hippocampal neurons. In M. Frotscher, P. Kugler, U. Misgeld and K. Zilles (Eds.), *Neurotransmission in the Hippocampus, Adv. Anat. Embryol. Cell Biol., Vol. 111,* Springer-Verlag, Berlin, pp. 20–39.

Misgeld, U. and Frotscher, M. (1982) Dependence of the viability of neurons in hippocampal slices on oxygen supply. *Brain Res. Bull.*, 8: 95–100.

Nafstad, P.H.J. (1967) An electron microscope study on the termination of the perforant path fibres in the hippocampus and the fascia dentata. *Z. Zellforsch.*, 76: 532–542.

Oertel, W.H., Schmechel, D.E., Mugnaini, E., Tappaz, M.L. and Kopin, I.J. (1982) Immunocytochemical localization of glutamate decarboxylase in the rat cerebellum with a new antiserum. *Neuroscience*, 6: 2715–2735.

Ramón y Cajal, S. (1911) *Histologie du Système Nerveux de l'Homme et des Vertébrés, Vol. I,* Maloine, Paris.

Ribak, C.E. and Anderson, L. (1980) Ultrastructure of the pyramidal basket cells in the dentate gyrus of the rat. *J. Comp. Neurol.*, 192: 903–916.

Ribak, C.E. and Seress, L. (1983) Five types of basket cell in the hippocampal dentate gyrus: a combined Golgi and electron microscopic study. *J. Neurocytol.*, 12: 577–597.

Ribak, C.E, Vaughn, J.E. and Saito, K. (1978) Immunocytochemical localization of glutamic acid decarboxylase in neuronal somata following colchicine inhibition of axonal transport. *Brain Res.*, 140: 315–332.

Sala, L. (1891) Zur feineren Anatomie des großen Seepferdefußes. *Z. Wiss. Zool.*, 52: 18–45.

Schaffer, K. (1892) Beitrag zur Histologie der Ammonshornformation. *Arch. Mikrosk. Anat.*, 39: 611–632.

Schlander, M. and Frotscher, M. (1986) Non-pyramidal neurons in the guinea pig hippocampus. A combined Golgi-electron microscope study. *Anat. Embryol.*, 174: 35–47.

Seifert, W. (Ed.) (1983) *Neurobiology of the Hippocampus,* Academic Press, London.

Seress, L. and Ribak, C.E. (1985) A combined Golgi-electron microscopic study of non-pyramidal neurons in CA1 area of the hippocampus. *J. Neurocytol.*, 14: 717–730.

Somogyi, P. and Takagi, H. (1982) A note on the use of picric acid-paraformaldehyde-glutaraldehyde fixative for correlated light and electron microscopic immunocytochemistry. *Neuroscience*, 7: 1779–1784.

Soriano, E., Cobas, A. and Fairén, A. (1989) Neurogenesis of glutamic acid decarboxylase immunoreactive cells in the hippocampus of the mouse. I: Regio superior and regio inferior. *J. Comp. Neurol.*, 281: 586–602.

Soriano, E., Nitsch, R. and Frotscher, M. (1990) Axo-axonic chandelier cells in the rat fascia dentata: Golgi-EM and immunocytochemical studies. *J. Comp. Neurol.*, in press.

Stephan, H. (1975) *Allocortex. Handbuch der mikroskopischen Anatomie des Menschen, Vol. IV/9,* Springer, Berlin.

Stephan, H. (1983) Evolutionary trends in limbic structures. *Neurosci. Biobehav. Rev.*, 7: 367–374.

Sternberger, L.A., Hardy, P.H., Curculis, J.J. and Meyer, H.G. (1970) The unlabelled antibody-enzyme method of immunocytochemistry. Preparation and properties of soluble antigen-antibody complex (horseradish peroxidase)) and its use in identification of spirochetes. *J. Cytochem.*, 18: 315–333.

Streit, P., Thompson, S.M. and Gähwiler, B.H. (1989) Anatomical and physiological properties of GABAergic neurotransmission in organotypic slice cultures of rat hippocampus. *Eur. J. Neurosci.*, 1: 603–615.

Zimmer, J. and Gähwiler, B.H. (1984) Cellular and connective organization of slice cultures of the rat hippocampus and fascia dentata. *J. Comp. Neurol.*, 228: 432–446.

J. Storm-Mathisen, J. Zimmer and O.P. Ottersen (Eds.)
Progress in Brain Research, Vol. 83
© 1990 Elsevier Science Publishers B.V. (Biomedical Division)

CHAPTER 25

Growth factors and growth factor receptors in the hippocampus. Role in plasticity and response to injury

Manuel Nieto-Sampedro and Paola Bovolenta

Laboratorio de Plasticidad Neural, Instituto Cajal, Doctor Arce 37, 28002 Madrid, Spain

Various growth factors are present in the hippocampal formation and appear responsible for the prominent plasticity of this brain area. Although hormone-like growth-promoting polypeptides are the best known, recent studies emphasize the importance in the growth response of molecules such as laminin proteoglycans, neurotransmitters and growth inhibitors. The progress and problems in the study of these substances are reviewed.

Introduction

The hippocampus is one of the mammalian brain structures more studied and perhaps, by any criterium, the best known. Over the years, the hippocampus has become the choice model to study CNS plasticity mechanisms. Not surprisingly, it was in this system where CNS growth factors and their probable relationship to CNS plasticity were first described (Crutcher and Collins, 1982; Nieto-Sampedro et al., 1982). Interest in CNS growth factors has now increased dramatically, and the hippocampal formation is at the center of much of this research. This article attempts to summarize some of the developments since 1982 and to point out areas in need of additional work.

Classes of growth factors

The increased interest in growth factor biology and the speed of this particular growth response, has caused a loss of sharpness in the meaning of the terms growth factor, trophic factor and the various activities included under these headings. Nature has contributed to further slur the issue by providing growth factors, such as NGF, FGF or EGF, with more than one kind of activity. At the mo-

ment, it may be useful to keep the meaning of the terms "growth factor" or "trophic factor" deliberately vague, to designate substances that promote survival and/or growth. However, it is also critical to make a clear assignation of specific names to specific activities.

As used in this review, the terms *neurotrophic or neuronotrophic* factor (NTF) refer to molecules required for neuronal survival, typically at hormone-like concentration. *Neurite-promoting or neuritogenic* factors (NPF) refer to factors capable of eliciting neurite outgrowth, typically from embryonic neurons in culture. *Sprouting* factors will be reserved for those molecules known to promote growth of sprouts from differentiated neurons, most frequently in vivo. *Mitogen* will be used for substances that promote cell division, although promotion of nucleotide incorporation into DNA is usually accepted as an alternative. Finally, *chemiotactic or chemiotropic* factors are molecules that attract neurite growth.

Culture of test neurons and growth factor assays

Quantitative measurement of CNS neurotrophic and neurite-promoting activities was initially carried out using as test cells dissociated peripheral neurons kept in low density culture. Sympathetic ganglion, ciliary ganglion and dorsal root ganglion cells are still in extensive use for a variety of reasons. Peripheral neurons can be easily purified away from non-neuronal cells, thus eliminating indirect effects, and assays for NTF and NPF activities have been carefully worked out (McCarthy and Partlow, 1976; Greene, 1977; Collins, 1978b).

Neurotrophic factor assays

Until recently, NTF assay involved labor-intensive, phase-contrast cell counting. The method required considerable experience and was quite subjective, in that it was not always obvious whether a given neuron was alive or dead. Recently, two different NTF assays have been developed. They are based on the ability of viable neurons to take up either radiolabeled aminoacids (Nieto-Sampedro et al., 1985) or a yellow tetrazolium derivative which living cells convert in an insoluble blue product (Manthorpe et al., 1986b). Both methods are objective and allow the processing of a large number of samples by comparatively inexperienced workers. However, of the two methods, that described by Manthorpe et al. (1986b) is cheaper, does not involve the use of radioactivity and is amenable to automation.

Neurite promoting factor assay

Neuritogenesis is a multi-step process and different molecules are probably responsible for neurite initiation, elongation and branching (Nishi and Berg, 1981; Collins and Dawson, 1983). Additionally, separate substances and different environmental influences may be involved in dendrite and axonal growth. Developmental growth, regenerative growth of damaged axons and reactive growth of undamaged axons may also have their individual requirements (Brown, 1984). The development of defined culture media has facilitated the use of CNS neurons in growth factor studies and low density cultures of hippocampal neurons, appropriate for growth factor assay, have

been described (Barbin et al., 1984b; Banker and Goslin, 1988). The description of specific markers for dendrites and axons in cultures of hippocampal cells (Garner et al., 1988; Goslin et al., 1988; Goslin and Banker, 1989) allows us to deal with these problems, but only the first steps have been initiated. Attempts to automate NPF assay, using image processing equipment, have not yet been successful and the assay still involves personal cell counting. Hopefully, this situation will soon improve.

Neurotrophic factors in the hippocampus

Evidence for the presence in brain of NTF and NPF activities was first presented by Nieto-Sampedro et al. (1982) and Crutcher and Collins (1982). These researchers suggested that these growth factor activities may be the basis for the neuronal plasticity observed at the histological level. However, since 1982 the characterization of the molecules involved has progressed very slowly.

A number of molecules probably contribute to both the NTF and NPF activities observed. Part of the central NTF activity is trypsin-resistant; it consists of small molecules, such as pyruvate, serine and Fe^{3+} and possibly other small molecular astrocyte metabolites (Müller et al., 1984; Selak et al., 1985; Manthorpe et al., 1986a). Another part of the activity is trypsin- and temperature-sensitive, and much of it consists of conventional hormone-like polypeptide growth factors. There is now overwhelming evidence that NGF is one of these factors, and the availability of pure NGF and specific antibodies has resulted in a great wealth of information on this growth factor. Several recent reviews provide up to date information on the subject (see, for example, Thoenen et al., 1987; Whittemore and Seiger, 1987). We will only mention that NGF concentration in hippocampus is the highest in the rat CNS. Although NGF is the model trophic agent and is receiving a great deal of attention, we cannot forget that the cholinergic cells addressed by this factor are only a very small proportion of the CNS cells. Even if other neuronal types were responsive to NGF, it would still be unlikely for this molecule to be the primary NTF for most CNS neurons.

Fibroblast growth factors

Other polypeptide growth factors are present in the hippocampus (Nieto-Sampedro et al., 1983; Ojika and Appel, 1984). Two of them, the fibroblast growth factors (acidic and basic, aFGF and bFGF) are well-characterized mitogens (Thomas and Giménez-Gallego, 1986) that exhibit potent NTF activity in vivo (Anderson et al., 1988) or on cultured neurons from many brain regions, including hippocampus (Morrison et al., 1986; Morrison, 1987; Walicke et al., 1986; Walicke, 1988). The two factors differ in neuronal specificity and, additionally, bFGF appears to be about 100 × more potent than aFGF (Walicke, 1988). It has been suggested that differences in stability in the absence of heparin may underlie this difference in potency (Thomas and Giménez-Gallego, 1986). In hippocampus and other forebrain areas, bFGF seems to be located exclusively within neurons (Pettmann et al., 1986), whereas a molecule very similar to aFGF, glia maturation factor (GMF), is located inside astrocytes (Lim et al., 1987). Since both factors are also glia mitogens, it has been suggested that FGFs may be involved in neuron – glia communication. However, the FGFs are not secreted and can directly support neuronal survival in the absence of astrocytes (Walicke and Baird, 1988). The fact that both FGFs are 2 – 4 orders of magnitude more abundant in brain than NGF (aFGF: about 10 μg/g brain and bFGF: 0.07 μg/g brain; calculated from data of Thomas et al., 1984, and Böhlen et al., 1985) makes them good candidates as neurotrophic factors for at least a major kind of hippocampal excitatory neurons, the pyramidal cells.

Other central neurotrophic factors

No doubt, other hormone-like neurotrophic factors for hippocampal and other CNS cells will be found in the near future. This will probably result both from the purification of new CNS factors and from testing well-known pure factors on appropriate target neurons. A small basic protein different from NGF, brain-derived neurotrophic factor (BDNF), was purified from pig brain (Barde et al., 1982). BDNF has NTF activity for sensory and retinal ganglion neurons, but not sympathetic or ciliary neurons (Johnson et al., 1986; Barde et al., 1987). Another non-NGF neurotrophic factor, the activity of which was defined using as target peripheral neurons, is the ciliary neuronotrophic factor (CNTF). Initially purified from chick eye (Barbin et al., 1984a), it was later purified from rat sciatic nerve (Manthorpe et al., 1986c). This 25 kDa acidic protein may also be present in brain, but no defined biological activities on central neurons have yet been described.

The specific location of EGF receptor immunoreactivity in select populations of probably GABAergic neurons (cerebellar Purkinje cells, some cortical basket cells) suggests than an EGF-like substance may be a deserving neurotrophic candidate for these cells (Gomez-Pinilla et al., 1988). The report that EGF supports a small proportion of brain neurons (Morrison et al., 1987) points in the same direction. Insulin-like factors, IGF I and II, seem to be neurotrophic for septal neurons, both directly and through non-neuronal cells (Hefti, 1989).

It has been suggested that neurotrophic factors may be involved in neurodegenerative pathology (Appel, 1981; Cotman and Nieto-Sampedro, 1983; Nieto-Sampedro et al., 1983). A recent report on the NTF activity for hippocampal pyramidal neurons of a peptide related to β-amyloid (Whitson et al., 1989), supports the idea that trophic factors may be involved in the generation of pathological growth in Alzheimer's disease.

Factors promoting neurite initiation, elongation and branching

Rat forebrain contains a variety of molecules, ranging in molecular weight from about 9 to higher than 200 kDa, capable of promoting neurite outgrowth from cultured ciliary ganglion neurons (Needels et al., 1986). All these molecules have a moderately acidic isoionic pH and those of highest molecular weight probably belong to the NPF class called PNPF, polycation bindable NPF. Typical members of this group are laminin and laminin-proteoglycan complexes.

Laminin and related molecules

Laminin and the laminin-heparan sulfate proteoglycan complexes of the extracellular matrix, have neurite-promoting activity in vitro on a wide variety of both peripheral and central neurons (Manthorpe et al., 1983b; Rogers et al., 1983; Lander et al., 1985a, b). Purified laminin, glia-derived laminin-proteoglycan and a polylysine bindable activity from injured entorhinal and hippocampal regions, are able to support the survival and growth of septal, hippocampal and striatal neurons in vitro (Manthorpe et al., 1986a; Pixley and Cotman, 1986; Gibbs et al., 1987). Laminin-related molecules are transiently expressed in the prospective pathway of ventral longitudinal axons in the hindbrain and spinal cord (Letourneau et al., 1987, 1988; Karagogeos et al., in preparation), on the surface of glial cells present in the pathway of ingrowing optic fibers, septal axons of the fimbria-fornix (Liesi and Silver, 1988) and in hippocampal neurons (Yamamoto et al., 1988). These observations raise the possibility that extracellular matrix components might in part be responsible for the observed brain NPF activity. Hippocampal cultures rapidly extend neurites in PNPF-treated substrate (Barbin et al., 1984b) but, at present, there is little evidence for a PNPF role in vivo, either in the CNS in general or in the hippocampus in particular.

Although the proportion of brain PNPF is probably lower than 10% of the total activity (Needels et al., 1986), the possibility of cooperative interactions between proteoglycans and smaller trophic polypeptides could make PNPF very important in the induction of central neurite outgrowth. In this respect, it is noteworthy that growth factors attached to heparan sulfate remain fully active (Roberts et al., 1988) and that heparin has high-affinity sites for a wide variety of growth factors including the FGFs (Gospodarowicz et al., 1984). Laminin and fibronectin greatly potentiate the neurotrophic and neurite-promoting activity of NGF on sensory neurons (Edgar and Thoenen, 1982; Millaruelo et al., 1988) and laminin itself has growth factor activity (Panayotou et al., 1989). Polypeptide growth factors are perhaps physiologically active in the form of complexes with proteoglycans (Gospodarowicz et al., 1987). NPFs and NTFs may in fact be presented to some of their physiological targets in a proteoglycan-bound form.

Hormone-like NPFs

Without any interaction with CNS proteoglycans, bFGF, but not aFGF (Walicke, 1988), is a powerful neurite-promoting agent for hippocampal neurons and is probably part of the activity described by Needels et al. (1986). The NPF activity of bFGF is selective for some central neurons but is not restricted to hippocampal neurons. Indeed, bFGF can promote neurite formation on cerebellar granule cells (Hatten et al., 1988) and mesencephalic neurons (Ferrari et al., 1989), as well as on PC12 cells (Togari et al., 1985; Rydel and Greene, 1987). The possible in vivo role of bFGF in hippocampal sprouting remains to be established.

A heat-stable protein with NPF activity for central neurons was purified from brain by Kligman and Marshak (1985). Tryptic and cyanogen bromide peptides from this protein had an aminoacid sequence identical to that of the β form of protein S100 (Moore, 1965; Isobe et al., 1981), a major brain protein located in glial cells. However, a commercial preparation of S100 protein had no detectable NPF activity. From the published data it seems clear that S100 is the major component of Kligman's NPF preparation. However, it is not clear that S100 is responsible for NPF activity. The biological activity of the protein purified by Kligman and Marshak (1985) was poorly described and not characterized in any detail. Conclusions about this protein must await further experimental evidence, such as development of inactivating antibodies.

Neurite initiation and polarity

From the few reports available, it seems that the initiation signal for axonal or dendritic growth, may be exogenous (Collins, 1978b), but the choice of neuronal polarity is made within the neuron. The progress of Gary Banker's team with hippocampal cultures is exemplary, in that it is showing the potential of a well-characterized culture system. After showing that cultured hippocampal neurons acquire their polarity following a stereotyped sequence of steps (Dotti et al., 1988), these workers showed that neuron polarity could be experimentally altered. Transected axons may become dendrites and vice-versa (Dotti and Banker, 1987). The possibility of polarity reversal by neuritomy was limited by the length of the neurite stump relative to that of the other neurites. Whichever neuronal process was more than 10 μm longer than the others, became the axon (Goslin and Banker, 1989). It remains to be discovered why this plasticity is not observed in vivo in more mature neurons, where short stumps after axotomy frequently lead to neuronal death rather than polarity reversal.

Neurite elongation and branching

Polypeptide growth factors seem to be involved in axonal elongation and axonal and dendritic branching. The data available, so far collected in the PNS, again emphasize the fact that the same factor may have (1) different types of activity when acting on different neuronal types and (2) various effects on the same neuronal type. Thus, NGF at concentrations around 1 ng/ml enhances the rate of neurite elongation from ciliary ganglion cells (a neuronal type for which NGF is not neurotrophic)

and dorsal root ganglion cells (a traditional neurotrophic target of NGF) (Collins and Dawson, 1983; Collins, 1988). On the other hand, on sympathetic ganglion cells, NGF is neurotrophic, neurite-promoting, capable of directing neurite growth and neurotransmitter phenotype (Thoenen et al., 1987), and also enhances dendritic arborization (Purves et al., 1988; Snider, 1988). The latter NGF effect has a parallel in developmental and reactive axonal branching of motor neurons, also promoted by target-derived, unidentified muscle factor/s (Brown, 1984). Specific neuron – astroglial interactions, possibly mediated by local neurotrophic factors, might also differentially regulate axonal and dendritic outgrowth. Mesencephalic dopaminergic neurons, in fact, display a long unbranched neurite when grown on striatal astrocytes, while they develop several branched neurites on local, mesencephalic astrocytes (Dennis-Donnini et al., 1984; Chamack et al., 1987).

Direction of neurite growth

As for the factors specifying the direction of neurite growth, few chemotropic activities have been described in the nervous system, possibly because, in vivo, it is difficult to discern if neurites are guided by cues present on the substrate or by chemoattractants secreted by distant targets. Evidence exists that growth cones of chick dorsal ganglion neurons orient themselves toward point sources of NGF in vitro (Gundersen and Barrett, 1979, 1980), and injections of NGF into the brainstem of neonatal rodents induces the ingrowth of peripheral sympathetic axons toward the site of injection (Montesini-Chen et al., 1978; Levi-Montalcini, 1982). In mammals, both in the PNS and in the CNS, intermediate or final targets have been shown to produce a gradient of diffusible molecule/s not yet identified but distinct from both NGF and laminin, which directs axonal outgrowth. Trigeminal sensory axons grow toward the maxillary arch, their peripheral target, when these structures are co-cultured in three dimensional collagen gel matrices which limit the diffusion of soluble factors (Lumdsen and Davis, 1986). With a similar experimental approach, Tessier-Lavigne et al. (1988) have shown that the growth cones of commissural neurons in the embryonic rat spinal cord project toward an intermediate target, the floor plate. To our knowledge, no chemotactic factor/s have yet been described in the hippocampus.

Growth factor receptors and second messages

All cell types that respond to growth factors must bear receptors for these molecules. The receptors for NGF and EGF have been purified, cloned, and characterized as far as interaction with their ligands and anatomical location is concerned, whereas there is much less information on the FGF receptor (see reviews by Carpenter, 1987, and Gospodarowicz et al., 1987; Whittemore and Seiger, 1987).

Growth factor receptors are membrane proteins with one or several transmembrane segments. Their extracellular moiety, that contains the ligand binding site, is called the receptor domain and is generally glycosylated. Typically, two kinds of K_d characterize the interaction of hormone-like trophic factors with their receptors. The so-called high-affinity receptors have K_d values in the range of 10^{-11} M, whereas low-affinity receptors have dissociation constants of the order of 10^{-9} M. It is not clear whether these receptors correspond in all cases to different molecular entities or glycosylation variants of the same molecule. In the case of the NGFRs, the two forms have very different molecular weights (low affinity, 80 kDa; high affinity, 159 kDa), although just a single mRNA, coding for low-affinity NGFR, has been observed. Low-affinity NGFR is converted to the high-affinity form by clustering with lectins or antibodies and the conversion probably involves association with another protein (Shooter, 1989). The physiological effects of NGF are thought to occur via the high-affinity form of the receptor.

NGF neurotrophic activity requires the internalization of the NGF – NGFR complex, which can occur only through the high-affinity form (Bernd and Greene, 1984; Hosang and Shooter, 1987).

The receptor domain is followed by an α-helical transmembrane segment/s (membrane domain) that terminate in a basic interface domain (about 13 amino acid residues) and leads to the cytoplasmic domain, where growth factor binding is translated into a second message. The nature of the membrane domain, the cytoplasmic domain, and the transmembrane signal of ligand binding into a second message is different for different growth factors. A categorization is not possible yet, but it will probably soon emerge.

The EGF receptor (EGFR) is one of the best known. It is a single chain glycoprotein of 170 kDa mol. wt., the cytoplasmic moiety of which has tyrosine kinase activity. EGF binding to the EGFR activates the kinase activity which, using ATP or GTP as phosphate donors, results in autophosphorylation and phosphorylation of other cytoplasmic proteins that finally result in eicosanoid product formation (Carpenter, 1987). The NGFR is a much smaller glycoprotein (42 kDa core protein, 41 kDa carbohydrate) and, like EGFR, has a single membrane spanning domain. Although no second message is known to mediate the physiological effects evoked by NGF binding, guanine nucleotide binding regulatory proteins (G-proteins; Gilman, 1987) or related molecules seem to be involved (Borasio et al., 1989).

The anatomical location of NGF receptors (NGFR) has been studied by autoradiography, using ^{125}I-NGF (Raivich and Kreutzberg, 1987; Richardson et al., 1986) and by immunohistochemistry (Hefti et al., 1986; Gómez-Pinilla et al., 1987; Springer et al., 1987). Both methods indicate that, in the brain, NGF receptors are generally associated to cholinergic neuronal somata, dendrites and axons. As for the EGF receptor, in adult rat brain strong EGFR immunoreactivity is present in cerebellar Purkinje cells and in a sparse population of cortical cells with the morphology of basket cells (Gómez-Pinilla et al., 1988).

Growth factor inhibitors

When measuring the NTF, NPF or glial mitogenic activities of brain extracts on CNS cells, a familiar observation is that of bell-shaped dose – response curves. Traditionally, the decrease in activity with increasing protein concentration has been interpreted as due to the simultaneous presence in the extract of high-affinity growth factors and lower affinity growth inhibitors (Manthorpe et al., 1983a). However, in comparison to growth factors, growth inhibitors or negative growth regulators have received comparatively little attention. Although tissue chalones were described long ago, the study of growth inhibitors faced the formidable problem of their isolation and chemical characterization. Consequently, most studies on cell growth and division concentrated on positive controllers, the growth factors. However, simultaneous growth control by means of both positive and negative regulators has obvious functional advantages and seems to be the actual mechanism used by nature. Triggered by the purification of several growth inhibitors, particularly transforming growth factor β (TGF-β), in the last few years there has been a revival of interest in negative regulators (reviewed by Wang and Hsu, 1986). In the CNS, two inhibitors closely concerned with injury repair have been recently described. One is an inhibitor of neurite outgrowth, associated to the oligodendrocyte membrane and CNS myelin (Caroni and Schwab, 1988a, b; Schwab and Caroni, 1988). Work in our laboratory led to the description of two other brain molecules, immunologically related to the EGF receptor (EGFR). One of them is a soluble astrocyte mitogen inhibitor, present in brain extracts and also produced by cultured astrocytes. Its concentration decreased after injury in parallel with the appearance of reactive astrocytes (Nieto-Sampedro, 1988; Nieto-Sampedro and Broderick, 1989). Another EGFR-immunoreactive molecule is present in the membrane of rat brain astrocytes in late development, is absent or present in very small amounts in the astrocytes of the adult, and re-appears after injury (Nieto-Sampedro et al., 1988a). The function of this membrane-bound molecule and its possible relationship to the EGFR and to the neurite inhibitor from oligodendrocytes, has not yet been examined.

Plasticity, growth factors and neurotransmitters

Excitatory aminoacid receptors, particularly of the NMDA type, seem to be involved in developmental plasticity, early learning, and long-term potentiation (reviewed by Monaghan et al., 1989). Because these phenomena have morphological correlates, it is logical to postulate a relationship between the effectors of growth factors and those of neurotransmitters at the level of ionic channels, metabolism of cytoskeletal elements and membrane recycling apparatus (Mattson, 1988). Some recent reports point directly in this direction.

Mattson et al. (1988) have shown that subtoxic doses of glutamate, quisqualate and kainate had a dose-dependent influence on dendritic outgrowth in cultured pyramidal cells. Increasing doses of glutamate reduced dendritic outgrowth rates or caused dendritic atrophy, whereas they had little or no effect on axonal elongation. The effect appeared to be caused by calcium influx, mediated by quisqualate/kainate type receptors. The calcium channel controlled by NMDA seems to have a more complex effect (Breuer and Cotman, 1989). In cultured dentate granule cells, glutamate and NMDA stimulated branching of neuronal processes, whereas MK-801, an antagonist acting on the NMDA-coupled calcium channel, blocked branching and promoted axonal elongation (Breuer and Cotman, 1989). Trophic effects of glutamate and NMDA have also been reported on cerebellar granule cells (Pearce et al., 1987; Balasz et al., 1988).

Growth effects of neurotransmitters are not restricted to the hippocampus or to excitatory neurotransmitters. Stimulation of D_1-type dopamine receptors inhibited growth cone motility in cultured retinal neurons (Lankford et al., 1988) and tetrodotoxin blockage of fetal retinal ganglion cell activity causes abnormally widespread terminal arborizations in the axons of these cells (Sretavan et al., 1988). Summarizing, the neurotransmitters themselves or the events linked to neurotransmission appear to have profound morphological and functional consequences. Research in this new field promises very exciting insights, uniting thus far separated areas of research in neuronal plasticity.

Hippocampal growth factors: response to injury

Cortical injury caused a large, time-dependent, increase in neurotrophic and neurite-promoting activity at the lesion site (Nieto-Sampedro et al., 1982; Needels et al., 1986). Similar activity enhancement was promoted by mechanical damage of the hippocampus, by deafferenting lesions of the entorhinal cortex (Nieto-Sampedro et al., 1983; Crutcher and Collins, 1986; Needels et al., 1986; Gibbs et al., 1987), damage to hippocampal areas CA3/CA4 by kainic acid injection (Nieto-Sampedro et al., 1983; Heacock et al., 1986), fimbria-fornix transection (Gage et al., 1984), medial septal lesion (Collins and Crutcher, 1985), and destruction of dorsal raphe afferents with 5,7-HT (Azmitia, 1987). The increase in NTF activity after a lesion, assayed in cultured peripheral and central neurons (Nieto-Sampedro et al., 1982, 1983; Manthorpe et al., 1983a; Whittemore et al., 1985; Needels et al., 1985), correlated in vivo with the enhanced survival of delayed implants in the wound cavity (Nieto-Sampedro et al., 1982, 1983, 1984; Manthorpe et al., 1983a). Although this is not evidence for a physiological role of the growth factors, it is a strong suggestion. A similar judgement applies to the strong correlation between the time-course of NPF induction after an entorhinal lesion and that of sprouting of septal and commissural/associational axons in the dentate molecular layer after a similar lesion (Needels et al., 1986). In this latter case, it is noteworthy that the observations of in vitro injury-induced NPF activity and in vivo sprouting response were made independently, at

different times, by different experimenters. We have proposed that one or more of the injury-induced NPFs is responsible for the observed sprouting. The increase in NTF and NPF activities after injury may be both quantitative and qualitative. There appears to be an increase in the basal trophic activity, but new factor/s also seem to appear after injury. The main difference between basal and injury-induced NPF activities seems to be the critical role of SH groups in the latter (Needels et al., 1986). The purification and molecular characterization of the growth factors involved has proven very difficult, in view of the scarcity and instability of the activities involved, and the labor-intensive nature of the preparation of the starting material. Some of the activities observed after injury may be produced by blood cells (Gurney et al., 1986a, 1986b; Chaput et al., 1988; Faik et al., 1988). However, the difficulty of the purification of new CNS growth factors appears to have channeled most researchers into the study of well-characterized factors, an area more productive in the short term. The response to injury of NGF in the hippocampus has been examined in some detail. In the neonate, both hippocampal NGF and NGF mRNA increased transiently by about 50% after fimbria transection but not after entorhinal ablation (Whittemore et al., 1987). In the adult, NGF levels appear to be regulated in a different manner, because elimination of septo-hippocampal afferents caused an increase in hippocampal NGF (Collins and Crutcher, 1985; Gasser et al., 1986; Korsching et al., 1986), but not in NGF mRNA (Goedert et al., 1986; Korsching et al., 1986; Whittemore et al., 1986). After entorhinal deafferentation, NGF mRNA levels were not affected, whereas NGF-like activity increased (Crutcher and Collins, 1986). Because low-affinity NGFR is transiently upregulated by NGF (Bernd and Greene, 1983; Cavicchioli et al., 1988; Shooter, 1989), the amount of hippocampal NGFR increases after an entorhinal lesion. This was particularly clear in the dentate molecular layer, where septal fiber sprouting was paralleled by an increase in NGFR immunoreactivity

(Gómez-Pinilla et al., 1987).

We have only hypothesized the initiation of the cascade of molecular and cellular events that follows brain injury. One of the earliest events, in terms of trophic factors, is the rapid release of aFGF. Brain FGFs are normally intracellular, but aFGF and the related GMF seem to be actively secreted less than one hour after injury (Nieto-Sampedro et al., 1988b). These factors, in turn, promote the secretion of interleukin-1 by macrophages (Fontana et al., 1983), a cytokine that is mitogenic for astrocytes (Nieto-Sampedro and Berman, 1987) and induces the synthesis of NGF (Thoenen, 1989). GMF and aFGF could also be mitogenic for macrophages, cells that may play a role in removing astrocyte mitogen inhibitors (Nieto-Sampedro, 1988). Astrocyte proliferation, in turn, would also lead to increased production of growth factors (see below).

Summarizing, in the last 7 years great progress has been made in understanding trophic factor response to injury. It is also clear that much further work is necessary to gain a satisfactory understanding of the systems involved.

Cellular origin of growth factors

The first physiological role proposed for non-neuronal cells of the CNS, was to provide trophic support to neurons (Ramón y Cajal, 1928). Since then, several lines of evidence have contributed to support the idea that non-neuronal cells, and astrocytes in particular, might be important cellular sources of NTF and NPF. The concentration of trophic factors released in rat brain after injury is maximal at the injury site, a location known to contain a large number of reactive astrocytes (Nieto-Sampedro et al., 1983). Astrocytes and astrocyte-conditioned medium can support the survival of hippocampal neurons in culture (Banker, 1980; Müller et al., 1984; Rudge et al., 1985). Furthermore, astrocytes have been proven to be a good substratum for neurite outgrowth of CNS neurons (Noble et al., 1984; Fallon et al., 1985). The introduction of defined culture conditions (i.e.

serum-free) have provided definitive proof that astrocytes are able to secrete several growth activities, including NGF, FGF, CNTF, pyruvate and related molecules and laminin and related molecules (Lindsay, 1979; Liesi et al., 1983; Lander et al., 1985a; Selak et al., 1985; Beckh et al., 1987; Varon et al., 1987; Hatten et al., 1988). Little direct evidence, however, exist that astrocytes are the in vivo sources of all these activities. Laminin immunoreactivity has been detected on the surface of reactive astrocytes after injury (Liesi, 1985). Immunosuppression with methotrexate, which reduces reactive gliosis, also reduced the hippocampal injury-induced neurotrophic activity, suggesting that astrocytes were responsible for NTF production (Heacock et al., 1986).

The cellular source of NGF in the hippocampus is better known, yet controversial. In vitro brain astrocytes synthesize and secrete a molecule very similar if not identical to NGF (Linsday, 1979; Furukawa et al., 1986). The use of a cDNA probe has localized the mRNA for NGF on astrocyte-like cells cultured from embryonic rat brains (Bandtlow et al., 1988). However, in vivo, cDNA probes for NGF have been shown to localize on neurons (Rennert and Heinrich, 1986; Ayer-LeLievre et al., 1988). The most intense labeling occurred on the hippocampal dentate gyrus and the pyramidal cell layer, which are the targets of the forebrain cholinergic neurons. Moreover, the destruction of these two regions with kainic acid and colchicine resulted in the loss of cells labelled with NGF probes, in spite of the local gliosis induced by the drugs, suggesting that in the hippocampus only neurons contained the NGF mRNA (Ayer-LeLievre et al., 1988). It is possible that astrocytes contain only low levels of NGF, undetectable by in situ hybridization. Also, astrocytes could function as storage sites for NGF through the low-affinity receptor probably localized on their surface (Bernd et al., 1988).

A further complexity arises from the possible role of monocytes/microglia. Recently, Mallat et al. (1989) have shown that ameboid microglial cells, purified from embryonic rat brains, release NGF upon stimulation with lipopolysaccharide. The direct neurotrophic role of brain macrophages needs further experimental support, but it has been proposed that they intervene in the initiation of the astroglial response to injury by removing mitogen inhibitors (Nieto-Sampedro, 1988).

Glial cells and target neurons seem to provide trophic support to the neuronal population. Conversely, neurons appear to release factors that influence the maturation and survival of astroglial cells (Pettmann et al., 1987), and glial cells can influence their own development. In this respect, the group of Raff has shown that, in the rat optic nerve, type-1 astrocytes are able to secrete two trophic factors, platelet derived growth factor (PDGF) and ciliary neuronotrophic factor (CNTF), which control the timed appearance of oligodendrocytes and type-2 astrocytes, respectively (Hughes et al., 1988; Lillien et al., 1988; Raff et al., 1988).

Acknowledgements

Supported by a grant from the CSIC, Spain. P.B. is a research fellow of the Ministerio de Educación y Ciencia.

References

Anderson, K.J., Dam, D., Lee, S. and Cotman, C.W. (1988) Basic fibroblast growth factor prevents death of lesioned cholinergic neurons in vivo. *Nature (Lond.)*, 332: 360 – 361.

Appel, S.H. (1981) A unifying hypothesis for the cause of amyotrophic lateral sclerosis, parkinsonism and Alzheimer's disease. *Ann. Neurol.*, 10: 499 – 505.

Ayer-LeLievre, C., Olson, L., Ebendal, T., Seiger, A. and Person, H. (1988) Expression of the β-nerve growth factor gene in hippocampal neurons. *Science*, 240: 1339 – 1341.

Azmitia, E.C. (1987) A serotonin hippocampal model indicates adult neurons survive transplantation and aged target may be deficient in a soluble serotonergic growth factor. *Ann. N.Y. Acad. Sci.*, 495: 362 – 377.

Balasz, R., Hack, N. and Jorgensen, O.S. (1988) Stimulation of the *N*-methyl aspartate receptor has a trophic effect on differentiating cerebellar granule cells. *Neurosci. Lett.*, 87: 80 – 86.

Bandtlow, C., Heumann, R., Schwab, M.E. and Thoenen, H. (1988) Cellular localization of nerve growth factor synthesis by *in situ* hybridization. *Soc. Neurosci. Abstr.*, 14: 1616.

Banker, G.A. (1980) Trophic interaction between astroglial cells and hippocampal neurons in culture. *Science*, 209: 809 – 810.

Banker, G.A. and Goslin, K. (1988) Developments in neuronal cell culture. *Nature (Lond.)*, 336: 185 – 186.

Barbin, G., Manthorpe, M. and Varon, S. (1984a) Purification of chick eye Ciliary Neuronotrophic Factor. *J. Neurochem.*, 43: 1468 – 1478.

Barbin, G., Selak, I., Manthorpe, M. and Varon, S. (1984b) Use of central neuronal cultures for the detection of neuronotrophic agents. *Neuroscience*, 12: 33 – 43.

Barde, Y.-A., Edgar, D. and Thoenen, H. (1982) Purification of a new neurotrophic factor from mammalian brain. *EMBO J.*, 1: 549 – 553.

Barde, Y.-A., Davies, A.M., Johnson, J.E., Lindsay, R.M. and Thoenen, H. (1987) Brain-derived neurotrophic factor. *Prog. Brain Res.*, 71: 185 – 189.

Beckh, S., Müller, H.W. and Seifert, W. (1987) Neurotrophic and neurite promoting activities in astroglial conditioned medium. In H. Althaus and W. Seifert (Eds.), *Glial-Neuronal Communication in Development and Regeneration*. Springer-Verlag, pp. 385 – 406.

Bernd, P. and Greene, L.A. (1983) Electron microscopic radioautographic localization of iodinated nerve growth factor bound to and internalized by PC12 cells. *Neuroscience*, 3: 631 – 643.

Bernd, P. and Greene, L.A. (1984) Association of 125-I nerve growth factor with PC12 pheochromocytoma cells. *J. Cell Biol.*, 259: 15509 – 15516.

Bernd, P., Martinez, H.J., Dreyfus, C.F. and Black, I.B. (1988) Localization of high-affinity and low-affinity nerve growth factor receptors in cultured rat basal forebrain. *Neuroscience*, 26: 121 – 129.

Böhlen, P., Esch, F., Baird, A. and Gospodarowicz, D. (1985) Acidic fibroblast growth factor (FGF) from bovine brain: amino-terminal sequence and comparison with basic FGF. *EMBO J.*, 4: 1951 – 1956.

Borasio, G.D., John, J., Wittinghoffer, A., Barde, Y-A., Sendtner, M. and Heumann, R. (1989) Ras p21 protein promotes survival and fiber outgrowth of cultured embryonic neurons. *Neuron*, 2: 1087 – 1096.

Breuer, G.J. and Cotman, C.W. (1989) NMDA receptor regulation of neuronal morphology in cultured hippocampal neurons. *Neurosci. Lett.*, 99: 268 – 273.

Brown, M.C. (1984) Sprouting of motor nerves in adult muscles: a recapitulation of ontogeny. *Trends Neurosci.*, 7: 10 – 14.

Caroni, P. and Schwab, M. (1988a) Two membrane protein fractions from rat central myelin with inhibitory properties for neurite outgrowth and fibroblast spreading. *J. Cell Biol.*, 106: 1281 – 1288.

Caroni, P. and Schwab, M. (1988b) Antibody against myelin-associated inhibitor of neurite outgrowth neutralizes nonpermissive substrate properties of CNS white matter. *Neuron,* 1: 85 – 96.

Carpenter, G. (1987) Receptors for EGF and other polypeptide mitogens. *Ann. Rev. Biochem.,* 56: 881 – 914.

Cavicchioli, L., Vantini, G., Flanigan, T., Walsh, F., Fusco, M., Bigon, E., Benvegnú, D. and Leon, A. (1988) NGF enhances the expression of NGF receptor messenger RNA *in vivo. Soc. Neurosci. Abstr.,* 14: 1248.

Chamak, B., Fellous, A., Glowinski, J. and Prochiantz, A. (1987) MAP-2 expression and neuritic outgrowth and branching are coregulated through region-specific neuro-astroglial interaction. *J. Neurosci.,* 7: 3163 – 3170.

Chaput, M., Claes, V., Portetelle, D., Cludts, I., Cravador, A., Burny, A., Gras, H. and Tartar, A. (1988) The neurotrophic factor neuroleukin is 90% homologous with phosphohexose isomerase. *Nature (Lond.),* 332: 454 – 455.

Collins, F. (1978a) Axon initiation by ciliary neurons in culture. *Dev. Biol.,* 65: 50 – 57.

Collins, F. (1978b) Induction of neurite outgrowth by a conditioned medium factor bound to culture substratum. *Proc. Natl. Acad. Sci. U.S.A.,* 75: 5210 – 5213.

Collins, F. (1988) Developmental time-course of the effect of nerve growth factor on parasympathetic ciliary ganglion. *Dev. Brain Res.,* 39: 111 – 116.

Collins, F. and Crutcher, K.A. (1985) Neurotrophic activity in the adult rat hippocampal formation: regional distribution and increase after septal lesion. *J. Neurosci.,* 5: 2809 – 2814.

Collins, F. and Dawson, A. (1983) An effect of nerve growth factor on parasympathetic neurite outgrowth. *Proc. Natl. Acad. Sci. U.S.A.,* 80: 2091 – 2094.

Cotman, C.W. and Nieto-Sampedro, M. (1983) Trophic influences on the *in vivo* survival of transplanted cholinergic neurons: a model system for the study of neuronal loss in Alzheimer's disease. In *Banbury Report 15: Biological Aspects of Alzheimer's Disease,* Cold Spring Harbour Laboratory, pp. 275 – 284.

Crutcher, K.A. and Collins, F. (1982) In vitro evidence for two distinct hippocampal growth factors: basis of neuronal plasticity? *Science,* 217: 67 – 68.

Crutcher, K.A. and Collins, F. (1986) Entorhinal lesions result in increased nerve growth factor-like activity in medium conditioned by hippocampal slices. *Brain Res.,* 399: 383 – 389.

Dennis-Donnini, S., Glowinski, J. and Prochiantz, A. (1984) Glial heterogeneity may define the three-dimensional shape of mouse mesencephalic neurons in culture. *Nature (Lond.),* 307: 641 – 643.

Dotti, C.G. and Banker, G.A. (1987) Experimentally induced alteration in the polarity of developing neurons. *Nature (Lond.),* 330: 254 – 256.

Dotti, C.G., Sullivan, C.A. and Banker, G.A. (1988) The establishment of polarity by hippocampal neurons in culture. *J. Neurosci.,* 8: 1454 – 1468.

Edgar, D. and Thoenen, H. (1982) Modulation of NGF-induced survival of chick sympathetic neurons by contact with a conditioned medium factor bound to the culture substrate. *Dev. Brain Res.,* 5: 89 – 92.

Faik, P., Walker, J.I.H., Redmill, A.A.M. and Morgan, M.J. (1988) Mouse glucose-6-phosphate isomerase and neuroleukin have identical 3′ sequences. *Nature (Lond.),* 332: 455 – 457.

Fallon, J.R. (1985) Preferential outgrowth of central nervous system neurites on astrocytes and Schwann cells as compared with non glial cells in vitro. *J. Cell Biol.,* 100: 198 – 207.

Ferrari, G., Minozzi, M.C., Toffano, G., Leon, A. and Skaper, S.D. (1989) Basic fibroblast growth factor promotes the survival and development of mesencephalic neurons in culture. *Dev. Biol.,* 133: 140 – 147.

Fontana, A., Weber, E., Grob, P.J., Lim, R. and Miller, J.F. (1983) Dual effect of glial maturation factor on astrocytes: differentiation and release of interleukin-1-like growth factors. *J. Neuroimmunol.,* 5: 261 – 269.

Furukawa, S., Furukawa, Y., Satoyoshi, E. and Hayashi, K. (1986) Synthesis and secretion of nerve growth factor by mouse atroglial cells in culture. *Biochem. Biophys. Res. Commun.,* 136: 57 – 63.

Gage, F.H., Björklund, A. and Stenevi, U. (1984) Denervation releases a neuronal survival factor in the hippocampus. *Nature (Lond.),* 308: 637 – 639.

Garner, C.C., Tucker, R.P. and Matus, A. (1988) Selective localization of mRNA for cytoskeletal protein MAP2 in dendrites. *Nature (Lond.),* 336: 674 – 677.

Gasser, U.E., Weskamp, G., Otten, U. and Dravid, A.R. (1986) Time course of the elevation of NGF content in the hippocampus and septum following lesions of the septohippocampal pathway in rats. *Brain Res.,* 376: 351 – 356.

Gibbs, R.B., Needels, J. Yu and Cotman, C.W. (1987) Effects of entorhinal lesions on trophic activities present in the rat entorhinal cortex and hippocampus as studied using primary cultures of entorhinal and septal tissue. *J. Neurosci. Res.,* 18: 274 – 288.

Gilman, A.G. (1987) G proteins: transducers of receptor generated signals. *Annu. Rev. Biochem.,* 56: 615 – 649.

Gómez-Pinilla, F., Cotman, C.W. and Nieto-Sampedro, M. (1987) NGF receptor immunoreactivity in rat brain: topographic distribution and response to entorhinal ablation. *Neurosci. Lett.,* 82: 260 – 266.

Gómez-Pinilla, F., Knauer, D.J. and Nieto-Sampedro, M. (1988) EGF receptor immunoreactivity in rat brain. Development and cellular localization. *Brain Res.,* 438: 385 – 390.

Goedert, M., Fine, A., Hunt, S.P. and Ullrich, U. (1986) Nerve growth factor mRNA in peripheral and central rat tissues and in the human central nervous system: lesion effects in the rat brain and levels in Alzheimer's disease. *Mol. Brain Res.,* 1: 85 – 92.

Goslin, K. and Banker, G.A. (1989) Experimental observations on the development of polarity by hippocampal neurons in culture. *J. Cell Biol.,* 108: 1507–1516.

Goslin, K., Schreyer, D.J., Skene, J.H.P. and Banker, G.A. (1988) Development of neuronal polarity: GAP-43 distinguishes axonal from dendritic growth cones. *Nature (Lond.),* 336: 672–674.

Gospodarowicz, D., Cheng, J., Lui, G.M., Baird, A. and Bohlent, P. (1984) Isolation and purification of brain fibroblast growth factor by heparin-sepharose affinity chromatography: identity with pituitary fibroblast growth factor. *Proc. Natl. Acad. Sci. U.S.A.,* 81: 6963–6967.

Gospodarowicz, D., Neufeld, G. and Schweigerer, L. (1987) Fibroblast growth factor: structural and biological properties. *J. Cell. Physiol.,* Suppl. 5: 15–26.

Greene, L.A. (1977) Quantitative *in vitro* studies on nerve growth factors (NGF) requirements of neurons. II. Sensory neurons. *Dev. Biol.,* 58: 106–113.

Gundersen, R.W. and Barrett, J.N. (1979) Neuronal chemotaxis: chick dorsal root axons turn towards high concentration of nerve growth. *Science,* 206: 1079–1080.

Gundersen, R.W. and Barrett, J.N. (1980) Characterization of the turning response of dorsal root neurites toward nerve growth factor. *J. Cell Biol.,* 87: 546–554.

Gurney, M.E., Apatoff, B.R., Spear, G.T., Baumel, M.J., Antel, J.P., Brown Bania, M. and Reder, A.T. (1986a) Neuroleukin: a lymphokine product of lectin-stimulated T cells. *Science,* 234: 574–581.

Gurney, M.E., Heinrich, S.P., Lee, M.R. and Yin, H.-S. (1986b) Molecular cloning and expression of neuroleukin, a neurotrophic factor for spinal and sensory neurons. *Science,* 234: 566–573.

Hatten, M.E., Lynch, M., Sanchez, J., Joseph-Silverstein, J., Moscatelli, M. and Rifkin D.B. (1988) *In vitro* neurite extension by granule neurons is dependent upon astroglial-derived fibroblast growth factor. *Dev. Biol.,* 125: 280–289.

Heacock, A.M., Schonfeld, A.R. and Katzman, R. (1986) Hippocampal neurotrophic factor: characterization and response to denervation. *Brain Res.,* 363: 299–306.

Hefti, F. (1989) Trophic control of forebrain cholinergic neurons. In A. Björklund, A. Aguayo and D. Ottoson (Eds.), *Brain Repair,* McMillan Press Ltd., London, in press.

Hefti, F., Hartikka, J., Salvatierra, A., Weiner, W.J. and Mash, D.C. (1986) Localization of NGF receptors in cholinergic neurons of the human basal forebrain. *Neurosci. Lett.,* 69: 37–41.

Hosang, M. and Shooter, E.M. (1987) The internalization of nerve growth factor by high-affinity receptors on pheochromocytoma PC12 cells. *EMBO J.,* 6: 1197–1202.

Hughes, S.M., Lillien, L.E., Raff, M.C., Rohrer, H. and Sendtner, M. (1988) Ciliary neurotrophic factor induces type-2 astrocyte differentiation in culture. *Nature (Lond.),* 335: 70–72.

Isobe, T., Ishioka, N. and Okuyama, T. (1981) Structural relation of two S100 proteins in bovine brain; subunit composi-

tion of S-100a protein. *Eur. J. Biochem.,* 115: 469–474.

Johnson, J.E., Barde, Y.-A., Schwab, M. and Thoenen, H. (1986) Brain-Derived Neurotrophic Factor supports the survival of cultured rat retinal ganglion cells. *J. Neurosci.,* 6: 3031–3038.

Kligman, D. and Marshak, D.R. (1985) Purification and characterization of a neurite extension factor from bovine brain. *Proc. Natl. Acad. Sci. U.S.A.,* 82: 7136–7139.

Korshing, S., Heumann, R., Thoenen, H. and Hefti, F. (1986) Cholinergic denervation of the rat hippocampus by fimbrial transection leads to a transient accumulation of NGF without change in mRNA^{NGF} content. *Neurosci. Lett.,* 66: 175–180.

Lankford, K.L., De Mello, F.G. and Klein, W.L. (1988) D1-type dopamine receptors inhibit growth cone motility in cultured retina neurons: evidence that neurotransmitters act as morphogenic growth regulators in the developing central nervous system. *Proc. Natl. Acad. Sci. U.S.A.,* 85: 4567–4571.

Lander, A.D., Fujii, D.K. and Reichardt, L.F. (1985a) Laminin is associated with the neurite outgrowth promoting factors in conditioned media. *Proc. Natl. Acad. Sci. U.S.A.,* 82: 2183–2187.

Lander, A.D., Fujii, D.K. and Reichardt, L.F. (1985b) Purification of a factor that promotes neurite outgrowth: isolation of laminin and associated molecules. *J. Cell Biol.,* 101: 893–913.

Levi-Montalcini, R. (1982) Developmental neurobiology and natural history of nerve growth factor. *Ann. Rev. Neurosci.,* 5: 341–362.

Letourneau, P.C., Rogers, S., Hammarback, J., Madsen, A., Palm, S., McCarthy, J., Furcht, L., Bozyczko, D. and Horowitz, A. (1987) The role of growth cone adhesion in neuronal morphogenesis, as demonstrated by interactions with fibronectin and laminin. In J.R. Wolff, J. Sievers and M. Berry (Eds.), *Mesenchymal-Epithelial Interactions in Neural Development,* Springer-Verlag, pp. 349–360.

Letourneau, P.C., Madsen, A., Palm, S. and Furcht, L. (1988) Immunoreactivity for laminin in the developing ventral longitudinal pathway of the brain. *Dev. Biol.,* 125: 135–144.

Liesi, P. (1985) Laminin-immunoreactive glia distinguish regenerative adult CNS systems from non-regenerative ones. *EMBO J.,* 4: 2505–2511.

Liesi, P. and Silver, J. (1988) Is astrocyte laminin involved in axonal guidance in the mammalian CNS? *Dev. Biol.,* 130: 774–785.

Liesi, P., Dahl, D. and Vaheri, A. (1983) Laminin is produced by early rat astrocytes in primary culture. *J. Cell Biol.,* 96: 920–924.

Lillien, L.E., Sendtner, M., Rohrer, H., Hughes, S.M. and Raff, M.C. (1988) Type-2 astrocyte development in rat brain cultures is initiated by a CNTF-like protein produced by type-1 astrocyte. *Neuron,* 1: 485–494.

Lim, R., Hicklin, D.J., Ryken, T.C. and Miller, J.F. (1987) Endogenous glia maturation factor-like molecule in astrocytes and glioma cells. *Dev. Brain Res.,* 33: 49–57.

Lindsay, R.M. (1979) Adult rat brain astrocytes support survival of both NGF-dependent and NGF-insensitive neurons. *Nature (Lond.),* 282: 80–82.

Lumsden, A.G.S. and Davies, A.M. (1986) Chemiotropic effect of specific target epithelium in the developing mammalian nervous system. *Nature (Lond.),* 323: 538–539.

Mallat, M., Houlgatte, R., Brachet, P. and Prochiantz, A. (1989) Lipopolysaccharide-stimulated rat brain macrophages releases NGF in vitro. *Dev. Biol.,* 133: 309–311.

Manthorpe, M., Nieto-Sampedro, M., Skaper, S.D., Lewis, E.R., Barbin, G., Longo, F.M., Cotman, C.W. and Varon, S. (1983a) Neuronotrophic activity in brain wounds of the developing rat. Correlation with implant survival in the wound cavity. *Brain Res.,* 267: 47–56.

Manthorpe, M., Evengall, E., Rouslahti, E., Longo, F.M., Davis, G.E. and Varon, S. (1983b) Laminin promotes neurite regeneration from cultured peripheral and central neurons. *J. Cell Biol.,* 97: 1882–1890.

Manthorpe, M., Rudge, J.S. and Varon, S. (1986a) Astroglial cell contributions to neuronal survival and neuritic growth. In S. Fedoroff and A. Vernadakis (Eds.), *Astrocytes, Vol. 2,* Academic Press, New York, pp. 315–376.

Manthorpe, M., Fagnani, R., Skaper, S.D. and Varon, S. (1986b) An automated colorimetric microassay for neuronotrophic factors. *Dev. Brain Res.,* 25: 191–198.

Manthorpe, M., Skaper, S.D., Williams, L.R. and Varon, S. (1986c) Purification of adult sciatic rat nerve ciliary neuronotrophic factor. *Brain Res.,* 367: 282–286.

Mattson, M.P. (1988) Neurotransmitters in the regulation of neuronal cytoarchitecture. *Brain Res. Rev.,* 13: 179–212.

Mattson, M.P., Dou, P. and Kater, S.B. (1988) Outgrowth-regulating actions of glutamate in isolated hippocampal pyramidal neurons. *J. Neurosci.,* 8: 2087–2100.

McCarthy, K.D. and Partlow, L.M. (1976) Preparation of pure neuronal and non-neuronal cultures from embryonic chick sympathetic ganglia. A new method based on differential cell adhesiveness and the formation of homotypic neuronal aggregates. *Brain Res.,* 114: 391–414.

Millaruelo, A.I., Nieto-Sampedro, M. and Cotman, C.W. (1988) Cooperation between nerve growth factor and laminin or fibronectin in promoting sensory neuron survival and neurite outgrowth. *Dev. Brain Res.,* 38: 219–228.

Monaghan, D.T., Bridges, R.J. and Cotman, C.W. (1989) The excitatory amino acid receptors: their classes, pharmacology, and distinct properties in the function of the central nervous system. *Annu. Rev. Pharmacol. Toxicol.,* 29: 365–402.

Montesini-Chen, G.M., Chen, J.S. and Levi-Montalcini, R. (1978) Sympathetic nerve fiber ingrowth in the central nervous system of neonatal rodents upon intracerebral NGF injection. *Arch. Ital. Biol.,* 116: 53–84.

Moore, B.W. (1965) A soluble protein characteristic of the nervous system. *Biochem. Biophys. Res. Commun.,* 19: 739–744.

Morrison, R.S. (1987) Fibroblast growth factors: potential neurotrophic agents in the central nervous system. *J. Neurosci. Res.,* 17: 99–101.

Morrison, R.S., Sharma, A., de Vellis, J. and Bradshaw, R.A. (1986) Basic fibroblast growth factor supports the survival of cerebral cortical neurones in primary culture. *Proc. Natl. Acad. Sci. U.S.A.,* 83: 7537–7541.

Morrison, R.S., Kornblum, H.I., Leslie, F.M. and Bradshaw, R.A. (1987) Trophic stimulation of cultured neurons from neonatal brain by epidermal growth factor. *Science,* 238: 72–75.

Müller, H.W., Beckh, S. and Seifert, W. (1984) Neurotrophic factor for central neurons. *Proc. Natl. Acad. Sci. U.S.A.,* 81: 1248–1252.

Needels, D.L., Nieto-Sampedro, M., Whittemore, S.R. and Cotman, C.W. (1985) Neuronotrophic activity for ciliary ganglion neurons. Induction following injury to the brain of neonatal, adult and aged rats. *Dev. Brain Res.,* 18: 275–284.

Needels, D.L., Nieto-Sampedro, M. and Cotman, C.W. (1986) Induction of a neurite-promoting factor in rat brain following injury or deafferentation. *Neuroscience,* 18: 517–526.

Nishi, R. and Berg, D.K. (1981) Two components from eye tissue that differentially stimulate the growth and development of ciliary ganglion neurons in culture. *J. Neurosci.,* 1: 505–513.

Nieto-Sampedro, M. (1988) Astrocyte mitogen inhibitor related to epidermal growth factor receptor. *Science,* 240: 1784–1786.

Nieto-Sampedro, M. and Berman, M. (1987) Interleukin-1-like activity in rat brain: sources, targets and effect injury. *J. Neurosci. Res.,* 17: 214–219.

Nieto-Sampedro, M. and Broderick, J.T. (1989) A soluble brain molecule related to epidermal growth factor receptor is a mitogen inhibitor for astrocytes. *J. Neurosci. Res.,* 22: 28–35.

Nieto-Sampedro, M., Lewis, E.R., Cotman, C.W., Manthorpe, M., Skaper, S.D., Barbin, G., Longo, F.L. and Varon, S. (1982) Brain injury causes a time-dependent increase in neuronotrophic activity at the lesion site. *Science,* 217: 860–861.

Nieto-Sampedro, M., Manthorpe, M., Barbin, G., Varon, S. and Cotman, C.W. (1983) Injury-induced neuronotrophic activity in adult rat brain: correlation with survival of delayed implants in the wound cavity. *J. Neurosci.,* 3: 2219–2229.

Nieto-Sampedro, M., Whittemore, S.R., Needels, D.L., Larson, J. and Cotman, C.W. (1984) The survival of brain transplants is enhanced by extracts from injured brain. *Proc. Natl. Acad. Sci. U.S.A.,* 81: 6250–6254.

Nieto-Sampedro, M., Needels, D.L. and Cotman, C.W. (1985) A simple, objective method to measure the activity of factors that promote neuronal survival. *J. Neurosci. Methods,* 15: 37–48.

Nieto-Sampedro, M., Gómez-Pinilla, F., Knauer, D.J. and Broderick, J.T. (1988a) Epidermal growth factor immunoreactivity in rat brain astrocytes. Response to injury. *Neurosci. Lett.,* 91: 276 – 282.

Nieto-Sampedro, M., Lim, R., Hicklin, D.J. and Cotman, C.W. (1988b) Early release of glia maturation factor and acidic fibroblast growth factor after rat brain injury. *Neurosci. Lett.,* 86: 361 – 365.

Noble, M., Fok-Seang, J. and Cohen, J. (1984) Glia are a unique substrate for the *in vitro* growth of central nervous system neurites. *J. Neurosci.,* 4: 1892 – 1903.

Ojika, K. and Appel, S.H. (1984) Neurotrophic effects of hippocampal extracts on medial septal nucleus in vitro. *Proc. Natl. Acad. Sci. U.S.A.,* 81: 2567 – 2571.

Panayotou, G., End, P., Aumailley, M., Timpl, R. and Engel, J. (1989) Domains of laminin with growth factor activity. *Cell,* 56: 93 – 101.

Pearce, I.A., Cambray-Deakin, M.A. and Burgoyne, R.D. (1988) Glutamate acting on NMDA receptors stimulates neurite outgrowth from cerebellar granule cells. *FEBS Lett.,* 223: 143 – 147.

Pettmann, B., Labourdette, G., Weibel, M. and Sensenbrenner, M. (1986) The brain fibroblast growth factor is localized in neurons. *Neurosci. Lett.,* 68: 175, 180.

Pettmann, B., Gensburger, C., Weibel, M., Perraud, F., Sensenbrenner, M. and Labourdette, G. (1987) Isolation of two astroglial growth factors from bovine brain: comparison with other growth factors; cellular localization. In H. Althaus and W. Seifert (Eds.), *Glial-neuronal Communication in Development and Regeneration,* Springer-Verlag, Berlin, pp. 451 – 478.

Pixley, S.K.R., and Cotman, C.W. (1986) Laminin supports short term survival of rat septal neurons in low density, serum-free cultures. *J. Neurochem. Res.,* 15: 1 – 17.

Purves, D., Snider, W.D. and Voyvodic, J.T. (1988) Trophic regulation of nerve cell morphology and innervation in the autonomic nervous system. *Nature (Lond.),* 336: 123 – 128.

Raff, M.C., Lillien, L.E., Richardson, W.D., Burne, J.F. and Noble, M.D. (1988) Platelet-derived growth factor from astrocytes drives a clock that times oligodendrocyte development in culture. *Nature (Lond.),* 333: 562 – 565.

Raivich, G. and Kreutzberg, G.W. (1987) The localization and distribution of high-affinity βNGF binding sites in the central nervous system in the adult rat. A light microscopic autoradiographic study using [125-I]β-NGF. *Neuroscience,* 20: 23 – 36.

Ramón y Cajal, S. (1928) *Degeneration and Regeneration of the Nervous System. Vol. 1,* Oxford University Press, pp. 329 – 396.

Rennert, P.D. and Heinrich, G. (1986) Nerve growth factor mRNA in brain: localization by in situ hybridization. *Biochem. Biophys. Res. Commun.,* 138: 813 – 818.

Richardson, P.M., Verge Issa, V.M.K. and Riopelle, R.J. (1986) Distribution of neuronal receptors for nerve growth factor in the rat. *J. Neurosci.,* 6: 2312 – 2321.

Roberts, R., Gallagher, J., Spooncer, E., Allen, T.D., Bloomfield, F. and Dexter, T.M. (1988) Heparan sulphate bound growth factor: a mechanism for stromal mediated hemopoiesis. *Nature (Lond.),* 332: 376 – 378.

Rogers, S.L., Letourneau, P.C., Palm, S., McCarthy, J.B. and Furcht, L.T. (1983) Neurite extension by peripheral and central nervous system neurons in response to substratum-bound fibronectin and laminin. *Dev. Biol.,* 98: 212 – 220.

Rudge, J.S., Manthorpe, M. and Varon, S. (1985) The output of neurotrophic and neurite promoting agents from rat brain astroglial cells: a microculture method for screening potential regulatory molecules. *Dev. Brain Res.,* 19: 161 – 172.

Rydel, R.E. and Grenee, L.A. (1987) Acid and basic fibroblast growth factors promote stable neurite outgrowth and neuronal differentiation in culture of PC12 cells. *J. Neurosci.,* 7: 3639 – 3653.

Schwab, M. and Caroni, P. (1988) Oligodendrocytes and CNS myelin are nonpermissive substrates for neurite growth and fibroblast spreading *in vitro. J. Neurosci.,* 8: 2381 – 2393.

Selak, I., Skaper, S.D. and Varon, S. (1985) Pyruvate participation in the low molecular weight trophic activity for central nervous system neurons in glia-conditioned media. *J. Neurosci.,* 5: 23 – 28.

Shooter, E.M. (1990) Factors involved in the regulation of NGF receptors. In A. Björklund, A. Aguayo and D. Ottoson (Eds.), *Brain Repair,* McMillan Press Ltd., London, in press.

Snider, W.D. (1988) Nerve growth factor enhances dendritic arborization of sympathetic ganglion cells in developing mammals. *J. Neurosci.,* 8: 2628 – 2634.

Springer, J.E., Koh, S., Tayrien, M.W. and Loy, R. (1987) Basal forebrain magnocellular neurons stain for NGF receptor: correlation with cholinergic cell bodies and effects of axotomy. *J. Neurosci. Res.,* 17: 111 – 118.

Sretavan, D.W., Shatz, C.J. and Stryker, M.P. (1988) Modification of retinal ganglion cell axon morphology by prenatal infusion of tetrodotoxin. *Nature (Lond.),* 336: 468 – 471.

Tessier-Lavigne, M., Placzeck, M., Lumsden, A.G.S., Dodd, J. and Jessell, T.M. (1988) Chemiotropic guidance of developing axons in the mammalian central nervous system. *Nature (Lond.),* 336: 775 – 778.

Thoenen, H. (1989) Regulation of NGF synthesis. Brain injury repair: growth factors. In A. Björklund, A. Aguayo and D. Ottoson (Eds.), *Brain Repair,* McMillan Press Ltd., London, in press.

Thoenen, H., Bandtlow, C. and Heumann, R. (1987) The physiological function of nerve growth factor in the central nervous system: comparison with the periphery. *Rev. Physiol. Biochem. Pharmacol.,* 109: 145 – 178.

Thomas, K. and Giménez-Gallego, G. (1986) Fibroblast growth factors: broad spectrum mitogens with potent angiogenic activity. *Trends Biochem. Sci.,* 11: 81 – 84.

Thoms, K., Rios-Candelore, M. and Fitzpatrick, S. (1984)

Purification and characterization of acidic fibroblast growth factor from bovine brain. *Proc. Natl. Acad. Sci. U.S.A.*, 81: 357 – 361.

Togari, A., Dickens, G., Kuzuya, H. and Guroff, G. (1985) The effect of fibroblast growth factor on PC12 cells. *J. Neurosci.*, 5: 341 – 362.

Varon, S., Skaper, S.D., Facci, L., Rudge, J.S. and Manthorpe, M. (1987) Trophic and metabolic coupling between astroglial cells and neurons. In H. Althaus and W. Seifert (Eds.), *Glial-Neuronal Communication in Development and Regeneration.* Springer-Verlag, Berlin, pp. 385 – 406.

Walicke, P. (1988) Basic and acidic fibroblast growth factors have trophic effects on neurons from multiple CNS regions. *J. Neurosci.*, 8: 2618 – 2627.

Walicke, P. and Baird, A. (1988) Neurotrophic effects of basic and acidic fibroblast growth factors are not mediated through glial cells. *Dev. Brain Res.*, 40: 71 – 79.

Walicke, P., Cowan, W.M., Ueno, N., Baird, A. and Guillemin, R. (1986) Fibroblast growth factor promotes survival of dissociated hippocampal neurons and enhances neurite extension. *Proc. Natl. Acad. Sci. U.S.A.*, 83: 3012 – 3016.

Wang, J.L. and Hsu, Y.-M. (1986) Negative regulators of cell growth. *Trends Biochem. Sci.*, 11: 24 – 26.

Whitson, J.S., Selkoe, D.J. and Cotman, C.W. (1989) Amyloid β protein enhances the survival of hippocampal neurons in vitro. *Science,* 243: 1488 – 1490.

Whittemore, S.R. and Seiger, Å. (1987) The expression, localization and functional significance of β-nerve growth factor in the central nervous system. *Brain Res. Rev.,* 12: 439 – 464.

Whittemore, S.R., Nieto-Sampedro, M., Needels, D.L. and Cotman, C.W. (1985) Neuronotrophic factors for mammalian brain neurons: injury induction in neonatal, adult and aged rat brain. *Dev. Brain Res.,* 20: 169 – 178.

Whittemore, S.R., Ebendal, T., Läkfors, L., Olson, L., Seiger, Å., Strömberg, I. and Persson, H. (1986) Developmental and regional expression of β NGF messenger RNA and protein in rat central nervous system. *Proc. Natl. Acad. Sci. U.S.A.,* 83: 817 – 821.

Whittemore, S.R., Läkfors, L., Ebendal, T., Holets, V.R., Ericsson, A. and Persson, H. (1987) Increased β-Nerve Growth Factor messenger RNA and protein levels in neonatal rat hippocampus following specific cholinergic lesions. *J. Neurosci.,* 7: 244 – 251.

Yamamoto, T., Iwasaki, Y., Yamamoto, H., Konno, H. and Isemura, M. (1988) Intraneuronal laminin-like molecule in the central nervous system: demonstration of its unique differential distribution. *J. Neurol. Sci.,* 84: 1 – 13.

J. Storm-Mathisen, J. Zimmer and O.P. Ottersen (Eds.)
Progress in Brain Research, Vol. 83
© 1990 Elsevier Science Publishers B.V. (Biomedical Division)

CHAPTER 26

NGF-dependent sprouting and regeneration in the hippocampus

Fred H. Gage, Gyorgy Buzsáki and David M. Armstrong

Department of Neurosciences, M-024, University of California, San Diego, La Jolla, CA 92093, U.S.A.

While a variety of sprouting and regenerative responses have been investigated in the hippocampus, the cellular and molecular events responsible for these plastic responses have not been determined. One transmitter system, the cholinergic system, shows several distinct responses to damage in the septohippocampal circuit. Present evidence strongly supports a role for nerve growth factor (NGF) in these responses. NGF is not only important for the survival of the adult cholinergic neurons, but can also induce regrowth of the damaged fibers given an appropriate substratum for growth. These reparative effects of NGF can manifest themselves in functional recovery in the aged rat and the young rat with fimbria-fornix lesions. Finally, a role for glia cells is proposed to clarify how NGF availability may be regulated during the degenerative and regenerative events. While all plasticity events certainly cannot be explained by the coincidence of NGF and the cholinergic system, their interaction may provide a template for other transmitter/trophic factor interactions.

Introduction

Experimental damage to the brain has been used as a tool to map the fiber pathways particularly in combination with degeneration stains (Blackstad, 1956, 1969). The effectiveness of the technique is in part dependent on the time following damage because of the propensity for the brain to try and reorganize itself following damage. This reorganization has resulted in the emergence of a separate area of investigation which revolves around the concepts of sprouting and regeneration which reflect morphological plasticity. This morphological plasticity can take the form of appropriate reorganization (homotypic) or inappropriate reorganization (heterotypic). The expectation is that homotypic plasticity will potentially result in functional recovery, while heterotypic plasticity will result in either delayed recovery or induction of further dysfunction. A current belief is that understanding the mechanisms underlying the morphological plasticity will lead to the development of strategies for brain repair. The hippocampus has proven to be a valuable region of the brain to investigate brain damage-induced morphological plasticity and reorganization.

Damage to selected pathways of the limbic circuitry results in some of the best characterized and most robust sprouting responses in the central nervous system. First, Raisman (1969) demonstrated that unilateral damage to the fimbria-fornix (FF) results in the elimination of ipsilateral hippocampal inputs to the dorsal lateral quadrant of the septum and that soon after this denervation the small input from the contralateral hippocampus will sprout and fill in the denervated terminal zones. Subsequently it was demonstrated that catecholamine fibers from the brainstem nuclei (Moore, 1975) and cholinergic fibers (Gage et al., 1986) from the remaining septal-diagonal band cells also sprout into this critical dorsal lateral quadrant of the septum. At present the mechanism responsible for this sprouting response is unknown.

In addition, when the FF is transected or medial septal area is lesioned, the aminergic and cholinergic fibers from the brainstem and basal forebrain which normally innervate the hippocampal formation degenerate (Gage et al., 1983). Furthermore the sympathetic fibers of the superior cervical ganglion (SCG) penetrate the central nervous system to innervate the terminal zone of the mossy fibers, which coincides with the terminal area of the cholinergic fibers eliminated by the FF lesion (Loy and Moore, 1977; Stenevi and Björklund, 1978). Nerve Growth Factor (NGF) has been implicated in this sprouting response (Crutcher, 1987), and recent evidence has confirmed that NGF exists in highest CNS concentration in the hippocampus and this high concentration and activity is further elevated by both FF lesions and perforant path (PP) lesions (Crutcher and Collins, 1982; Collins and Crutcher, 1985). Furthermore, the ingrowth of sympathetic fibers from the SCG can be retarded by infusions of anti-NGF (Springer and Loy, 1985), presumably as a result of the NGF receptors on the SCG fibers which sprout into the hippocampus (Blaker et al., 1988; Batchelor et al., 1989). Thus, it is reasonable to assume that the NGF accumulation in the hippocampus following FF transection or medial septal lesions plays a role in the sprouting of the catecholamine-containing fibers of the SCG into the hippocampus.

The emerging consensus is that NGF is synthesized in the hippocampus (Ayer-LeLievre et al., 1983; Korsching et al., 1985; Shelton and Reichardt, 1986; Whittemore et al., 1986) and retrogradely transported to the cholinergic neurons of the basal forebrain (Schwab et al., 1979; Seiler and Schwab, 1984), similar to that which occurs in the SCG and its respective target tissues. Transection of these ascending cholinergic fibers blocks the retrograde transport of NGF, resulting in an accumulation of NGF in the hippocampus (Gage et al., 1984; Collins et al., 1985; Korsching et al., 1986; Springer et al., 1987). This accumulation sets up a gradient which promotes the growth of the sympathetic fibers toward the source of the NGF. These cholinergic neurons are thought to be depen-

dent on NGF for their health even as adults. Thus the transection of the fibers results in retrograde degeneration of the cholinergic neurons which can be reversed by exogenous application of NGF (Hefti, 1986; Williams et al., 1986; Kromer, 1987; Gage et al., 1988a).

At the temporal pole of the hippocampus, PP transection which destroys the entorhinal inputs to the outer two thirds of the molecular zone of the dentate granular cells, results in a dramatic "reactive synapto-genesis" exemplified by sprouting of the cholinergic fibers from the inner one third of the molecular zone to fill in the deafferented outer molecular zone (Lynch et al., 1972). This heterotypic innervation is one of the best characterized sprouting responses in the central nervous system, though at present the mechanisms responsible for this sprouting response are unknown. Recent evidence, however, has shown that NGF-like activity is increased in the dentate gyrus following PP lesions (Crutcher, 1987). Thus it is reasonable to suggest that the cholinergic sprouting observed in the outer molecular zone could be elicited by an increase in NGF activity in this zone.

Paralleling this emerging story of a dependence of cholinergic sprouting on NGF, astrocytes have been identified as a possible functional source of the NGF, through evidence that shows that fetal, neonatal, and hypertrophic adult astrocytes can release NGF as well as other neuronotrophic and neuritic promoting factors in vitro (Lindsay, 1979; Banker, 1980; Hatten and Liem, 1981; Liesi et al., 1984; Fallon, 1985; Nieto-Sampedro et al., 1983; Furukawa et al., 1986; Tarris et al., 1986). The proliferative and hypertrophic response of astrocytes to damage has been well documented, while the importance of these responses in either degenerative or regenerative changes in the CNS is less clear. However, Rose et al. (1976) demonstrated that astrocytes were hypertrophied and increased in number selectively in the outer molecular zone during degeneration of the PP and sprouting of the septal cholinergic fibers following entorhinal lesions. Subsequently, several investigators have observed that microglia (Gall et al., 1979) and lysosomal enzymes (Vijayan, 1983) are also elevated during these critical periods in the outer molecular area following PP lesions, and these latter markers of phagocytosis may precede the increase in astrocytes. This sequential relationship between microglia and astrocytes is further supported by the finding that reactive microglia secrete factors or peptides which can induce the proliferation of astrocytes (Giulian and Baker, 1985).

In the following sections we will review the evidence supporting a role for NGF in the plastic events summarized above, that occur in the septohippocampal system following deafferentation.

Degeneration of NGF-dependent neurons

The cholinergic projection from the adult rat septum and diagonal band to the ipsilateral hippocampus has been a useful model for examining CNS plasticity. Neurons of the medial septum and the vertical limb of the diagonal band project dorsally to the hippocampus mainly through the

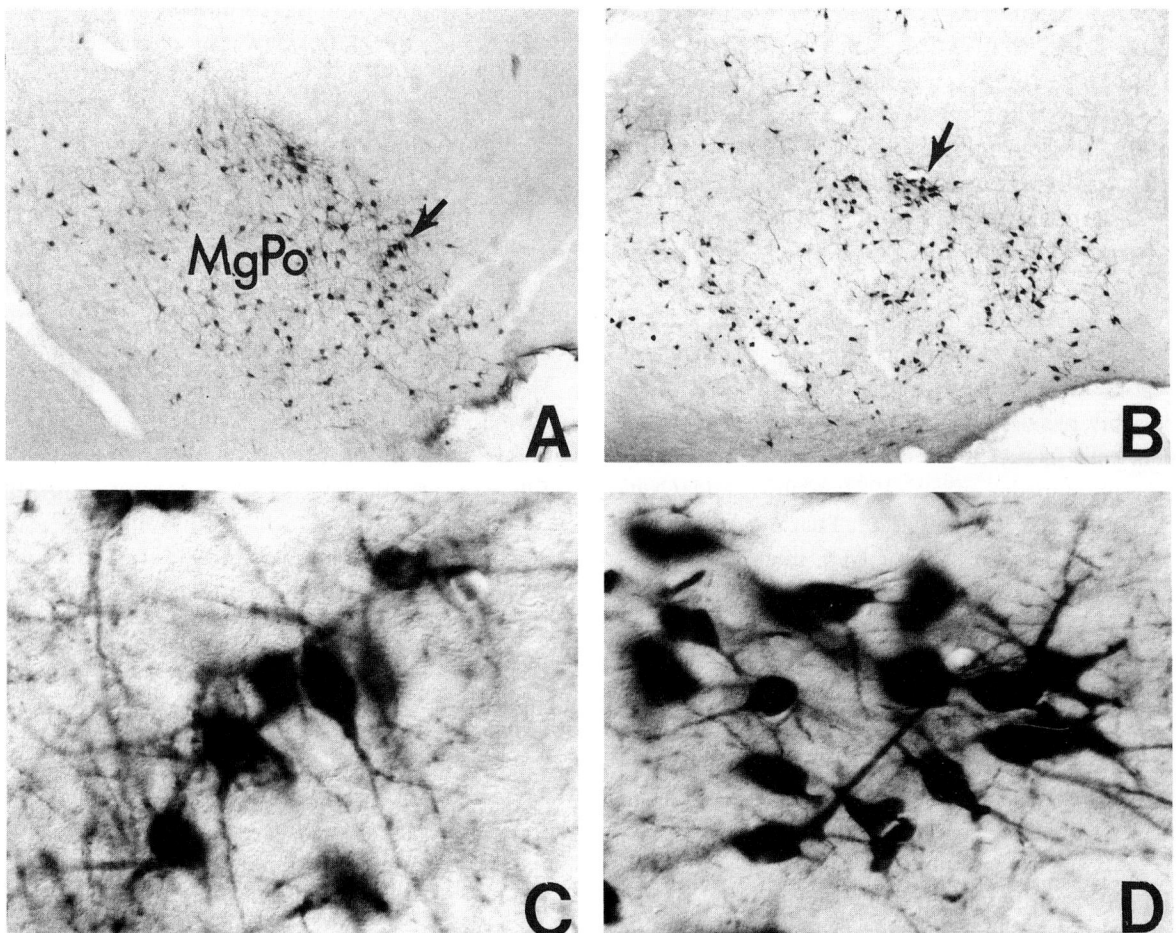

Fig. 1. Low- and high-power photomicrographs showing (A and B) ChAT- and (C and D) NGFr-labeled neurons in the magnocellular preoptic area. Magnification = 106× (A and C); 388× (B and D). Arrows in A and B indicate regions shown in C and D. MgPo = magnocellular preoptic area.

fimbria-fornix (Lewis et al., 1967; Gage et al., 1983; Gage and Björklund, 1986a). About 50% of the septal/diagonal band neurons sending fibers through the fimbria-fornix are cholinergic (Amaral and Kurz, 1985; Wainer et al., 1985) and provide the hippocampus with about 90% of its total cholinergic innervation (Storm-Mathisen, 1974).

Complete transection of the fimbria/fornix pathway in adult rats results in the retrograde degeneration and death of many of the septal/diagonal band neurons which contribute axons through this pathway (Amaral and Kurz, 1985). Markers of cell survival, including retrogradely transported fluorescent dyes and Nissl stains (Gage et al., 1986; Tuszynski et al., 1988), transmitter enzyme expression (AChE, ChAT) (Gage et al., 1986; Armstrong et al., 1987; Otto et al., 1989), and NGFr expression on cells of the MS (Springer et al., 1978; Montero and Hefti, 1988; Tuszynski et al., 1988) demonstrate a loss of 50–90% of cells in this region depending on the location and completeness of the lesion (Sofroniew and Isacson, 1988).

One explanation for this axotomy-induced cell dysfunction or death is that the septal neurons become deprived of a critical supply of NTF possibly provided by the postsynaptic neurons or glial cells in the target areas of the hippocampus (Nieto-Sampedro et al., 1983; Collins and Crutcher, 1985; Gage et al., 1986). That this hippocampal NTF might be NGF or NGF-like is supported by the previously listed studies from several laboratories reporting an NGF presence within the septohippocampal system, and the presence of NGF receptors on the cholinergic cell bodies and processes (Fig. 1).

NGF protects cholinergic neurons from degeneration

The above observations raise the question whether exogenous administration of NGF to neuronal populations in the adult showing NGF regulation might prevent lesion-induced neuronal degeneration and atrophy.

Within the septohippocampal circuit, for example, NGF administration to axotomized septal neurons might prevent the normally ensuing retrograde cell degeneration and death. This rescue by NGF might then allow the axotomized neurons to regenerate their cut axons, or extend new axons, back to the hippocampal formation. Recently, several groups (Hefti et al., 1986; Williams et al., 1986; Kromer, 1987; Gage et al., 1988a) have independently reported that intraventricular administration of purified NGF into adult rats from the time of fimbria/fornix transection onward prevents the loss of most of the axotomized cholinergic septum/diagonal band neurons. Complete unilateral fimbria/fornix lesions usually result in a loss of 60–90% of cholinergic cell bodies depending on the location of the lesion (Gage et al., 1984; Armstrong et al., 1987; Sofroniew and Isacson, 1988) compared to the contralateral, unlesioned side, but NGF infusion can rescue 90–100% of the cell population (Hefti et al., 1986; Williams et al., 1986; Kromer, 1987; Gage et al., 1988a). Although various lesion and NGF infusion paradigms have been used in these studies, the results are consistent and comparable.

Recently, transient infusions of NGF have been shown to be insufficient to permanently save septal cholinergic neurons (Montero and Hefti, 1988). Thus work is currently directed toward inducing the regeneration of lesioned axons from saved septal cells back to their hippocampal target in an attempt to restore an endogenous, continuous supply of NGF. NGF infusions could then be discontinued when axons have reconnected with their target, thus permanently saving the projecting septal neurons (see below). The ability of NGF to induce axonal regeneration in the adult CNS in vivo has already been evidenced by the presence of robust sprouting of cholinergic fibers into the dorsolateral quadrant of the septum two weeks following fimbria/fornix lesions (Gage et al., 1986, 1988a).

NGF effects on cells other than cholinergic neurons in the adult CNS have received less attention. GABAergic cells in addition to cholinergic cells of the medial septum degenerate after fimbria/fornix lesions (Peterson et al., 1987), and one recent study reports a failure of NGF to save these GABAergic neurons (Montero and Hefti, 1988). The identification of NGF-responsive cell populations in the CNS depends in part upon the visualization of NGF receptors with immunocytochemical methods. However, since immunocytochemistry currently employs antibodies that appear to identify only the low-affinity NGF receptor (Taniuchi and Johnson, 1985), future studies may require methods that detect the active, high-affinity receptor as well (e.g. autoradiography).

NGF regulates its own receptor

The ability of neurons to respond to NGF seems to depend on the presence of cell surface receptors, which in the PNS mediate the binding, internalization and transport of NGF from the terminals to the parent cell bodies (see Thoenen and Barde, 1985, for review). Such NGF receptors have also been demonstrated on the NGF-responsive cholinergic neurons in the CNS both during development and in the adult animal (see Fig. 1 and Taniuchi et al., 1986; Richardson et al., 1986).

The cholinergic neurons of the striatum appear to represent a special case. In contrast to the neurons in the septal-diagonal band area and the nucleus basalis, these neurons possess very low or undemonstrable levels of NGFr in the adult, and their responsiveness to NGF has been reported to decline dramatically during postnatal development (Martinez et al., 1985; Mobley et al., 1985; Johnston et al., 1987). Nevertheless, our previous findings have shown that chronic infusion of NGF into the lateral ventricle of adult animals following fimbria/fornix lesion not only spared the medial septal neurons from degeneration, but also resulted in hypertrophy of the cholinergic neurons of the ipsilateral striatum (Gage et al., 1988). Similarly, chronic infusions of NGF into the lateral ventricle of aged rats ameliorated the age-related atrophy of the cholinergic neurons of the striatum, as well as the basal forebrain (Fischer et al., 1987). The in vivo effects of NGF on the striatal cholinergic neurons are in apparent contradiction with the lack of demonstrable NGFr immunoreactivity in these neurons normally. However, Taniuchi et al. (1986) have recently reported that peripheral nerve damage will induce the expression of NGFr on Schwann cells within the denervated distal portion of the nerve, raising the possibility that the ability of striatal neurons to respond to NGF depends on the up-regulation of the NGFr, and that this up-regulation is induced by the tissue damage. In a recent experiment we tested this hypothesis. Chronic NGF infusion into the adult neostriatum resulted in re-expression of the NGFr such that many cholinergic interneurons become immunoreactive for NGFr. This effect was seen also after striatal damage induced by infusion of vehicle alone, whereas infusion of anti-NGF serum partially inhibited the receptor's re-expression. Infusion of NGF, but not vehicle alone, dramatically increased the size and the intensity of ChAT-immunoreactivity of these same cholinergic neurons (Gage et al., 1989).

These findings indicate that these central cholinergic neurons, which lose their NGFr during postnatal development, will resume their NGF responsiveness when the tissue is damaged. Such a damage-induced mechanism may act to enhance the action of trophic factors, including NGF, released at the site of injury, and enhance the responsiveness of damaged CNS neurons to exogenously administered trophic factors.

Although damage produces an emergence of NGFr protein-*immunoreactivity* in adult striatal cholinergic neurons, in situ hybridization of NGFr mRNA shows that vehicle infusion by itself will not increase the number of NGFr mRNA-positive neurons in the striatum as compared to non-treated animals (Gage et al., 1989). Thus, only NGF treatment, but not vehicle, induces NGFr *gene expression* within striatal neurons, suggesting the possibility that *lesion-induced* damage increases NGFr level through non-transcriptional mechanisms, such as the "un-masking" of existing stores of NGFr protein. Additionally, these findings are in agreement with our recent in situ hybridization studies which show that chronic NGF administration, but not vehicle infusions, induce NGFr gene expression within those basal forebrain cholinergic neuronal populations that normally express NGFr protein in adult rat brain (Higgins et al., 1989). NGF not only produced neuronal hypertrophy, as we had demonstrated in earlier studies (Fischer et al., 1987), but also increased NGFr mRNA abundance per cell and induced the expression of NGFr message within basal forebrain neurons that had previously not contained a detectable level of NGFr mRNA. These findings provide strong evidence that NGF can induce expression of its own receptor within the central nervous system.

In vitro evidence also supports the concept that NGF can induce the expression of its own receptor. When NGF is applied to cultures of septal neurons, striatal neurons, or PC-12 cells (Bernd and Greene, 1984; Hefti, 1986), the number of NGF receptors on the cells increase. In addition, the exposure of cultured chick sensory neurons to long-term NGF treatment will prevent the normal disappearance of receptors on these cells (Rohrer and Barde, 1982).

NGF functions as a tropic factor

In addition to its function of maintaining the normal integrity of the central cholinergic basal forebrain neurons and of peripheral sympathetic and neural crest-derived sensory neurons (*neurotrophic*), NGF has also been postulated to have a role in the axonal growth of these neurons after damage to the nervous system (*neurotropic*). Two forms of axonal growth are commonly observed in the mature hippocampus: *regeneration*, or the regrowth of axons previously damaged, and *collateral sprouting,* or the new growth of remaining (intact) axons (Gage and Björklund, 1986a). Collateral sprouting occurs within the hippocampus from two distinct populations of neurons following fimbria/fornix transection.

Superior cervical ganglion (SCG) derived sympathetic axons, which normally surround the hippocampal vasculature, undergo a robust sprouting response into the dentate gyrus and CA3 pyramidal cell region of the hippocampal parenchyma after fimbria/fornix lesions (Loy and Moore, 1977; Stenevi and Björklund, 1978). In addition, the magnocellular septal-midline cholinergic neurons on the dorsal hippocampal formation sprout into the dorsal subiculum and CA1 pyramidal cell layers in response to fimbria/fornix lesion (Blaker et al., 1988). To test the postulate that NGF has tropic effects on cholinergic axons in the hippocampus and that the lesion-induced increase in NGF in the hippocampal formation may serve as a chemo-attractant of NGF-responsive axons towards the source of its production (Crutcher, 1987), we examined the fimbria/fornix lesioned hippocampal formation to determine whether the sprouting neurons stain positively for NGFr. We found that the 2 populations of neurons within the hippocampus that undergo collateral sprouting, namely the septal-midline magnocellular cholinergic neurons of the dorsal hippocampus and the sympathetic neurons of the SCG, stain strongly for NGFr with a monoclonal antibody (Taniuchi et al., 1986). In contrast, the small intrinsic cholinergic neurons of the hippocampus exhibited neither sprouting response nor staining for NGFr (Batchelor et al., 1989).

In the dentate gyrus and CA4 and CA3 (but not CA1) pyramidal cell fields, a sprouting response was observed. Large-diameter, coarse, varicose, NGFr-positive (but AChE-negative) fibers appeared both above and below the granule cell layer and in the stratum lucidum and inner third of the stratum oriens of the pyramidal cell layer. These fibers had the distribution and morphological appearance of sympathetic fibers known to invade the hippocampal formation following FF transection (Loy and Moore, 1977) (see Fig. 2). That these fibers were indeed of sympathetic origin was subsequently confirmed in two ways. First, immunohistochemistry in adjacent sections demonstrated that these fibers stained strongly for tyrosine hydroxylase (TH). Second, unilateral superior cervical ganglionectomy (performed on 4 animals) resulted in a loss of TH (and NGFr)-immunoreactive fibers on the lesion side. Taken together, these results suggest the possibility that the differing sprouting responses exhibited by the various neuronal populations to FF transection may be due to the presence or absence of NGFr

(and presumably the accompanying intracellular machinery required to respond to the elevation of intrahippocampal NGF known to accompany septohippocampal denervation). This hypothesis, that increases in NGF beyond the concentrations that are normally required for neuronal homeostasis are capable of initiating and directing the sprouting of populations of neurons with NGFr, is

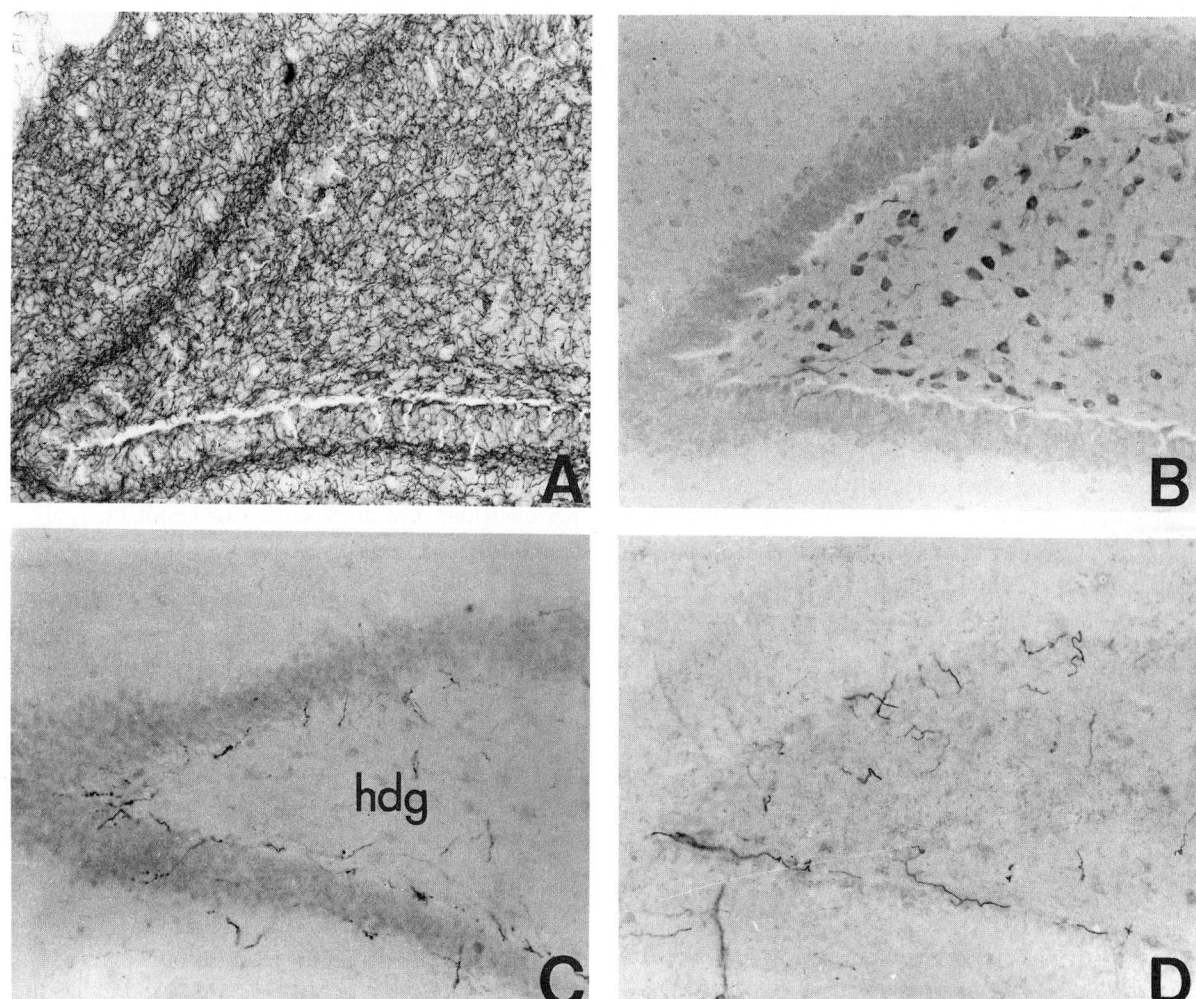

Fig. 2. A: photomicrographs of AChE in the dorsal hippocampus of an unlesioned brain. B: the same region is devoid of AChE 2 weeks following complete lesioning of the fimbria-fornix. C: photomicrograph of tyrosine hydroxylase (TH) in the dorsal hippocampus 8 weeks following fimbria-fornix transection. Note TH-positive fibers in the infragranular zone and through the granular layer. D: when adjacent sections to C are stained with antibodies against NGFr a very similar pattern of immunolabelling is detected. Again, note the NGFr-positive fibers in the infragranular zone and through the granular layer. Magnifications: ×37 (A,C); ×183 (B,D); hdg, hilus of the dentate gyrus.

supported by several lines of evidence. Firstly, intracephalic injections of NGF into the locus coeruleus of neonatal rats results in the ingrowth of SCG-derived sympathetic fibers into the region surrounding the injection site (Menesini-Chen et al., 1978). Secondly, the sprouting fibers are not randomly distributed within the hippocampal formation, but are localized to the dentate-CA3 region (sympathetic fibers) and the medial subicular region (midline fibers), areas which undergo a significant increase in NGF-like activity after medial septal lesion (Collins and Crutcher, 1985). This increase in NGF presumably results from the lesion-induced interruption of retrograde axonal transport in magnocellular NGFr-positive basal forebrain neurons. Thirdly, granule cell axons (mossy fibers), which stain strongly for zinc, an element believed to be complexed with the 7S form of NGF, are distributed together with sympathetic fibers in the dentate gyrus and CA3 regions, areas with the highest pre- and postlesion NGF-like activities. Lesioning of these presumptive NGF-producing cells by injections of colchicine into the hippocampus prevents sympathetic sprouting (Crutcher, 1987). Fourth, intrahippocampal injections of antiserum to NGF following lesioning of the FF pathway severely stunts the sympathetic sprouting around the injection site (Springer and Loy, 1985).

Overall, this evidence supports the above hypothesis that neuronal populations which are normally trophically dependent on NGF for survival can be stimulated to undergo collateral sprouting by greater than normal levels of NGF.

NGF induces regeneration into the denervated hippocampus

Attempts to restore this severed fimbria/fornix pathway have been made by grafting fetal tissue (Kromer et al., 1981; Buzsáki et al., 1987a, b; Gage et al., 1988b) which may act as a bridge between the disconnected septo-hippocampal pathway. Increases in ChAT activity and AChE fiber innervation in the host hippocampus have been consistent-

ly reported in these studies, but the extent of reinnervation is small.

A possible explanation for the limited restoration of the cholinergic circuitry may be that the majority of the cholinergic neurons in the medial septum and diagonal band of Broca degenerate, become dysfunctional, and die within a month following the transection (Daitz and Powell, 1954; Gage et al., 1986; Armstrong et al., 1987). These results led to the prediction that the exogenous delivery of NGF could not only promote the survival of septal neurons but also would then promote the cholinergic axons to extend across a bridge of hippocampal fetal tissue placed in the fimbria/fornix cavity. Thus, in a recent study we combined the exogenous infusion of NGF to the lateral ventricle adjacent to the denervated septum with the simultaneous grafting of fetal hippocampal tissue to the fimbria-fornix cavity, as a set of procedures that may more fully and functionally restore the severed septo-hippocampal circuitry (Buzsáki et al., 1987b). Imbedded in the design of this study were two additional related questions: (1) does the transient two-week NGF infusion period which has been shown to result in significant cholinergic cell rescue have an enduring effect on the medial septal cells 6–8 months following termination of the NGF infusion and (2) will fetal hippocampal grafts alone, in the absence of exogenous NGF infusion, support the survival of the axotomized cholinergic neurons of the medial septum?

A combination of intracerebral grafting and intraventricular infusion of NGF was used to attempt the reconstruction of the cholinergic component of the septo-hippocampal pathway following fimbria/fornix lesions. Four groups were used: lesion only (FF); lesion and fetal hippocampal graft (FF-HPC); lesion and NGF (FF-NGF); and lesion, graft and NGF (FF-HPC-NGF). Choline acetyltransferase immunoreactivity (ChAT-IR), acetylcholinesterase (AChE) fiber staining, and behavior-dependent theta electrical activity were used to assess the extent of pathway reconstruction. The NGF infusion only lasted the first two weeks following the FF lesion, while theta activity and histological analysis were conducted 6–8 months after the lesion. Only the FF-HPC-NGF group had long-term savings of ChAT-IR cells as

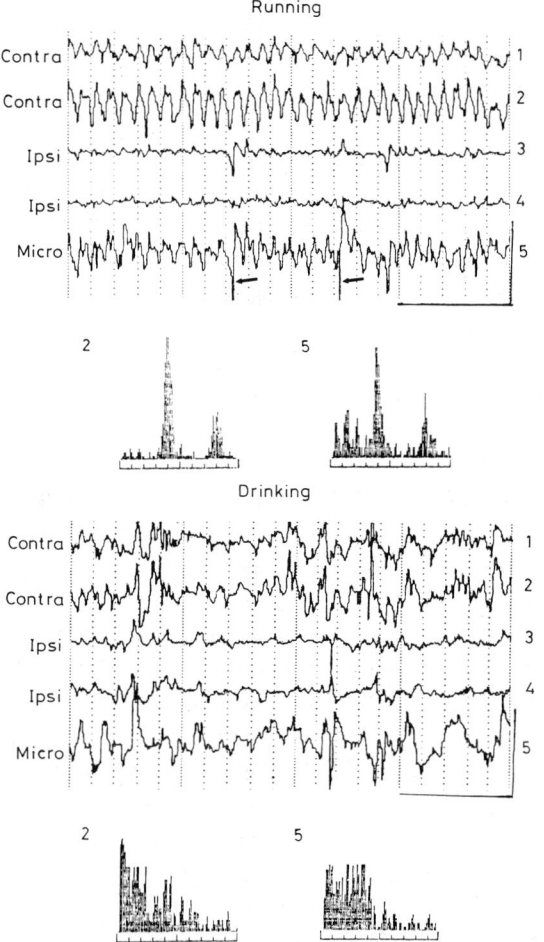

Fig. 3. EEG recordings and power spectra obtained during running and drinking in a rat with HPC graft and transient NGF treatment. Traces 1–4 were recorded with fixed microelectrodes from the hippocampus contralateral (contra) and ipsilateral (ipsi) to the fimbria-fornix lesion. Micro: EEG recorded with the movable microelectrode from near the hippocampal fissure. Subsequent histological analysis revealed that the electrode penetrated an AChE-dense area of the septal pole of the reinnervated hippocampus. Power spectra calculated from 20 s segments of traces 2 and 5 (micro) indicated power peaks at 8–9 Hz during running and absence of rhythmicity during drinking. Arrows indicate large amplitude sharp transients typical in grafted animals. Calibrations: 1 s, 2 mV.

compared to the FF and FF-HPC group. In addition the FF-HPC-NGF group had more extensive re-innervation of the hippocampus than any other group. Further, the FF-HPC-NGF group had the most complete evidence of behavior-dependent theta activity restoration (see Fig. 3). These results demonstrate clearly that a combination of short-term intraventricular NGF infusion and fetal hippocampal grafts can result in a more complete reconstruction of the damaged septo-hippocampal circuit. However complete long-term cholinergic cell survival or cholinergic fiber re-innervation of the denervated hippocampus was not achieved with the study described above.

Glial cells may mediate NGF influences in damaged hippocampus

Damage to the fimbria-fornix, and separately to the perforant path, leads to distinct and dramatic time-dependent increases in glial fibrillary acidic protein immunoreactivity (GFAP-IR) in specific areas of the hippocampal formation (Gage et al., 1988c). Specifically, FF lesions resulted in an increase in the GFAP-IR in the pyramidal and stratum oriens layers of the CA3 region, as well as in the inner molecular layer of the dentate gyrus. In addition, in the septum ipsilateral to the lesion, there was a rapid and robust increase in GFAP-IR in the dorsal lateral quadrant of the septum, but not in the medial septal region. Only after 30 days did the GFAP-IR reach the medial septum. Following perforant path lesions, there was a selective increase in GFAP-IR in the outer molecular layer of the dentate gyrus (see Fig. 4). Most of these changes were transient, and had disappeared by 30 days postlesion. We speculate that the increase in GFAP-IR, reflecting activation of astrocytic cells in these target areas, is a necessary requirement for sprouting responses (Gage et al., 1988c).

Considerable in vitro and in vivo evidence supports the presumption that astrocytes make and secrete neurotrophic factors that can subsequently support the survival and/or axonal outgrowth of a

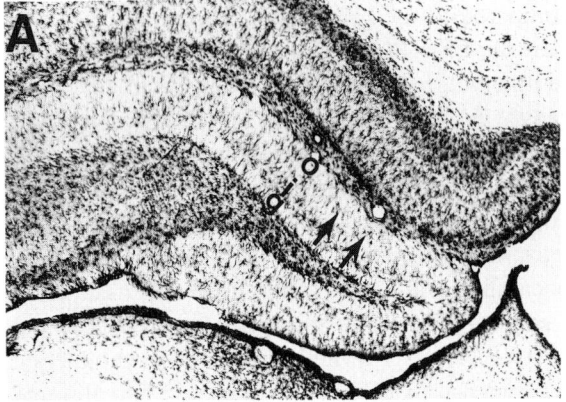

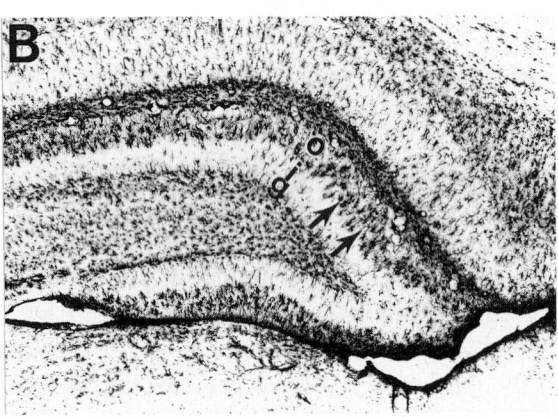

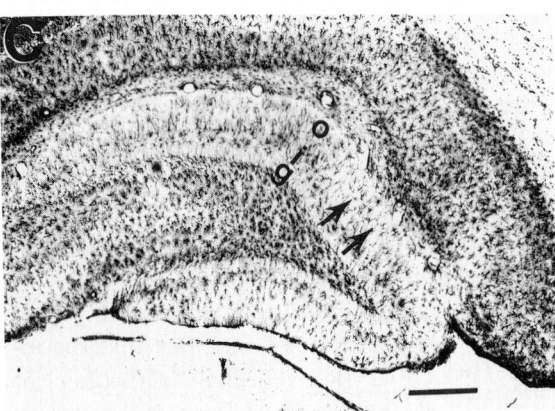

Fig. 4. Photomicrographs of GFAP-positive stained dorsal hippocampus. A: control; B: 8 days following perforant path lesion; C: 8 days following fimbria-fornix lesion. g, granule layer; i, inner molecular layer; o, outer molecular layer. Arrows indicate distinct border of increased GFAP staining. Magnification bar = 200 μm.

variety of central and peripheral neurons (Lindsay, 1977; Banker, 1980; Hatten and Liem, 1981; Liesi et al., 1984; Tarris et al., 1986). At present, when a new putative factor is tested in vitro for its neurotrophic activity, rigorous controls must be used to establish that the neuronal population is not contaminated with glia and that the presumed neurotrophic factor is not acting through the glial cell population in vitro. To date the evidence supports the notion that only reactive and/or proliferating astrocytes secrete trophic and tropic substances, thus it is essential to understand the signals for this activation in vivo. Microglial proliferation often precedes the astrocytic proliferation (Gall et al., 1979; Vijayan, 1983). Recently, Giulian et al. (1986) showed that activated microglia produce IL-1 in vitro, and that IL-1 stimulates astrocyte proliferation in vitro and in vivo (Giulian et al., 1988). Very recently it has been shown that IL-1 regulates the synthesis of NGF in non-neuronal cells of the damaged rat sciatic nerve (Lindholm et al., 1987), and that IL-1 is most likely secreted from activated macrophages in the vicinity of the damaged nerve (Heumann et al., 1987).

Work in the CNS has demonstrated time-dependent changes in microglial and astrocytic populations in the outer molecular layer of the dentate gyrus denervated by perforant path transection (Fagan et al., 1988). Reactive microglia stained with the monoclonal antibody OX-42 appear in this area within 24 h after transection. The appearance of cells immunostained for IL-1 in this area parallels that of microglia, suggesting that the reactive microglia themselves produce IL-1 in vivo in response to deafferentation. The astrocyte response, as indexed by GFAP immunoreactivity, is not observed until a later time point coincident with the disappearance of IL-1 staining. These observations provide suggestive evidence that reactive microglia produce IL-1 in vivo in response to injury, and that IL-1 may be the signal responsible for the documented astrocyte response in the outer molecular layer of the dentate gyrus observed after damage to the entorhinal input to the hippocampus.

Hypothetical steps for sprouting

The results of data summarized in the previous sections suggest (1) a role of IL-1 in the proliferation of astrocytes, (2) activated microglia and macrophages can secrete IL-1, and (3) IL-1 can activate NGF synthesis in non-neuronal cells. We have made the following suggestion for the outline of the events that lead to the NGF-sensitive sprouting responses in the hippocampus and septum following fimbria/fornix and PP lesions: perforant pathway damage induces terminal degeneration of the axons of cells which were transected in the entorhinal cortex. This terminal degeneration in the outer molecular layer of the dentate gyrus activates microglia to phagocytize in the restricted zone of terminal degeneration. These activated microglia release IL-1 into the surrounding environment, which induces the proliferation of astrocytes. The activated astrocytes in turn secrete NGF which results in the attraction of cholinergic fibers that express NGFr on their membrane surfaces.

Similarly, following fimbria/fornix lesions, cholinergic terminals are disconnected from their cell bodies in the septum and once again there is terminal degeneration, this time in the areas of heaviest cholinergic innervation in the CA3 region and dentate gyrus. This degeneration leads to a microglial proliferation, IL-1 secretion, and an astrocytic mitogenic reaction in CA3 and inner molecular layer of the dentate gyrus. The activated astrocytes secrete NGF and promote the ingrowth of NGFr-bearing sympathetic fibers of the superior cervical ganglia.

This working hypothesis generates several specific testable predictions, which when examined should reveal more about the mechanism underlying survival, growth and function of normal and damaged cholinergic afferents to the hippocampal formation.

Acknowledgements

We thank Sheryl Christenson for typing the manuscript. The research presented in this chapter was supported by NIA AG 06088, Office of Naval Research; the Pew, Whitehall; and Sandoz Foundations.

References

Amaral, D.G. and Kurz, J. (1985) An analysis of the origins of the cholinergic and non-cholinergic septal projections to the hippocampal formation of the rat. *J. Comp. Neurol.*, 240: 37 – 59.

Armstrong, D.M., Terry, R.D., Deteresa, R.M., Bruce, G., Hersh, L.B. and Gage, F.H. (1987) Response of septal cholinergic neurons to axotomy. *J. Comp. Neurol.*, 264: 421 – 436.

Assouline, J.G., Bosch, P., Lim, R., Kim, I.S., Jensen, R. and Pantazis, N.J. (1987) Rat astrocytes and Schwann cells in culture synthesize nerve growth factor-like neurite-promoting factors. *Dev. Brain Res.*, 31: 103 – 118.

Ayer LeLievre, C.S., Ebendal, T., Olsen, L. and Seiger, A. (1983) Localization of NGF-like immunoreactivity in rat neuron tissue. *Med. Biol.*, 61: 296 – 304.

Banker, G.A. (1980) Tropic interactions between astroglial cells and hippocampal neurons in cultures. *Science*, 209: 809 – 810.

Batchelor, P.E., Armstrong, D.M., Blaker, S.M. and Gage, F.H. (1989) Nerve growth factor receptor and choline acetyltransferase colocalization in neurons within the rat forebrain: response to fimbria-fornix transection. *J. Comp. Neurol.*, 284: 187 – 204.

Bernd, P. and Greene, L.A. (1984) Association of 125 I-nerve growth factor with PC12 pheochromocytoma cells. Evidence for internalization via high-affinity receptors only and for long term regulation by nerve growth factor. *J. Biol. Chem.*, 259: 15509 – 15516.

Blackstad, T. (1956) Commissural connections of the hippocampus region in the rat, with special reference to their mode of termination. *J. Comp. Neurol.*, 105: 417 – 537.

Blackstad, T. (1969) Studies on the hippocampus: methods of analysis. In M. Brazier (Ed.), *The Interneuron*, UCLA Forum in Medical Sciences, Los Angeles, pp. 319 – 414.

Blaker, S.N., Armstrong, D.M. and Gage, F.H. (1988) Cholinergic neurons within the rat hippocampus: response to fimbria/fornix transection. *J. Comp. Neurol.*, 272: 127 – 138.

Buzsáki, G., Gage, F.H., Kellenyi, L. and Björklund, A. (1987a) Restoration of rhythmic slow activity (theta) in the subcortically denervated hippocampus by embryonic CNS transplants. *Brain Res.*, 400: 321 – 333.

Buzsáki, G., Bickford, R.G., Varon, S., Armstrong, D.M. and Gage, F.H. (1987b) Reconstruction of the damaged septohippocampal circuitry by a combination of fetal grafts and tran-

368

sient NGF infusion. *Soc. Neurosci. Abstr.*, 13: 568.

Collins, F. and Crutcher, K.A. (1985) Neurotrophic activity in the adult rat hippocampal formation: regional distribution and increase after septal lesion. *J. Neurosci.*, 5: 2809–2814.

Collins, F. and Dawson, A. (1983) An effect of nerve growth factor on parasympathetic neurite outgrowth. *Proc. Natl. Acad. Sci. U.S.A.*, 80: 2091–2094.

Cowan, W.M., Fawcett, J.W., O'Leary, D.D. and Stanfield, B.B. (1984) Regressive events in neurogenesis. *Science*, 225: 1258–1265.

Coyle, J.T., Price, P.H. and Delong, M.R. (1983) Alzheimer's disease: a disorder of cortical cholinergic innervation. *Science*, 219: 1184–1189.

Crain, S.M. (1975) Physiology of CNS tissue in culture. In S. Berl, D.D. Clarke, and D.D. Schneider (Eds.) *Metabolic Compartmentation and Neurotransmission. Relation to Brain Structure and Function.* Plenum, New York, pp. 273–303.

Crain, S.M. and Peterson, E.R. (1974) Enhanced afferent synaptic functions in fetal mouse spinal cord-sensory ganglion explants following NGF-induced ganglion hypertrophy. *Brain Res.*, 79: 145–152.

Crutcher, K.A. (1987) Sympathetic sprouting in the central nervous system: a model for studies of axonal growth in the mature mammalian brain. *Brain Res. Rev.*, 12: 203–233.

Crutcher, K.A. and Collins, F. (1982) In vitro evidence for two distinct hippocampal growth factors: basis of neuronal plasticity. *Science,* 217: 67–68.

Daitz, H.M. and Powell, T.P.S. (1954) Studies on the connexions of the fornix system. *J. Neurol. Neurosurg. Psychiatry*, 7: 75–82.

Fagan, A.M., Robertson, R. and Gage, F.H. (1988) Degeneration and regeneration in the outer molecular layer of the dentate gyrus after perforant path lesions: role of astrocytes, microglia and Interleukin-1. *Soc. Neurosci. Abstr.*, 14: 116.

Fallon, J.R. (1985) Preferential outgrowth of central nervous system neurites on astrocytes and Schwann cells as compared with nonglial cells in vitro. *J. Cell. Biol.*, 100: 198–207.

Fischer, W., Wictorin, K., Björklund, A., Williams, L.R., Varon, S. and Gage F.H. (1987) Amelioration of cholinergic neuron atrophy and spatial memory impairment in aged rats by nerve growth factor. *Nature (Lond.)*, 329: 65–68.

Furukawa, S., Furukawa, Y., Satoyoshi, E. and Hayashi, K. (1986) Synthesis and secretion of nerve growth factor by mouse astroglial cells in culture. *Biochem. Biophys. Res. Commun.,* 136: 57–63.

Gage, F.H. and Björklund, A. (1986a) Compensatory collateral sprouting of aminergic systems in the hippocampal formation following partial deafferentation. In R.L. Isaacson and K.H. Pribram (Eds.), *The Hippocampus, Vol. 3*, Plenum Publishing Corp., New York.

Gage, F.H. and Björklund, A. (1986b) Enhaced graft survival in the hippocampus following selective denervation. *Neuroscience*, 17: 89–98.

Gage, F.H. and Björklund, A. (1986c) Cholinergic septal grafts into the hippocampal formation improve spatial learning and memory in aged rats by an atropine sensitive mechanism. *J. Neurosci.*, 2837–2847.

Gage, F.H., Björklund, A. and Stenevi, U. (1984) Denervation releases a neuronal survival factor in adult rat hippocampus. *Nature (Lond.)*, 308: 637–639.

Gage, F.H., Wictorin, K., Fischer, W., Williams, L.R., Varon, S. and Björklund, A. (1986) Life and death of cholinergic neurons: in the septal and diagonal band region following complete fimbria fornix transection. *Neuroscience*, 19: 241–255.

Gage, F.H., Armstrong, D.M., Williams, L.R. and Varon, S. (1988a) Morphologic response of axotomized septal neurons to nerve growth factor. *J. Comp. Neurol.*, 269: 147–155.

Gage, F.H., Blaker, S.N., Davis, G.E., Engvall, E., Varon, S. and Manthorpe, M. (1988b) Human amnion membrane matrix as a substratum for axonal regeneration in the central nervous system. *Exp. Brain Res.*, 72: 371–380.

Gage, F.H., Olinechek, P. and Armstrong, D.M. (1988c) Astrocytes are important for NGF-mediated hippocampal sprouting. *Exp. Neurol.*, 102: 2–13.

Gage, F.H., Batchelor, P., Chen, K.S., Chin, D., Higgins, G.A., Koh, S., Deputy, S., Rosenberg, M.B., Fischer, W. and Björklund, A. (1989) NGF receptor re-expression and NGF mediated cholinergic neuronal hypertrophy in the damaged adult neostriatum. *Neuron*, 2: 1177–1184.

Gall, C., Rose, G. and Lynch, G. (1979) Proliferative and migratory activities of glial cells in the partially deafferented hippocampus. *J. Comp. Neurol.*, 183: 539–550.

Giulian, D. and Baker, T.J. (1985) Peptides released by ameloid microglia regulate astroglial proliferation. *J. Cell. Biol.*, 101: 2411–2415.

Giulian, D., Baker, T.J. Shih, L.N. and Lachman, L.B. (1986) Interleukin-1 of the central nervous system is produced by ameboid microglia, *J. Exp. Med.*, 164: 594–604.

Giulian, D., Woodward, J., Young, D.G., Krebs, J.F. and Lachman, L.B. (1988) Interleukin-1 injected into mammalian brain stimulates astrogliosis and neovascularization, *J. Neurosci.*, 8: 2485–2490.

Gnahn, H. Hefti, F., Heumann, R., Schwab, M.E. and Thoenen, H. (1983) NGF-mediated increase in choline acetyltransferase (ChAT) in the neonatal rat forebrain; evidence for physiological role of NGF in the brain? *Dev. Brain Res.*, 9: 45–52.

Hatten, M.E. and Liem, R.H.K. (1981) Astrogial cells provide a template for the positioning of developing cerebellar neurons in vitro. *J. Cell. Biol.*, 90: 622–630.

Hayes, R.C., Rosenberg, M.B., Higgins, G.A., Chen, K.S., Gage, F.H. and Armstrong, D.M. (1988) In situ hybridization of NGF mRNA in adult rat brain. *Soc. Neurosci. Abstr.*, 14: 684.

Hefti, F. (1986) Nerve growth factor (NGF) promotes survival of septal cholinergic neurons after fimbria transection. *J.*

Neurosci., 6: 2155 – 2162.

Hefti, F., Hartikka, J. and Knusel, B. (1986) Function of neurotrophic factors in the adult and aging brain and their possible use in the treatment of neurodegenerative diseases. *Neurobiol. Aging*, 6: 2155 – 2162.

Heumann, R., Korshing, S. and Thoenen, H. (1987) Changes of nerve growth factor synthesis in nonneuronal cells in response to sciatic nerve transection. *J. Cell. Biol.*, 104: 1623 – 1631.

Higgins, G.A., Koh, S., Chen, K.S. and Gage, F.H. (1989) Nerve growth factor induces NGF-receptor gene expression in basal forebrain neurons of adult rat. *Brain. Exp. Neurol.*, in press.

Johnson, D.G., Silberstein, S.D., Hanbauer, I. and Kopin, I.J. (1972) The role of nerve growth factor in the ramification of sympathetic nerve fibers into the iris in organ culture. *J. Neurochem.*, 19: 2025 – 2029.

Johnston, M.V., Rutkowski, J.L., Wainer, B.H., Long, J.B. and Mobley, W.C. (1987) NGF effects on developing forebrain cholinergic neurons are regionally specific. *Neurochem. Res.*, 12: 985 – 994.

Korsching, S., Heumann, R., Thoenen, H. and Hefti, F. (1986) Cholinergic denervation of the rat hippocampus by fimbrial transection leads to a transient accumulation of nerve growth factor (NGF) without change in mRNA (NGF) content. *Neurosci. Lett.*, 66: 175 – 180.

Kromer, L.F. (1987) Nerve growth factor treatment after brain injury prevents neuronal death. *Science*, 235: 214 – 216.

Kromer, L.F., Björklund, A. and Steveni, U. (1981) Regeneration of the septo-hippocampal pathways in adult rats is promoted by utilizing embryonic hippocampal implants with bridges. *Brain Res.*, 210: 173 – 200.

Landmeser, L. and Pilar, G. (1978) Interactions between neurons and their targets during in vivo synaptogenesis. *Fed. Proc.*, 37: 2016 – 2021.

Lewis, P.R., Shute, C.C.D. and Silver, A. (1967) Confirmation from cholineacetylase of a massive cholinergic innervation to the rat hippocampus. *J. Physiol. (Lond.)*, 191: 215 – 224.

Levi-Montalcini, R. and Angeletti, P.U. (1963) Essential role of the nerve growth factor on the survival and maintenance of dissociated sensory and sympathetic embryonic nerve cells in vitro. *Dev. Biol.*, 7: 653 – 659.

Liesi, P., Kaakkola, S., Dahl, D. and Vaheri, A. (1984) Laminin is induced in astrocytes of adult brain injury. *EMBO J.*, 683 – 686.

Lindholm, D., Heumann, R., Meyer, M. and Thoenen, H. (1987) Interleukin-1 regulates synthesis of nerve growth factor in non-neuronal cells of rat sciatic nerve. *Nature (Lond.)*, 330: 658 – 660.

Lindsay, R.M. (1979) Adult rat brain astrocytes support survival of both NGF-dependent and NGF-insensitive neurons. *Nature (Lond.)*, 282: 80 – 82.

Loy, R. and Moore, R.Y. (1977) Anomalous innervation of the hippocampal formation by peripheral sympathetic axons following mechanical injury. *Exp. Neurol.*, 57 : 645 – 650.

Lynch, G., Matthews, D.A., Mosko, S., Parks, T. and Cotman, C.W. (1972) Induced acetylcholinesterase-rich layer in rat dentate gyrus following entorhinal lesions. *Brain Res.*, 42: 311 – 318.

Martinez, H.J., Dreyfus, C.F., Jonakait, G.M. and Black, I.B. (1985) Nerve growth factor promotes cholinergic development in brain striatal cultures. *Proc. Natl. Acad. Sci. U.S.A.*, 82: 7777 – 7781.

Menesini-Chen, M.G., Chen, J.S. and Levi-Montalcini, R. (1978) Sympathetic nerve fibers ingrowth in the central nervous system of neonatal rodents upon intracerebral NGF injections. *Arch. Ital. Biol.*, 116: 53 – 84.

Mobley, W.C., Rutkowski, J.L., Tennekoon, G.I., Buchanan, K. and Johnston, M.W. (1985) Choline acetyltransferase activity in striatum of neonatal rats increased by nerve growth factor. *Science*, 229: 284 – 287.

Mobley, W.C., Rutkowski, J.L., Tennekoon, G.I., Gemski, J., Buchanan, K. and Johnston, M.V. (1986) Nerve growth factor increases choline acetyltransferase activity in developing basal forebrain neurons. *Mol. Brain Res.*, 1: 53 – 62.

Montero, C.N. and Hefti, F. (1988) Rescue of lesioned septal cholinergic neurons by nerve growth factor: specificity and requirement for chronic treatment. *J. Neurosci.*, 8: 2986 – 2999.

Moore, R.Y. (1975) Monoamine neurons innervating the hippocampal formation and septum. Organization and response to injury. In R.L. Isaacson and K.H. Pribram (Eds.), *The Hippocampus, Vol. 1, Structure and Development*, Plenum, New York, pp. 215 – 238.

Nieto-Sampedro, M., Manthorpe, M., Barbin, G., Varon, S. and Cotman, C.W. (1983) Injury-induced neuronotrophic activity in adult rat brain: correlation with survival delayed implants in the wound cavity. *J. Neurosci*, 3: 2219 – 2229.

Otto, D., Frotscher, M. and Unsicker, K. (1989) Basic fibroblast growth factor and nerve growth factor administered in gel foam rescue medial septal neurons after fimbria fornix transection. *J. Neurosci. Res.*, 83: 159 – 168.

Peterson, G.M., Williams, L.R., Varon, S. and Gage, F.H. (1987) Loss of GABAergic neurons in the medial septum after fimbria-fornix transection. *Neurosci. Lett.*, 76: 140 – 144.

Raisman, G. (1969) Neuronal plasticity in the septal nuclei of the adult rat. *Brain Res.*, 14: 25 – 48.

Richardson, P.M., Verge Isse, V.M.K. and Riopelle, R.J. (1986) Distribution of neuronal receptors for nerve growth factor in the rat. *J. Neurosci.*, 6: 2312 – 2321.

Rohrer, H. and Barde, Y.A. (1982) Presence and disappearance of nerve growth factor receptors on sensory neurons in culture. *Dev. Biol.*, 89: 309 – 315.

Rohrer, H. and Sommer, I. (1983) Simultaneous expression of neuronal and glial properties by chick ciliary ganglion cells during development. *J. Neurosci.*, 3: 1683 – 1699.

Rose, G., Lynch, G. and Cotman, C.W. (1976) Hypertrophy

370

and redistribution of astrocytes in the deafferented dentate gyrus. *Brain Res. Bull.*, 1: 87–92.

Schwab, M.E., Otten, U., Agid, Y. and Thoenen, H. (1979) Nerve growth factor (NGF) in the rat CNS: absence of specific retrograde axonal transport and tyrosine hydroxylase induction of locus coeruleus and substantia nigra. *Brain Res.*, 168: 473–483.

Scott, S.M., Tarris, R., Eveleth, D., Mansfield, H., Weichsel, M.E. and Fisher, D.A. (1981) Bioassay detection of mouse nerve growth factor (mNGF) in the brain of adult mice. *J. Neurosci. Res.*, 6: 653–658.

Seiler, M. and Schwab, M.E. (1984) Specific retrograde transport of nerve growth factor (NGF) from cortex to nucleus basalis in the rat. *Brain Res.*, 300: 33–39.

Shelton, D.L. and Reichardt, L.F. (1986) Studies on the expression of beta NGF gene in the central nervous system: level and regional distribution of NGF mRNA suggest that NGF functions as a trophic factor for several neuronal populations. *Proc. Natl. Acad. Sci. U.S.A.*, 83: 2714–2718.

Sofroniew, M.V. and Isacson, O. (1988) Distribution of degeneration of cholinergic neurons in the septum following axotomy in different portions of the fimbria-fornix; a correlation between degree of cell loss and proximity of neuronal somata to the lesion. *J. Chem. Neuroanat.*, 1: 6.

Springer, J.E. and Loy, R. (1985) Intrahippocampal injections of antiserum to nerve growth factor inhibit sympathohippocampal sprouting. *Brain Res. Bull.*, 15: 629–634.

Springer, J.E., Koh, S., Tayrien, M.W. and Loy, R. (1987) Basal forebrain magnocellular neurons stain for nerve growth factor receptor: correlation with cholinergic cell bodies and effects of axotomy. *J. Neurosci. Res.*, 17: 111–118.

Stenevi, U. and Björklund, A. (1978) Growth of vascular sympathetic axons into the hippocampus after lesions of the septo-hippocampal pathway: a pitfall in brain lesion studies. *Neurosci. Lett.*, 7: 219–224.

Storm-Mathisen, J. (1974) Choline acetyltransferase and acetylcholinesterase in fascia dentata following lesions of the entorhinal afferent. *J. Brain Res.*, 80: 119–181.

Taniuchi, M. and Johnson, E.M. (1985) Characterization of the binding properties and retrograde axonal transport of monoclonal antibody directed against the rat nerve growth factor receptor. *J. Cell. Biol.*, 101: 1100–1106.

Taniuchi, M., Schweizer, J.B. and Johnson, E.M. (1986) Nerve growth factor receptor molecules in rat brain. *Proc. Natl. Acad. Sci. U.S.A.*, 83: 1950–1954.

Tarris, R.H., Wieschsel, M.E.J. and Fisher, D.A. (1986) Synthesis and secretion of a nerve growth-stimulating factor by neonatal mouse astrocyte cells in vitro. *Ped. Res.*, 20: 367–372.

Thoenen, H. and Barde, Y.A. (1980) Physiology of nerve growth factor. *Physiol. Rev.*, 60: 1284–1335.

Tuszynski, M.H., Buzsáki, G., Stearns, G. and Gage, F.H. (1988) Septal cell death following fimbria/fornix transection, and hippocampal cholinergic regeneration following nerve growth factor infusion plus grafting of synthetic and neuronal bridges. *Soc. Neurosci. Abstr.* 14: 587.

Vijayan, V.K. (1983) Lysosomal enzyme changes in young and aged control and entorhinal-lesioned rats. *Neurobiol. Aging*, 4: 13–23.

Wainer, B.H., Levey, A.I., Rye, D.B., Mesulam, M. and Mufson, E.J. (1985) Cholinergic and non-cholinergic septohippocampal pathways. *Neurosci. Lett.*, 54: 45–52.

Wainer, B.H., Hsiang, J., Hoffman, P.C., Heller, A. and Mobley, W.C. (1986) Nerve growth factor enhances central cholinergic cell survival and fiber proliferation in reaggregate cultures. *Neurosci. Lett.*, S17.

Whittemore, S.R., Ebendal, T., Larkfors, L., Olson, L., Seiger, A., Stromberg, I. and Persson, H. (1986) Developmental and regional expression of B nerve growth factor messenger RNA and protein in the rat central nervous system. *Proc. Natl. Acad. Sci. U.S.A.*, 83: 817–821.

Williams, L.R., Varon, S., Peterson, G.M., Wictorin, K., Fisher, W., Björklund, A. and Gage, F.H. (1986) Continuous infusion of nerve growth factor prevents basal forebrain neuronal death after fimbria-fornix transection. *Proc. Natl. Acad. Sci. U.S.A.*, 83: 9231–9235.

Wujek, J.R. and Akeson, R.A. (1987) Extracellular matrix derived from astrocytes stimulates neuritic outgrowth from PC12 cells in vitro. *Dev. Brain Res.*, 34: 87–97.

J. Storm-Mathisen, J. Zimmer and O.P. Ottersen (Eds.)
Progress in Brain Research, Vol. 83
© 1990 Elsevier Science Publishers B.V. (Biomedical Division)

CHAPTER 27

Seizures, neuropeptide regulation, and mRNA expression in the hippocampus

Christine Gall[1], Julie Lauterborn[1], Paul Isackson[1] and Jeffrey White[2]

[1]*Department of Anatomy and Neurobiology, University of California, Irvine, CA 92717, U.S.A. and* [2]*Division of Endocrinology, Department of Medicine, State University of New York, Stony Brook, NY 11794, U.S.A.*

Recent studies have demonstrated that the regulation of neuropeptide expression in forebrain neurons is responsive to external influences including changes in physiological activity. This has been demonstrated most clearly in studies of hippocampus where the synthesis and resting levels of several neuropeptides, localized within well-characterized components of hippocampal circuitry, have been shown to be selectively influenced by seizure activity. In studies described here, we examined the influence of recurrent limbic seizures on the expression of enkephalin, dynorphin, cholecystokinin, and neuropeptide Y (NPY) in rat and mouse hippocampus using immunohistochemical, in situ hybridization and blot hybridization techniques. The data demonstrate that seizures differentially influence the expression of each peptide as a part of a broader cascade of changes in genomic expression within individual hippocampal neurons. In particular, seizures increase preproenkephalin mRNA and enkephalin peptide but decrease dynorphin peptide in the dentate gyrus granule cell/mossy fiber system. Seizure-induced decreases in the concentration of preprodynorphin mRNA in the granule cells have been reported by others. Immunoreactivity for CCK, which is codistributed with the opioid peptides in the mossy fiber system of mouse, is also dramatically reduced in the granule cell axons by seizure. Recurrent seizures induce two temporally distinct changes in NPY expression in hippocampus. First, there is an increase in hybridization to preproNPY mRNA within scattered, probable local circuit neurons in all subfields. This is followed by the seemingly novel appearance of preproNPY mRNA within the dentate gyrus granule cells and pyramidal cells of field CA1. Clues about mechanisms of neuropeptide regulation have come from observations of other, more rapid, transcriptional events induced by seizure. Most notably, our results and those of others demonstrate that seizures increase the expression of messenger RNAs from immediate-early genes (*c-fos, c-jun,* and NGFI-A) which encode proteins that may mediate neuropeptide gene regulation. In addition, mRNA for nerve growth factor is dramatically increased in the dentate gyrus granule cells by seizure; increased production of this trophic factor might mediate the more delayed changes in genomic expression and growth responses observed to occur in hippocampus and other forebrain areas following seizure activity.

Introduction

Because of its anatomical simplicity, the hippocampus is frequently used as a "model" system for the analysis of fundamental neurobiological properties of forebrain neurons and, in particular, their capacity for changing their form and function. The focus of the greater portion of these studies has been on plasticity at the level of the synapse and, somewhat more broadly considered, the intrinsic plasticity of pre- and postsynaptic elements. For example, studies of hippocampus have demonstrated that developing and mature

central nervous system (CNS) axons have the capacity for growth and reactive synaptogenesis in response to the loss of neighboring axonal systems (Gall et al., 1986b). Mature dendrites can lose and elaborate new dendritic spines in response to deafferentation and re-innervation, respectively (Parnavelas et al., 1974; Caceres and Steward, 1983). Repetitive afferent activation can lead to a permanent change in synaptic efficacy in the form of long-term potentiation (LTP) (Bliss and Lømo, 1973; Larson and Lynch, 1988) and this physiological change is associated with alterations in spine shape and, quite possibly, the formation of synapses (Lee et al., 1980; Chang and Greenough, 1984).

With the advent and popular use of immunochemical and molecular biological techniques we are now rapidly coming to appreciate that beyond these capacities for local structural and functional plasticity, mature CNS neurons exhibit whole cell changes in response to a variety of environmental cues in the form of changes in genomic expression. The virtual explosion of research on this topic has given rise to demonstrations that the expression of messenger molecules and their biosynthetic enzymes is responsive to (1) circulating hormones (Davis et al., 1986; Sawchenko, 1987; Harlan, 1988), (2) growth factors (Gnahn et al., 1983; Mobley et al., 1985), (3) the activation of particular neurotransmitter receptors (Romano et al., 1987) and, possibly as a consequence of the latter, (4) the presence of intact innervation by particular afferent systems (Young et al., 1986). Central to any discussion of the regulation of genomic expression is the question of the contributions of normal and abnormal physiological activity and this is the topic of the present review. As will be discussed, studies using brief seizures indicate that physiological activity does in fact have a pervasive influence on the biosynthetic activities of neurons in hippocampus and other forebrain regions.

Hippocampal neurons contain numerous neuropeptides which, in most instances, are considered to be co-localized with classical neurotransmitters (e.g. GABA, glutamate) (Crawford and Connor, 1973; Gall, 1984a; Altschuler et al., 1985; Kosaka et al., 1985). We have examined the effect of recurrent limbic seizure activity on the expression of the opioid peptides enkephalin and dynorphin, cholecystokinin (CCK), and neuropeptide Y (NPY) in rat and mouse hippocampus and have found that seizures differentially influence the expression of each of these neuropeptides as part of a broader cascade of changes in genomic expression. As demonstrated by the results to be described below, these studies provide clues as to the normal mechanisms which regulate neuropeptide ex-

pression by forebrain neurons and reveal more fully the phenotypic capacities and limitations for different classes of neurons within the hippocampus.

Limbic seizures and hippocampal neuropeptide expression

The opioid peptides: enkephalin and dynorphin

The synthetically distinct opioid peptides methionine enkephalin and dynorphin are both contained within well-characterized aspects of hippocampal circuitry and have been demonstrated to be influenced by seizure activity. Of the two, the normal distribution of dynorphin immunoreactivity is by far the simplest including localization within the dentate gyrus granule cells, their mossy fiber axons, and very few scattered neurons within the dentate gyrus molecular layer (McGinty et al., 1983; Gall, 1988). In contrast to this restricted distribution, enkephalin-like immunoreactivity (ENK-I) has been localized within a variety of morphological cell types sparsely scattered across all major hippocampal subfields including the granule cells of dentate gyrus. Moreover, in rat ENK-I has been localized within at least 3 distinct axonal systems: the mossy fiber axons of dentate gyrus granule cells; the perforant path and temporoammonic afferents from the lateral entorhinal and perirhinal cortices (which innervate the outer dentate gyrus molecular layer and hippocampal stratum lacunosum-moleculare, respectively); and a third population of axons which line the interface between stratum radiatum and stratum lacunosum-moleculare of region CA1 (Gall et al., 1981). Immunostaining for enkephalin is quite light in these axonal systems within the septal third of rat hippocampus but increases in density across the middle to temporal thirds of the structure. With the exception of species differences in the localization of ENK-I within perforant path afferents to the dentate gyrus molecular layer (Stengaard-Pedersen et al., 1983; Gall, 1990), the distribution of enkephalin and dynorphin described here for rat hippocampus is, by and large, representative of the distributions of these neuropeptides in the hippocampus of other mammals thus far studied including guinea pig, monkey, and most particularly the mouse which has served, in addition to rat, as an experimental subject in the studies of neuropeptide regulation to be described below.

Although the co-distribution of enkephalin- and dynorphin-like immunoreactivities within the mossy fiber system originally raised concern as to possible cross-reactivity between enkephalin antisera and the dynorphin peptides (McGinty et al., 1983), subsequent immunochemical, biochemical, and in situ hybridization studies have determined that both peptide families are, in fact, present within this one axonal system. The distribution of dynorphin immunoreactivity described above has been replicated using a number of antisera which react with distinct peptide products of prodynorphin (dynorphin A(1 − 8), dynorphin B, α-neoendorphin) (Weber and Barchas, 1983; Gall, 1988) whereas the distribution of ENK-I has been observed with antisera to leucine enkephalin as well as with antisera to the proenkephalin products methionine enkephalin, Met-enkephalin-ArgPhe and Met-enkephalin-ArgGlyLeu (Gall, 1984b; McGinty et al., 1984) which exhibit no cross-reactivity with the dynorphin peptides. Moreover, the techniques of in vivo radiolabeling and chromatographic purification have been used to demonstrate that the dentate gyrus granule cells synthesize, and the mossy fiber axons contain, each of these proenkephalin products as well as BAM18 (White et al., 1986).

In immunohistochemical studies it has been observed consistently that, in the normal rat, immunoreactivity for dynorphin is present in large numbers of mossy fiber boutons which fill the hilus and stratum lucidum. In contrast, peptides of the enkephalin family normally are immunohistochemically detectable within what is clearly a small minority of the mossy fiber boutons. This disparity in normal distribution, and the seeming independent localization of enkephalin and dynorphin peptides in granule cell perikarya of colchicine-treated rats (McGinty,

1985), led to the suggestion that there are distinct enkephalin- and dynorphin-containing subpopulations of granule cells. As will be described below, more recent in situ hybridization studies, particularly those involving analysis of animals who have experienced seizure activity, argue against there being subpopulations of granule cells which can be distinguished on the basis of their neuropeptide content.

In situ hybridization analyses of the distribution of mRNAs encoding enkephalin and dynorphin have corroborated and extended the understanding of the distribution of these neurochemical systems in hippocampus. Although not evaluated at the level of cellular resolution, other laboratories have reported that mRNA encoding the dynorphin peptides is most prominently, and seemingly solely, localized within the layer of dentate gyrus granule cells (Morris et al., 1987, 1988). As expected, the distribution of preproenkephalin (PPE) mRNA is much more complex. In in situ hybridization studies using a ^{35}S-labeled cRNA probe to PPE mRNA (Yoshikawa et al., 1984) and both film and emulsion autoradiographic techniques, we have observed hybridization-labeled cells very sparsely scattered across all subfields of the hippocampus proper, within the central dentate gyrus hilus, as well as within stratum granulosum. In the latter two fields, greater numbers of neurons are labeled autoradiographically in the temporal than in the more septal aspects of hippocampus (Fig. 2). With the exception of cellular labeling within stratum granulosum, the number and distribution of cells which contain hybridizable PPE mRNA is in good agreement with the very best immunohistochemical preparations for the localization of ENK-I. However, in regard to the dentate gyrus granule cells it is clear that the in situ hybridization localization of PPE mRNA provides a much higher estimate of the proportion of these neurons which are engaged in enkephalin synthesis. In both normal and colchicine-treated adult rats, only a very small number of granule cells contain detectable quantities of ENK-I. However, by in situ hybridization it is clear that, most particularly in the temporal dentate gyrus, the greater proportion of the granule cells contain at least low levels of PPE mRNA although there is a great deal of variability in the density of hybridization across neurons within this population.

Hong and colleagues (1980) first reported that seizures influenced peptide levels in hippocampus as they observed an increase in ENK-I following treatment with kainic acid or repeated electroconvulsive shock (ECS). Since that time, hippocampal ENK-I and, in fewer studies, PPE mRNA have consistently been observed to increase in paradigms which involve *recurrent* hippocampal seizures including intracerebroventricular (i.c.v.) kainic acid (Kanamatsu et al., 1986b; Gall, 1988), ECS (Kanamatsu et al., 1986a), chemical and electrical stimulation-induced kindling (Iadarola et al., 1986; McGinty et al., 1986), focal lesion placement (White et al., 1987; Gall, 1988), and intense electrical stimulation (Morris et al., 1988). Our own studies of the influence of seizure activity on the expression of enkephalin, and other hippocampal neuropeptides, primarily have made use of a paradigm of recurrent seizure induction by unilateral electrolytic lesion placement in the dentate gyrus hilus with an insulated stainless steel wire. The placement of such a hilus lesion (HL) in rat or mouse induces recurrent behavioral seizures of the limbic kindling type (Racine, 1972) and electrographic seizures within hippocampus which begin 1.5 – 2 h postlesion and recur for a period of approximately 8 h, with the vast majority of full paroxysmal discharges in hippocampus clustered within the first 3 h of seizure activity (Baudry et al., 1986; Gall et al., 1988b). This paradigm of recurrent seizure induction has proven advantageous for studies of neuropeptide regulation in that it is highly replicable, does not induce secondary neuronal degeneration within the contralateral hippocampus, and stimulates very large bilateral changes in the expression of hippocampal neuropeptides and other, possibly associated, substances as will be described below. For corroboration of the results obtained with the HL paradigm, we have also evaluated the effect of

convulsant doses of i.c.v. kainic acid on hippocampal neuropeptides. Kainic acid induces limbic seizure activity which is of rapid onset and continues for several hours postinjection (Sloviter and Damiano, 1981). One limitation to seizure induction with kainic acid or other convulsant drugs is the neurotoxic properties of these compounds. The doses of kainic acid used in our experiments result in the degeneration of neurons within rostral hippocampal region CA3 which is most pronounced ipsilateral to injection placement; higher doses, as used in other published reports, lead to the degeneration of neurons in superficial layers of olfactory cortical areas as well. Due to traumatic and neurotoxic damage to hippocampus ipsilateral to the HL and kainic acid injection, respectively, our analyses have focused on seizure-induced changes in neuropeptide immunoreactivity and mRNA expression contralateral to treatment. Moreover, all of the alterations in expression reported here to be induced by seizure activity have been demonstrated, via appropriate controls, to be dependent upon seizure activity as opposed to other aspects of each particular treatment (e.g. anesthesia, neuronal degeneration, deafferentation).

As seen in immunohistochemical preparations, the influence of HL and kainic acid-induced seizures on hippocampal ENK-I are most striking in the mossy fiber system (Fig. 1). At both 6 and 12 h after a seizure-producing HL in rat or mouse, ENK-I is entirely depleted from mossy fiber axons. By 18 h post-HL, ENK-I can be seen to have returned to the more proximal aspects (hilar region, CA3c) of the system and by 24 h mossy fiber ENK-I appears to have returned to normal. However, ENK-I continues to increase in this system to reach maximal levels by 3 – 5 days postlesion. During this period, stratum lucidum appears to be filled with densely enkephalin-immunoreactive mossy fiber terminal boutons, bilaterally (White and Gall, 1987a; White et al., 1987; Gall, 1988). Similarly large, bilateral increases in the density of immunostaining and the number of mossy fiber boutons containing ENK-I have been observed following limbic seizure induction by i.c.v. kainic acid (Kanamatsu et al., 1986b; Gall, 1988).

While most prominent in the mossy fiber system, ENK-I is also elevated in other axonal systems in response to HL-induced seizures in rats and mice. Most notably, at 4 days post-HL ENK-I is increased in entorhinal cortex and the temporoammonic and perforant path afferents to the hippocampus which arise from this area. Outside the hippocampal formation, increases in ENK-I can be seen in portions of the amygdaloid complex and septum. However, as described below, it has become clear from the results of in situ hybridiza-

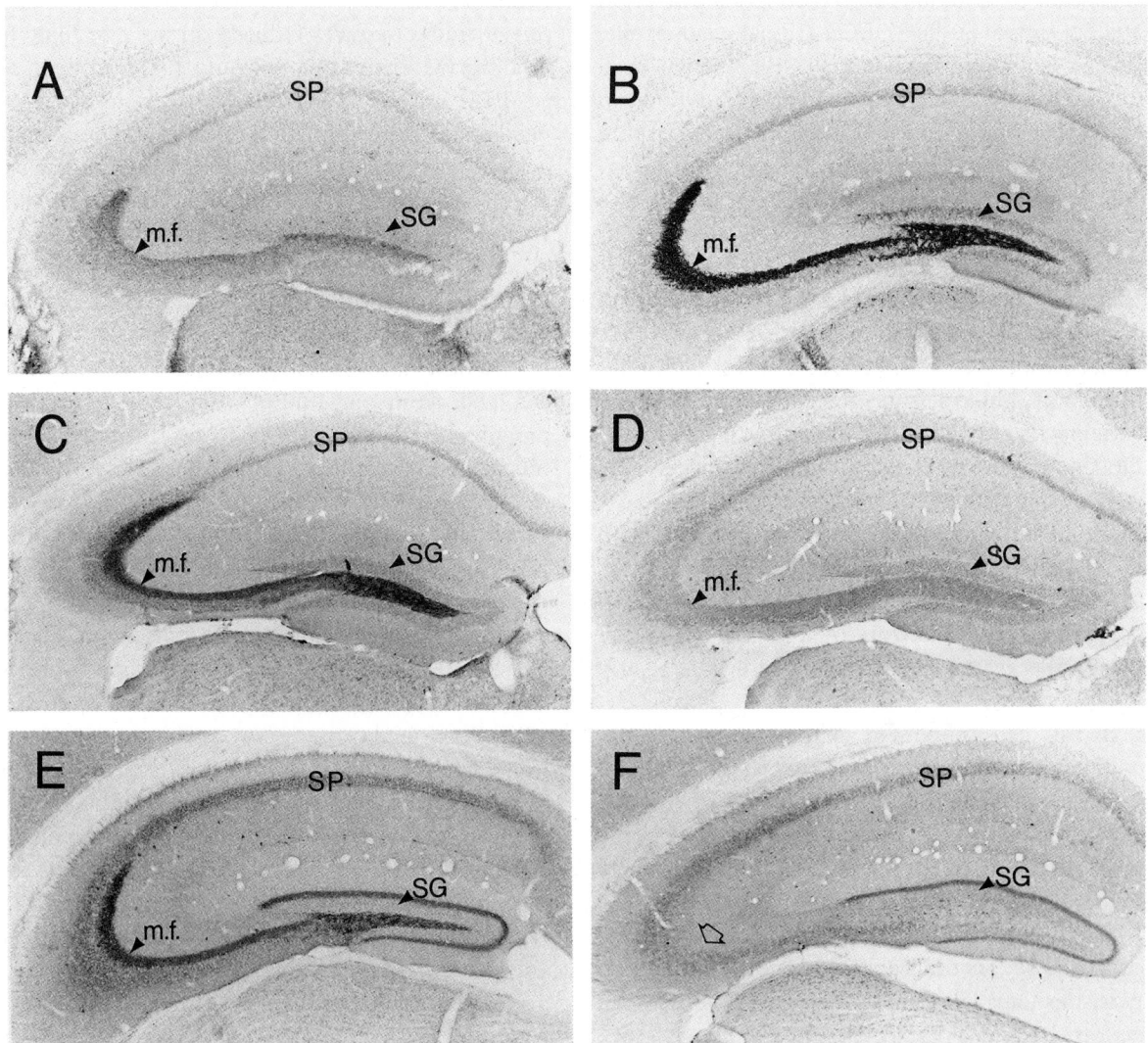

Fig. 1. Low-magnification, light-field photomicrographs of coronal sections through rostral hippocampus showing peroxidase antiperoxidase immunostaining for ENK-I (A, B), dynorphin-I (C, D) and CCK-I (E, F) in control mice (A, C, E) and paired experimental mice (B, D, F) sacrificed 4 days after a contralateral, seizure-producing HL. Note the dramatic increase in ENK-I (B), the reduced density of dynorphin immunoreactivity (D), and the complete loss of CCK-I (F, open arrow) within the mossy fiber system (m.f.) of the HL mice relative to controls (A, C, and E, respectively). Abbreviations: SG, stratum granulosum; SP, stratum pyramidale.

tion studies that HL seizure-induced changes in enkephalin expression are much more broadly distributed across the structures of the limbic and olfactory forebrain than can be appreciated in immunohistochemical preparations.

In sharp contrast to the influence of recurrent limbic seizures on ENK-I, seizures induced by i.c.v. kainic acid (Kanamatsu et al., 1986b; Gall, 1988), amygdaloid kindling (Iadarola et al., 1986; McGinty et al., 1986), ECS (Kanamatsu et al., 1986a), and hilus lesion (Gall, 1988) have been found to *reduce* immunoreactivity for dynorphin within the mossy fibers. Like ENK-I, dynorphin immunoreactivity is strikingly depleted during, and near the termination of, a recurrent seizure episode. However, in most HL and kainic acid-treated rats and mice, immunostaining for dynorphin remains well below normal during the period of maximal enkephalin elevation 3–5 days postseizure (Fig. 1). In further contrast to the influence of limbic seizures on ENK-I, which is invariably increased in HL and kainic acid treated rats that exhibited behavioral seizures, the decrease in dynorphin immunoreactivity is variable across experimental animals; in some rats and mice with HL-induced increases in mossy fiber ENK-I the amount of dynorphin immunoreactivity appeared normal 4 days postseizure, whereas in others the mossy fiber dynorphin immunostaining was clearly reduced.

In rat, seizure-induced changes in enkephalin and dynorphin immunoreactivity are transient. By 2 weeks following either the HL or i.c.v. kainic acid both immunoreactivities have returned to normal levels as seen in immunohistochemical preparations (White and Gall, 1987a; Gall et al., 1988b) or measured by RIA (Hong et al., 1980). In contrast, we have observed changes in ENK-I to persist as long as 6 months in a few HL and kainic acid-treated mice that exhibited particularly severe behavioral seizures during the initial episode (Gall et al., 1988b). It is unclear whether the seizure episode induced permanent changes in the relative balance of opioid peptide expression in these animals or whether seizures recurred in these mice

to, in effect, provide recent stimulation for increased enkephalin expression prior to sacrifice.

These seizure-induced changes in hippocampal opioid peptide levels are most probably due to changes in transcriptional activity. In situ hybridization studies have demonstrated that preprodynorphin mRNA levels are dramatically reduced within stratum granulosum following either intense electrical stimulation of hippocampus or limbic seizures induced during amygdaloid kindling (Morris et al., 1987 and 1988). Conversely, PPE mRNA levels are increased in rat hippocampus following seizures induced by kainic acid (Kanamatsu et al., 1986b), ECS (Kanamatsu et al., 1986a), amygdaloid kindling (Naranjo et al., 1986) and intense electrical stimulation (Morris et al., 1988).

The only information as to both the temporal parameters and cellular localization of seizure-induced increases in hippocampal PPE mRNA is available from our studies using the hilus lesion paradigm (Gall et al., 1987). In agreement with the time course of changes in PPE mRNA levels induced by kainic acid, Northern blot analysis demonstrates that following HL seizures PPE mRNA levels in the dentate gyrus subfield are slightly elevated by 1.5 h following seizure onset, rise to a maximum of 15- to 30-fold control levels by 18–30 h postlesion, and then decline to near-control values by 96 h postlesion (White et al., 1987; White and Gall, 1987a). By in situ hybridization analysis it is clear that PPE mRNA expression is elevated dramatically within the dentate gyrus granule cells at the earliest of these time points. The density of hybridization to this mRNA species increases further within stratum granulosum to reach maximal levels by 17–24 h postlesion at which time it appears that all of the granule cells, across the full septotemporal extent of the structure, contain high concentrations of PPE mRNA (Fig. 2B and F). Using in vivo radiolabeling techniques we have determined that enkephalin synthesis in the rat dentate gyrus granule cells has increased 14-fold above control levels at these post-HL intervals (White et al., 1987).

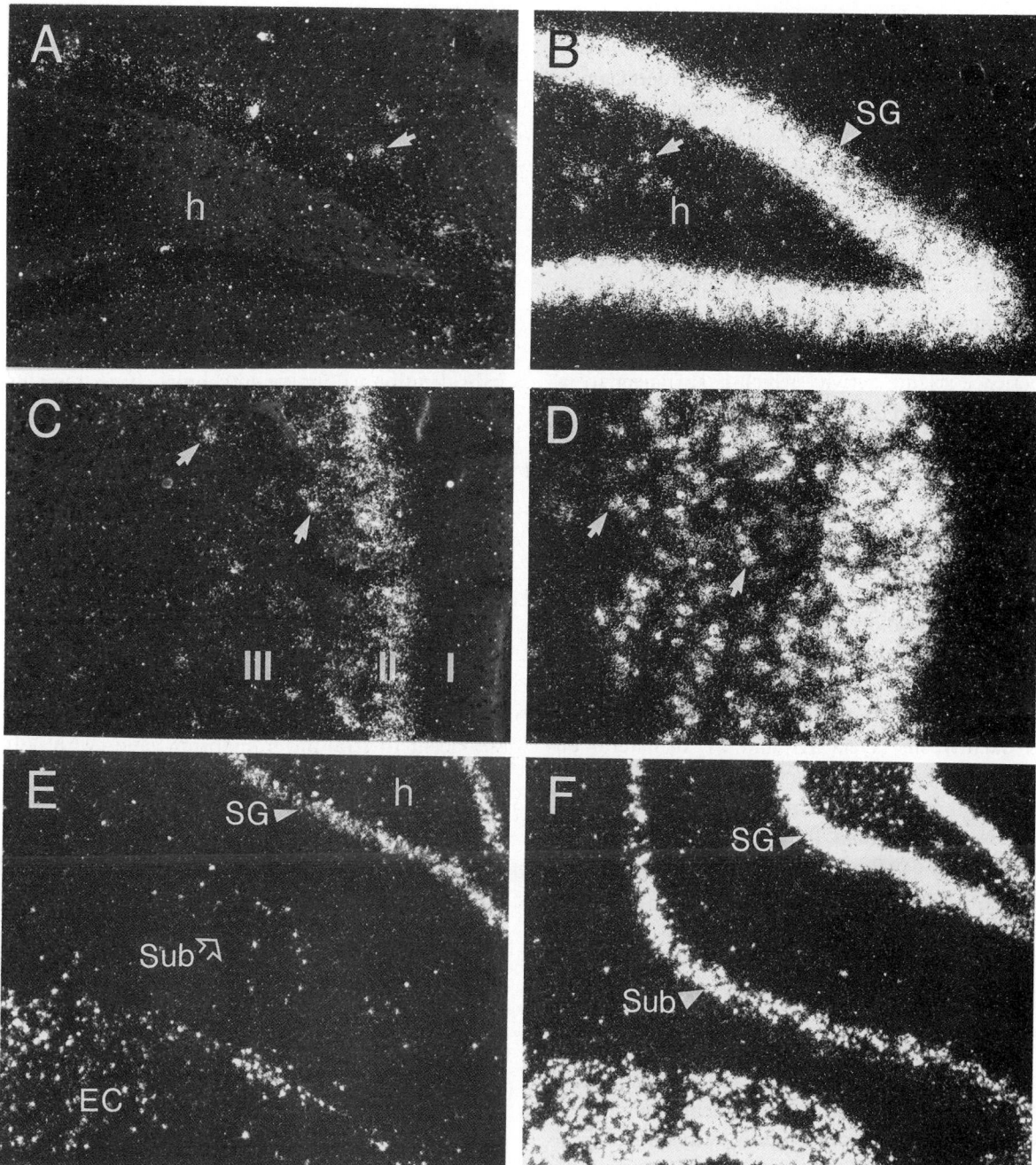

Fig. 2. Dark-field photomicrographs illustrating the autoradiographic localization of in situ hybridization to PPE mRNA in coronal sections through the septal dentate gyrus (A, B), lateral entorhinal cortex (EC) (C, D), and temporal subiculum (Sub) (E, F) in untreated rats (A, C, E) and paired experimental rats sacrificed either 24 h (B, D) or 2 days (F) post-HL. Arrows indicate a few of the ^{35}S-cRNA labeled neurons (seen as white). Note that only a small number of labeled neurons are evident within septal aspects of stratum granulosum (SG) in the untreated rat (A) whereas 24 h following a seizure-inducing HL the full population of neurons in this layer appear densely labeled (B). Also at 24 h post-HL, a dramatic increase in the number of cells showing hybridization to PPE mRNA can be seen in layers II and III of entorhinal cortex (D). At 2 days postlesion (F), hybridization to PPE mRNA is still elevated within stratum granulosum and entorhinal cortex and is clearly increased within the subiculum of the HL rat relative to the paired control (E). Abbreviations: h, dentate gyrus hilus.

Outside stratum granulosum, the distribution of seizure-induced increases in hybridization of PPE cRNA reveals populations of hippocampal neurons with the capacity for enkephalin expression which were not fully appreciated from studies of the untreated rat. Most particularly, cells within superficial aspects of the prosubicular and subicular cell layers (Figs. 2E and F), and large neurons within stratum pyramidale of region CA3c and the central hilus are well labeled in HL rats. Although, as will be described below, the pyramidal cells of regions CA1 through CA3b experience seizure activity which is sufficient to induce changes in the concentrations of other mRNA species, no change is observed in the number of neurons which exhibit hybridization to PPE cRNA.

As expected from increases in ENK-I in the perforant path and temporoammonic afferents to hippocampus, hybridization to PPE mRNA in entorhinal cortical neurons is increased following HL seizures as well. In the normal rat, cells which exhibit light-to-moderate densities of hybridization to PPE cRNA are observed in layer IIb and, less frequently, in layers III and IV of lateral entorhinal cortex. Increases in hybridization are evident in entorhinal cortex by 6 h post-HL, somewhat later than the increase in the dentate gyrus (Fig. 5). By 24 h post-HL, there is an increase in the number of cells, and the density of individual cell labeling, in both superficial and deeper layers of lateral entorhinal cortex as well as within the adjacent medial and perirhinal fields (Fig. 2).

As mentioned above, it is evident from the in situ hybridization material that HL-induced seizures stimulate increases in enkephalin synthesis which are much more broadly distributed across olfactory/limbic forebrain than was anticipated from immunocytochemical studies. As such, at 24 h post-HL, hybridization to PPE mRNA is increased several-fold within layers II and III across the full rostrocaudal extent of the piriform cortex, the lateral and posterior corticomedial amygdaloid nuclei, the medial olfactory tubercle, the intermediate lateral septum, and the granule cell layer of the olfactory bulb. More modest increases in hybridization are evident in the nucleus accumbens and the inferior half of the caudate nucleus.

These increases in PPE mRNA expression are all transient but abate with different latencies across brain regions. At 48 h post-HL, hybridization to PPE mRNA is still elevated well above control levels in all regions mentioned above. By 4 days post-HL, hybridization within the hippocampus has declined to normal levels. In contrast, hybridization within the entorhinal cortex remains elevated at post-HL day 4 but returns to normal by one week postlesion.

Cholecystokinin (CCK)

Like enkephalin, the neuropeptide CCK has been localized within a number of different cell types and axonal systems in hippocampus. In all mammals examined thus far, CCK-like immunoreactivity (CCK-I) has been localized within perikarya distributed within and around stratum pyramidale, subjacent to stratum granulosum, and, with colchicine treatment, in the central hilus (Greenwood et al., 1981; see Gall, 1990 for review). Neurons in the former two loci give rise to local CCK-I axons that form varicose pericellular arborizations within stratum pyramidale, and that most probably innervate the supragranular molecular layer and stratum granulosum, respectively. Considerable species differences have been observed in the localization of CCK-I in long axonal systems. In rat and mouse, CCK-I neurons of the central hilus have been found to contribute to the commissural and associational systems which innervate the dentate gyrus inner molecular layer, although CCK-I is much denser within this terminal field and much more evenly distributed across the septotemporal axis of this lamina, in mouse than in rat (Gall et al., 1986a; Fredens et al., 1987). In addition, in rat CCK-I has been localized within medial perforant path afferents to the dentate gyrus middle molecular layer (Fredens et al., 1984). Finally,

CCK-I has been localized immunohistochemically within a seemingly large proportion of dentate gyrus granule cells and mossy fiber boutons in mouse, guinea pig, and monkey but not within mossy fibers of rat, cat, or rabbit (Gall, 1990).

The influence of seizure activity on CCK expression by hippocampal neurons in the rat remains unclear. We have not observed conspicuous changes in the density or distribution of immunostaining for CCK in rat hippocampus following HL- or i.c.v. kainic acid-induced seizures although Meyer et al. (1986) have reported a modest but significant increase in total hippocampal CCK-I measured by RIA 10 days following an intraperitoneal injection of kainic acid. Furthermore, two groups have examined alterations in hippocampal CCK-I in association with amygdaloid kindling with conflicting results: Iadarola et al. (1986) observed a 162% increase whereas Harris et al. (1988) found no kindling- or seizure-induced change in total hippocampal CCK-I as measured by RIA.

In contrast, we have observed consistent, discrete changes in immunostaining for CCK in mouse hippocampus following either HL- or kainic acid-induced seizures. The mouse was selected for study because the co-distribution of CCK-I with both enkephalin and dynorphin immunoreactivities in mouse mossy fibers afforded the opportunity to determine whether these immunoreactivities were differentially regulated in this one axonal system by epileptiform physiological activity. Indeed, this proved to be the case. As with the opioid peptides, CCK-I was depleted from the mossy fibers during both HL- and kainic acid-induced seizures in adult Swiss–Webster mice (Gall et al., 1988b). Four days following the seizure episode, CCK-I was generally still completely absent from these granule cell axons (Fig. 1). Like the seizure-induced increase in mossy fiber ENK-I, this loss of CCK-I was a reliable outcome of behaviorally verified limbic seizure activity. Moreover, this seizure-induced loss of CCK-I appeared specific to the mossy fiber system; immunostaining for CCK

within the dentate gyrus inner molecular layer (commissural and associational afferents) and scattered local circuit neurons was not clearly affected when examined 4 days postseizure (Gall, 1988).

Further work is needed before definitive statements can be made as to the influence of seizure activity on CCK expression in hippocampus. In situ hybridization analysis should be particularly helpful in resolving a number of outstanding questions. Specifically, is there in fact no change in the expression of CCK by local circuit and dentate gyrus commissural/associational neurons following hippocampal seizure? If so, is it appropriate to conclude that CCK synthesis in these neurons is not influenced by the pattern or intensity of physiological activity experienced during seizure? Is the postseizure decrease in CCK-I within mouse mossy fibers associated with a decrease in mRNA for preproCCK in the dentate gyrus granule cells? The answers to these questions must await further analysis.

Neuropeptide Y (NPY)

Recent in situ hybridization studies in our laboratories have demonstrated that HL- and kainic acid-induced seizures stimulate changes in the expression of NPY by hippocampal neurons. In hippocampus of untreated rat and monkey, NPY-like immunoreactivity (NPY-I) is primarily localized within scattered local circuit neurons and their intrahippocampal axonal arborizations (Köhler et al., 1986). Perikarya containing NPY-I are most numerous within the dentate gyrus hilus and stratum oriens although immunoreactive neurons are less densely distributed within stratum pyramidale and the apical pyramidal dendritic fields. Immunocytochemical studies have not detected NPY-I within the dentate gyrus granule cells, or any other population of "projection neurons" in hippocampus of the normal rat. In situ hybridization analysis of the distribution of preproNPY mRNA in rat hippocampus is in good agreement with these immunocytochemical results.

As seen in emulsion autoradiograms, a ^{35}S-labeled RNA probe complementary to rat preproNPY (Higuchi et al., 1988) labels neurons scattered across all hippocampal subfields with greatest numbers of labeled cells in the dentate gyrus hilus and surrounding stratum pyramidale. Within stratum granulosum, extremely few individual labeled neurons are observed. In further agreement with immunocytochemical data (Köhler, 1986), the few neurons containing detectable preproNPY mRNA within the retrohippocampal cortex are most numerous in deeper cell layers; virtually no neurons labeled with the cRNA probe were seen in more superficial layers which give rise to the principal efferent projections to hippocampus.

We have analyzed the influence of both HL- and kainic acid-induced seizure activity on the abundance of preproNPY mRNA in rat with nuclease protection and in situ hybridization analyses

(Yount et al., 1989). Although there are some differences in the time course of NPY-induction between these treatments, the results are largely in agreement. As such, only the influence of HL-induced seizures on preproNPY contralateral to treatment will be described here.

By nuclease protection analysis the total amount of preproNPY mRNA in the combined dentate gyrus and CA1 subfields was normal 3 h post-HL, had increased only slightly by 6 h, and then increased dramatically to approximately 30-fold and 50-fold normal values by 12 and 18 h post-HL, respectively. By 30 h, total preproNPY mRNA in these fields had begun to decline but did not return to baseline values until after 4 days post-HL. In situ hybridization studies have demonstrated that this seizure-induced increase in total preproNPY mRNA reflects changes in NPY expression in a number of different hippocampal cell types and

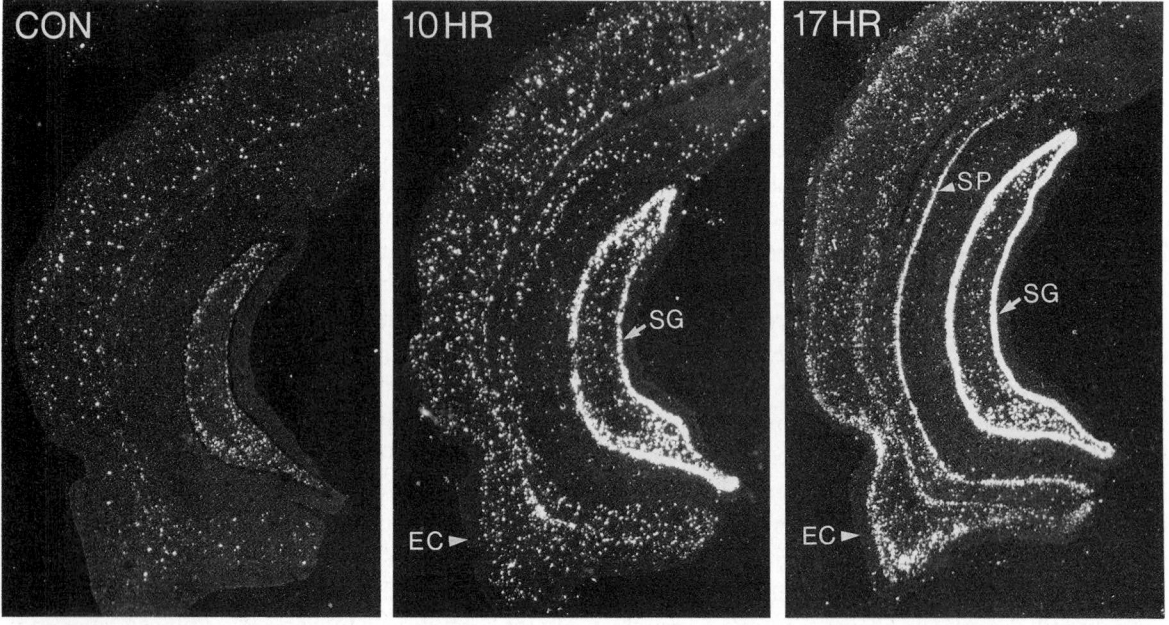

Fig. 3. Low-magnification dark-field photomicrographs of coronal sections through caudal hippocampus illustrating the autoradiographic localization of in situ hybridization to preproNPY mRNA in tissue from a control (CON) rat and rats sacrificed 10 h and 17 h following a contralateral HL. In the control tissue, neurons labeled with the preproNPY cRNA probe (seen as white dots) are scattered throughout the dentate gyrus hilus, neocortex, and deep entorhinal cortex (EC). In the 10 h HL rat, seizure-induced increases in preproNPY mRNA are evident in stratum granulosum (SG), superficial entorhinal cortex, and virtually all layers of neocortex. By 17 h post-HL, hybridization has appeared within stratum pyramidale (SP) of region CA1 and has increased further within SG and superficial layers of entorhinal cortex and neocortex.

that the period of elevated preproNPY expression differs between groups (Fig. 3).

In agreement with the nuclease protection data, and in contrast to seizure-induced changes in enkephalin expression, no change in hybridization to preproNPY mRNA was observed in rats sacrificed 3 h post-HL. However, by 6 h there was an increase in the density of autoradiographic labeling of neurons scattered throughout hippocampus although there was no clear change in the numbers or distribution of labeled cells relative to paired control rats. Further changes in the pattern of hybridization were evident by 10 h post-HL with the appearance of clusters of densely labeled granule cells. By 17 h post-HL the full stratum granulosum was heavily labeled and an even density of autoradiographic grains was first evident overlying the entirety of stratum pyramidale in region CA1 (Fig. 3). At this time point, the density of grains overlying the greater part of CA1 stratum pyramidale was lower than that overlying cells in the adjacent strata oriens and radiatum. This disparity was lost by 24 h postlesion at which time hybridization labeling was elevated far above normal over stratum granulosum, CA1 stratum pyramidale, and neurons scattered within the hippocampal dendritic fields and the dentate gyrus hilus. As in the case of seizure-induced increases in the abundance of PPE mRNA, the HL-induced increases in mRNA for NPY were not limited to the hippocampus. Most particularly, there was a large increase in the hybridization labeling of neurons in the superficial layers of piriform and entorhinal cortex, including the fields which give rise to the perforant path projections to hippocampus, which became evident after 6 h post-HL and appeared maximal by 24 h. By 2 days postlesion, the dentate gyrus granule cells were no longer autoradiographically labeled whereas hybridization remained elevated in region CA1 and entorhinal cortex. By 4 days hybridization appeared normal in all fields.

These data demonstrate that seizure-induced increases in NPY expression by hippocampal neurons are more delayed, relative to seizure onset, than increases in enkephalin expression and differ in duration across the various neuronal populations affected. Moreover, these data demonstrate that several different populations of hippocampal and entorhinal cortical neurons which were not previously considered to contain NPY can be stimulated to express this neuropeptide in response to epileptiform activity.

Early gene responses and the regulation of neuropeptide expression

The cellular proto-oncogene c-fos and the "immediate early" genes

As described above, recurrent seizure activity induces changes in the expression of neuroactive peptides within hippocampus that are specific both with respect to the particular neuropeptide genes induced and with respect to the neuronal populations affected. These results raise obvious questions as to the cellular mechanisms responsible for differential control of neuropeptide gene expression. Pertinent to this, an emerging concept in molecular and cellular biology is that the expression of phenotype-specific genes may be controlled, at least in part, by prior transcription of genes encoding trans-acting transcriptional activation factors (Maniatis et al., 1987). These so-called "immediate-early" genes are induced in response to activation of cell surface receptors and intracellular second messenger systems, and are transcribed in the absence of new protein synthesis. Many immediate-early genes have been found to encode proteins that bind specific DNA sequences and enhance transcription of reporter, or "target", genes. An example of this phenomenon is the cascade of changes in genomic expression induced in pheochromocytoma cells, and other responsive cell lines, to treatment with growth factors (Quantin and Breathnach, 1988). Should similar regulatory mechanisms exist in adult CNS neurons, one might expect seizure-induced alterations in the expression of neurotransmitter molecules to be embedded in a broad genomic response which begins with the

382

transcription of immediate-early genes (Curran and Morgan, 1987).

In agreement with this prediction, seizure activity has been found to stimulate rapid increases in the abundance of mRNAs and proteins encoded by several immediate-early genes including *c-fos, c-jun, jun-B* and *zif*/268 (Dragnow and Robertson, 1987; Morgan et al., 1987; White and Gall, 1987b; Le Gal La Salle, 1988; Saffen et al., 1988). Among these, the ability to stimulate transcription of reporter genes has been demonstrated for the Fos and Jun proteins, which form a heterodimer as part of the AP-1 transcriptional activation factor (Chiu et al., 1988). Interestingly, the promoter region of the PPE gene is among the most extensively studied gene promoters and has been found to contain DNA sequences which bind several transcriptional activation factors including AP-1, AP-2, and AP-4, and contains sequences which confer inducibility by cAMP and phorbol esters (Comb et al., 1988; Hyman et al., 1989). Although no studies have been conducted using purified transcription factors, the preproNPY promoter region contains consensus DNA sequences for SP1 binding (McKnight and Tjian, 1986) and partial consensus sequences for AP-1 binding and phorbol ester inducibility. However, despite these intriguing correlations, activation of PPE or preproNPY gene transcription by "immediate early" genes remains to be demonstrated directly.

One prediction of the hypothesis that immediate-early genes mediating activity-dependent changes in the transcription of neuropeptide genes is that *c-fos* mRNA levels should rise prior to alterations in neuropeptide gene expression and should be observable in all neuronal populations which exhibit changes in neuropeptide synthesis. This prediction has been confirmed with regard to

HL-induced increases in PPE and preproNPY mRNA expression (Figs. 4 and 5). We have observed increases in *c-fos* mRNA within hippocampal neurons following seizures induced by HL, kainic acid, amygdaloid kindling, and acute perforant path stimulation using in situ hybridization techniques (Gall and Isackson, 1989) and an 805 base ^{35}S-labeled RNA probe complementary to *v-fos*

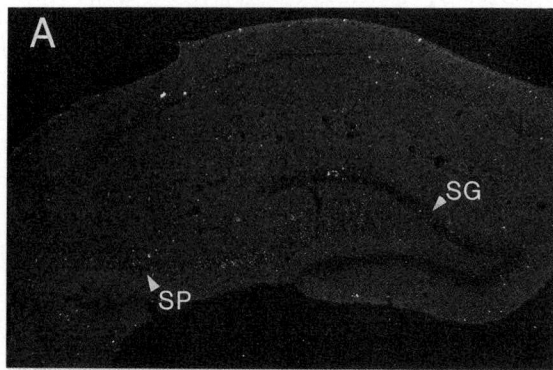

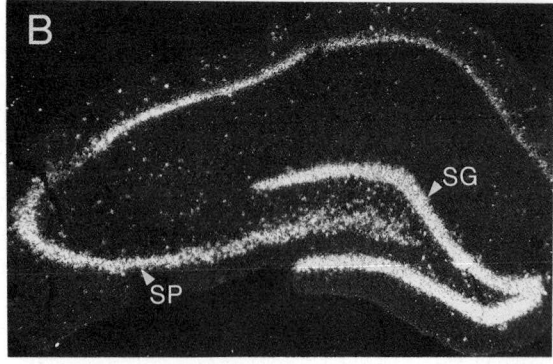

Fig. 4. Low-magnification dark-field photomicrographs illustrating the autoradiographic localization of in situ hybridization labeling of *c-fos* mRNA in tissue sections through the rostral hippocampus of an untreated rat (A) and a paired rat sacrificed 3 h post-HL (B). Note the large seizure-induced increase in hybridization within stratum granulosum (SG), stratum pyramidale (SP), and neurons scattered outside these principal cell layers in the HL rat relative to the paired control.

Fig. 5. Low-magnification dark-field photomicrographs of coronal sections through caudal hippocampus illustrating the correspondence between the distribution of HL seizure-induced increases in mRNAs for *c-fos* (A, B) and PPE (C, D) in control rats (A, C) and rats sacrificed 3 h (B) and 6 h (D) post-HL. As can be seen in panel B, hybridization to *c-fos* mRNA is strikingly elevated in neurons of stratum granulosum (SG), entorhinal cortex (EC) as well as the subiculum and CA1 stratum pyramidale at 3 h post-HL. In panel D one can see that the abundance of PPE mRNA is also most strikingly increased within stratum granulosum and entorhinal cortex of the HL rat (relative to its paired control) but, unlike the pattern of *c-fos* induction, PPE mRNA is not increased within stratum pyramidale.

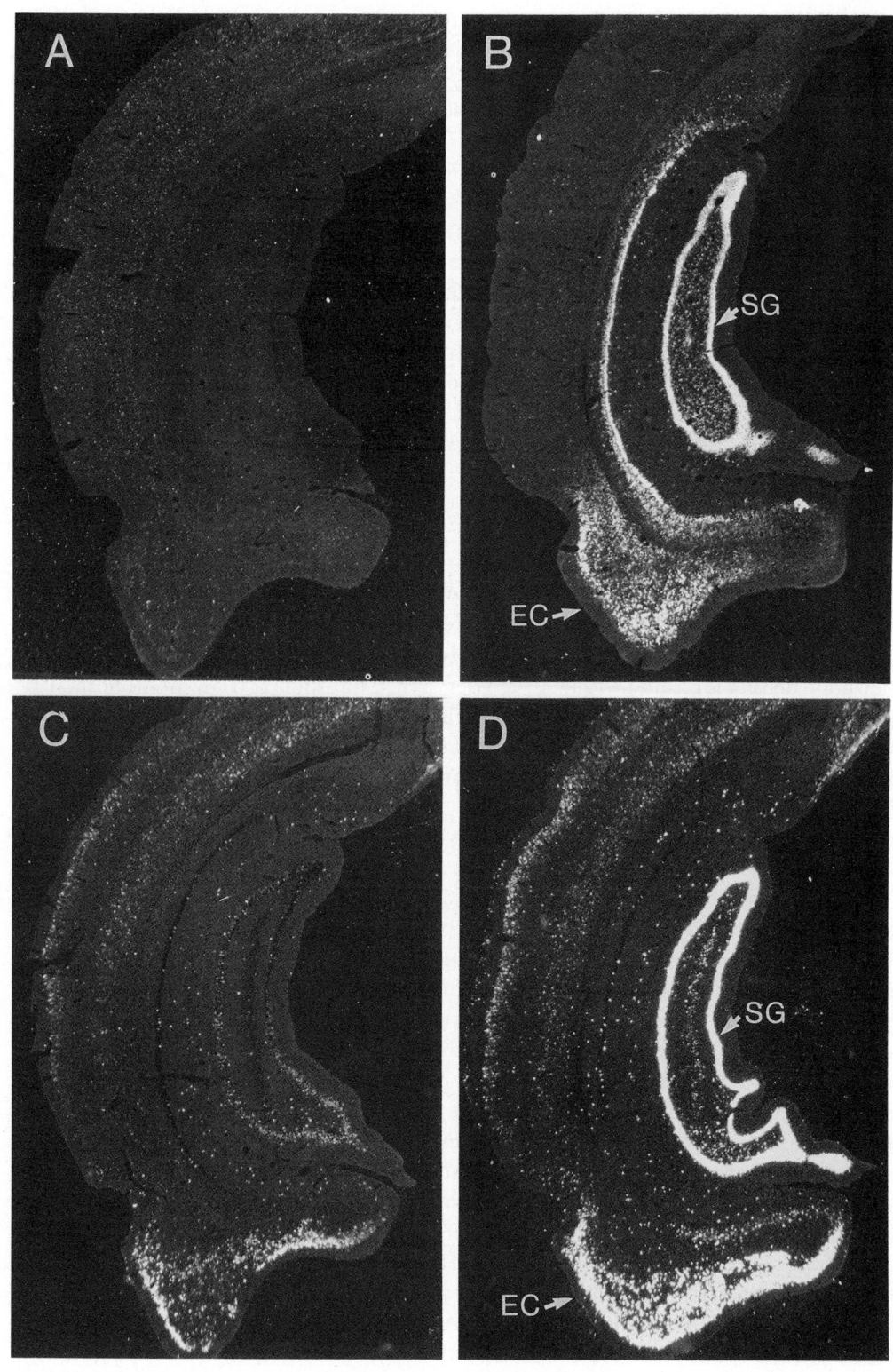

mRNA (White and Gall, 1987b; Gall et al., 1988a). Extremely low levels of hybridization to *c-fos* mRNA are observed in tissue from untreated rats with lightly labeled cells most frequently seen in neocortex, superficial layers of olfactory cortex, and both stratum granulosum and stratum pyramidale of hippocampus. Following hippocampal afterdischarges induced by 10 Hz stimulation of the perforant path in the anesthetized rat, *c-fos* mRNA is increased dramatically within both ipsilateral and contralateral stratum granulosum within 15 min of the first afterdischarge whereas PPE mRNA is not increased until approximately 1 h following stimulation onset.

With HL-induced seizures, the abundance of *c-fos* mRNA is dramatically elevated across what appears to be all populations of hippocampal neurons (Fig. 4). By 3 h following HL, hybridization is elevated in neurons throughout hippocampus, subiculum, entorhinal cortex, piriform cortex, anterior olfactory nucleus, and subnuclei of the amygdaloid complex (Fig. 5). At these early time points, hybridization density is greatest within stratum granulosum where densitometric measures of film autoradiograms indicate *c-fos* mRNA levels are 30 to 50 fold higher than in paired control rats. From 3 to 6 h postlesion, the density of hybridization within the aforementioned extrahippocampal loci increases further. Moreover, from 3 to 6 h post-HL there is a lesser, but nevertheless robust, increase in *c-fos* mRNA expression in neocortex, nucleus accumbens, and the granule cell layer of the olfactory bulb. The greater portion of the seizure-induced increases in hybridization to *c-fos* mRNA is lost from stratum granulosum by 10 h following the hilus lesion, and from region CA1, entorhinal cortex, and neocortex during the interval from 10 to 18 h postlesion. In rats sacrificed 27 h after the HL, extremely low levels of hybridization are observed throughout the forebrain.

Although these increases in hybridization density are broadly distributed, they remain topographically specific; the absence of increased hybridization to *c-fos* mRNA in regions of the thalamus and hypothalamus argue against non-specific induc-tion, independent of circuit relationships with limbic structures. Furthermore, the HL-induced increase in hybridization appears restricted to neurons. Hybridization to glial cells in white matter or the dendritic fields of hippocampus was negligible in both control and HL rats up to 27 h postlesion. Finally, the HL-induced increases in *c-fos* mRNA levels are arguably dependent upon seizure activity, as opposed to the damage and/or trauma associated with surgery and lesion placement, in that equivalent-sized lesions placed in the dentate gyrus hilus with a platinum-iridium wire, that do not induce seizure activity (Campbell et al., 1984), do not stimulate changes in neuronal *c-fos* mRNA expression within tissue contralateral to the lesion.

Nerve growth factor (NGF)

One of the more surprising outcomes of our analyses of early genomic responses to seizure activity is that limbic seizures stimulate dramatic increases in the expression of NGF. In the normal rat forebrain, NGF mRNA is most abundant in hippocampus and, at lesser concentrations, in olfactory cortex and neocortex (Shelton and Reichardt, 1986). As seen in tissue sections processed for in situ hybridization localization of β-NGF mRNA, within hippocampus of the naive adult rat this message is most abundant in neurons scattered within the dentate gyrus hilus and within and around stratum pyramidale. In addition, variable but low levels of hybridizable NGF mRNA are observed within the dentate gyrus granule cells. Following seizure activity induced by HL, i.c.v. kainic acid, acute electrical stimulation of the perforant path, or perforant path kindling there is a large increase in hippocampal NGF mRNA expression that is primarily localized within stratum granulosum (Gall and Isackson, 1989; Gall et al., 1989).

In HL rats sacrificed 1–4 h following seizure onset a large increase in hybridization to β-NGF mRNA is evident within stratum granulosum; at these time points virtually all of the granule cells

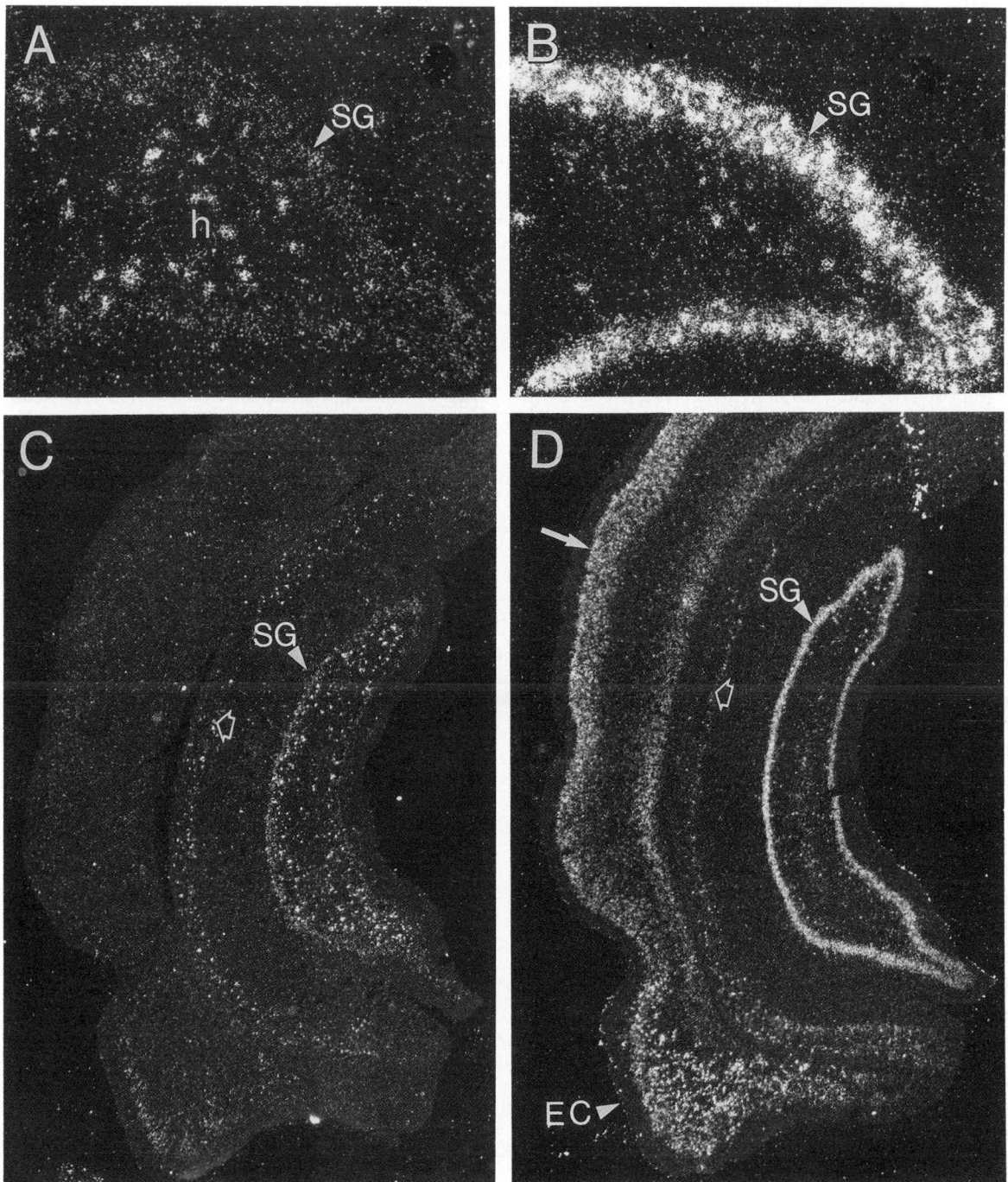

Fig. 6. Dark-field photomicrographs showing the autoradiographic localization of in situ hybridization to β-NGF mRNA in tissue sections through the dentate gyrus (A, B) and caudal hippocampus (C, D) of untreated rats (A, C) and paired HL rats sacrificed either at 3 h (B) or 24 h (D) following contralateral HL placement. Note the large increase in density of autoradiographic labeling of stratum granulosum (SG) in HL rats (B, D) as compared to controls (A, C). Seizure-dependent increases are also observed in the entorhinal cortex (EC) and the superficial and deep layers of neocortex (arrow) at 24 h postlesion (D). Open arrow (C, D) indicates the hippocampal pyramidale cell layer which does not appear to be affected by HL-induced seizures. Abbreviations: h, dentate gyrus hilus.

are heavily labeled and no increase in hybridization is evident in other populations of hippocampal neurons (Fig. 6). By 17 – 24 h post-HL, hybridization has declined somewhat within stratum granulosum but has increased slightly within stratum pyramidale, dramatically in entorhinal and piriform cortices and, most particularly in rats which exhibited a protracted behavioral seizure episode, is evident within layers II, III and VI of broad fields of neocortex. In densitometric measures of film autoradiograms from one experiment, the density of hybridization within stratum granulosum was elevated 22-fold in a rat sacrificed 3 h post-HL and 7-fold in a rat sacrificed 24 h post-HL relative to the density of hybridization in a paired control rat. In contrast, hybridization within layers II and III of neocortex remained at normal levels in the 3-h HL animal but had increased to 28-fold the control values in the 24-h HL rat. In a separate experiment, the density of hybridization to β-NGF cRNA within stratum granulosum was elevated 22-fold and 7-fold above control levels in rats sacrificed 2 and 5.5 h, respectively, following an i.c.v. injection of 0.5 μg kainic acid. These in situ hybridization results have been replicated using 3 different RNA probes complementary to β-NGF mRNA of guinea pig (Schwarz et al., 1989), mouse (Scott et al., 1983) and rat (Whittemore et al., 1988). Furthermore, nuclease protection analysis has demonstrated the increase in hybridization within hippocampus following both HL and kainic acid-induced seizures is associated with an mRNA transcript which is indistinguishable from transcript B of murine β-NGF (Selby et al., 1987; Gall and Isackson, 1989).

The seizure-induced increase in hippocampal β-NGF mRNA content exhibits characteristics of an immediate-early gene response in that it is rapid in both onset and decay. However, Mocchetti et al. (1989) have reported evidence that β-adrenergic stimulation of increased NGF mRNA expression in C6 astrocytoma may be dependent upon intermediate increases in the abundance of c-fos mRNA and Fos protein. This suggests that increases in NGF expression by hippocampal neurons following seizure might also be activated by an earlier seizure-induced increase in Fos protein. Regardless of mechanism, the observation that seizures induce a rapid increase in β-NGF mRNA within hippocampus raises the possibility that increased production of this trophic factor may play a role in more delayed neuroplastic phenomena observed in hippocampus following seizures. NGF receptor mRNA has recently been identified in rat hippocampus by nuclease protection analysis (Buck et al., 1988). As described above, the seizure-induced increase in NPY expression within hippocampus occurs much later than alterations in the c-fos, β-NGF, or PPE mRNAs and NGF has been found to stimulate the expression of neuropeptides, including NPY, in PC12 cells in vitro (Allen et al., 1987). Moreover, seizures have been found to result in the elaboration of new somatic spines (Bundman et al., 1988) and in the growth of exuberant supragranular collaterals of the mossy fibers (Sutula et al., 1988). Thus, the suggestion that seizure-induced NGF expression may regulate local changes in genomic expression and growth by hippocampal neurons is consistent with the known localization, seizure response, and trophic action of this protein.

Concluding comments

As described above, work using seizure paradigms has revealed several fundamental principles about the regulation of neuropeptide expression in hippocampus and other forebrain regions. First, these studies provide evidence that physiological activity differentially regulates the expression of synthetically distinct neuropeptide families. This "peptide specificity" is amply illustrated by the seizure-induced changes in neuropeptide expression in dentate gyrus granule cells. Results from studies using a variety of experimental paradigms indicate that seizures induce increased concentrations of enkephalin peptide and PPE mRNA, decreased concentrations of dynorphin peptide and preprodynorphin mRNA, and the novel appearance of detectable levels of preproNPY mRNA in this one population of neurons. The observation that seemingly all granule cells contain high levels of the PPE and preproNPY mRNAs one day following HL-induced seizures forces the conclusion that these peptide families co-exist and are indeed differentially regulated within individual granule cells. Moreover, differences in the temporal parameters of these seizure-induced changes in neuropeptide mRNA expression are indicative of differences in the mechanism and/or effective stimulus for induction. Again, this contrast is most clearly illustrated by consideration of changes in mRNA expression in the granule cells; the abundance of PPE mRNA is dramatically elevated within 1 h of HL-induced seizure onset whereas preproNPY mRNA is not detectably elevated until 8–10 h post-HL, well after the period of most frequent electrographic seizures in this paradigm.

Consideration of these changes in neuropeptide expression in the context of the fuller genomic response to seizure activity has provided insight into normal mechanisms of neuropeptide regulation. It is now clear from our work and that of others that the most rapid genomic response to seizure activity is increased transcription of the c-fos proto-oncogene and other immediate-early genes which encode known and putative transcriptional activation factors. The c-fos gene product is involved in transcriptional activation of what might be considered a family of genes associated with AP-1 binding sites, including preproenkephalin. Our observation of rapid seizure-induced increases in c-fos mRNA concentrations in all neuronal populations which exhibit more delayed increases in PPE mRNA is consistent with Fos-associated activation of the PPE gene in these paradigms. However, the fact that seizures induce large increases in c-fos mRNA content in neuronal groups which do not exhibit PPE mRNA expression, such as the pyramidal cells of hippocampal region CA3, demonstrates that the consequence of c-fos induction is phenotype-specific. Models of Fos action would suggest that other, yet to be identified,

phenotype-specific "target" genes may be activated by seizure in these neurons.

Finally, the results described above have significantly expanded our appreciation of the capacities and limitations of the biosynthetic activities in different populations of hippocampal neurons. It has been seen that granule cells and CA1 pyramidal cells can express NPY mRNA at high levels in response to an "appropriate" stimulus; the synthesis of NPY had not been considered a phenotypic characteristic of these neurons from studies of untreated animals. Similarly, we have seen that seizures stimulate the expression of enkephalin by all granule cells and a subpopulation of subicular neurons. In addition, the response to seizure activity has afforded the identification of specific neuronal populations which synthesize nerve growth factor and has provided the first demonstration that the expression of this trophic substance is responsive to changes in physiological activity.

In conclusion, the studies described above have demonstrated that physiological activity, in the form of recurrent electrographic seizures, leads to dramatic changes in the expression of two classes of messenger molecules: neuromodulatory peptides and at least one well-characterized neurotrophic factor. The more important issues raised by this work, which must now be addressed, are whether physiological activity within the normal range of experience similarly regulates the expression of these substances and whether such regulation represents a functionally consequential mechanism through which normal physiological activity might have an enduring effect on synaptic physiology and trophic interactions in the adult brain.

References

Allen, J.M., Martin, J.B. and Heinrich, G. (1987) Neuropeptide Y gene expression in PC12 cells and its regulation by nerve growth factor: a model for developmental regulation. *Brain Res.*, 427: 39–43.

Altschuler, R.A., Monaghan, D.T., Hasser, W.G., Wenthold, R.J., Curthoys, N.P. and Cotman, C.W. (1985) Immunocytochemical localization of glutaminase-like and aspartate aminotransferase-like immunoreactivities in the rat and guinea pig hippocampus. *Brain Res.,* 330: 225 – 233.

Baudry, M., Lynch, G. and Gall, C. (1986) Induction of ornithine decarboxylase as a possible mediator of seizure-induced changes in genomic expression in rat hippocampus. *J. Neurosci.,* 6: 3430 – 3435.

Bliss, T. and Lømo, T. (1973) Long-lasting potentiation of synaptic transmission in the dentate area of the anaesthetized rabbit following stimulation of the perforant path. *J. Physiol. (Lond.),* 232: 331 – 356.

Buck, C.R., Martinez, H.J., Chao, M.V. and Black, I.B. (1988) Differential expression of the nerve growth factor receptor gene in multiple brain areas. *Dev. Brain Res.,* 44: 259 – 268.

Bundman, M., Pico, R.M., Athanikar, J. and Gall, C.M. (1988) Novel morphological changes in hippocampal dentate granule cell perikarya following recurrent limbic seizures. *Soc. Neurosci. Abstr.,* 14: 833.

Caceres, A. and Steward, O. (1983) Dendritic reorganization in the denervated dentate gyrus of the rat following entorhinal cortical lesions: a golgi and electron microscopic analysis. *J. Comp. Neurol.,* 214: 387 – 403.

Campbell, K.A., Bank, B. and Milgram, N.W. (1984) Epileptogenic effects of electrolytic lesions in the hippocampus: role of iron deposition. *Exp. Neurol.,* 86: 506 – 514.

Chang, F.-L.F. and Greenough, W.T. (1984) Transient and enduring morphological correlates of synaptic activity and efficacy change in the rat hippocampal slice. *Brain Res.,* 309: 34 – 46.

Chiu, R., Boyle, W.J., Meek, J., Smeal, T., Hunter, T. and Karin, M. (1988) The c-Fos protein interacts with c-Jun/AP-1 to stimulate transcription of AP1 responsive genes. *Cell,* 54: 541 – 552.

Comb, M., Mermod, N., Hyman, S.E., Pearlberg, J., Ross, M.E. and Goodman, H.M. (1988) Proteins bound at adjacent DNA elements act synergistically to regulate human pro-enkephalin cAMP inducible transcription. *EMBO J.,* 7: 3793 – 3805.

Crawford, I.L. and Connor, J.D. (1973) Localization and release of glutamic acid in relation to the hippocampal mossy fibre pathway. *Nature (Lond.),* 244: 442 – 443.

Curran, T. and Morgan, J.I. (1987) Memories of fos. *Bio Essays,* 7: 255 – 258.

Davis, L.G., Arentzen, R., Reid, J.M., Manning, R.W., Wolfson, B., Lawrence, K.L. and Baldino, Jr., R. (1986) Glucocorticoid sensitivity of vasopressin mRNA levels in the paraventricular nucleus of the rat. *Proc. Natl. Acad. Sci. U.S.A.,* 83: 1145 – 1149.

Dragunow, M. and Robertson, H.A. (1987) Kindling stimulation induces *c-fos* protein(s) in granule cells of the rat dentate gyrus. *Nature (Lond.),* 329: 441 – 442.

Fredens, K., Stengaard-Pedersen, K. and Larsson, L.-T. (1984) Localization of enkephalin and cholecystokinin im-

munoreactivities in the perforant path terminal fields of the rat hippocampal formation. *Brain Res.,* 304: 255 – 263.

Fredens, K., Stengaard-Pederson, K. and Wallace, M.N. (1987) Localization of cholecystokinin in the dentate commissural-associational system of the mouse and rat. *Brain Res.,* 401: 68 – 78.

Gall, C. (1984a) The distribution of cholecystokinin-like immunoreactivity in the hippocampal formation of the guinea pig: localization in the mossy fibers. *Brain Res.,* 306: 73 – 83.

Gall, C. (1984b) Ontogeny of dynorphin-like immunoreactivity in the hippocampal formation of the rat. *Brain Res.,* 307: 327 – 331.

Gall, C. (1988) Seizures induce dramatic and distinctly different changes in enkephalin, dynorphin, and cholecystokinin immunoreactivities in mouse hippocampal mossy fibers. *J. Neurosci.,* 8: 1852 – 1862.

Gall, C. (1990) Comparative anatomy of the hippocampus with special reference to differences in the distributions of neuroactive peptides. In E.G. Jones and A. Peters (Eds.), *The Cerebral Cortex, Vol. 8,* Plenum Publishing Corp., New York, in press.

Gall, C. and Isackson, P. (1989) Limbic seizures increase neuronal production of mRNA for nerve growth factor. *Science.,* 245: 758 – 761.

Gall, C., Brecha, N., Karten, H.J. and Chang, K.-J. (1981) Localization of enkephalin-like immunoreactivity in identified axonal and neuronal populations in the rat hippocampus. *J. Comp. Neurol.,* 198: 335 – 350.

Gall, C., Berry, L. and Hodgson, L. (1986a) Cholecystokinin in the mouse hippocampus: localization in the mossy fiber and dentate commissural system. *Exp. Brain Res.,* 62: 431 – 437.

Gall, C., Ivy, G. and Lynch, G. (1986b) Neuroanatomical plasticity: its role in organizing and reorganizing the central nervous system. In F. Falkner and J.M. Tanner (Eds.), *Human Growth, Vol. 2,* Plenum Publishing Corp., New York, pp. 411 – 436.

Gall, C., White, J.D. and Lauterborn, J.C. (1987) In situ hybridization analyses of increased preproenkaphalin mRNA following seizures. *Soc. Neurosci. Abstr.,* 13: 1277.

Gall, C., Arai, A. and White, J. (1988a) Localization of increased *c-fos* mRNA content in rat CNS following recurrent seizures. *Soc. Neurosci. Abstr.,* 14: 1161.

Gall, C., Pico, R. and Lauterborn, J. (1988b) Seizures induce distinct long-lasting changes in mossy fiber peptide immunoreactivity. *Peptides,* 9: 79 – 84.

Gall, C.M., Murray, K.D. and Isackson, P.J. (1989) Kainic acid-induced seizures stimulate increased expression of β-NGF mRNA in adult rat forebrain. *Soc. Neurosci. Abstr.,* 15: 864.

Gnahn, H., Hefti, F., Heumann, R., Schwab, M.E. and Thoenen, H. (1983) NGF-mediated increase of choline acetyltransferase (ChAT) in the neonatal rat forebrain: evidence for a physiological role of NGF in the brain? *Dev.*

Brain Res., 9: 45 – 52.

Greenwood, R.S., Godar, S., Reaves Jr., T.A. and Wayward, J. (1981) Cholecystokinin in hippocampal pathways. *J. Comp. Neurol.,* 203: 335 – 350.

Harlan, R.E. (1988) Regulation of neuropeptide gene expression by steroid hormones. *Mol. Neurobiol.,* 2: 183 – 200.

Harris, Q.L.G., Lewis, S.J., Shulkes, A., Vajda, F.J.E. and Jarrott, B. (1988) Regional brain concentrations of cholecystokinin in the rat: the effects of kindled and non-kindled seizures. *Neuropharmacology,* 27: 547 – 550.

Higuchi, H., Yang, H.-Y.T. and Sabol, S.L. (1988) Rat neuropeptide Y precursor gene expression. *J. Biol. Chem.,* 263: 6288 – 6295.

Hong, J.S., Wood, P.L., Gillin, J.C., Yang, H.Y.T. and Costa, E. (1980) Changes of hippocampal Met-enkephalin content after recurrent motor seizures. *Nature (Lond.),* 285: 231 – 232.

Hyman, S.E., Comb, M., Pearlberg, J. and Goodman, H.M. (1989) An AP-2 element acts synergistically with the cyclic AMP- and phorbol ester-inducible enhancer of the human proenkephalin gene. *Mol. Cell. Biol.,* 9: 321 – 324.

Iadarola, M.J., Shin, C., McNamara, J.O. and Yang, H.Y.T. (1986) Changes in dynorphin, enkephalin and cholecystokinin content of hippocampus and substantia nigra after amygdala kindling, *Brain Res.,* 365: 181 – 191.

Kanamatsu, T., McGinty, J.F., Mitchell, C.L. and Hong, J.S. (1986a) Dynorphin- and enkephalin-like immunoreactivity is altered in limbic-basal ganglia regions of rat brain after repeated electroconvulsive shock. *J. Neurosci.,* 6: 644 – 649.

Kanamatsu, T., Obie, J., Grimes, L., McGinty, J.F., Yoshikawa, K., Sabol, S. and Hong, J.S. (1986b) Kainic acid alters the metabolism of Met^5-enkephalin and the level of dynorphin A in the rat hippocampus. *J. Neurosci.,* 6: 3094 – 3102.

Köhler, C. (1986) Cytochemical architecture of the entorhinal area. In R. Schwarcz and Y. Ben-Ari (Eds.), *Excitatory Amino Acids and Epilepsy,* Plenum Press, New York, pp. 83 – 98.

Köhler, C., Eriksson, L., Davies, S. and Chan-Palay, V. (1986) Neuropeptide Y innervation of the hippocampal region in the rat and monkey brain. *J. Comp. Neurol.,* 244: 384 – 400.

Kosaka, T., Kosaka, K., Teteishi, K., Hamaoka, Y., Yanaihara, N., Wu, J.-Y. and Hama, K. (1985) Gabaergic neurons containing CCK-I-like and/or VIP-like immunoreactivities in the rat hippocampus and dentate gyrus. *J. Comp. Neurol.,* 239: 420 – 430.

Larson, J. and Lynch, G. (1988) Role of N-methyl-D-aspartate receptors in the induction of synaptic potentiation by burst stimulation patterned after the hippocampal theta rhythm. *Brain Res.,* 441: 111 – 118.

Lee, K.S., Schottler, F., Oliver, M. and Lynch, G. (1980) Brief bursts of high-frequency stimulation produce two types of structural change in rat hippocampus. *J. Neurophysiol.,* 44: 247 – 257.

Le Gal La Salle, G. (1988) Long-lasting and sequential increase of *c-fos* oncoprotein expression in kainic acid-induced status epilepticus. *Neurosci. Lett.,* 88: 127 – 130.

Maniatis, T., Goodbourn, S. and Fischer, J.A. (1987) Regulation of inducible and tissue-specific gene expression. *Science,* 236: 1237 – 1244.

McGinty, J.F. (1985) Prodynorphin immunoreactivity is located in different neurons than proenkephalin immunoreactivity in the cerebral cortex of rats. *Neuropeptides,* 5: 465 – 468.

McGinty, J.F., Henriksen, S.J., Goldstein, A., Terenius, L. and Bloom, F.E. (1983) Dynorphin is contained within hippocampal mossy fibers: immunohistochemical alterations after kainic acid administration and colchicine-induced cytotoxcity. *Proc. Natl. Acad. Sci. U.S.A.,* 80: 589 – 593.

McGinty, J.F., Van Der Kooy, D. and Bloom, F.E. (1984) The distribution of opioid peptide immunoreactive neurons in the cerebral cortex of rats. *J. Neurosci.,* 4: 1104 – 1117.

McGinty, J.F., Kanamatsu, T., Obie, J., Dyer, R.S., Mitchell, C.L. and Hong, J.S. (1986) Amygdaloid kindling increases enkephalin-like immunoreactivity but decreases dynorphin A-like immunoreactivity in rat hippocampus. *Neurosci. Lett.,* 71: 31 – 36.

McKnight, S. and Tjian, R. (1986) Transcriptional selectivity of viral genes in mammalian cells. *Cell,* 46: 795 – 805.

Meyer, D.K., Widmann, R. and Sperk, G. (1986) Increased brain levels of cholecystokinin octapeptide after kainic acid-induced seizures in the rat. *Neurosci. Lett.,* 69: 208 – 211.

Mobley, W.C., Rutkowski, J.L., Tennekoon, G.I., Buchanan, K. and Johnston, M.V. (1985) Choline acetyltransferase activity in striatum of neonatal rats increased by nerve growth factor. *Science,* 229: 284 – 287.

Mocchetti, I., De Bernardi, M.A., Szekely, A.M., Alho, H., Brooker, G. and Costa, E. (1989) Regulation of nerve growth factor biosynthesis by β-adrenergic receptor activation in astrocytoma cells: a potential role of c-Fos protein. *Proc. Natl. Acad. Sci. U.S.A.,* 86: 3891 – 3895.

Morgan, J.I., Cohen, D.R., Hempstead, J.L. and Curran, T. (1987) Mapping patterns of *c-fos* expression in the central nervous system after seizure. *Science,* 237: 192 – 197.

Morris, B.J., Moneta, M.E., Bruggencate, G. ten and Hollt, V. (1987) Levels of prodynorphin mRNA in rat dentate gyrus are decreased during hippocampal kindling. *Neurosci. Lett.,* 80: 298 – 302.

Morris, B.J., Feasley, K.J., Bruggencate, G. ten, Herz, A. and Hollt, V. (1988) Electrical stimulation in vivo increases the expression of proenkephalin mRNA and decreases the expression of prodynorphin mRNA in rat hippocampal granule cells. *Proc. Natl. Acad. Sci. U.S.A.,* 85: 3226 – 3230.

Naranjo, J.R., Iadarola, M.J. and Costa, E. (1986) Changes in the dynamic state of brain proenkephalin-derived peptides during amygdaloid kindling. *J. Neurosci. Res.,* 16: 75 – 87.

Parnavelas, A.J., Lynch, G., Brecha, N., Cotman, C.W. and Globus, A. (1974) Spine loss and regrowth in hippocampus

390

following deafferentation. *Nature (Lond.),* 248: 71 – 73.

Quantin, B. and Breathnach, R. (1988) Epidermal growth factor stimulates transcription of the *c-jun* proto-oncogene in rat fibroblasts. *Nature (Lond.),* 334: 538 – 539.

Racine, R. (1972) Modulation of seizure activity by electrical stimulation: II. Motor seizure. *Electroenceph. Clin. Neurophysiol.,* 32: 281 – 294.

Romano, G.J., Shivers, B.D., Harlan, R.E., Howells, R.D. and Pfaff, D.W. (1987) Haloperidol increases preproenkephalin mRNA levels in the caudate-putamen of the rat: a quantitative study at the cellular level using *in situ* hybridization. *Mol. Brain Res.,* 2: 33 – 41.

Saffen, D.W., Cole, A.J., Worley, P.F., Christy, B.A., Ryder, K. and Baraban, J.M. (1988) Convulsant-induced increase in transcription factor messenger RNAs in rat brain. *Proc. Natl. Acad. Sci. U.S.A.,* 85: 7795 – 7799.

Sawchenko, P.E. (1987) Adrenalectomy-induced enhancement of CRF and vasopressin immunoreactivity in parvocellular neurosecretory neurons: anatomic, peptide and steroid specificity. *J. Neurosci.,* 7: 1093 – 1106.

Schwarz, M.A., Fisher, D., Bradshaw, R.A. and Isackson, P.J. (1989) Isolation and sequence of a cDNA clone of β-nerve growth factor from the guinea pig prostate gland. *J. Neurochem.,* 52: 1203 – 1209.

Scott, J., Selby, M., Urdea, M., Quiroga, M., Bell, G.I. and Rutter, W.J. (1983) Isolation and nucleotide sequence of a cDNA encoding the precursor of mouse nerve growth factor. *Nature (Lond.),* 302: 538 – 540.

Selby, M.J., Edwards, R., Sharp, F. and Rutter, W.J. (1987) Mouse nerve growth factor gene: structure and expression. *Mol. Cell. Biol.,* 7: 3057 – 3064.

Shelton, D.L. and Reichardt, L.F. (1986) Studies on the expression of the beta nerve growth factor (NGF) gene in the central nervous system; level and regional distribution of NGF mRNA suggest that NGF functions as a trophic factor for several distinct populations of neurons. *Proc. Natl. Acad. Sci. U.S.A.,* 83: 2714 – 2718.

Sloviter, R.S. and Damiano, B.P. (1981) On the relationship between kainic acid-induced epileptiform activity and hippocampal neuronal damage. *Neuropharmacology,* 20: 1003 – 1011.

Stengaard-Pederson, K., Fredens, K. and Larsson, L.-I. (1983) Comparative localization of enkephalin and cholecystokinin immunoreactivities and heavy metals in the hippocampus. *Brain Res.,* 273: 81 – 96.

Sutula, T., He, X.X., Cavazos, J. and Scott, G. (1988) Synaptic reorganization in hippocampus induced by abnormal functional activity. *Science,* 239: 1147 – 1150.

Weber, E. and Barchas, J.D. (1983) Immunohistochemical distribution of dynorphin B in rat brain: relation to dynorphin A and α-neo-endorphin systems. *Proc. Natl. Acad. Sci. U.S.A.,* 80: 1125 – 1129.

White, J.D. and Gall, C.M. (1987a) Increased enkephalin gene expression in hippocampus following seizures. In J.W. Holliday, P.Y. Law, and A. Herz (Eds.), *Progress in Opioid Research.,* NIDA Research Monograph, pp. 393 – 396.

White, J.D. and Gall, C.M. (1987b) Differential regulation of neuropeptide and proto-oncogene mRNA content in the hippocampus following recurrent seizures. *Mol. Brain Res.,* 3: 21 – 29.

White, J.D., Gall, C.M. and McKelvy, J.F. (1986) Evidence for projection-specific processing of proenkephalin in the rat central nervous system. *Proc. Natl. Acad. Sci. U.S.A.,* 83: 7099 – 7103.

White, J.D., Gall, C.M. and McKelvy, J.F. (1987) Enkephalin biosynthesis and enkephalin gene expression are increased in hippocampal mossy fibers following a unilateral lesion of the hilus. *J. Neurosci.,* 7: 753 – 759.

Whittemore, S.R., Friedman, P.L., Larhammar, D., Persson, H., Gonzalez-Carvajal, M. and Holets, V.R. (1988) Rat β-nerve growth factor sequence and site of synthesis in the adult hippocampus. *J. Neurosci. Res.,* 20: 403 – 410.

Yoshikawa, K., Williams, C. and Sabol, S.L. (1984) Rat brain preproenkephalin mRNA. *J. Biol Chem.,* 259: 14301 – 14308.

Young, S.W., III, Bonner, T.I. and Brann, M.R. (1986) Mesencephalic dopamine neurons regulate the expression of neuropeptide mRNAs in the rat forebrain. *Proc. Natl. Acad. Sci. U.S.A.,* 83: 9827 – 9831.

Yount, G.L., Gall, C.M. and White, J.D. (1989) Stimulation of hippocampal preproneuropeptide Y expression following recurrent seizure. *Soc. Neurosci. Abstr.,* 15: 1274.

J. Storm-Mathisen, J. Zimmer and O.P. Ottersen (Eds.)
Progress in Brain Research, Vol. 83
© 1990 Elsevier Science Publishers B.V. (Biomedical Division)

CHAPTER 28

Grafting of fetal CA3 neurons to excitotoxic, axon-sparing lesions of the hippocampal CA3 area in adult rats

Niels Tønder, Torben Sørensen and Jens Zimmer

PharmaBiotec, Institute of Neurobiology, University of Aarhus, DK-8000 Aarhus C, Denmark

Hippocampal CA3 neurons from fetal rats were grafted to excitotoxic lesions in the CA3 subfield of the adult rat hippocampus and the formation of graft – host brain nerve connections examined. The excitotoxic lesions were induced by localized, stereotaxic injection of ibotenic acid (IA), a glutamic acid agonist, into CA3 of the dorsal hippocampus. The result was a so-called axon-sparing lesion with localized degeneration of nerve cells, but preservation of the extrinsic afferent fibers, now deprived of their targets. One week after the lesion a suspension of embryonic (E18 – 20) CA3 cells was grafted to the lesion site. Six weeks or more later the recipient brains were processed and analyzed by ordinary cell stains, histochemistry for acetylcholinesterase (AChE) and heavy metals (Timm staining), immunohistochemistry for the neuropeptides cholecystokinin and somatostatin and glial fibrillary acidic protein (GFAP) for astroglia, electron microscopy, and axonal tracing with retrogradely axonal transported fluorescent dyes or lesion-induced, anterograde degeneration combined with silver staining or electron microscopy. More than 90% of the grafts survived. They contained the normal types of CA3 neurons, which are mainly pyramidal cells, in addition to some normal, peptidergic, cholecystokinin- and somatostatin-reactive neurons. The grafts were innervated by AChE-positive, host cholinergic fibers, Timm-positive mossy fiber terminals from the host fascia dentata, and host commissural fibers traced by axonal degeneration. Efferent transplant projections were traced to the ipsilateral host CA1 (Schaffer collaterals) and the contralateral host hippocampus by retrograde axonal transport of fluorochromes injected into these host brain areas. All grafts analyzed by electron microscopy contained axonal varicosities resembling axonal growth cones even after long survival times. The results demonstrate that fetal rat hippocampal neurons, grafted to excitotoxic, axon-sparing lesions in the adult brain, can become both structurally and connectively well incorparated in the mature host central nervous system.

Introduction

Intracerebral transplantation of hippocampal and fascia dentata tissue has been used to study the development, plasticity and regenerative capacity of central nervous neurons and nerve connections (Sunde and Zimmer, 1983; Sunde et al., 1984; Zimmer and Sunde, 1984; Zimmer et al., 1985, 1986, 1987, 1988a, b, c). This includes repair of an induced maldevelopment of the neuronal circuitry in both newborn (Sunde et al., 1984, 1985) and adult rats (Sunde et al., 1985). Granule cells in the fascia dentata damaged by X-irradiation at birth can thus partly be replaced by homotypic

transplants of immature fascia dentata (Sunde et al., 1984, 1985). The exchange of connections depends, however, on the age of the recipient animal. In animals X-irradiated and grafted at birth there is a higher degree of nerve fiber exchange than in animals X-irradiated at birth, but with a delay of grafting into adulthood (Sunde et al., 1985). We have, however, recently shown that homotypic grafts placed in so-called axon-sparing lesions of the hippocampal subfield CA1, induced by transient cerebral ischemia (Tønder et al., 1989a), or corresponding lesions of the fascia dentata, induced by localized injection of the excitotoxic glutamate analogue, ibotenic acid (IA)

(Tønder et al., 1989b), can receive extensive nerve connections from the adult host brain. The growth of host brain perforant path fibers into fascia dentata transplants placed in the IA-lesioned host fascia dentata was thus alsmost as extensive as the ingrowth observed after grafting to newborn, X-irradiated animals (Tønder et al., 1989b). We suggest that the axon-sparing lesion promotes the ingrowth of adult host fibers into the grafts, presumably by priming the growth capacity of these fibers. To extend these experiments and further validate our suggestion we now describe and discuss the exchange of nerve connections between graft and host brain after transplantation of cell suspensions of late embryonic CA3 tissue into ibotenic acid lesions of the adult hippocampal CA3 area.

Materials and methods

Young adult 150 g Wistar rats of both sexes were used. For ibotenic acid lesion Nembutal-anesthetized rats were fixed in a Kopf stereotaxic apparatus with the incisor bar at 3.3 mm below the interaural line. A bore hole was made unilaterally in the skull 3 mm posterior to Bregma and 3.2 mm lateral (right) to the midline. At this position the needle of a 5 μl Hamilton syringe was lowered vertically, to a position 3.3 mm below the dura, and 0.5 μl of a 1% w/v solution of ibotenic acid (IA) (Sigma) dissolved in phosphate buffer, pH 7.4, was injected for 5 min. The needle was kept in place for an additional 5 min to allow for diffusion of the drug and prevent reflux through the needle tract. A total of 66 rats were injected and afterwards subjected to one of three procedures. After one week 43 rats were injected with a cell suspension of fetal hippocampal CA3 tissue into the IA lesion (see below). Six other rats were sacrificed at this time for examination of the appearance of the IA lesion at the time of transplantation. A further 17 non-grafted rats were allowed to survive for another 2 – 9 months for examination of the long-term appearance of the IA-lesion, including the possible reorganization of the remaining tissue and neuronal pathways.

At sacrifice the lesion-control rats were deeply anesthetized with Nembutal and processed according to one of three methods: (1) after perfusion through the heart for 4 – 5 min with a sulfide solution (0.5% Na_2S and 0.5% NaH_2PO_4, H_2O) brains ($n = 15$) were frozen and sectioned frontally at 30 μm on a cryostat and mounted on glass slides. Parallel series of sections were processed with the Timm method to monitor the distribution of major hippocampal and dentate afferent projections (Timm, 1958; Haug, 1973), acetylcholinesterase staining for cholinergic projections (Geneser-Jensen and Blackstad, 1971) and thionine cell staining; (2) after 4 – 5 min perfusion with a phosphate-buffered 4% paraformaldehyde solution brains ($n = 8$) were sectioned at 50 μm in the frontal plane on a Vibratome. These sections were stained immunocytochemically with antibodies against cholecystokinin (CCK) (1 : 1200; gift from Prof. Rehfeld, Copenhagen), somatostatin (SS) (1 : 4000; from Ferring, Kiel, F.R.G.), and an astroglial marker, glial fibrillary acidic protein (GFAP) (1 : 3000; DAKOPATTS, Copenhagen), using the unlabelled antibody peroxidase-antiperoxidase method by Sternberger (1979) as previously reported (Zimmer and Sunde, 1984). Some sections were counterstained with Toluidine blue; (3) after 15 min perfusion with a mixture of 1% glutaraldehyde and 1% paraformaldehyde in 0.1 M phosphate buffer (pH 7.4) brains ($n = 7$) were processed for conventional electron microscopy (Sørensen and Zimmer, 1988a, b).

Transplantation

The *donor* tissue was obtained from Wistar rat embryos of gestational age 18 – 20. The embryos were removed from Nembutal-anesthetized dams and their brains removed in toto and placed in a solution of 0.6% glucose and 0.9% NaCl. By separating the two hemispheres in the midline the hippocampal regions were exposed in the medial wall of the hemispheres. After dissecting out the entire hippocampal region, tissue blocks containing the CA3 subfield were separated from the CA1 subfield and the fascia dentata. Blocks of CA3 tissue from 5 – 8 fetuses were collected in a small well until further processing involving the preparation of a cell suspension essentially as described by Björklund et al. (1983). The tissue was incubated for 20 min at 37°C in 250 µl of a glucose-saline solution containing 0.025% w/v of trypsin (Sigma type 3). After 4 – 5 changes with glucose-saline a final volume of 5 – 10 µl of this solution was added per tissue block and the tissue tritiated with cannulas of gradually smaller diameters. This resulted in a milky fluid with suspended single cells, and occasional small cell blocks. The viability of the cells in suspension was estimated by the Trypan blue test. A drop of 0.5% Trypan blue in distilled water was mixed with 5 µl of the cell suspension on a glass slide, coverslipped and examined microscopically. Using the criterion that only dead cells take up the dye and stain, a viability of approximately 70% of the cells in suspension was estimated.

For transplantation 43 IA-lesioned rats were reanesthetized with Nembutal one week after the IA injection and placed in a Kopf stereotaxic apparatus. The borehole in the skull overlying the dorsal hippocampus was re-opened and 5 µl of the freshly prepared cell suspension injected over 5 min by a 5 µl Hamilton syringe into the IA injection site in the dorsal hippocampus. The needle was left in place for an extra 5 min to minimize reflux of the suspension in the needle track.

The rats were sacrificed between 6 weeks and 1 year after grafting, most after 6 – 8 weeks. Twenty-four of them were perfused with the sulfide solution and parallel series of 30 µm thick cryostat sections of the brain were processed for (1) *Timm staining* in order to visualize possible Timm-stained mossy fiber terminals of host rat origin in the grafts, (2) *AChE staining* in order to trace host AChE-positive cholinergic afferents to the grafts, and (3) ordinary cell stains to show the cellular organization of the grafts. Ten rats were used for *axonal tracing by retrograde axonal transport of fluorochromes*. Four rats were injected stereotaxically with 0.1 µl of a 2% Fluoro-Gold (FG) solution in distilled water into the dorsal hippocampus contralateral to the transplants at a position 4 mm posterior to Bregma, 3 mm lateral to the midline and 3 mm ventral to the dura. Six rats received an injection of 0.1 – 0.2 µl of a 2% FG solution into posterior and temporal parts of the hippocampus on the transplanted side using a lateral approach through the temporal bone. All fluorochrome injections were made 6 – 7 days before the rats were deeply anesthetized with Nembutal and perfused for 10 min with 400 ml of a 4% formaldehyde solution containing 4% sucrose and 4% magnesium sulfate. After removal from the skull the brains were soaked in 30% sucrose overnight, frozen in gaseous CO_2 and cut in the frontal plane in serial 30 µm thick cryostat sections. Adjacent sets of serial sections were stained with Toluidine blue, stained for AChE or coverslipped in Entellan for fluorescent microscopy of the fluorescent dye tracer. Two rats were perfused with the phosphate-buffered 4% paraformaldehyde solution 6 weeks after transplantation, and their brains sectioned at 50 µm on a Vibratome. Sections through the lesion and graft site were immunohistochemically stained for CCK, SS, and GFAP (see lesion controls).

Seven rats were perfused for 15 min with a mixture of 1% paraformaldehyde and 1% glutaraldehyde in 0.1 M phosphate buffer (pH 7.4) and processed for electron microscopy 2 – 4 months after grafting. Three days before sacrifice 5 rats had the hippocampal commissures transected next to the midline on the non-grafted side in order to trace host hippocampal commissural connections to the grafts by anterograde electron dense, axonal degeneration.

Results

The cell and neuropil layers of the dorsal hippocampus in the normal rat are shown in Fig. 1a, together with the normal laminar distribution of the major hippocampal connections shown in

Timm staining (Fig. 1b) and the normal distribution of AChE-positive, cholinergic septo-hippocampal projection (Fig. 1c). The major hippocampal nerve connections of the CA3 region are shown schematically in Fig. 1d. The normal distribution of CCK- and SS-immunoreactive nonpyramidal neurons and terminal fields are shown in Figs. 3a and c, respectively.

Lesion controls with IA injections only

The damage caused by the focal IA injections was examined after one week (Fig. 2a–c) and 2 months (Fig. 2d–f). With the dose injected the damage affected an approximately 3 mm long segment of the dorsal hippocampus. At its maximum the lesion included not only CA3 but also adjacent parts, or in a few cases all, of CA1 and the dentate granule cell layer.

After one week an almost total loss of neurons was seen in and around the injection site (Fig. 2a) with a dinstict transition zone towards the intact areas. This transition zone sharpened with increasing survival time (Fig. 2d). In addition to the pyramidal cells (Fig. 2a and d) also the CCK- and SS-immunoreactive cells disappeared (Fig. 3b and d), leaving few, if any, neuron-like cells in the IA-injected area. Accompanying the loss of neurons there was heavy gliosis of both cell and neuropil layers as shown by the hypertrophy and increased

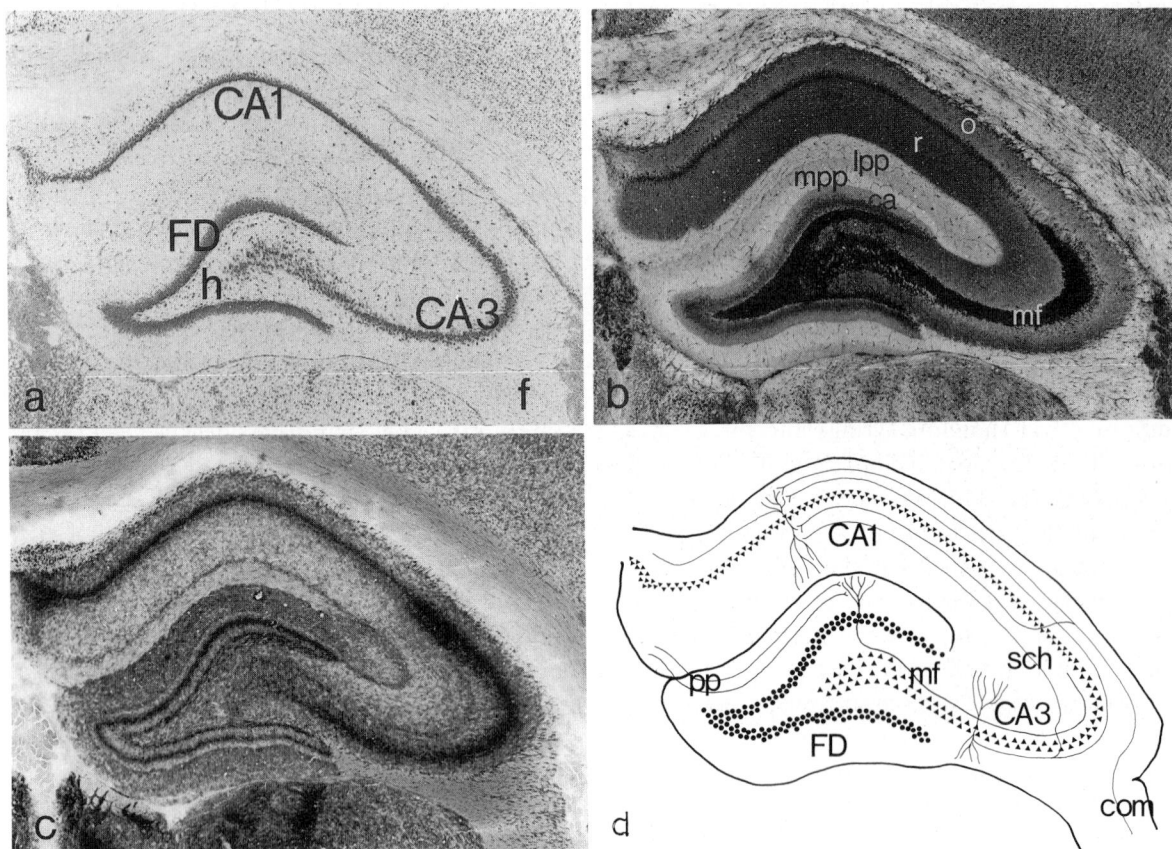

Fig. 1. The dorsal part of the normal adult hippocampus in frontal thionine- (a), Timm- (b) and AChE-stained (c) sections. d: schematic presentation of major intrinsic hippocampal pathways. Note distinct laminar organization of both cell layers (a) and afferent pathways (a–d). ×18.4.

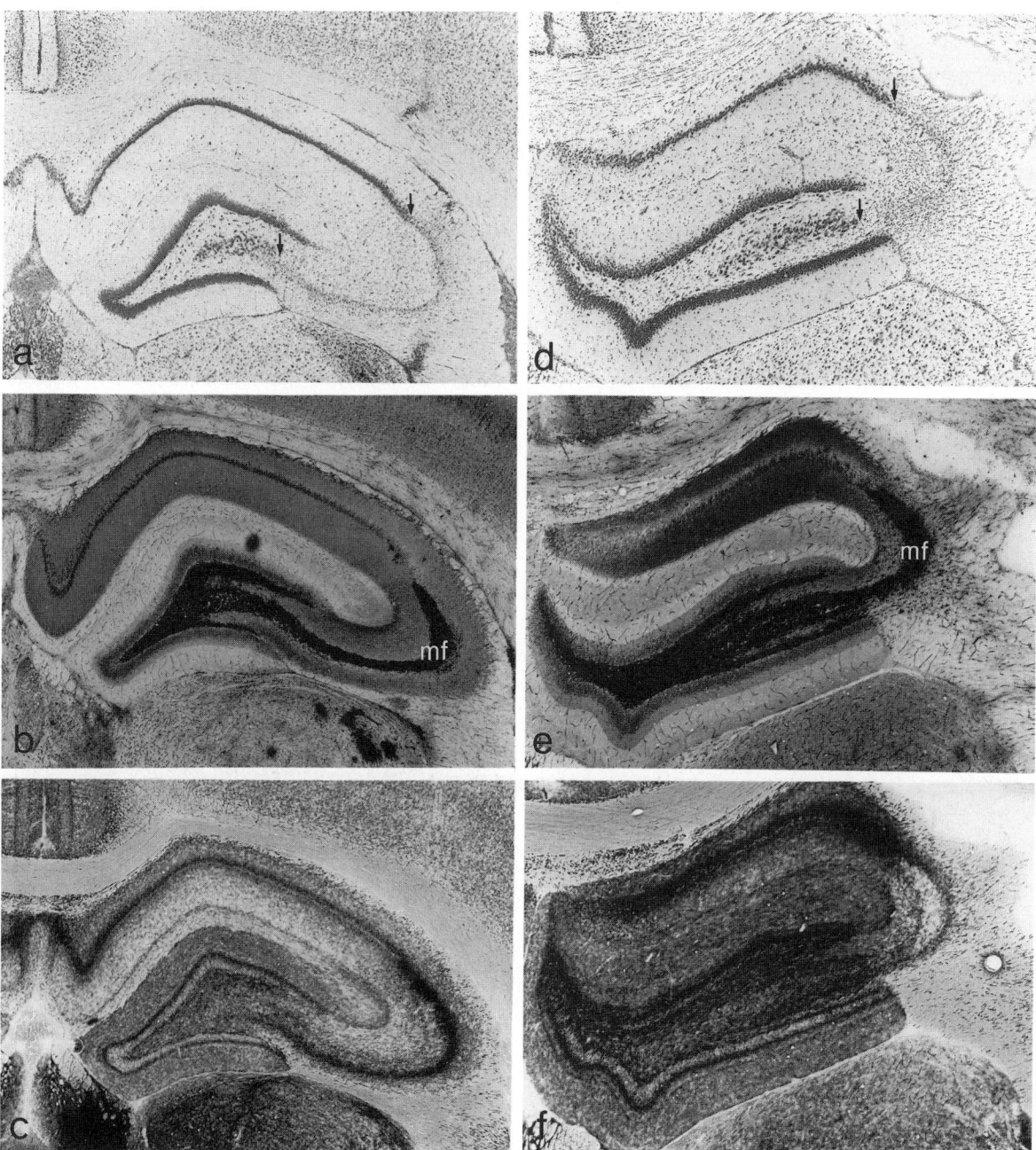

Fig. 2. Thionine- (a, d), Timm- (b, e) and AChE-stained (c, f) sections through 1- (a – c) and 8-week-old (d – f) ibotenic acid lesion of the CA3 region. The pyramidal cells are lost after 1 week (between arrows; a), but Timm-stained mossy fiber terminals (mf, b) and AChE-positive cholinergic afferents (c) persist. Note also persistence of other terminal-related Timm staining in CA3 (b). After 8 weeks the lesioned area is atrophic, with only slight decrease in terminal field, Timm- and AChE-staining (e, f). ×18 (a – c), ×26 (d – f).

GFAP reactivity (Fig. 4) and Timm stainability (Fig. 2b) of astrocytes. The damaged CA3 pyramidal cell layer was infiltrated by cells with small, densely stained nuclei seen in cell staining (Fig. 2a). A reactive gliosis, although slightly weaker, was also observed in the contralateral CA3 at corresponding septo-temporal levels, i.e., the levels most heavily innervated by the lesioned CA3 pyramidal cells.

After *one week* there was no apparent change in the distribution of afferents in the lesioned area as observed in Timm staining for hippocampal afferents (Fig. 2b) and AChE staining for septohippocampal afferents (Fig. 2c). The Timm staining displayed its normal laminar pattern, corresponding to the distribution of the major afferent associational and commissural connections,

although the colors were slightly altered with a reddish hue of the staining in str. radiatum, str. oriens and str. moleculare. This indicates some ongoing degenerative reaction in the terminal fields (Haug et al., 1971). As observed in the Timm staining the mossy fiber zone stood out as a normal, densely stained band along the damaged pyramidal cell layer (Fig. 2b). Also the staining for AChE showed a near normal lamination in the neuropil with highest activity as normally around the now damaged pyramidal cell layer, in the mossy fiber zone and in the str. oriens (Fig. 2c). Despite the total loss of neurons, afferents to the area were accordingly still present (axon-sparing lesion). After longer survival times of *2 – 9 months* there was a pronounced atrophy of the lesioned CA3 area (Fig. 2d – f) with heavy, condensed gliosis. A distinct

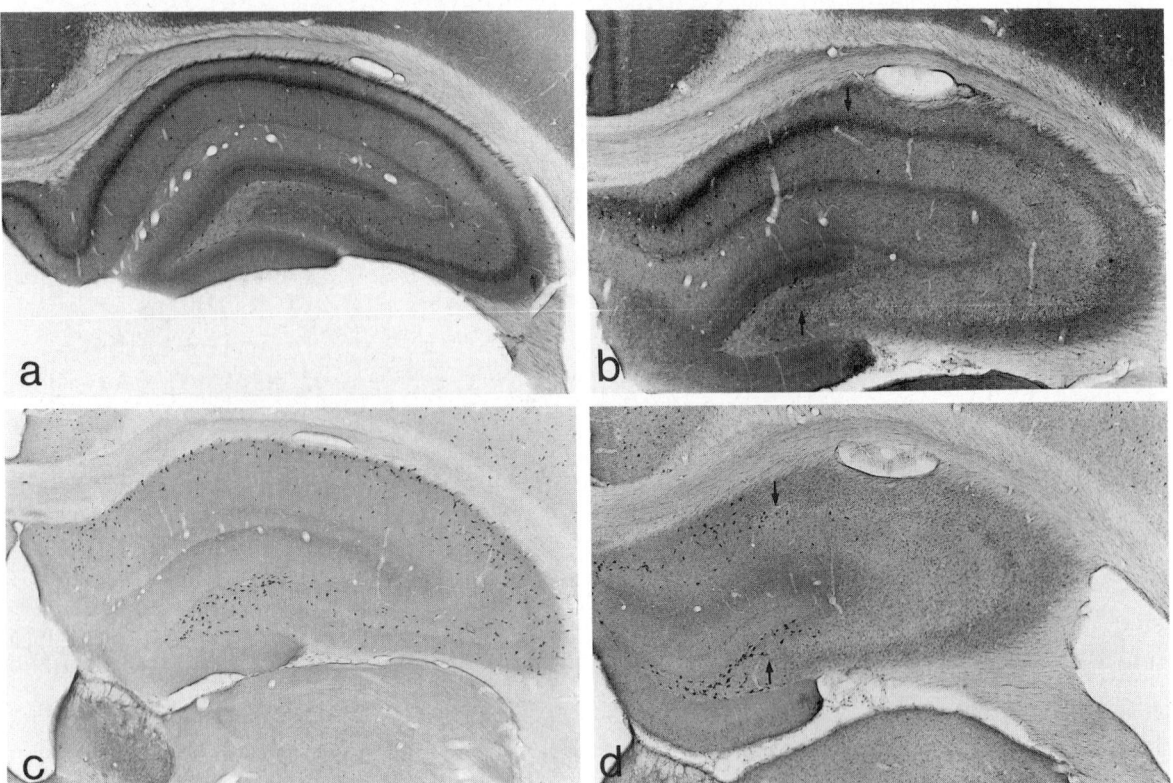

Fig. 3. Cholecystokinin- (CCK) (a, b) and somatostatin- (SS) (c, d) immunohistochemically stained sections through the dorsal part of the normal hippocampus (a, c), and one week after IA injection damaging CA3 and part of CA1 (between arrows) (b – d). Note loss of CCK- (b) and SS-stained neurons (d) in lesioned area. × 19.

laminar Timm staining of the neuropil was still present, although there was a decrease in the density of the terminal-like staining (Fig. 2e). This staining was also to some degree obscured by the Timm staining of cell bodies and processes of reactive astrocytes. Also the AChE staining retained a normal laminar distribution, but again the density was lower than normal in all layers (Fig. 2f). The observations after longer survival times accordingly indicate that afferents remain in the lesioned area, although they may have gone through some kind of reorganization.

General histological organization of CA3 transplants

Transplants were recovered in 40 of the 43 IA-lesioned and grafted rats, although the size of the grafts did vary considerably. Some grafts only consisted of a few groups of pyramidal-like neurons located within the lesioned host hippocampus. Others were very large and filled out the entire IA lesion, sometimes causing distortion of the surrounding, normal host brain tissue. Most grafts were centered within the lesioned area (Fig. 5), but some extended dorsally through the corpus callosum into the overlying neocortex or ventrally in the thalamus, or both.

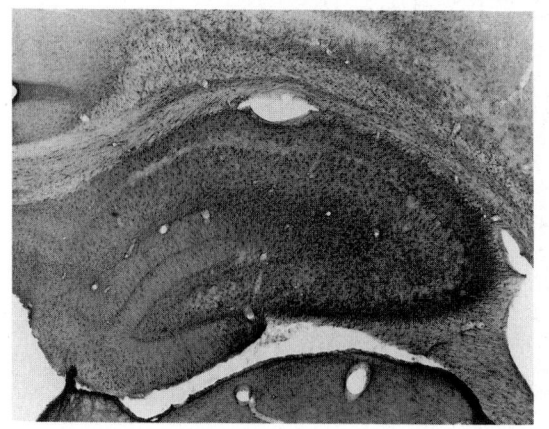

Fig. 4. GFAP-stained section showing reactive astrogliosis in 1-week-old IA lesion of the dorsal hippocampus. The section is adjacent to sections shown in Fig. 3b and d. ×17.5.

All grafts contained large pyramidal-like neurons which tended to be arranged in small clusters separated by neuropil. In some of the smaller grafts the pyramidal cells seemed to arrange themselves around the damaged host pyramidal cell layer (Fig. 5a and b). In addition to pyramidal cells the grafts also contained neuropeptidergic, non-pyramidal neurons, which reacted immunohistochemically for CCK and SS (Fig. 6a and b). Such neurons are normally present in CA3. In the grafts they were not arranged in special patterns, but were scattered throughout the transplants with a higher density of SS- than CCK-reactive neurons. *Dentate granule cells were not observed in any of the grafts.*

In general the grafts showed a near normal astroglial staining density for GFAP (Fig. 6c), but a slight gliosis was commonly observed next to and at the host – graft interface. A reactive gliosis with a density of GFAP-staining equal to that in the IA-lesioned host CA3 was never observed in the grafts. Also the distribution and density of small cells with densely stained nuclei appeared normal (Fig. 5b).

Apart from a variable content of mossy fiber staining attributed to ingrown host mossy fiber terminals (see below), the neuropil of the CA3 grafts displayed a Timm staining similar to that found in situ in str. radiatum and str. oriens of the normal CA3 or transplanted parts of CA3 observed in other studies (Sunde and Zimmer, 1983). Terminal-like CCK immunoreactivity was seen throughout the grafts (Fig. 6a), suggesting innervation of the graft pyramidal cells by intrinsic graft CCK-immunoreactive neurons, similar to what is observed in the normal CA3 area (Fig. 3a).

Ultrastructure of CA3 transplants

In all 7 rats processed for electron microscopy the CA3 transplants had survived. Most neurons in the grafts were pyramidal cells with large spiny dendrites. Synaptic contacts of both symmetric and asymmetric types were present on the shafts. Synapses on the spines were of the asymmetric

398

type, and they were of both the *complex type* with W- and U-shaped synaptic configurations as previously described for the fascia dentata (Sørensen and Zimmer, 1988a) and the more *simple type* with a straight synaptic contact, usually with a small spine head. Only when large mossy fiber-like terminals were present (see below), spines arising from the proximal parts of the dendrites resembled the very complex excrescences, characteristic of the normal CA3 pyramidal cells (Blackstad, 1963, 1967). In two grafts we observed large dendritic expansions filled with mitochondria, similar to those found in isolated grafts of fascia dentata (Sørensen and Zimmer, 1988a).

In the neuropil of all grafts we observed large varicosities with a spherical or elongated shape and a diameter of $1-5$ μm, which in a few cases could be up to 8 μm. The varicosities, resembling *growth*

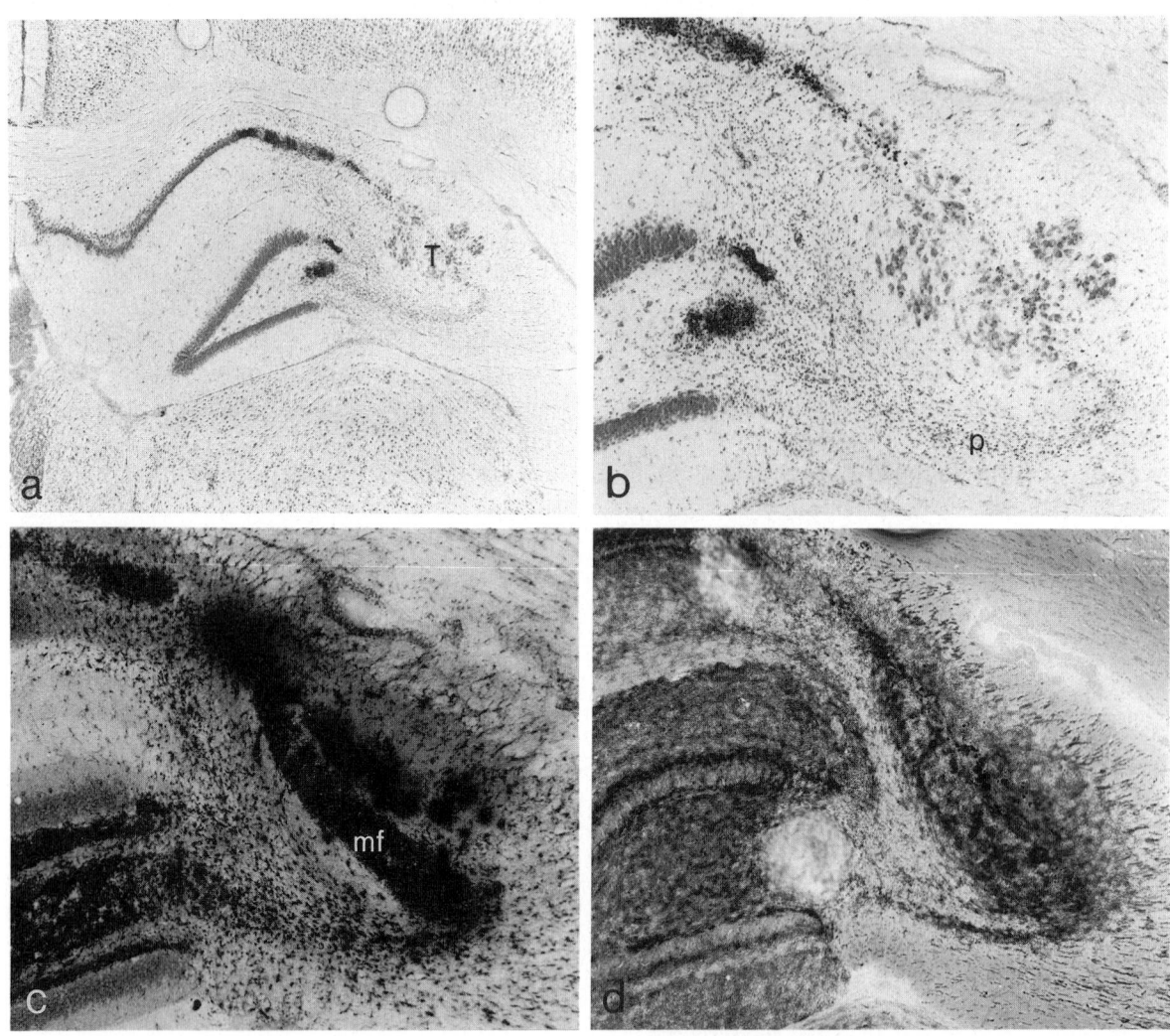

Fig. 5. Thionine- (a, b), Timm- (c) and AChE-stained (d) sections through CA3 transplant 6 weeks after grafting to 1-week-old IA lesion. The neurons in the small transplant (T) are arranged in clusters around the damaged host pyramidal cell layer (p). Note the layer of Timm-stained mossy fiber terminals (mf) in the transplant (c), as well as the positive AChE staining (d). ×21 (a), ×47 (b–d).

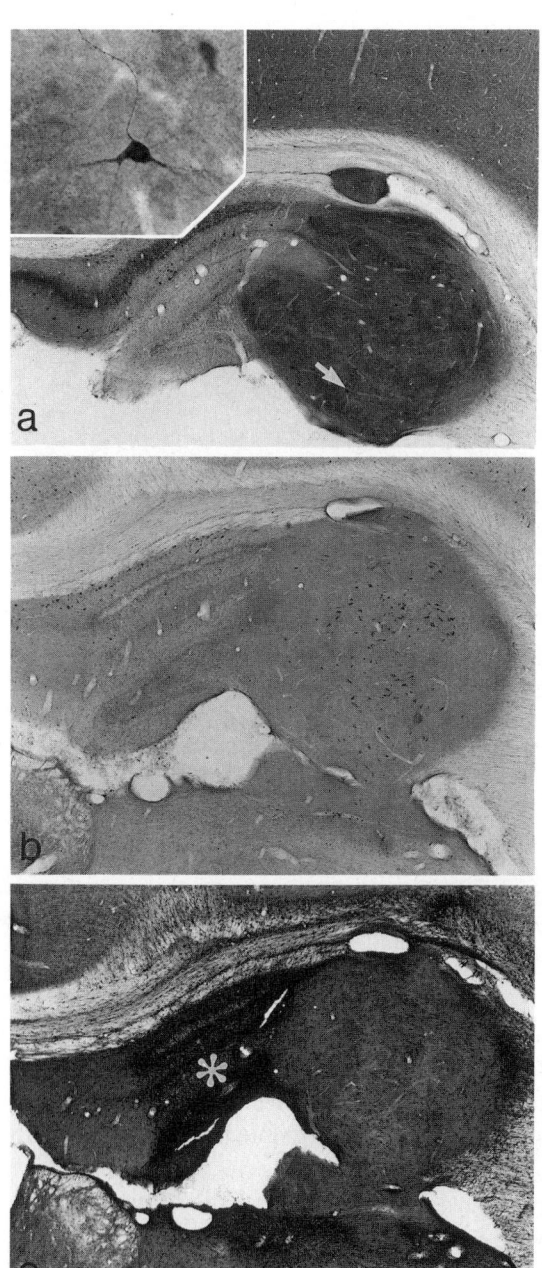

Fig. 6. CCK- (a), SS- (b) and GFAP- (c) immunohistochem
ly stained sections through large CA3 transplant 8 weeks after
grafting. Note CCK- (a and inset corresponding to arrow), and
SS-stained (b) neurons and dense CCK terminal field staining
(a) in the transplant. The density of GFAP staining is normal
in transplant (c) compared with increased staining in the lesioned host neuropil (asterisk). ×24.

cones, were often found as single structures
although "bundles" of more elongated varicosities
were seen. The varicosities often arose from the
end of a myelinated axon or from a node of Ranvier (Fig. 7b) (as observed in the peripheral nervous system (McQuarrie, 1985)), and they were
often partially covered by myelin. In most cases a
direct structural continuity with an axon was not
evident in the ultrathin section. The varicosities
were filled with different organelles and with
neurotubules and neurofilaments dispersed in between these or arranged in bundles near the center
of the varicosity. Mitochondria were numerous
and usually centrally placed. Vesicles ranging in
size from that of synaptic vesicles to large
vacuoles, and sometimes filled with electron-dense
material, were seen in all varicosities. The most
common structure in most of the varicosities was
in fact these vesicles, which in part or totally were
filled with electron-dense material (Fig. 7). They
sometimes resembled lysosomes. The "inclusions"
in the vesicles could be laminated, as in residual
bodies or degenerating mitochondria. Multi-
vesicular bodies were also present, in particular
near the center of the varicosities. A few small
dense core vesicles, resembling those commonly
found in catecholaminergic nerve terminals, and a
few ordinary lysosomes also appeared in the
varicosities. A few other varicosities were dominated by tubular structures, resembling smooth endoplasmic reticulum or dilated neurotubules.
Some of the varicosities made asymmetric synaptic
contacts on dendritic shafts and spines (Fig. 7).
Varicosities of similar appearance were also found
outside the graft in the IA-lesioned host CA3.
Compared with the unensheathed varicosities
described by Peschanski and Besson (1987) we saw
very few protrusions from the varicosities, and
when present they were filled with synaptic
vesicles.

Nerve connections from host brain to transplant

Host cholinergic fibers

All grafts stained for AChE (Fig. 5d), indicating

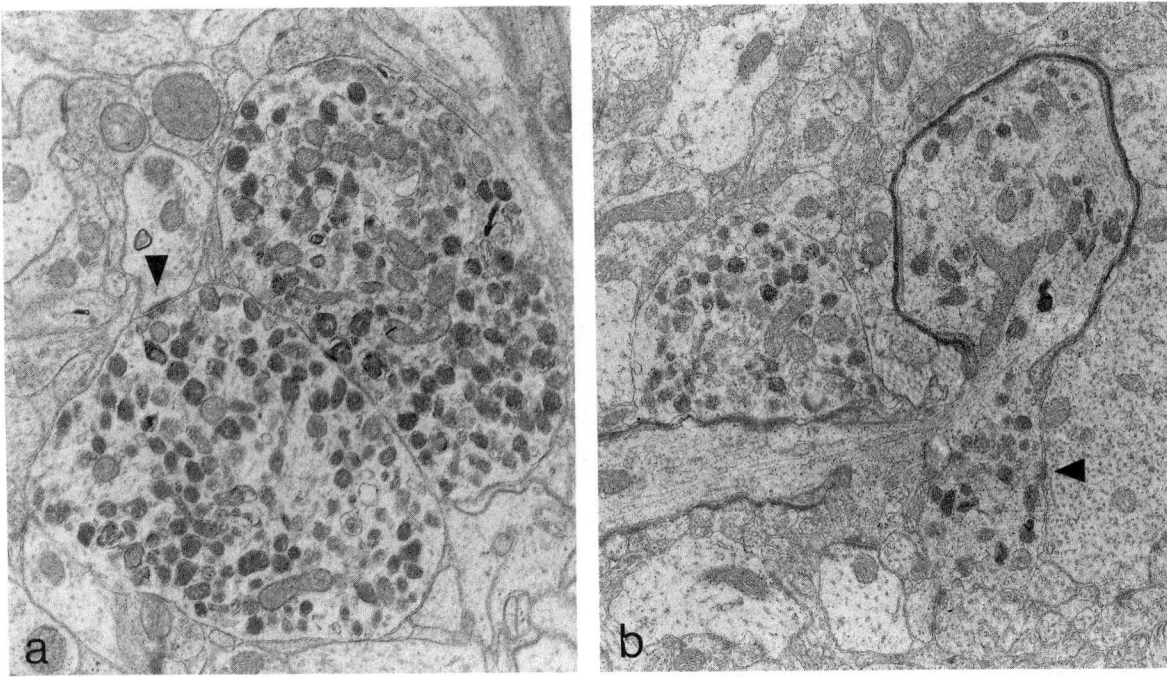

Fig. 7. Large varicosities observed from the center of the two CA3 grafts. a: two adjacent varicosities containing many vacuoles with inclusions of electron-dense material as well as several mitochondria. One of the varicosities is presynaptic to an asymmetric synaptic contact with short broadnecked spine (arrowhead). b: two organelle-filled varicosities. One of the varicosities arises at a node of Ranvier. The organelle content is the same type as in (a), but less densely packed. An asymmetric synaptic contact is formed with dendritic shaft at arrowhead. Graft survival a: 108 days. b: 58 days, a: ×14,000, b: ×13,500.

an innervation by cholinergic host, septo-hippocampal fibers. The AChE staining was in particular found near pyramidal cell bodies as in CA3 in situ. In grafts, heavily innervated by host mossy fibers (see below), the AChE staining had a preference for the mossy fiber layer, like in the normal hippocampus.

Host mossy fibers

Sixteen of the 27 grafts processed for Timm staining contained characteristically stained mossy fiber terminals, suggesting an innervation by host mossy fibers. Some grafts only contained a few scattered, large and densely stained terminals, whereas others displayed a densely stained, normal-looking mossy fiber zone (Fig. 5c). The pyramidal cells in this graft were arranged in a layer almost corresponding to the position of the

former, lesioned host pyramidal cell layer.

In 6 of the 7 grafts, studied at the ultrastructural level, large mossy fiber-like terminals were found. While a couple of the grafts were heavily innervated, others only contained a few clusters. The large mossy fiber-like terminals were filled with clear spherical synaptic vesicles with a few dense core vesicles in between, and they formed asymmetric synapses with dendritic shafts and spines (Fig. 8). The spines were of the very complex type forming the earlier mentioned characteristic excrescences with spinulae invaginating the terminals. Non-synaptic, desmosome-like membrane specializations or junctions were as normally present both between the mossy fiber terminals and the dendritic shafts and between the mossy fiber terminals themselves. The terminals were always located near the cell bodies of pyramidal cells, cor-

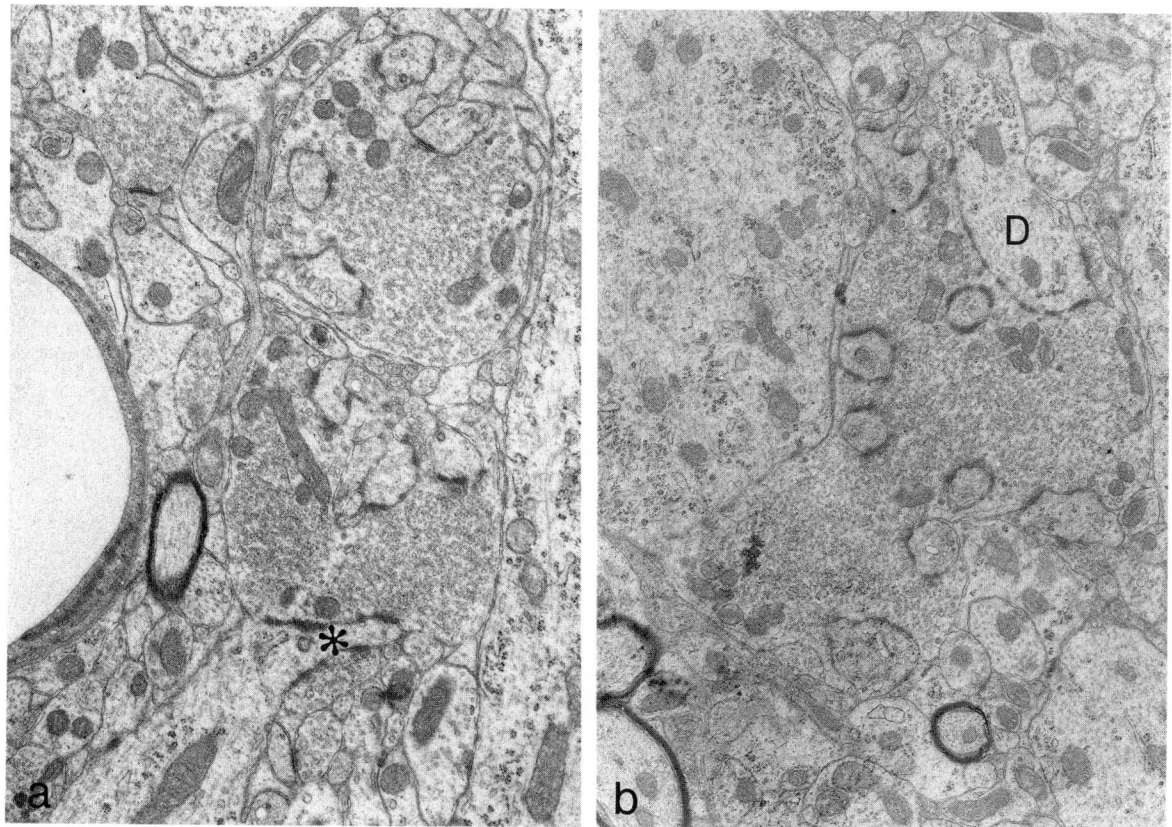

Fig. 8. Host mossy fiber innervation of CA3 grafts. a: two large mossy fiber terminals close to pyramidal cell body (right part of the picture) form multiple asymmetric synaptic contacts with complex dendritic spines. One spine originates from dendritic shaft (asterisk). b: large mossy fiber terminal forms multiple asymmetric synaptic contacts with complex spines and a dendritic shaft (D). Non-synaptic desmosome-like junctions are also formed with the dendritic shaft (D). Graft survival: 53 days. a: ×11,700, b: ×9 900.

responding to their location in the normal CA3.

In the mossy fiber layer of the IA-lesioned host CA3, where CA3 pyramidal cells were absent, mossy fibers were present as large bundles of un-myelinated axons *without* large mossy fiber terminals.

Host hippocampal commissural fibers

In the 5 rats with commissural lesions 3 grafts had close relations to the host fimbria. Despite this proximity to the normal trajectory of hippocampal commissural fibers only one graft contained electron-dense, degenerating terminals. They were located in those parts of the graft nearest to the host fimbria. The same graft for some unknown reason did not appear to contain host mossy fibers. The degenerating terminals of contralateral hip-pocampal origin contacted dendritic spines in par-ticular along the more distal parts of the dendritic arbors. The synapses were asymmetric and of both simple straight and more complex types. In the lat-ter the terminals contacted a cup-formed indenta-tion in the spine head and the membrane with synaptic contact displayed either a U- or W-form (Fig. 9) (Sørensen and Zimmer, 1988a).

Nerve connections from transplant to host brain

Commissural connections

In 3 of the 4 rats which received a contralateral injection of FG, retrogradely labeled neurons were found in the graft (Fig. 10a, b), demonstrating that these graft neurons had developed axonal projections to the injected part of the contralateral host hippocampus. The FG filled out the cell body and proximal dendrites of the labeled pyramidal-like neurons. When the number of labeled neurons was counted in every 4th section through the grafts, 7, 12 and 55 labeled neurons were counted in the 3 grafts, respectively. The neurons were located throughout the septotemporal extent of the grafts, but with a tendency to be located at the level just opposite the fluorochrome injection site. Retrogradely labeled neurons were also found in the host CA3 and dentate hilus outside the lesion area. In the last rat the injection was placed too far rostrally in the host brain, and neither graft nor host hippocampal neurons were labeled.

Associational connections

In 4 of the 6 rats with ipsilateral FG injections retrogradely labeled neurons were found in the graft (Fig. 10c, d). Since FG had spread from the host hippocampal injection site to the lateral ventricle in 3 of the cases, labeling of graft neurons by diffusion from the ventricle could not be entirely excluded in those animals, although such labeling by diffusion seemed unlikely. When the number of labeled neurons was counted in every 4th section of the graft in the 4th animal a total of 49 labeled graft neurons was found. These neurons were distributed throughout the graft.

Discussion

Cerebral lesions induced by focal injection of the excitotoxic, glutamate analogue ibotenic acid (IA) are of the so-called *axon-sparing type* with degeneration of the neurons in the area, but sparing of extrinsic presynaptic afferents and fibers en passage (Köhler et al., 1979, Schwarcz et al., 1979;

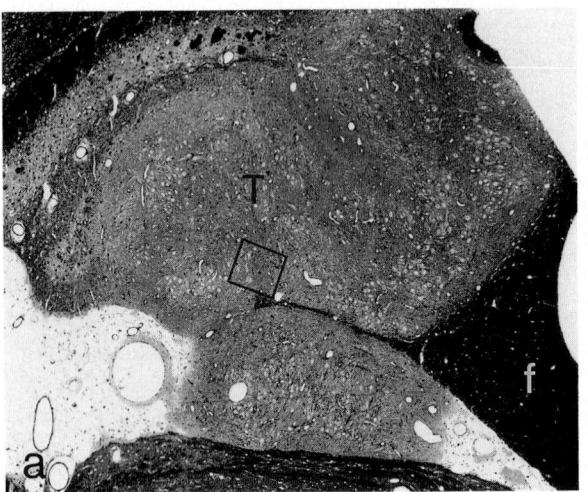
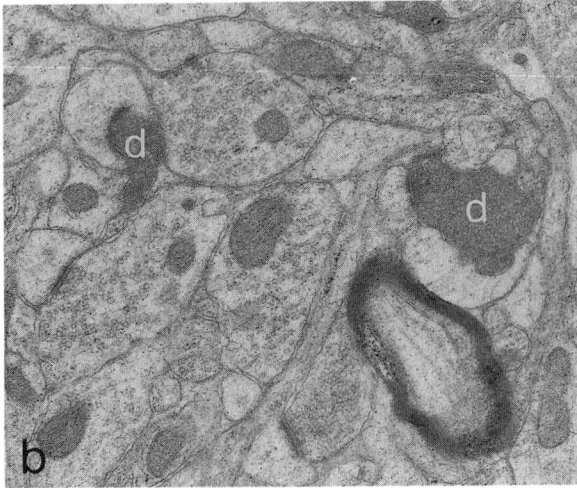

Fig. 9. Innervation of CA3 graft by host hippocampal commissural fibers. a: semithin section of large, lobulated CA3 graft (T) replacing most of the host hippocampus at this level. Note the intimate relation between the graft and the host fimbria (f). Electron micrograph in (b) is from framed area. b: electron-dense, degenerating terminals of contralateral host hippocampal origin 3 days after transection of the contralateral host fimbria. The degenerating terminals form asymmetric synaptic contacts with dendritic spines in graft neuropil. Graft survival 108 days. a: ×36, b: ×17,500.

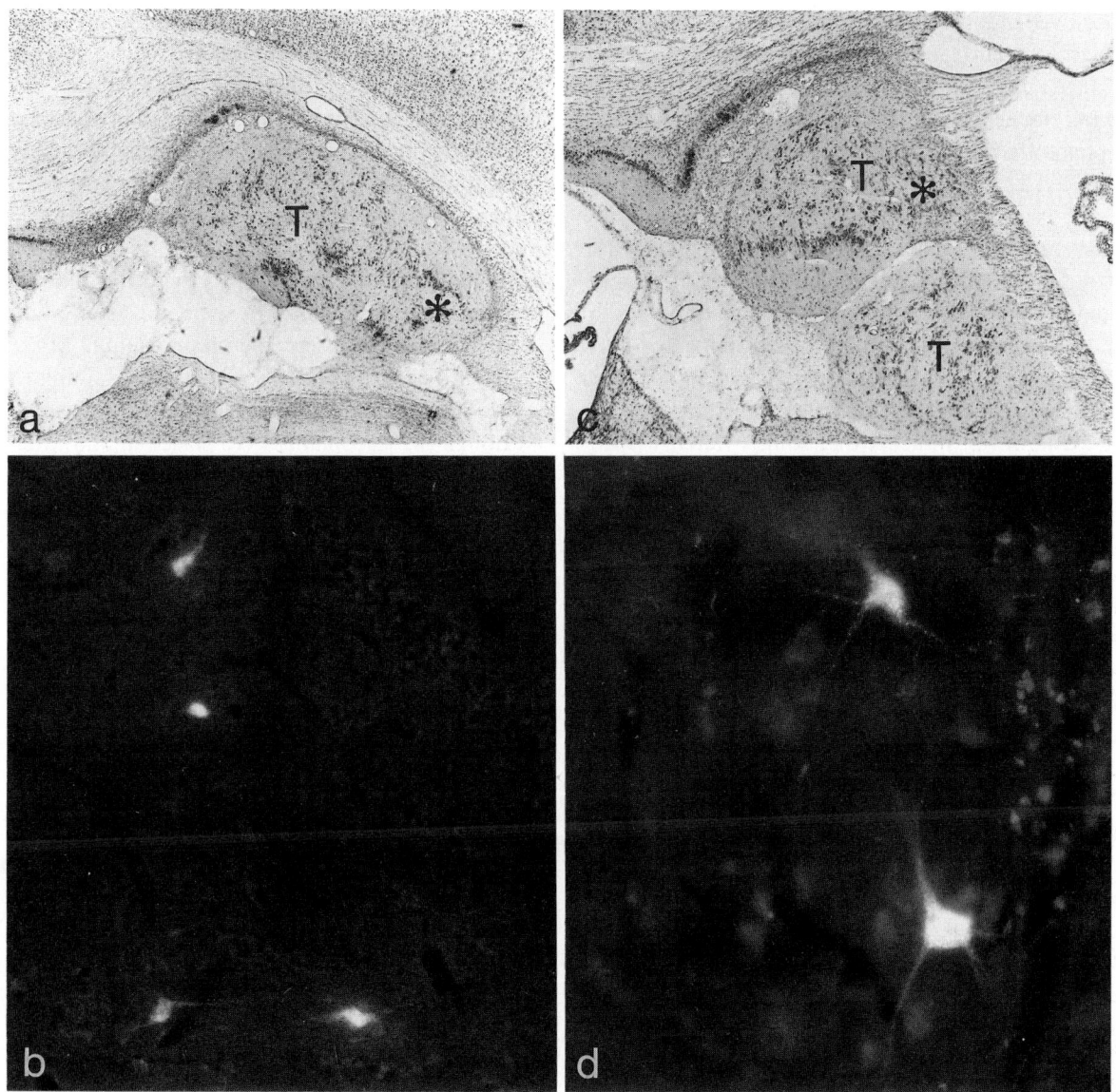

Fig. 10. a – d: graft commissural and associational projections. a – b: commissural projection from CA3 graft, shown in Toluidine blue-stained section in (a), demonstrated in (b) by retrograde axonal transport of Fluoro-Gold injected into the contralateral host hippocampus. The fluorescent graft neurons (b) are photographed in the adjacent section at the area marked with asterisk in (a). c – d: projection from CA3 graft, shown in Toluidine blue-stained section in (c), to more temporal levels of ipsilateral host hippocampus. Retrogradely labelled, Fluoro-Gold fluorescent graft neurons (d) photographed in the adjacent section at the area marked with asterisk in (c). a: ×24, b: ×54, c: ×29, d: ×76.

Coyle and Schwarcz, 1983; Köhler, 1983). Following IA-injections into CA3 of the adult rat the sparing of extrinsic afferent axons was shown by the persistence of Timm-stained mossy fiber terminals in the mossy fiber layer and the persistence of the characteristic terminal-related Timm staining in str. oriens and str. radiatum one week after the IA injection. At this timepoint all CA3 pyramidal cells and CCK- and SS-immunoreactive non-pyramidal cells had degenerated. The AChE-positive, cholinergic septo-hippocampal fibers also retained their characteristic distribution in the lesioned area, as also observed by Köhler (1983). After longer survival times some reorganization apparently did take place, as described after IA-induced lesions in the neostriatum (Schwarcz et al., 1979; Isacson et al., 1985) and after kainic acid lesions in the hippocampus (Nadler et al., 1981). Besides atrophy of the lesioned area, there was some reduction of the terminal field staining in CA3 as observed in both Timm staining for hippocampal afferents and AChE staining for cholinergic fibers. The persistence of some staining does, however, indicate that some afferents (with or without specialized terminals) remained in the lesioned area (see discussion of ultrastructural results below).

The IA-lesioned CA3 area was heavily gliotic at the time of grafting, but this did not affect the *transplant survival*. The survival rate was thus the same or higher than after grafting of developing hippocampal tissue to normal newborn and adult rats (Sunde and Zimmer, 1983; Zimmer and Sunde, 1984; Sørensen et al., 1986). As discussed in a previous study (Tønder et al., 1989b), the good survival and the higher degree of nerve fiber exchange between graft and host after transplantation to IA-induced and ischemic lesions might indicate that the reactive gliosis is in fact beneficial to the grafts. As shown by others (Lindsay et al., 1982; Nieto-Sampedro et al., 1984, and this volume; Cotman and Nieto-Sampedro, 1985; Whittemore et al., 1985; Heacock et al., 1986; Kesslak et al., 1986) reactive glial cells can produce neurotrophic factors, and the presence of those might enhance the graft survival and growth.

As shown previously by Tønder et al. (1989a) and Mudrick et al. (1988) cell suspension grafts of hippocampal tissue contain the neurons typical for the area, including pyramidal cells and non-pyramidal CCK- and SS-immunoreactive neurons. Both in the present and the previous studies the graft CA3 and CA1 pyramidal cells in some cases tended to arrange themselves around the empty host pyramidal cell layer. Often they were,

however, scattered throughout the grafts as single cells or in smaller or larger clusters. This variability in cellular organization might relate to the differences observed in the ingrowth of host mossy fiber into the CA3 transplants, because mossy fibers normally, as well as after lesions and from transplants with dentate granule cells (Sunde and Zimmer, 1981; Sunde et al., 1984), preferentially grow along cell layers, close to the cell bodies of their target cells. Regarding the organization of intrinsic fiber connections, the Timm staining of the CA3 grafts corresponded to the Timm staining of str. radiatum and str. oriens in the normal CA3. Although the transplants were placed in and often surrounded by heavily gliotic host brain tissue, there was a near normal GFAP reactivity in the transplant.

Axonal growth cones

Structures resembling axonal growth cones were observed in all CA3 cell suspension grafts. Similar structures were observed by Peschanski and Besson (1987) in the adult rat thalamus 30 days after kainic acid lesion. The structures resembled the axonal growth cones previously observed both in vitro and in vivo, displaying a high content of mitochondria, elements of smooth endoplasmic reticulum more or less filled with dense material, lysosomes, neurotubules and neurofilaments (Tennyson, 1970; Yamada et al., 1971; Bunge, 1973; Landis, 1983). Structures like that have also been described in the regenerating proximal stump of the transected rat sciatic nerve (Morris et al., 1972). With their high content of organelles the presently observed growth cones more resembled the regenerative growth cones seen in tissue cultures (Bunge, 1973; Landis, 1983), after ischiatic nerve transection (Morris et al., 1972) and in other excitotoxic lesion studies (Peschanski and Besson, 1987; Nothias et al., 1988), than the growth cones with electron-lucent cytoplasm and few organelles found in the developing cerebellum and spinal cord (Del Cerro and Snider, 1968; Nordlander and Singer, 1982). The many vesicles more or less filled with electron-dense material could be early secondary lysosomes engaged in the degradation of either material taken up by pinocytosis or intrinsic mitochondria and other organelles. The increase in degradation products in the growth cones could, however, also be the result of an increased anterograde transport of membrane-bound proteins in regenerating nerves (Peters et al., 1976; Cancalon et al., 1982). Vesicle-filled protrusions extending from the growth cone-like structures were very rare. Microspikes, i.e. filament-filled, thin protrusions arising from the growth cones, were not observed in our material. Peschanski and Besson observed a few of these, and both in vivo and in vitro they are regularly seen (Tennyson, 1970; Yamada et al., 1971; Bunge, 1973) and correlated to the motility of the growth cones (Argiro et al., 1984). This could indicate that the growth cones observed in our material are rather immobile, possibly because of the age of the graft at the time of examination (all older than 7 weeks). The presence of other large and mitochondria-filled expansions arising from dendrites (dendritic growth cones; Sotelo and Palay, 1968; Sørensen and Zimmer, 1988a) in addition to the axonal growth cones, indicates that plastic, dendritic and axonal changes occur in the grafts more than 100 days after transplantation.

Exchange of nerve connections

Nerve fibers belonging to the so-called *global systems,* that is the cholinergic and cate-cholaminergic systems in the brain, grow quite readily into and out of neural transplants placed in newborn as well as adult recipients (discussed in Zimmer et al., 1987). In contrast graft – host exchange of nerve fibers belonging to the so-called *point-to-point systems,* which form the majority of projections in the central nervous system, clearly depends on the age of the recipient. These fibers normally grow well into and out of transplants placed in developing recipient brains, but their growth from the *adult* brain into grafts is usually limited in both extent and density. The results of

the present study support previous findings showing that transplants of immature neurons grafted to an *axon-sparing lesion* also can exchange precise and extensive connections of the point-to-point type with the adult recipient brains and thus at least structurally and in terms of connections replace some of the damaged host brain neurons (Pritzel et al., 1986; Sotelo and Alvarado-Mallart, 1988; Tønder et al., 1989a, b).

In particular the ingrowth of host fibers into the grafts has been studied (Tønder et al., 1989b), and a preceding axon-sparing lesion clearly seems to stimulate the growth of host point-to-point fibers. In the present experimental paradigm these fibers, which mainly consisted of dentate mossy fibers and host hippocampal CA3 associational and commissural fibers, had been devoid of their normal CA3 pyramidal target cells for about a week. At the time of transplantation they might accordingly have been primed into a regenerative state, ready for growth. This would allow them to do better in the competition with the intrinsic graft fibers for available synaptic sites within the grafts than they would do for example after direct grafting into a fresh lesion.

The ingrowth of host commissural fibers and dentate mossy fibers was confirmed at the ultrastructural level. Host mossy fibers thus innervated most of the grafts placed in the IA lesions of the host CA3 region. As normally the fibers contacted the most proximal part of the pyramidal cell dendrites and formed the normal characteristic type of complex mossy fiber synapses.

Not all graft pyramidal cells were contacted by mossy fibers and the dendrites of these pyramidal cells did not display large complex spines (excrescences). The role of mossy fibers as the presynaptic element in inducing these spines has also been observed in other studies. We know that an aberrant collateral projection of mossy fibers induced to grow into the inner part of the dentate molecular layer, by either denervation of the fascia dentata in situ or transplantation of the fascia dentata with incomplete restoration of the major extrinsic afferent connections (Laurberg and Zimmer, 1981; Frotscher and Zimmer, 1983, 1986; Sørensen and Zimmer, 1988a, b; Tønder et al., 1989b), results in the formation of larger than normal, complex spines on the proximal part of the granule cell dendrites. Mossy fibers also induce similar changes on CA1 pyramidal cells when they are manipulated to innervate these cells, which they otherwise not normally contact in the rat (Raisman and Ebner, 1983). In contrast to this inductive role of mossy fibers on the postsynaptic element stands the observation that interneurons in CA3, which also are contacted by mossy fibers, do not have large complex spines (Ribak and Seress, 1983; Frotscher, 1985, 1989). The presently available information therefore indicates that differentiation of complex spines of the excrescence type in CA3 and other excrescence-like spines in CA1 and fascia dentata is regulated as an interaction between pre- and postsynaptic elements where the CA3 and CA1 pyramidal cells and dentate granule cells need the mossy fibers as presynaptic elements to form such spines. This is in contrast to the situation in the auditory thalamus were the postsynaptic neurons are the main determining factor in the regulation of the spine configuration, as well as the size of the presynaptic terminals and the location of synapses on the target neurons themselves (Campbell and Frost, 1988).

Efferent graft connections

Recently we have demonstrated that CA1 pyramidal neurons grafted to an ischemic lesion in the adult rat can project to the ipsilateral host hippocampus (Tønder et al., 1989a), and that CA3 pyramidal neurons and dentate hilar (CA4) neurons transplanted to the normal newborn (Tønder et al., 1988) and the normal adult rat hippocampus (unpublished results) can project to the contralateral hippocampus. (The neurons projecting after grafting to normal adult rats are few in number.) Together with the present observation of contralateral and ipsilateral projections from CA3 neurons grafted to IA lesions, this demonstrates that grafted neurons, at least of the normal projec-

ting type, can extend axons for considerable distances into the adult host brain. In this relation it is of interest that the axons growing to the contralateral hippocampus at least part of the way must pass through white matter, which in other studies has been shown to impede fiber growth (Caroni et al., 1988).

In a previous study of fascia dentata transplants placed in IA lesions of the adult rat fascia dentata we did not observe outgrowth of mossy fibers from the graft granule cells to the intact host CA3 (Tønder et al., 1989b). This lack of outgrowth of mossy fibers was explained by improper orientation of the fascia dentata transplants or lack of direct contact between the graft hilar region, through which the mossy fibers normally are funneled out, and the host CA3 pyramidal cell layer. Other studies with transplantation of dentate granule cells to adult rats have thus demonstrated outgrowth of mossy fibers to both CA3 (Sunde et al., 1985; Sørensen et al., 1986) and CA1 (Raisman and Ebner, 1983). Seen in relation to the observed projection of graft CA3 pyramidal cells in this study and CA1 pyramidal cells after grafting to ischemic lesions (Tønder et al., 1989a) it may, however, be worth noting that the pyramidal cells are projection neurons, normally with long and often many collateral projections, while the mossy fibers from the dentate granule cells normally are shorter and intrinsic to the hippocampus. Besides preservation of a characteristic terminal morphology and specialized terminal-spine configurations, preservation of the general projection pattern may accordingly be another normal characteristic of grafted neurons.

The *functional aspects* of the nerve connections formed between the CA3 grafts and the host hippocampus are at present unknown. Studies on transplantation of embryonic striatal tissue into the adult rat IA-lesioned neostriatum have, however, suggested that a differentiated functional restitution following grafting is dependent on the formation of nerve connections between graft and host (Pritzel et al., 1986; see also Dunnett and Isacson, 1989). Ongoing attempts to combine IA-lesioning with and without subsequent homotypic grafting of fetal CA3 neurons with appropriate electrophysiological and behavioral testing should, however, help us clarify whether this also applies to repair of hippocampal lesions by neural transplantation.

Acknowledgements

Support from the Aarhus University Research Foundation, the Danish MRC, the International Spinal Research Trust, the Lundbeck Foundation, the NOVO Foundation and the Sv.Aa. Wacherhausen Foundation is gratefully acknowledged, together with the help from Ms. P.K. Møller, Mr. B. Krunderup, Ms. D. Jensen, Ms. A. Schmidt, Ms.K. Wiedemann, Mr. A. Meier and Mr. T.A. Nielsen.

References

Argiro, V., Bunge, M.B. and Johnson, M.I. (1984) Correlation between growth form and movement and their dependence on neuronal age. *J. Neurosci.*, 4: 3051 – 3062.

Björklund, A., Stenevi, U., Schmidt, R.H., Dunnett, S.B. and Gage, F.H. (1983) Intracerebral grafting of neuronal cell suspensions. I. Introduction and general methods of preparation. *Acta Physiol. Scand.*, Suppl. 522: 1 – 7.

Blackstad, T.W. (1963) Ultrastructural studies on the hippocampal region. *Prog. Brain Res.*, 3: 122 – 148.

Blackstad, T.W. (1967) Cortical grey matter. Correlation of light and electron microscopic data. In H. Hydén (Ed.) *The Neuron*, Elsevier, Amsterdam, pp. 49 – 118.

Bunge, M.B. (1973) Fine structure of nerve fibers and growth cones of isolated sympathetic neurons in culture. *J. Cell Biol.*, 56: 713 – 735.

Campbell, G. and Frost, D.O. (1988) Synaptic organization of anomalous retinal projections to the somatosensory and auditory thalamus: target-controlled morphogenesis of axon terminals and synaptic glomeruli. *J. Comp. Neurol.*, 272: 383 – 408.

Cancalon, P., Cole, G.J. and Elam, J.S. (1982) The role of axonal transport in the growth of the olfactory nerve axons. In D.G. Weiss and A. Gorio (Eds.), *Axoplasmic Transport in Physiology and Pathology*, Springer, Berlin, pp. 62 – 69.

Caroni, P., Savio, T. and Schwab, M.E. (1988) Central nervous system regeneration: oligodendrocytes and myelin as nonpermissive substrates for neurite growth. *Prog. Brain Res.*, 78: 363 – 371.

Cotman, C.W. and Nieto-Sampedro, M. (1985) Progress in facilitating the recovery of function after central nervous system trauma. *Ann. N.Y. Acad. Sci.*, 457: 83 – 104.

Coyle, J.T. and Schwarcz, R. (1983) The use of excitatory amino acids as selective neurotoxins. In A. Björklund and T. Hökfelt (Eds.), *Handbook of Chemical Neuroanatomy, Vol. 1: Methods in Chemical Neuroanatomy*, Elsevier, Amsterdam, pp. 508 – 527.

del Cerro, M.P. and Snider, R.S. (1968) Studies on the developing cerebellum. Ultrastructure of the growth cones. *J. Comp. Neurol.*, 133: 341 – 362.

Dunnett, S. and Isacson, O. (1989) Trophic mechanisms are not enough. *Trends Neurosci.*, 12: 257.

Frotscher, M. (1985) Mossy fibres form synapses with identified pyramidal basket cells in the CA3 region of the guinea-pig hippocampus: combined Golgi-electron microscope study. *J. Neurocytol.*, 14: 245 – 259.

Frotscher, M. (1989) Mossy fiber synapses on glutamate decarboxylase-immunoreactive neurons: evidence for feedforward inhibition in the CA3 region of the hippocampus. *Exp. Brain Res.*, 75: 441 – 445.

Frotscher, M. and Zimmer, J. (1983) Lesion-induced mossy fibers to the molecular layer of the rat fascia dentata: identification of postsynaptic granule cells by the Golgi-EM technique. *J. Comp. Neurol.*, 215: 299 – 311.

Frotscher, M. and Zimmer, J. (1986) Intracerebral transplants of the rat fascia dentata: a Golgi/electron microscope study of dentate granule cells. *J. Comp. Neurol.*, 246: 181 – 190.

Geneser-Jensen, F.A. and Blackstad, T.W. (1971) Distribution of acetyl cholinesterase in the hippocampal region of the guinea pig. I. Entorhinal area, parasubiculum, and presubiculum. *Z. Zellforsch.*, 114: 460 – 481.

Haug, F.-M.S. (1973) Heavy metals in the brain. A light microscope study of the rat with Timm's sulphide silver method: methodological considerations and cytological and regional staining patterns. *Adv. Anat. Embryol. Cell Biol.*, 45: 1 – 71.

Haug, F.-M.S., Blackstad, T.W., Simonsen, A.H. and Zimmer, J. (1971) Timm's sulfide silver reaction for zinc during experimental anterograde degeneration of hippocampal mossy fibers. *J. Comp. Neurol.*, 142: 23 – 32.

Heacock, A.M., Schonfeld, A.R. and Katzman, R. (1986) Hippocampal neurotrophic factor: characterization and response to denervation. *Brain Res.*, 363: 299 – 306.

Isacson, O., Brundin, P., Gage, F.H. and Björklund, A. (1985) Neural grafting in a rat model of Huntington's disease: progressive neurochemical changes after neostriatal ibotenate lesions and striatal tissue grafting. *Neuroscience*, 16: 799 – 817.

Kesslak, J.P., Nieto-Sampedro, M., Globus, J. and Cotman, C.W. (1986) Transplants of purified astrocytes promote behavioral recovery after frontal cortex ablation. *Exp. Neurol.*, 92: 377 – 390.

Köhler, C. (1983) Neuronal degeneration after intracerebral injections of excitotoxins. A histological analysis of kainic acid, ibotenic acid and quinolinic acid lesions in the rat brain. In K. Fuxe, P. Roberts and R. Schwarcz (Eds.) *Excitotoxins,* Macmillan Press, London, pp. 99–111.

Köhler, C., Schwarcz, R. and Fuxe, K. (1979) Intrahippocampal injections of ibotenic acid provide histological evidence for a neurotoxic mechanism different from kainic acid. *Neurosci. Lett.,* 15: 223–228.

Landis, S.C. (1983) Neuronal growth cones. *Ann. Rev. Physiol.,* 45: 567–580.

Laurberg, S. and Zimmer, J. (1981) Lesion-induced sprouting of hippocampal mossy fiber collaterals to the fascia dentata in developing and adult rats. *J. Comp. Neurol.,* 200: 433–459.

Lindsay, R.M., Barber, P.C., Sherwood, M.R.C., Zimmer, J. and Raisman, G. (1982) Astrocyte cultures from adult rat brain. Derivation, characterization and neurotrophic properties of pure astroglial cells from corpus callosum. *Brain Res.,* 243: 329–343.

McQuarrie, I.G. (1985) Effect of a conditioning lesion on axonal sprout formation at nodes of Ranvier. *J. Comp. Neurol.,* 231: 239–249.

Morris, J.H., Hudson, A.R. and Weddell, G. (1972) A study of degeneration and regeneration in the divided rat sciatic nerve based on electron microscopy. III. changes in the axons of the proximal stump. *Z. Zellforsch.,* 124: 131–164.

Mudrick, L.A., Leung, P.P.-H., Baimbridge, K.G. and Miller, J.J. (1988) Neuronal transplants used in the repair of acute ischemic injury in the central nervous system. *Prog. Brain Res.,* 78: 87–93.

Nadler, J.V., Evenson, D.A. and Cuthbertson, G.J. (1981) Comparative toxicity of kainic acid and other acidic amino acids toward rat hippocampal neurons. *Neuroscience,* 6: 2505–2517.

Nieto-Sampedro, M., Whittemore, S.R., Needels, D.L., Larson, J. and Cotman, C.W. (1984) The survival of brain transplants is enhanced by extracts from injured brain. *Proc. Natl. Acad. Sci. U.S.A.,* 81: 6250–6254.

Nordlander, R.H. and Singer, M. (1982) Morphology and position of growth cones in the developing *Xenopus* spinal cord. *Dev. Brain Res.,* 4: 181–193.

Nothias, F., Wictorin, K., Isacson, O., Björklund, A. and Peschanski, M. (1988) Morphological alteration of thalamic afferents in the excitotoxically lesioned striatum. *Brain Res.,* 461: 349–354.

Peschanski, M. and Besson, J. -M. (1987) Structural alteration and possible growth of afferents after kainate lesion in the adult rat thalamus. *J. Comp. Neurol.,* 258: 185–203.

Peters, A., Palay, S.L. and Webster, H. deF. (1976) *The Fine Structure of the Nervous System. The Neurons and Supporting Cells,* W.B. Saunders Company, Philadelphia, PA, 406 pp.

Pritzel, M., Isacson, O., Brundin, P., Wiklund, L. and Björklund, A. (1986) Afferent and efferent connections of striatal grafts implanted into the ibotenic acid lesioned

neostriatum in adult rats. *Exp. Brain Res.,* 65: 112–126.

Raisman, G. and Ebner, F.F. (1983) Mossy fibre projections into and out of hippocampal transplants. *Neuroscience,* 9: 783–801.

Ribak, C.E. and Seress, L. (1983) Five types of basket cells in the hippocampal dentate gyrus: a combined Golgi and electron microscopic study. *J. Neurocytol.,* 12: 577–597.

Schwarcz, R., Hökfelt, T., Fuxe, K., Jonsson, G., Goldstein, M. and Terenius, L. (1979) Ibotenic acid-induced neuronal degeneration: a morphological and neurochemical study. *Exp. Brain Res.,* 37: 199–216.

Sotelo, C. and Alvarado-Mallart, R.-M. (1988) Integration of grafted Purkinje cell into the host cerebellar circuitry in Purkinje cell degeneration mutant mouse. *Prog. Brain Res.,* 78: 141–155.

Sotelo, C. and Palay, S.L. (1968) The fine structure of the lateral vestibular nucleus in the rat. I. Neurons and neuroglial cells. *J. Cell Biol.,* 36: 151–179.

Sternberger, L.A. (1979) *Immunocytochemistry,* Wiley, New York.

Sunde, N. Aa. and Zimmer, J. (1981) Transplantation of central nervous tissue. An introduction with results and implications. *Acta Neurol. Scand.,* 63: 323–335.

Sunde, N. and Zimmer, J. (1983) Cellular, histochemical and connective organization of the hippocampus and fascia dentata transplanted to different regions of immature and adult rat brains. *Dev. Brain Res.,* 8: 165–191.

Sunde, N., Laurberg, S. and Zimmer, J. (1984) Brain grafts can restore irradiation-damaged neuronal connections in newborn rats. *Nature (Lond.),* 310: 51–53.

Sunde, N., Zimmer, J. and Laurberg, S. (1985) Repair of neonatal irradiation-induced damage to the rat fascia dentata. Effects of delayed intracerebral transplantation. In A. Björklund and U. Stenevi (Eds.), *Neural Grafting in the Mammalian CNS,* Elsevier, Amsterdam, pp. 301–308.

Sørensen, T. and Zimmer, J. (1988a) Ultrastructural organization of normal and transplanted rat fascia dentata: I. A qualitative analysis of intracerebral and intraocular grafts. *J. Comp. Neurol.,* 267: 15–42.

Sørensen, T. and Zimmer, J. (1988b) Ultrastructural organization of normal and transplanted rat fascia dentata: II. A quantitative analysis of the synaptic organization of intracerebral and intraocular grafts. *J. Comp. Neurol.,* 267: 43–54.

Sørensen, T., Jensen, S., Møller, A. and Zimmer, J. (1986) Intracephalic transplants of freeze-stored rat hippocampal tissue. *J. Comp. Neurol.,* 252: 468–482.

Tennyson, V.M. (1970) The fine structure of the axon and growth cone of the dorsal root neuroblast of the rabbit embryo. *J. Cell Biol.,* 44: 62–79.

Timm, F. (1958) Zur Histochemie der Schwermetalle: Das Sulfid-Silber-Verfahren. *Dtsch. Z. Gerichtl. Med.,* 46: 706–711.

Tønder, N., Sørensen, J.C., Bakkum, E., Danielsen, E. and

Zimmer, J. (1988) Hippocampal neurons grafted to newborn rats establish efferent commissural connections. *Exp. Brain Res.,* 72: 577 – 583.

Tønder, N., Sørensen, T., Zimmer, J., Jørgensen, M.B., Johansen, F.F. and Diemer, N.H. (1989a) Neural grafting to ischemic lesions of the adult rat hippocampus. *Exp. Brain Res.,* 74: 512 – 526.

Tønder, N., Sørensen, T. and Zimmer, J. (1989b) Enhanced host perforant path innervation of neonatal dentate tissue after grafting to axon sparing, ibotenic acid lesions in adult rats. *Exp. Brain Res.,* 75: 483 – 496.

Whittemore, S.R., Nieto-Sampredro, M., Needels, D.L. and Cotman, C.W. (1985) Neuronotrophic factors for mammalian brain neurons: injury induction in neonatal, adult and aged rat brain. *Dev. Brain Res.,* 20: 169 – 178.

Yamada, K.M., Spooner, B.S. and Wessels, N.K. (1971) Ultrastructure and function of growth cones and axons of cultured nerve cells. *J. Cell Biol.,* 49: 614 – 635.

Zimmer, J. and Sunde, N. (1984) Neuropeptides and astroglia in intracerebral hippocampal transplants: an immunohistochemical study in the rat. *J. Comp. Neurol.,* 227: 331 – 347.

Zimmer, J., Sunde, N., Sørensen, T., Jensen, S., Møller, A.G. and Gähwiler, B.H. (1985) The hippocampus and fascia dentata. An anatomical study of intracerebral transplants and intraocular and in vitro cultures. In A. Björklund and U. Stenevi (Eds.), *Neural Grafting in the Mammalian CNS,* Elsevier, Amsterdam, pp. 285 – 299.

Zimmer, J., Laurberg, S. and Sunde, N. (1986) Non-cholinergic afferents determine the distribution of the cholinergic septohippocampal projection: a study of the AChE staining pattern in the rat fascia dentata and hippocampus after lesions, X-irradiation, and intracerebral grafting. *Exp. Brain Res.,* 64: 158 – 168.

Zimmer, J., Finsen, B., Sørensen, T. and Sunde, N. (1987) Hippocampal transplants: synaptic organization, their use in repair of neuronal circuits and mouse to rat xenografting. In H.H. Althaus and W. Seifert (Ed.) *NATO ASI Series H, Vol. 2: Glial-Neuronal Communication in Development and Regeneration,* Springer, Heidelberg, pp. 547 – 564.

Zimmer, J., Finsen, B., Sørensen, T. and Poulsen, P.H. (1988a) Xenografts of mouse hippocampal tissue. Exchange of laminar and neuropeptide specific nerve connections with the host rat brain. *Brain Res. Bull.,* 20: 369 – 379.

Zimmer, J., Finsen, B., Sørensen, T. and Poulsen, P.H. (1988b) Xenografts of mouse hippocampal tissue. Formation of nerve connections between the graft fascia dentata and the host rat brain. *Prog. Brain Res.,* 78: 271 – 280.

Zimmer, J., Finsen, B., Sørensen, T., Sunde, N.A. and Poulsen, P.H. (1988c) Brain grafts: a survey with examples of repair and xenografting of hippocampal tissue. In F. Cohadon and J. Lobo Antunes (Eds.), *Recovery of Function in the Nervous System, Fidia Research Series,* 13: 161 – 184.

J. Storm-Mathisen, J. Zimmer and O.P. Ottersen (Eds.)
Progress in Brain Research, Vol. 83
© 1990 Elsevier Science Publishers B.V. (Biomedical Division)

CHAPTER 29

Reafferentation of the subcortically denervated hippocampus as a model for transplant-induced functional recovery in the CNS

Anders Björklund, Ola G. Nilsson and Peter Kalén

Department of Medical Cell Research, Section of Neurobiology, University of Lund, Biskopsgatan 5, S-223 62 Lund, Sweden

Subcortical deafferentation of the hippocampal formation is known to induce profound behavioural deficits. Transplants of fetal septal or brainstem tissue are capable of restoring some aspects of normal physiological and behavioural function in subcortically deafferented (i.e. fimbria-fornix or septal lesioned) rats. Such grafts have been shown to re-establish extensive new afferent inputs to the denervated hippocampal formation. As shown for grafted cholinergic and noradrenergic neurons, the ingrowing axons form laminar innervation patterns which closely mimic those of the normal cholinergic and noradrenergic innervations. The ingrowth appears to be very precisely regulated by the denervated target: each neuron type produces distinctly different innervation patterns; the growth is inhibited by the presence of an intact innervation of the same type; and it is stimulated by additional denervating lesions. Both ultrastructurally and electrophysiologically the graft-derived fibres have been seen to form extensive functional synaptic contacts. Biochemically, cholinergic septal grafts and noradrenergic locus coeruleus grafts restore transmitter synthesis and turnover in the reinnervated hippocampus. Intracerebral microdialysis has revealed that acetylcholine and noradrenaline release is restored to normal or supranormal levels in the graft-reinnervated hippocampus, and that the grafted neurons can be activated in a normal way from the host through behavioural activation induced by sensory stimulation or electrical stimulation of the lateral habenula. These results indicate that the grafted monoaminergic neurons can restore tonic regulatory neurotransmission at previously denervated synaptic sites even when they are implanted into the ectopic brain sites. Such functional reafferentation may be sufficient for at least partial restoration of function in the subcortically deafferented hippocampus.

Introduction

The hippocampal formation is reciprocally connected with the neocortex via the subicular complex and the entorhinal area, and with the diencephalon and the lower brainstem via the fimbria-fornix (FF) pathways and the septal area (Swanson et al., 1987). FF transection, which disconnects the hippocampus from its brainstem and septal regulatory inputs, has provided a highly useful model for the study of morphological and functional aspects of intracerebral neural transplants. This lesion produces a behavioural syndrome in the rat, characterized, e.g., by severe and long-lasting learning and memory deficits which has allowed both electrophysiological and behavioural analysis of graft – host interactions. Moreover, the discretely laminated terminal fields of the hippocampal afferent systems are ideal for morphological analyses of the specificity of graft – host connectivity.

The studies summarized here are focussed on the ability of transplanted fetal CNS neurons to functionally reinnervate the subcortically denervated hippocampus in adult FF-lesioned rats. This reafferentation paradigm is based on the idea that grafted neurons, particularly those of the monoaminergic types, can at least to some extent replace the normal regulatory inputs in order to achieve functional reactivation of a previously denervated target.

Grafts of fetal cholinergic neurons to the FF-lesioned hippocampus

The cholinergic innervation of the hippocampal formation is known to originate in the septal-diagonal band area (see Swanson et al., 1987, for review). A complete FF lesion, which includes both the fimbria and fornix as well as the supracallosal striae, removes approximately 90% of the hippocampal cholinergic innervation (Björklund and Stenevi, 1977; Gage et al., 1983). The residual 10% reaches the hippocampus via the so-called ventral route and is confined to the temporal pole of the hippocampal formation. With time, this spared portion expands and will result in a partial reinnervation of the temporal 1/3 of the hippocampus. The dorsal-septal two-thirds, however, will remain permanently denervated (Gage et al., 1983).

Fetal cholinergic neurons, obtained from the developing septal-diagonal band area of 14-to 17-day-old rat fetuses, have been grafted either as a solid piece into the FF lesion cavity (Björklund and Stenevi, 1977), or as a cell suspension directly into the host hippocampus (Björklund et al., 1983b) (Fig. 1). The grafts provide within a few weeks an extensive acetylcholinesterase (AChE)-positive reinnervation of the host hippocampus. The pattern of the AChE-positive innervation established from the graft mimicked very closely that of the normal intrinsic cholinergic innervation. The cholinergic nature of the ingrowing fibres has been confirmed by choline acetyltransferase (ChAT) biochemistry (Björklund and Stenevi, 1977; Björklund et al., 1983a) and ChAT immunocytochemistry (Clarke et al., 1986). Combined light- and electronmicroscopic immunocytochemistry (Anderson et al., 1986; Clarke et al., 1986) have shown that the graft-derived cholinergic fibres form synaptic contacts with neuronal elements in the host hippocampus and dentate gyrus.

The extension of ingrowing cholinergic axons into the terminal fields of the normal cholinergic innervation depends on the presence or absence of the intrinsic cholinergic afferent input. With septal suspension grafts, the graft-derived ChAT level is 4-fold greater in the cholinergically denervated hippocampus as compared to grafts implanted into the non-denervated hippocampus. Morphologically, this is reflected in a considerably more extensive AChE-positive innervation of the host hippocampus when the grafts are placed in a previously denervated target (Gage and Björklund, 1986b). In an experiment with solid septal grafts placed in the retrosplenial cortex (overlying the dorsal aspect of the hippocampus) (Björklund and Stenevi, 1977; Björklund et al., 1979a) we observed that the extension of AChE-positive fibres into the normal cholinergic terminal zones was greatly reduced if the intrinsic septo-hippocampal pathway was left intact. Instead, the fibres terminated heavily in the outer part of the dentate molecular layer (the terminal zone of the entorhinal perforant path fibres) which was denervated of its non-cholinergic input by the transplantation lesion. These various observations indicate that the ingrowing graft-derived axons compete with the intrinsic system and that the presence of an intact cholinergic input will inhibit or greatly reduce the growth of the grafted cholinergic neurons into the normal cholinergic terminal zones. From the ultrastructural observations of Clarke et al. (1986) and Anderson et al. (1986) it seems likely that the vast majority of the synapses formed by the grafted cholinergic neurons in the denervated hippocampus represent filling of vacated terminal sites on the denervated target neurons (e.g. dentate granule cells and hippocampal pyramidal neurons). It is evident, however, that anomalous connections can be induced as well, such as when grafts are placed in a hippocampus with combined septal and entorhinal deafferentation (Björklund and Stenevi, 1977; Björklund et al., 1979a).

Specificity of the graft-derived fibre ingrowth

There is considerable evidence that the extent of fibre ingrowth and the patterning of the ingrowing axons from implanted neurons depend on the nature of the grafted neurons. This is seen both

413

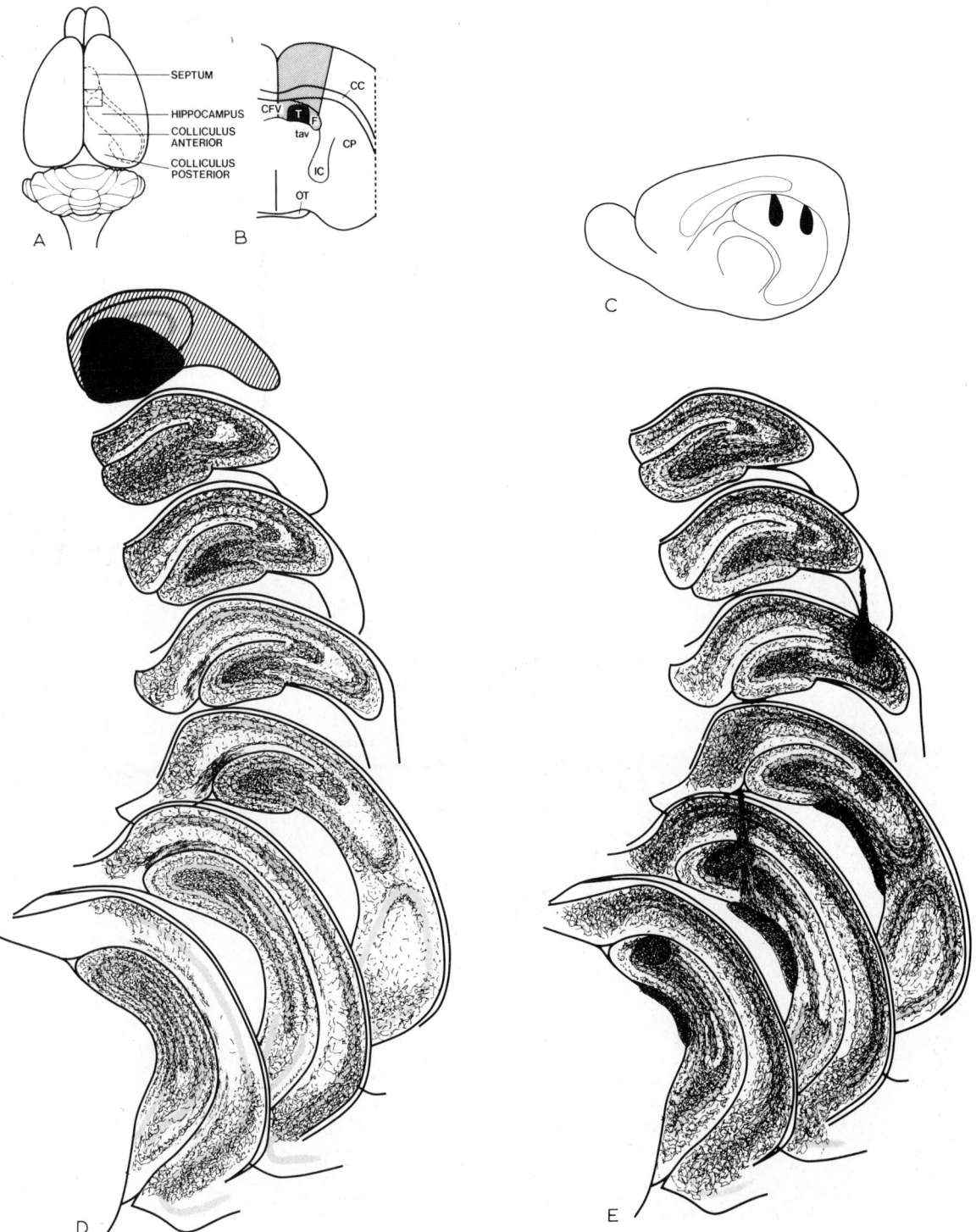

Fig. 1. A and B: extent and position of the fimbria-fornix cavity and the transplant (T) when placed as a solid piece in the lesion cavity. C: placement of the cell suspension transplants (black) in the dorsal hippocampal formation. D and E: semi-schematic camera lucida drawings illustrating the extent of cholinergic (AChE-positive) innervation from a solid septal graft (D; 6 months post-transplantation) and two deposits of septal cell suspensions (E; 14 months postgrafting). (Data compiled from Björklund and Stenevi, 1977, and Björklund et al., 1983).

when comparing neurons of different transmitter types, and when comparing grafts of different types of cholinergic neurons.

Björklund et al. (1976, 1979a, b) compared the fibre outgrowth from noradrenergic neurons (from the locus coeruleus region of the pons) (Figs. 2 and 3), serotonergic neurons (from the mesencephalic raphe region) and dopaminergic neurons (from the ventral mesencephalon) after transplantation to the hippocampus cortex, and the outgrowth patterns were compared to those seen after transplantation of cholinergic neurons from the septal-diagonal band area (Fig. 3). The different types of grafted neurons formed distinctly different terminal patterns. When grafted to the retrosplenial cortex, the noradrenergic axons were seen to avoid, and even grow through the denervated ter-minal zone of the entorhinal perforant path (which innervates the outer half of the dentate molecular layer). Instead, they grew into those areas which normally receive dense noradrenergic innervation (e.g. the dentate hilar zone). By contrast, the serotonergic and dopaminergic axons (like the cholinergic ones) ramified extensively in the dener-vated perforant path zone, and the dopaminergic neurons, in particular showed no tendency to grow into the normal terminal zones of the noradrenergic afferents (e.g. the dentate hilus) (Björklund et al., 1976).

More recently, Nilsson et al. (1988a) and Clarke et al. (1990) compared grafts of cholinergic neurons obtained from 5 different fetal CNS regions; the septal-diagonal band area, the nucleus basalis (NBM) region, the striatum, the mesen-

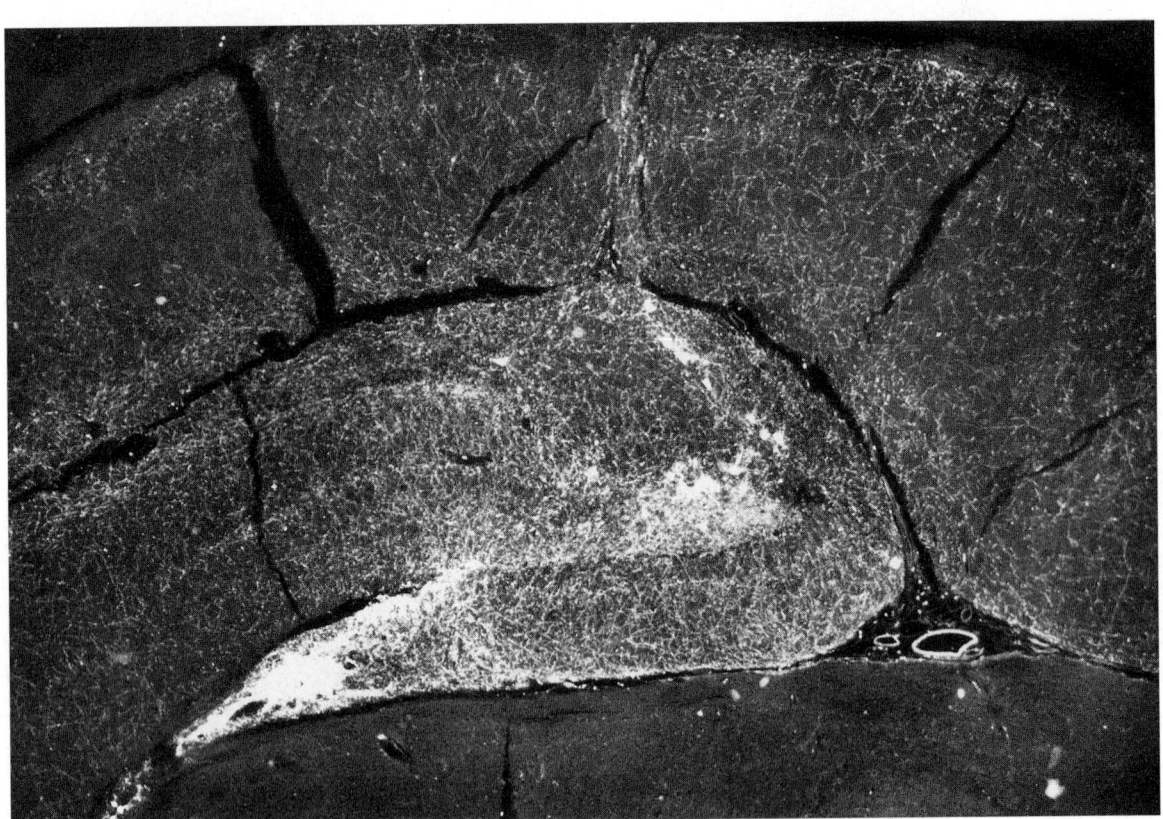

Fig. 2. Histofluorescence picture showing the noradrenaline-containing cell bodies and associated fibre growth into the host hip-pocampus and dentate gyrus (3 months postgrafting). The rat was completely denervated of its intrinsic noradrenergic innervation by an i.v. 6-OHDA injection prior to transplantation (From Björklund et al., 1986).

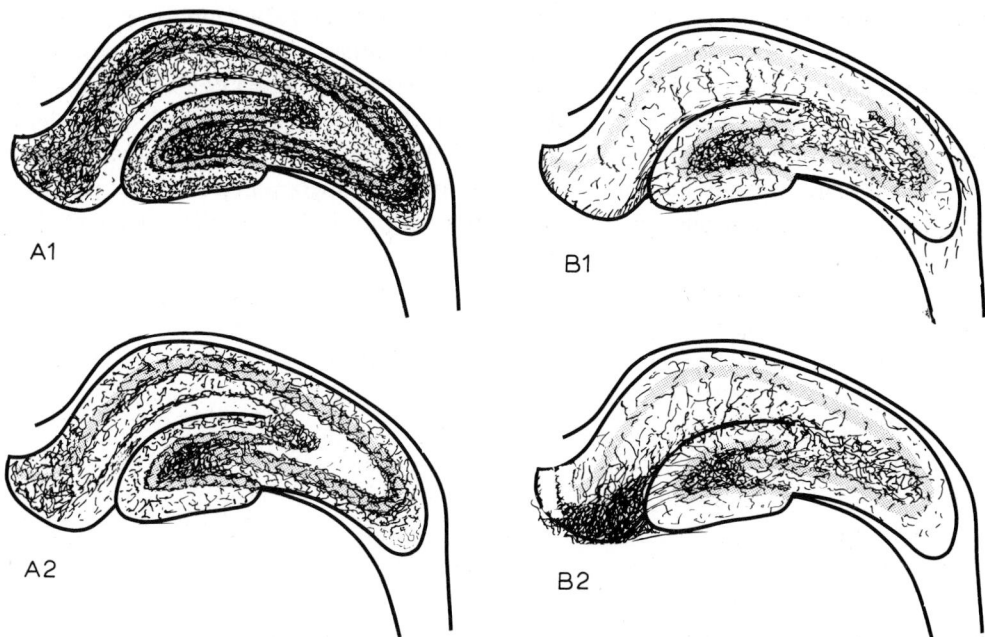

Fig. 3. Semischematic camera-lucida drawings showing the normal patterning of cholinergic (i.e. AChE-positive) and noradrenergic (noradrenaline histofluorescent) afferents in the intact brain (A1 = AChE; B1 = noradrenaline). Below are given for comparison examples of graft-derived cholinergic (A2) and noradrenergic (B2) innervations in the subcortically deafferented (fimbria-fornix lesioned) hippocampus. A2 is from a solid septal graft and B2 is from a solid locus coeruleus graft. The animal in B2 had, in addition, received an i.v. 6-OHDA lesion to remove all intrinsic noradrenergic innervation. Note that the noradrenergic and cholinergic innervation patterns are distinctly different, and that the graft-derived innervations resemble closely those of the intact animal.

cephalic brainstem, and the spinal cord (see inset in Fig. 4). The tissue was prepared as a cell suspension and approximately the same number of viable cells was implanted into the hippocampus of FF-lesioned rats. As summarized in Fig. 4, the results obtained from the 5 graft types differed in 3 different aspects: with respect to the size of the surviving grafts, with respect to their total AChE-positive fibre outgrowth, and with respect to the patterning of the ingrowing AChE-positive fibres. Interestingly, all three types of forebrain grafts – the septal, NBM and striatal tissues – formed essentially normal innervation patterns, although the overall fibre outgrowth and graft survival differed considerably. The spinal cord cholinergic neurons grew very poorly into the hippocampus, although the grafts survived well, and the brainstem grafts exhibited a clearly abnormal innervation pattern (Figs. 5 and 6).

These various observations, as well as similar studies from other laboratories (Lewis and Cotman, 1983; Zhou et al., 1985; Gibbs et al., 1986), demonstrate a high degree of specificity in the growth of different types of grafted neurons into the hippocampal formation. The results, moreover, suggest that the ingrowth and patterning of axons from the grafted neurons are regulated by the target tissue and that this target influence plays an important role in the regulation of both neuronal survival and fibre outgrowth from different types of neurons. It seems likely that this neuron–target interaction, here observed in the lesioned adult hippocampus, reflects the same mechanisms which regulate the formation of axonal connections during ontogenetic development.

416

Graft-induced effects on behaviour

The hippocampus has a special role in learning and memory. Subcortical deafferentation of the hippocampal formation by bilateral FF lesions or lesions of the septal-diagonal band area are known to result in severe memory and learning impairments (Olton et al., 1979; Dunnett et al., 1982; Morris, 1983). Since similar (though less pronounced) effects are obtained by pharmacological blockade of cholinergic transmission (Sutherland et al., 1982; Wishaw, 1985), it appears that damage to the cholinergic septo-hippocampal pathway contributes importantly to the memory im-

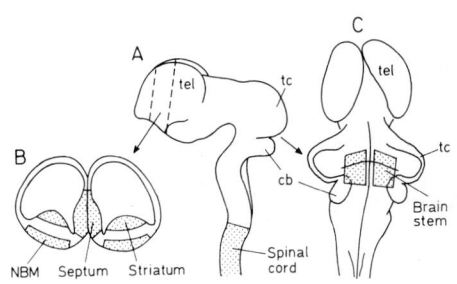

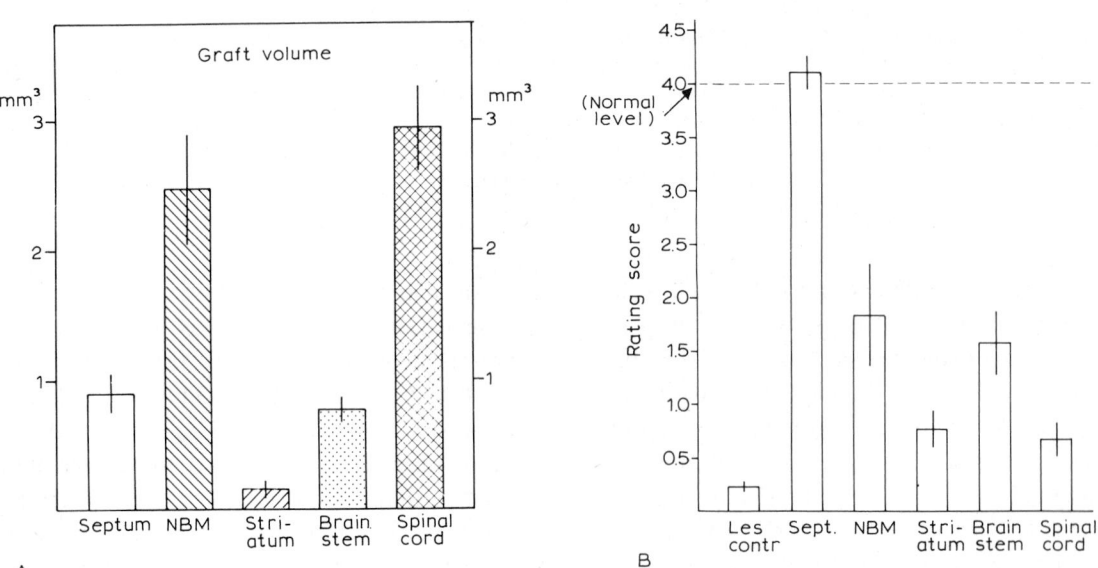

Fig. 4. Final graft volumes (A) and total extent of graft-derived AChE-positive fibre outgrowth (B) from different types of cholinergic-rich grafts. Five different regions were dissected from 14-to 15-day-old rat fetuses, as illustrated in the inset, and the same amount of cell suspensions from each region (35 × 10⁴ cells) was injected into the fimbria-fornix lesioned hippocampus. Only the appropriate graft types (i.e. the septal-diagonal band neurons) were capable of a complete reinnervation of the denervated hippocampal target. (From Nilsson et al. (1988a). *J. Comp. Neurol.*, 268: 204 – 222. Reprinted with permission.)

Fig. 5. Pictures of AChE-stained sections from a normal rat (A) and fimbria-fornix lesioned rats with suspension grafts from the fetal brainstem (B) and cervical spinal cord (C). While the brainstem graft has formed a clearly abnormal innervation pattern in the host hippocampus, the fibre growth from the spinal cord transplant into the host is very sparse. (From Nilsson et al. (1988a). *J. Comp. Neurol.*, 268: 204 – 222. Reprinted with permission.)

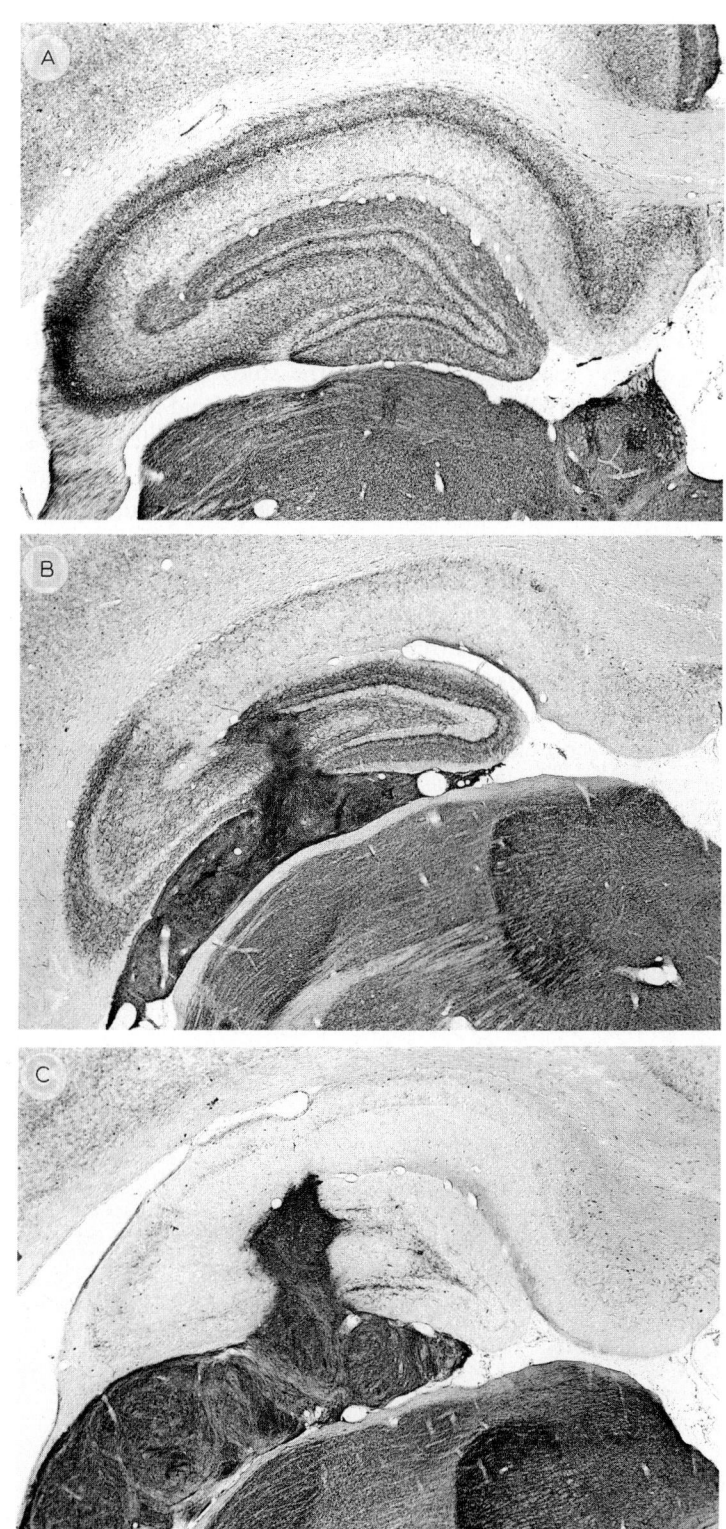

pairments seen after such lesions.

Septal solid or suspension grafts can ameliorate the learning and memory impairments in rats with FF or medial septal lesions, although the behavioural recovery is variable and often incomplete. The graft-induced effects have been observed on spatial working memory in a forced-choice alternation task in the T-maze (Dunnett et al., 1982; Daniloff et al., 1985), in the radial 8-arm maze (Low et al., 1982; Pallage et al., 1986; Hodges et al., 1990), and on spatial working and reference memory in different place-navigation tasks in the Morris water maze (Nilsson et al., 1987; Segal et al., 1987). In the study of Dunnett et al. (1982) there was a significant correlation between T-maze performance of the grafted rats and the extent of graft-derived cholinergic reinnervation in the host hippocampus, and in the studies of Nilsson et al. (1987) and Hodges et al. (1990), the graft-induced recovery was abolished by central muscarinic cholinergic receptor blockade. Ameliorative effects of intrahippocampal septal grafts on maze-learning impairments have been observed also in behaviourally impaired aged rats (Gage et

al., 1984; Gage and Björklund, 1986a; Schenk et al., 1988; Dunnett et al., 1989). Also in this case the graft-induced behavioural recovery was abolished by atropine (Gage and Björklund, 1986a).

The specificity of the transplant effect in the hippocampal deafferentation model has been addressed in several studies. In FF-lesioned rats, Dunnett et al. (1982) observed that rats with grafts of fetal locus coeruleus performed just as bad as rats with lesions alone, and in the study of Hodges et al. (1990), using combined ibotenic acid lesions of the septal-diagonal band area and the nucleus basalis, grafts of non-cholinergic tissue (fetal hippocampus) had no effect. In the latter study, septal transplants implanted into the basal forebrain (in contrast to grafts placed in the target areas in the hippocampus or cortex) were ineffective, too. A similar difference in effectiveness between cholinergic-rich (basal forebrain tissue) and cholinergic-poor (hippocampal tissue) transplants on lesion-induced learning and memory impairments has been observed in rats with ibotenic acid lesions of the nucleus basalis (Fine et al.,

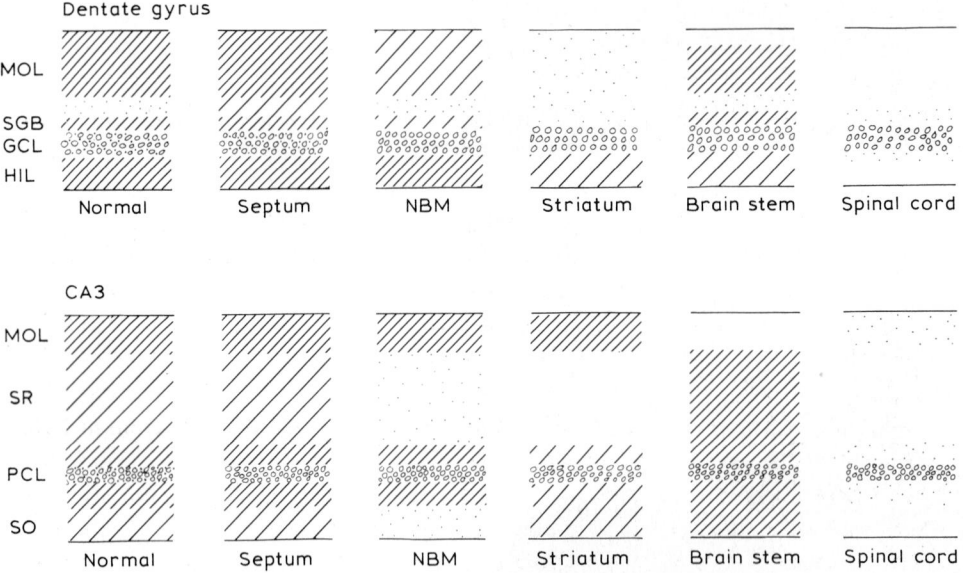

Fig. 6. Schematic illustration of the differences in laminar distribution of graft-derived AChE-positive fibre in the host dentate gyrus and CA3 area from the 5 different types of cholinergic-rich grafts (shown in Fig. 4). (From Nilsson et al. (1988a). *J. Comp. Neurol.*, 268: 204 – 222. Reprinted with permission.)

1985; Dunnett et al., 1985) and in rats subjected to chronic alcohol exposure (Arendt et al., 1988). In these various models the transplanted effect is thus both tissue- and site-specific.

Transplant specificity has been studied also in rats with combined lesions to the cholinergic and serotonergic afferent systems. Rats with such combined lesions show more profound impairments in learning and memory than rats subjected to a cholinergic or a serotonergic lesion alone (Nilsson et al., 1988b; Richter-Levin and Segal, 1989). Intrahippocampal grafts of serotonin-rich raphe tissue (Richter-Levin and Segal, 1989) or grafts of mixed septal and raphe tissue (Nilsson et al., 1990a) had significant ameliorative effects in this situation. Interestingly, in the study of Nilsson et al. (1990a), improved performance in the water maze task was seen only with mixed septal-raphe transplants but not with identical grafts of septal or raphe tissue when transplanted individually.

Electrophysiological studies of graft – host connectivity

These various observations indicate that the ability of the septal grafts to reverse spatial learning and memory impairments in rats with lesions of the septo-hippocampal system may at least partly depend on the re-establishment of functional cholinergic graft – host connections.

This interpretation finds support in the electrophysiological studies of Segal et al. (1985, 1987). In these experiments the connections of septal suspension implants in FF-lesioned rats were analyzed using intracellular recordings in hippocampal slices at 4 – 8 weeks after grafting. Stimulation of the septal graft contained within the slice produced a slow and long-lasting, voltage-dependent depolarization in some host CA1 neurons located up to about 2 mm from the graft. This was associated with an increase in spontaneous action potential discharges and in spontaneous postsynaptic potentials. These responses were similar to those seen after topical application of acetylcholine. Topical application of atropine

attenuated, and physostigmine potentiated, the graft-induced depolarizing responses. In combination with the electron microscopic data of Clarke et al. (1986) and Anderson et al. (1986) these observations provide compelling evidence for the formation of cholinergic synapses with normal functional properties by the ingrowing axons onto the previously denervated neuronal elements of the host.

In vivo studies using single unit or EEG recordings suggest that some aspects of normal hippocampal electrophysiological function, which are disrupted in the subcortically deafferented hippocampus, are normalized in the graft-reinnervated hippocampi. Buzsáki et al. (1987) have reported restoration of behaviour-dependent theta rhythm in FF-lesioned rats with septal solid grafts (but not septal suspension grafts) implanted into the fimbrial lesion cavity, and Low et al. (1982) observed partial recovery of so-called paired-pulse potentiation in the dentate gyrus granule cells in such animals. More recently, Shapiro et al. (1989) have shown that place unit firing, recorded in a radial maze, which is disrupted in FF-lesioned rats are partially recovered in behaviourally recovered animals where the hippocampus had been reinnervated by septal suspension grafts.

Functional effects as assessed by the [^{14}C]2-deoxyglucose technique

Kelly et al. (1985) studied the magnitude of FF lesion-induced functional alterations in different regions of the hippocampal formation using the autoradiographic [^{14}C]2-deoxyglucose technique. As summarized schematically in Fig. 7, transection of the septo-hippocampal pathway by a unilateral FF lesion resulted in a 30 – 50% reduction in 2-DG utilization throughout the ipsilateral hippocampal formation, and this depressed function still persisted by 6 months after the lesion (i.e. the time point illustrated in Fig. 7). Interestingly, the areas of depressed 2-DG utilization within the lesioned hemisphere were largely coextensive with the areas of the cingulate cortex and the hippocampal formation that had been substantially cholinergically denervated as a consequence of the FF transection (left panel in Fig. 7). FF-lesioned rats that had received solid septal grafts displayed a significant recovery in hippocampal 2-DG use, as compared to the rats with lesion alone. The graft-induced recovery in 2-DG utilization was significantly correlated with the recovery in AChE staining density in adjacent sections from the same brains

$(r = 0.84; P < 0.01)$, thus suggesting a relationship between the cholinergic reinnervation from the septal grafts and the restoration of functional glucose utilization. Indeed, the areas of the host hippocampus and dentate gyrus that showed a complete restoration of AChE-positive innervation was normalized with respect to 2-DG utilization rate (cross-hatching in Fig. 7, right), whereas the areas with only partial AChE-positive reinnerva-

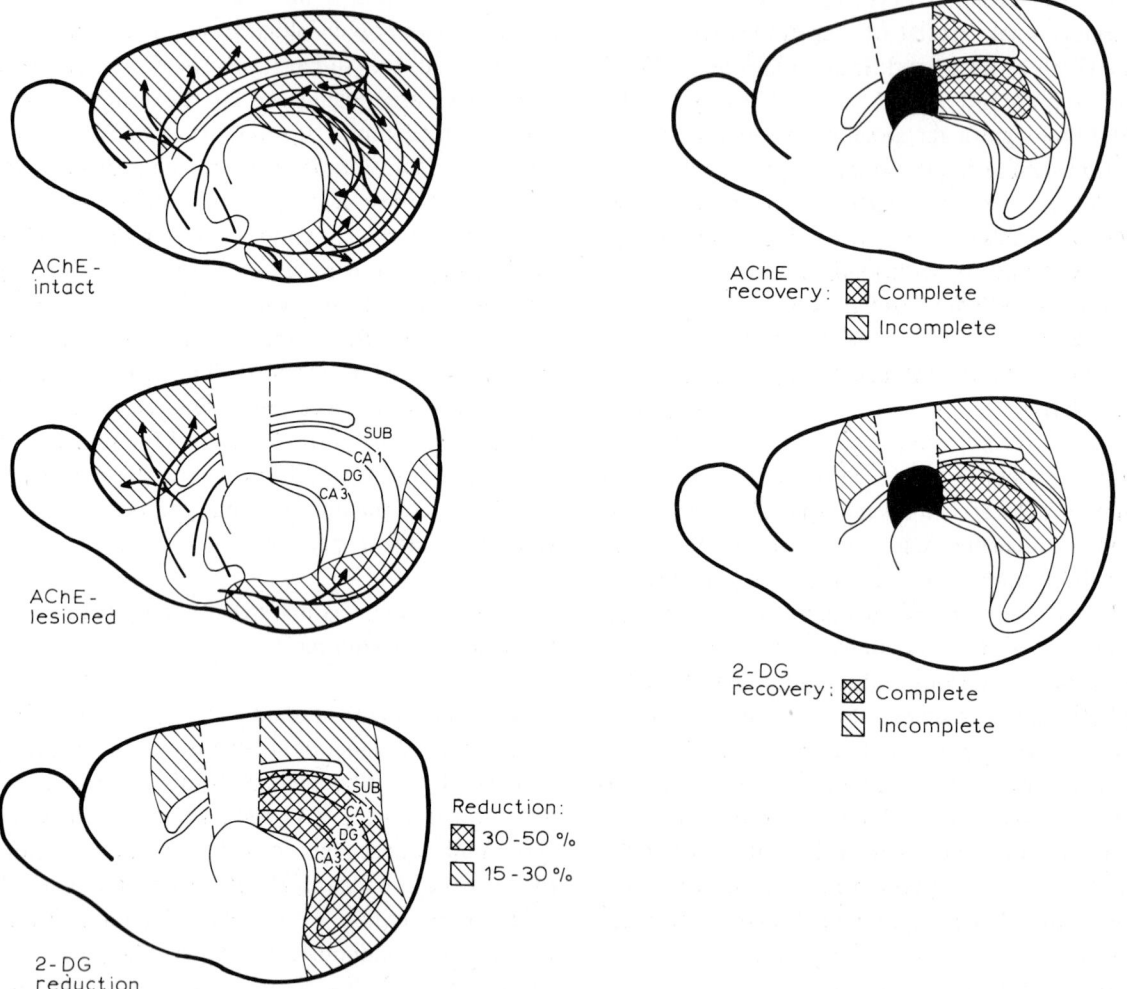

Fig. 7. Changes in 2-deoxyglucose (2-DG) utilization rates after subcortical deafferentation by a fimbria-fornix lesion (left) and after reinnervation of the hippocampus by a solid septal graft (right). The fimbria-fornix lesion removed the cholinergic (i.e. AChE-positive) input to the dorsal two-thirds of the hippocampal formation (middle left) and this was accompanied by a 15 – 50% reduction in hippocampal 2-DG utilization (bottom left). The septal grafts restored both the cholinergic afferent input (top right) and the 2-DG utilization rate (bottom right). The analysis was made 6 months after lesion and grafting. (Based on data from Kelly et al., 1985.)

tion showed a partial and incomplete recovery of 2-DG use (hatching in Fig. 7). These results strongly suggest that the cholinergic component of the grafts is functional at the biochemical level and influences, or normalizes, the overall functional performance of the deafferented hippocampal formation.

Monitoring of transplant function by means of intracerebral microdialysis

The extracellular levels of transmitters, such as acetylcholine (ACh), noradrenaline (NA) and serotonin (5-HT) as measured by the microdialysis technique have been shown to reflect ongoing neuronal activity, and changes in the extracellular transmitter levels are closely related to changes in synaptic transmitter release in the area surrounding the probe (see e.g. Kalén et al., 1988a, b; Nilsson et al., 1990b). In the hippocampal formation, the extracellular levels of ACh, NA and 5-HT depend on the integrity of the septo-hippocampal, coeruleo-hippocampal and raphe-hippocampal pathways, respectively. Transmitter overflow is sharply increased by K^+-induced depolarization and greatly decreased by addition of the sodium channel blocker tetrodotoxin (TTX) to the perfusion fluid (Kalén et al., 1988a, b; Nilsson et al., 1990b). In awake freely moving rats, the extracellular NA and 5-HT levels change with the day – night cycle, and they correlate overall with the activity state of the animal (Kalén et al., 1989b). Behavioural activation by sensory stimulation (handling), tail-pinch, or electrical stimulation of the lateral habenula are accompanied by increased extracellular levels of NA and ACh in the hippocampus (Kalén et al., 1989a; Nilsson et al., 1990b), indicating that the monoaminergic afferents to the hippocampal formation are generally activated by such stimuli.

Recently, we have adopted the microdialysis method to monitor transmitter release from intracerebrally grafted monoaminergic neurons (Fig. 8). In particular, we have been interested to use this in vivo method as a tool to explore mechanisms of regulation of grafted fetal monoaminergic neurons reinnervating the previously denervated hippocampus in adult recipient rats (Daszuta et al., 1989; Kalén et al., 1990; Nilsson et al., 1990c).

Consistent with previous biochemical studies performed on postmortem tissue (Björklund et al., 1983a, 1986; Daszuta et al., 1989), the microdialysis results indicate that the grafted serotonergic, noradrenergic and cholinergic neurons are spontaneously active despite their ectopic location. The grafts restore extracellular 5-HT, NA and ACh levels in the graft-reinnervated area to levels close to or even above that seen in normal intact rats (Fig. 9). As in the intact hippocampus, depolarization by high K^+, or pharmacological blockade of transmitter elimination by either reuptake blockers (indalpine for 5-HT and desipramine for NA) or AChE inhibition (by neostigmine) causes a several-fold increase in transmitter overflow from the grafts. The ability of TTX to reduce the extracellular 5-HT, NA and ACh down to the levels seen after acute axotomy in the normal hippocampus, indicates that transmitter release in the graft-reinnervated hippocampus depends on tonic impulse activity in the grafted neurons.

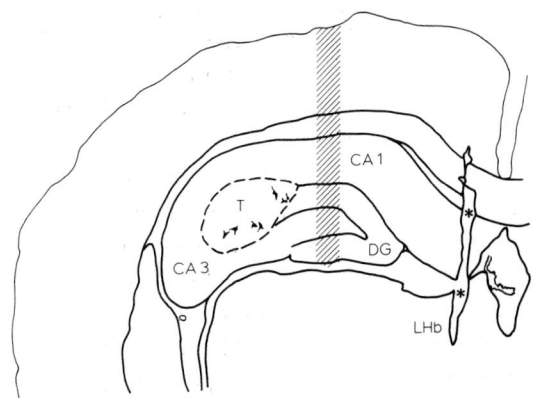

Fig. 8. Position of the dialysis probe (hatched area) in relation to the septal or locus coeruleus suspension transplants (T) in the dorsal hippocampus. In addition, the figure shows the track of the stimulating electrode in the lateral habenula (LHb) (asterisks).

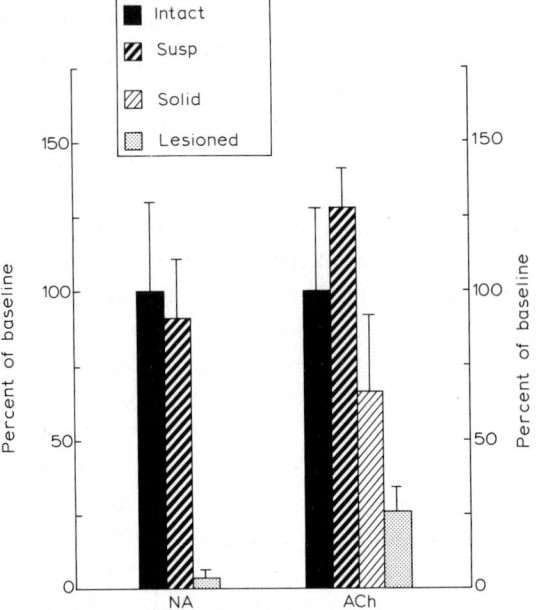

Fig. 9. Hippocampal baseline levels of noradrenaline (NA) and acetylcholine (ACh) in intact, lesioned (6-OHDA, or FF lesion), suspension-grafted (locus coeruleus or septum) and solid-grafted (septum) rats as measured by microdialysis. (Data from Nilsson et al., 1990b and Kalén et al., 1990).

The results obtained with grafted serotonergic raphe neurons (Daszuta et al., 1989) suggest that autoregulatory mechanisms, operating on the terminal level, may play an important role in the maintenance of transmitter-release in the graft-reinnervated hippocampus. Thus, in the postmortem biochemical analysis 5-HT turnover (5-HIAA:5-HT ratio) was found to be inversely related to the density of reinnervation (as assessed by the tissue concentration of 5-HT in the area around the probe). The grafted serotonin neurons produced in most cases a pronounced hyperinnervation pattern in the hippocampus. Despite this, the extracellular 5-HT levels, as measured by microdialysis in vivo, were close to normal. Thus, similar to what has been observed for monoaminergic neurons in situ, local feedback mechanisms are likely to operate at the terminal

level to compensate for abnormalities in innervation density in the area. Such local (possibly autoreceptor-mediated) control has previously been proposed as an important regulatory mechanism in intrastriatal grafts of mesencephalic dopamine neurons (Bolam et al., 1987; Strecker et al., 1987). The present results indicate that this autoregulatory principle may be of general importance for the maintenance of a physiologically adequate functional level in grafted monoaminergic neurons.

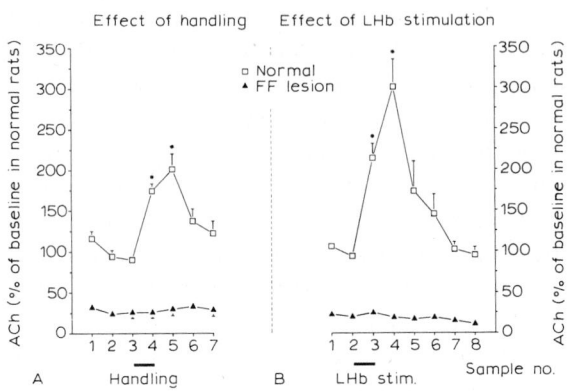

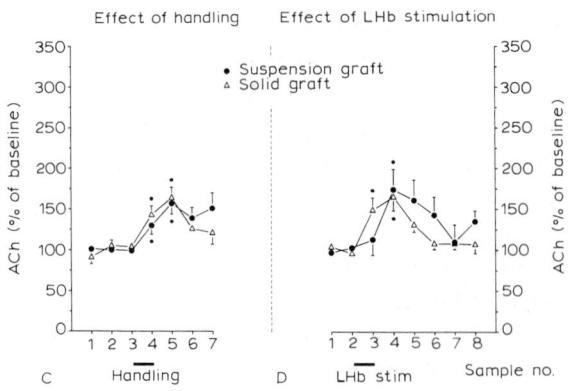

Fig. 10. Baseline acetylcholine release and effect of handling and LHb stimulation in the normal and fimbria-fornix lesioned hippocampus (top panel A and B), and in the fimbria-fornix lesioned hippocampus reinnervated by solid septal grafts (open triangles) and septal suspension grafts (filled circles) (bottom panel C and D). The baseline acetylcholine release was restored to near-normal levels in the graft-reinnervated hippocampi and the acetylcholine release responded to handling and LHb stimulation in a normal way, although the response was, on the average, smaller in magnitude. (From Nilsson et al., 1990c.)

The microdialysis data have provided evidence that the grafted neurons are, at least to some extent, integrated with the host neuronal circuitry. In awake rats, ACh release from septal grafts can be activated by both sensory stimulation by gentle handling, as well as by electrical stimulation of the lateral habenula (Fig. 10; Nilsson et al., 1990c). These effects were seen both in rats with solid septal grafts, implanted into the FF lesion cavity, as well as in FF-lesioned rats with septal suspension grafts implanted into the deafferented hippocampal formation. Stimulation of the lateral habenula, which projects extensively to the brainstem reticular formation (Sutherland, 1982), has been found to offer an effective route for the activation of the ascending brainstem monoaminergic systems, including the septal cholinergic projections. Transection of the output pathway of the lateral habenula, which is confined to the fasciculus retroflexus, abolished the effects of habenula stimulation both in the normal and the septal grafted rats.

Grafts of noradrenergic locus coeruleus neurons, grafted as a cell suspension into the 6-hydroxydopamine-denervated hippocampus, was similarly activated by lateral habenula stimulation, whereas the effects of sensory stimulation by handling was more variable: while 2 of the 6 grafted rats showed a marked response to handling, the other 4 showed essentially no response, despite that the same grafts responded to the habenular stimulation (Kalén et al., 1990). This indicates that the underlying mechanisms, or the anatomical pathways may be different for the two types of activation.

Mechanisms of action of intrahippocampal grafts

The profound functional influence of the subcortical afferents on the hippocampus is illustrated by the fact that the behavioural deficits induced by a complete FF transection is as severe as those seen after removal of the hippocampus itself (Olton et al., 1979). The subcortical inputs have been estimated to contribute only about 5% of all extrinsic inputs to the hippocampus (Buzsáki and Gage, 1989). This quantitatively modest subcortical input is generally conceived of as a regulatory system which is necessary to maintain normal function in the cortico-cortical transmission pathway which passes through the dentate gyrus, hippocampus proper, and subiculum. Both acetylcholine, noradrenaline and serotonin have been shown to regulate excitability at the granule cell and pyramidal cell synapses (Bliss et al., 1983; Segal et al., 1989). The aminergic systems are thus likely to play a permissive role in the function of the cortico-hippocampo-cortical loop. In addition, Buzsáki and Gage (1989) have reported that subcortical deafferentation leaves the hippocampus in a state of apparent disinhibition which makes the hippocampus susceptible to seizure-inducing stimuli.

The combined morphological, biochemical and electrophysiological data, summarized above, provide substantial evidence that grafted cholinergic and monoaminergic neurons can reinstate functional synaptic neurotransmission in the subcortically deafferented hippocampal formation and there is compelling, albeit largely indirect, evidence that such graft-induced reafferentation is sufficient to restore some aspects of normal hippocampal function in the subcortically deafferented animal. The functional and behavioural effects of intrahippocampal transplants should be viewed from the perspective of the non-specific modulatory nature of these systems. It is likely that some of their normal effects are tonic modulatory in nature, and thus that certain aspects of cholinergic and monoaminergic function at the synaptic level are quite non-specific. It seems likely, however, that different types of grafted neurons can influence different aspects of hippocampal dysfunction. While the cholinergic-rich septal grafts have been seen to reinstate hippocampal EEG rhythmicity and influence memory-related functions such as heterosynaptic facilitation or paired-pulse potentiation (Low et al., 1982) and firing properties of hippocampal place units

(Shapiro et al., 1989), the noradrenaline-rich locus coeruleus grafts have been observed to normalize hyperexcitability in the subcortically deafferented hippocampus (Buzsáki et al., 1988), as well as seizure development during kindling in the noradrenergically denervated animal (Barry et al., 1987).

The reafferentation paradigm summarized in this chapter assumes that the grafted monoaminergic modulatory neurons can function in a tonic, autoregulated manner, in the absence of any extrinsic afferent control. However, the more recent electrophysiological studies and in vivo transmitter release experiments indicate that the intrahippocampal grafts, despite their ectopic position, can become functionally integrated with the host brain, and that both neuronal firing properties and transmitter release can be modulated from the host brain during ongoing behaviour. Dunnett (1989) and Hodges et al. (1990) have compared the effects of cholinergic-rich septal suspension grafts with those obtained after different doses of cholinergic agonists (arecoline and physostigmine) in aged rats and in young rats with ibotenic acid lesions of the basal forebrain cholinergic system. In both cases the effects of systemically administered agonists did not match the improvements seen in the grafted animals. This further suggests that the function of the intrahippocampal grafts is not limited to a pharmacological "minipump" type of mechanism. The degree of physiological and behavioural recovery seen in the reafferentation paradigm is thus likely to depend on synaptic mechanisms and partial restoration of regulatory neuronal circuits.

Acknowledgements

The research reviewed here was supported by grants from the Swedish MRC (04X-3874), the National Institutes of Health (NS-06701) and the Greta and Johan Kock Foundation.

References

Anderson, K.J., Gibbs, R.B., Salvaterra, P.M. and Cotman, C.W. (1986) Ultrastructural characterization of identified cholinergic neurons transplanted to the hippocampal formation of the rat. *J. Comp. Neurol.,* 249: 279–292.

Arendt, T., Allen, Y., Sinden, J., Schugens, M.M., Marchbanks, R.M., Lantos, P.L. and Gray, J.A. (1988) Cholinergic-rich brain transplants reverse alcohol-induced memory deficits. *Nature (Lond.),* 332: 448–450.

Barry, D.I., Kikvadze, I., Brundin, P., Bolwig, T.M., Björklund, A. and Lindvall, O. (1987) Grafted noradrenergic neurons suppress seizure development in kindling-induced epilepsy. *Proc. Natl. Acad. Sci. U.S.A.,* 84: 8712–8715.

Björklund, A. and Stenevi, U. (1977) Reformation of the severed septohippocampal cholinergic pathway in the adult rat by transplanted septal neurones. *Cell Tissue Res.,* 185: 289–302.

Björklund, A., Stenevi, U. and Svendgaard, N.-A. (1976) Growth of transplanted monoaminergic neurons into the adult hippocampus along the perforant path. *Nature (Lond.),* 262: 787–790.

Björklund, A., Kromer, L.F. and Stenevi, U. (1979a) Cholinergic reinnervation of the rat hippocampus by septal implants is stimulated by perforant path lesion. *Brain Res.,* 173: 57–64.

Björklund, A., Segal, M. and Stenevi, U. (1979b) Functional reinnervation of rat hippocampus by locus coeruleus implants. *Brain Res.,* 170: 409–426.

Björklund, A., Gage, F.H., Schmidt, R.H., Stenevi, U. and Dunnett, S.B. (1983a) Intracerebral grafting of neuronal cell suspensions. VII. Recovery of choline acetyl-transferase activity and acetylcholine synthesis in the denervated hippocampus reinnervated by septal suspension implants. *Acta Physiol. Scand.,* Suppl. 522: 59–66.

Björklund, A., Gage, F.H., Stenevi, U. and Dunnett, S.B. (1983b) Intracerebral grafting of neuronal cell suspensions. VI. Survival and growth of intrahippocampal implants of septal cell suspensions. *Acta Physiol. Scand.,* Suppl. 522: 49–58.

Björklund, A., Nornes, H. and Gage, F.H. (1986) Cell suspension grafts of noradrenergic locus coeruleus neurons in rat hippocampus and spinal cord: reinnervation and transmitter turnover. *Neuroscience,* 18: 685–698.

Bliss, T.V.P., Goddard, G.V. and Riives, M. (1983) Reduction of long-term potentiation in the dentate gyrus of the rat following selective depletion of monoamines. *J. Physiol. (Lond.),* 232: 331–356.

Bolam, J.P., Freund, T.F., Björklund, A., Dunnett, S.D. and Smith, A.D. (1987) Synaptic input and local output of dopaminergic neurons in grafts that functionally reinnervate the host neostriatum. *Exp. Brain Res.,* 68: 131 – 146.

Buzsáki, G. and Gage, F.H. (1989) Pathophysiology of the subcortically deafferented hippocampus: improvement and deterioration of function by fetal grafts. In F. Gage, A. Privat and Y. Christen (Eds.), *Neuronal Grafting and Alzheimer's Disease,* Springer-Verlag, Berlin, pp. 103 – 119.

Buzsáki, G., Gage, F.H., Czopf, J. and Björklund, A. (1987) Restoration of rhythmic slow activity (theta) in the subcortically denervated hippocampus by fetal CNS transplants. *Brain Res.,* 400: 321 – 333.

Buzsáki, G., Ponomareff, G.L., Bayardo, F., Ruiz, R. and Gage, F.H. (1988) Suppression and induction of epileptic activity by neuronal grafts. *Proc. Natl. Acad. Sci. U.S.A.,* 85: 9327 – 9330.

Clarke, D.J., Gage, F.H. and Björklund, A. (1986) Formation of cholinergic synapses by intra-hippocampal septal grafts as revealed by choline acetyltransferase immunocytochemistry. *Brain Res.,* 369: 151 – 162.

Clarke, D.J., Nilsson, O.G., Brundin, P. and Björklund, A. (1990) Synaptic connections formed by grafts of different types of cholinergic neurons in the host hippocampus. *Exp. Neurol.,* 107: 11 – 22.

Daniloff, J.K., Bodony, R.P., Low, W.C. and Wells, J. (1985) Cross-species embryonic septal transplants: restoration of conditioned learning behavior. *Brain Res.,* 346: 176 – 180.

Daszuta, A., Kalén, P., Strecker, R.E., Brundin, P. and Björklund, A. (1989) Serotonin neurons grafted to the adult rat hippocampus. II. 5-HT release as studied by intracerebral microdialysis. *Brain Res.,* 498: 323 – 333.

Dunnett, S.B. (1989) Short-term memory in rodent models of ageing: effects of cortical cholinergic grafts. In F. Gage, A. Privat and Y. Christen (Eds.), *Neuronal Grafting and Alzheimer's Disease.* Springer-Verlag, Berlin, pp. 85 – 102.

Dunnett, S.B., Low, W.C., Iversen, S.D., Stenevi, U. and Björklund, A. (1982) Septal transplants restore maze learning in rats with fornix-fimbria lesions. *Brain Res.,* 251: 335 – 348.

Dunnett, S.B., Toniolo, G., Fine, A., Ryan, C.N., Björklund, A. and Iversen, S.D. (1985) Transplantation of embryonic ventral forebrain neurons to the neocortex of rats with lesions of nucleus basalis magnocellularis. II. Sensorimotor and learning impairments. *Neuroscience,* 16: 787 – 797.

Dunnett, S.B., Badman, F., Rogers, D.C., Evenden, J.L. and Iversen, S.D. (1989) Cholinergic grafts in the neocortex or hippocampus of aged rats: reduction of delay-dependent deficits in the delayed non-matching to position task. *Exp. Neurol.,* 102: 57 – 64.

Fine, A., Dunnett, S.B., Björklund, A. and Iversen, S.D. (1985) Cholinergic ventral forebrain grafts into the neocortex improve passive avoidance memory in a rat model of Alzheimer's disease. *Proc. Natl. Acad. Sci. U.S.A.,* 82: 5227 – 5230.

Gage, F.H. and Björklund, A. (1986a) Cholinergic septal grafts into the hippocampal formation improve spatial learning and memory in aged rats by an atropine sensitive mechanism. *J. Neurosci.,* 6: 2837 – 2847.

Gage, F.H. and Björklund, A. (1986b) Enhanced graft survival in the hippocampus following selective denervation. *Neuroscience,* 17: 89 – 98.

Gage, F.H., Björklund, A. and Stenevi, U. (1983) Reinnervation of the partially deafferented hippocampus by compensatory collateral sprouting from spared cholinergic and noradrenergic neurons. *Brain Res.,* 268: 27 – 39.

Gage, F.H., Björklund, A., Stenevi, U., Dunnett, S.B. and Kelly, P.A.T. (1984) Intrahippocampal septal grafts ameliorate learning impairments in aged rats. *Science,* 225: 533 – 536.

Gibbs, R.B., Anderson, K. and Cotman, C.W. (1986) Factors affecting innervation in the CNS: comparison of three cholinergic cell types transplanted to the hippocampus of adult rats. *Brain Res.,* 383: 362 – 366.

Hodges, H., Allen, Y., Sinden, J., Lantos, P.L. and Gray, J.A. (1990) Cholinergic-rich transplants alleviate cognitive deficits in lesioned rats but exacerbate response to cholinergic drugs. *Prog. Brain Res.,* in press.

Kalén, P., Kokaia, M., Lindvall, O. and Björklund, A. (1988a) Basic characteristics of noradrenaline release in the hippocampus of intact and 6-hydroxydopamine lesioned rats as studied by in vivo microdialysis. *Brain Res.,* 474: 374 – 379.

Kalén, P., Strecker, R.E., Rosengren, E. and Björklund, A. (1988b) Endogenous release of neuronal serotonin and 5-hydroxyindoleacetic acid in the caudate-putamen of the rat as revealed by intracerebral dialysis coupled to high-performance liquid chromatography with fluorimetric detection. *J. Neurochem.,* 51: 1422 – 1435.

Kalén, P., Lindvall, O. and Björklund, A. (1989a) Electrical stimulation of the lateral habenula increases hippocampal noradrenaline release as monitored by in vivo microdialysis. *Exp. Brain Res.,* 76: 239 – 245.

Kalén, P., Rosengren, E., Lindvall, O. and Björklund, A. (1989b) Hippocampal noradrenaline and serotonin release over 24 hours as measured by the dialysis technique in freely moving rats: correlation to behavioral activity state, effect of handling and tail-pinch. *Eur. J. Neurosci.,* 1: 181 – 188.

Kalén, P., Cenci, M.A., Daszuta, A., Lindvall, O. and Björklund, A. (1990) In vivo microdialysis: a new approach for the study of functional activity of grafted monoaminergic neurons and their interaction with the host brain. *Prog. Brain Res.,* in press.

Kelly, P.A.T., Gage, F.H., Ingvar, M., Lindvall, O., Stenevi, O. and Björklund, A. (1985) Functional reactivation of the deafferented hippocampus by embryonic septal grafts as assessed by measurements of local glucose utilization. *Exp. Brain Res.,* 58: 570 – 579.

Lewis, E.R. and Cotman, C.W. (1983) Neurotransmitter characteristics of brain grafts: striatal and septal tissues form the same laminated input to the hippocampus. *Neuroscience,* 8: 57 – 66.

426

Low, W.C., Lewis, P.R., Bunch, S.T., Dunnett, S.B., Thomas, S.R., Iversen, S.D., Björklund, A. and Stenevi, U. (1982) Functional recovery following neural transplantation of embryonic septal nuclei in adult rats with septohippocampal lesions. *Nature (Lond.)*, 300: 260 – 262.

Morris, R.G.M. (1983) An attempt to dissociate "spatial mapping" and "working memory" theories of hippocampal function. In W. Seifert (Ed.), *The Neurobiology of the Hippocampus*, Academic Press, London.

Nilsson, O.G., Shapiro, M.L., Gage, F.H., Olton, D.S. and Björklund, A. (1987) Spatial learning and memory following fimbria-fornix transection and grafting of fetal septal neurons to the hippocampus. *Exp. Brain Res.*, 67: 195 – 215.

Nilsson, O.G., Clarke D.J., Brundin, P. and Björklund, A. (1988a) Comparison of growth and reinnervation properties of cholinergic neurons from different brain regions grafted to the hippocampus. *J. Comp. Neurol.*, 268: 204 – 222.

Nilsson, O.G., Strecker, R.E., Daszuta, A. and Björklund, A. (1988b) Combined cholinergic and serotonergic denervation of the forebrain produces severe deficits in spatial learning in the rat. *Brain Res.*, 453: 235 – 246.

Nilsson, O.G., Brundin, P. and Björklund, A. (1990a) Amelioration of spatial memory impairment by intrahippocampal grafts of mixed septal and raphe tissue in rats with combined cholinergic and serotonergic denervation of the forebrain. *Brain Res.*, in press.

Nilsson, O.G., Kalén, P., Rosengren, E. and Björklund, A. (1990b) Acetylcholine release in the rat hippocampus as studied by microdialysis is dependent on axonal impulse flow and increases during behavioural activation. *Neuroscience*, in press.

Nilsson, O.G., Kalén, P., Rosengren, E. and Björklund, A. (1990c) Acetylcholine release from intrahippocampal septal grafts is under the control of the host brain. *Proc. Natl. Acad. Sci. U.S.A.*, in press.

Olton, D.D., Becker, J.T. and Handelman, G.E. (1979) Hippocampus, space and memory. *Behav. Brain Sci.*, 2: 313 – 365.

Pallage, V., Toniolo, G., Will, B. and Hefti, F. (1986) Long-term effects of nerve growth factor and neural transplants on behavior of rats with medial septal lesions. *Brain Res.*, 386: 197 – 208.

Richter-Levin, G. and Segal, M. (1989) Raphe cells grafted into the hippocampus can ameliorate spatial memory deficits in rats with combined serotonergic/cholinergic deficiencies.

Brain Res., 478: 184 – 186.

Schenk, F., Contant, B. and Werffeli, P. (1988) Intrahippocampal grafts in aged rats effects response patterning in the radial maze and exploration on a hole board task. *Eur. J. Neurosci.*, Suppl. 1, Abstract no. 78.21.

Segal, M., Björklund, A. and Gage, F.H. (1985) Transplanted septal neurons make viable cholinergic synapses with a host hippocampus. *Brain Res.*, 336: 302 – 307.

Segal, M., Greenberger, V. and Milgram, N.W. (1987) A functional analysis of connections between grafted septal nuclei and a host hippocampus. *Prog. Brain Res.*, 71: 349 – 357.

Segal, M., Richter-Levin, G., Greenberger, V. and Shpiegelman (1989) Neural grafts and neurotransmitters interactions in cognitive deficits. In F. Gage, A. Privat and Y. Christen (Eds.), *Neuronal Grafting and Alzheimer's Disease*, Springer-Verlag, Berlin, H, pp. 141 – 149.

Shapiro, M.L., Simon, D.K., Olton, D.S., Gage, F.H., Nilsson, O.G. and Björklund, A. (1989) Intrahippocampal grafts of fetal basal forebrain tissue influence the place fields of complex-spike units in the hippocampus of behaving rats with fimbria-fornix lesions. *Neuroscience*, 32: 1 – 18.

Strecker, R.E., Sharp, T., Brundin, P., Zetterström, T., Ungerstedt, U. and Björklund, A. (1987) Autoregulation of dopamine release and metabolism by intrastriatal nigral grafts as revealed by intracerebral dialysis. *Neuroscience*, 22: 169 – 178.

Sutherland, R.J. (1982) The dorsal diencephalic conduction system: a review of the anatomy and functions of the habenular complex. *Neurosci. Behav. Rev.*, 6: 1 – 13.

Sutherland, R.J., Whishaw, I.Q. and Regeher, J.C. (1982) Cholinergic receptor blockade impairs spatial localization using distal cues in the rat. *J. Comp. Physiol. Psychol.*, 96: 563 – 573.

Swanson, L.W., Köhler, C. and Björklund, A. (1987) The limbic region. I. The septohippocampal system. In A. Björklund, T. Hökfelt and L.W. Swanson (Eds.), *Handbook of Chemical Neuroanatomy. Vol. 5: Integrated Systems of the CNS, Part I*, Elsevier, Amsterdam, pp. 125 – 277.

Whishaw, I.Q. (1985) Cholinergic receptor blockade impairs locale but not taxon strategies for place navigation in a swimming pool. *Behav. Neurosci.*, 99: 979 – 1005.

Zhou, C.F., Raisman, G. and Morris, R.J. (1985) Specific patterns of fibre outgrowth from transplants to host mice hippocampi, shown immunohistochemically by the use of allelic forms of thy-1. *Neuroscience*, 16: 819 – 833.

J. Storm-Mathisen, J. Zimmer and O.P. Ottersen (Eds.)
Progress in Brain Research, Vol. 83
© 1990 Elsevier Science Publishers B.V. (Biomedical Division)

CHAPTER 30

Axon sprouting in the rodent and Alzheimer's disease brain: a reactivation of developmental mechanisms?

Carl W. Cotman[1], James W. Geddes[2] and Jennifer S. Kahle[1]

[1]*Department of Psychobiology and* [2]*Division of Neurosurgery, University of California, Irvine, CA 92717, U.S.A.*

Research over the past 15 years has led to a comprehensive description of the processes of axonal sprouting and synaptic reorganization in the hippocampus. Previous studies on axonal sprouting have now been supplemented with recent studies on excitatory amino acid receptor plasticity. These and related studies pave the way to research strategies which detail the molecular mechanisms of the sprouting response. The re-expression of the fetal form of α-tubulin mRNA in rat after entorhinal lesions was found to be similar to the re-expression of the human fetal form of α-tubulin in Alzheimer's brain. This result suggests that the sprouting process may involve a reactivation of certain developmental mechanisms and that this may possibly contribute to the etiology of Alzheimer's disease.

Introduction

Synaptic neural plasticity has become an important new concept in neurobiology in recent years based to a large degree on studies carried out in the hippocampus. Studies of the hippocampus have demonstrated that axons in the developing and mature brain have the capacity for growth and reactive synaptogenesis in response to the loss of neighboring axons (for review see Cotman and Lynch, 1976; Cotman and Anderson, 1988). Blackstad and colleagues' careful description and characterization of the cytoarchitectonics, lamination, and projections to and from the various regions of the hippocampus (Blackstad, 1956; Blackstad, 1958; Blackstad and Kjaerheim, 1961; Blackstad, 1963; Storm-Mathisen and Blackstad, 1964) have helped lay the foundation for the studies involving in-depth analysis of the synaptic re-organization which occurs in response to neuronal damage or disease. Indeed, Blackstad (1963) accurately described the future importance of his early studies when he wrote:

"So far, only the normal histology [of the hippocampus] has been investigated, and a great amount of work along the same lines seems useful and required. When the normal histology of the region has become sufficiently known, this part of the cerebral cortex should be eminently suited for investigations of other types as well, including experimental modifications of glia and neurons."

The study of hippocampal anatomy and cytoarchitectonics has since progressed explosively. Hippocampal anatomy is very well characterized at all stages of development and to a large degree in various disease states (for review see Swanson, 1983; Amaral, 1987). In addition to classical morphological techniques, the hippocampus has been comprehensively studied using biochemical methods at an anatomical level. Such methods include receptor autoradiography, immunocytochemistry, metabolic stains, etc. Detailed histological analysis of excitatory amino acid (EAA) binding sites, uptake sites, neurotransmitter pools, and EAA localization has established a more complete description of the EAA transmitter systems in the hippocampus (Cotman et al., 1987).

428

The highly laminated organization and the well-characterized anatomy and biochemistry of the hippocampus has, as Blackstad suggested, made many studies on the neuronal and glial response of the hippocampus to modifications possible.

Thus, sprouting of both cholinergic and glutamatergic fibers in response to entorhinal lesions has also been well characterized (Cotman and Nieto-Sampedro, 1984; Cotman and Anderson, 1988).

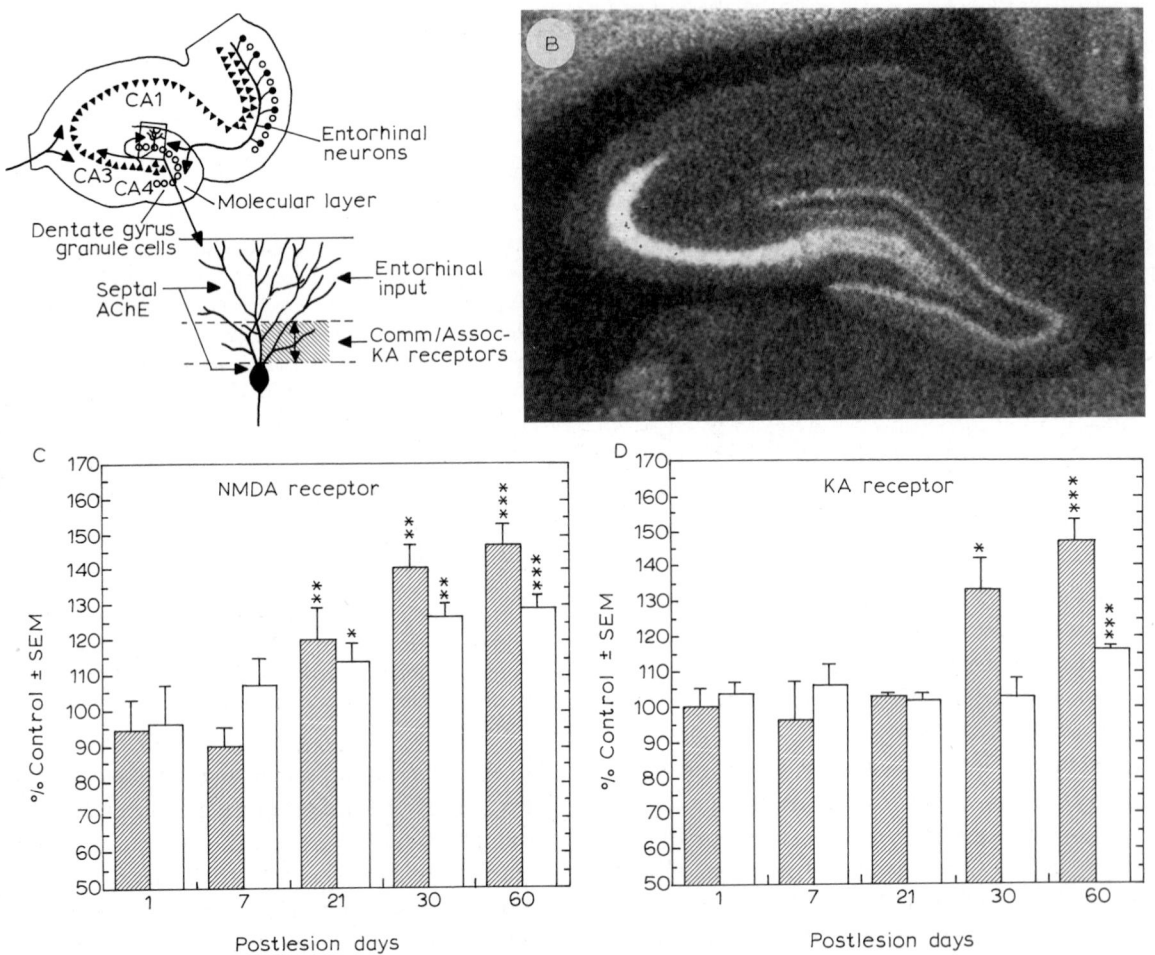

Fig. 1. Dentate gyrus molecular layer anatomy and excitatory amino acid receptor distribution. A: diagram illustrating the normal projections involved in the sprouting response after entorhinal lesions. The entorhinal perforant pathway innervates the outer two-thirds of the molecular layer, whereas the commissural/associational (Comm/Assoc) pathways project to the inner one-third. Kainate (KA) receptors are normally relatively dense in the inner one-third. Septal inputs, as stained for AChE, project to the outer two-thirds and to the supragranule layer. B: autoradiogram showing the normal distribution of KA binding sites in the rat hippocampus. Lighter shades indicate higher binding densities. Note high KA binding levels in CA3 (mossy fiber zone) and the inner molecular layer of the dentate gyrus. C and D: graphs illustrating the time-course of changes in KA and N-methyl-D-aspartate (NMDA) binding levels in the ipsilateral dentate molecular layer after unilateral entorhinal lesions in the rat. At later postoperative times, KA and NMDA binding levels increase over control values in both the outer and inner molecular layer. *, $P < 0.05$; **, $P < 0.01$; ***, $P < 0.001$ in comparison to unoperated controls; ▨, outer two-thirds of the dentate gyrus molecular layer; □, inner one-third of the molecular layer. (Data for NMDA receptors taken from Ulas et al., 1990a and data for KA receptors taken from Ulas et al., 1990b.)

In this chapter, we will discuss recent advances in the study of axonal sprouting in the hippocampus with the use of new molecular markers. It is suggested that the etiology of Alzheimer's disease may involve the reinstatement of developmental processes during the sprouting response.

Properties of axon sprouting after entorhinal lesions

The entorhinal cortex provides a major input to the dentate gyrus, terminating primarily on the outer 2/3 of the dendrites of the granule cells (Blackstad, 1958; Steward, 1976; Fig. 1A). A variety of other inputs also synapse on the dentate granule cells including the basal forebrain cholinergic and non-cholinergic systems (Mosko et al., 1973; Wainer et al., 1985) and the commissural and associational (C/A) inputs (Blackstad, 1956; Laurberg, 1979). Like the entorhinal input, these appear to be highly laminated (Gottlieb and Cowan, 1973). This precise pattern is rearranged following entorhinal lesions.

In 1972, Lynch, Cotman and coworkers reported that following unilateral lesions of the entorhinal cortex in adult rats, the cholinergic forebrain inputs showed an intensification of staining for the enzyme acetylcholinesterase (AChE) within the denervated molecular layer. The increased staining density was interpreted as reflecting the sprouting and proliferation of axons which contained the enzyme AChE. The increase in staining was accompanied by a decrease in staining in the inner molecular layer which may have indicated a selective retraction of fiber input into that region. Entorhinal lesions in the developing brain also caused cholinergic input to be reorganized and form new synapses (Cotman et al., 1973). It is now clear that these observations provided the initial demonstration of the widespread capacity of the adult and developing brain to reform and turn over its synapses in response to disturbances of its circuitry such as lesions.

Quantitative electron microscopic analyses following unilateral ablation of the entorhinal cor-

tex showed that over 80% of the synapses in the outer molecular layer degenerate (Matthews et al., 1976; Hoff et al., 1982; Steward and Vinsant, 1983). Normal synapses disappear, while degenerative debris accumulates in the denervated zone. New synapses begin to form within 4–7 days following the lesion while debris is still being removed. The maximum rate of synapse replacement occurs between 10 and 30 days postlesion and synaptic density is restored to prelesion levels within a few weeks.

The variety of reactive fibers which participate in the reinnervation of the denervated zone have been described in detail (Cotman and Nieto-Sampedro, 1984). Afferents from the ipsilateral and contralateral hilar neurons (the C/A pathway), which do not normally synapse in the denervated zone, over time occupy the inner one-half of the molecular layer. The development of autoradiographic methods to localize EAA receptors has allowed a description of the response of the various receptors (Fig. 1B; Cotman et al., 1987). As the fibers sprout, their corresponding receptors (particularly the kainate (KA) and N-methyl-D-aspartate subtypes) also increase where the new fibers have grown (Fig. 1C, D).

Fibers from the contralateral entorhinal cortex, normally sparse in the molecular layer, also sprout extensively in the denervated zone after unilateral lesions. These new synapses can drive the previously denervated dentate gyrus granule cells. Since the sprouted input from the contralateral cortex is essentially homologous to the lost entorhinal input, these sprouted fibers may thereby participate in the functional recovery following unilateral entorhinal ablation (Scheff and Cotman, 1977; Reeves and Steward, 1988).

Molecular correlates of axon sprouting

Early work at a cellular level from a variety of groups provided the solid foundation upon which to examine the molecular events of the sprouting reaction. The molecular programs underlying sprouting remain largely undefined, but may involve a selective reactivation of developmental mechanisms. This is consistent with early observations showing that new synapses associated with the formation of a new postsynaptic site appear to be formed during the sprouting process (Matthews et al., 1976; Cotman and Kelly, 1980). Thus, sprouting does not simply involve the replacement of vacated postsynaptic densities but requires the rebuilding of the dendritic spine and synapse. Also consistent is evidence from recent studies showing that the developmental or fetal forms of certain cytoskeletal proteins are re-expressed in adult animals under conditions that produce sprouting (Busciglio et al., 1987). Most recently, it has been shown that fetal forms of cytoskeletal proteins are also re-expressed in the Alzheimer's brain (Kosik et al., 1989; Wolozin et al., 1989; Geddes et al., 1990).

In particular, one form of α-tubulin mRNA (Tα1 in rat; Miller et al., 1987, 1989) has been shown to be highly abundant in fetal brain and is specifically expressed during neonatal morphological differentiation (Lewis et al., 1985; Miller et al., 1987, 1989). In contrast, a second form of α-tubulin mRNA, T26, is under less developmental regulation and is expressed at similar levels in both the fetal and adult brain (Miller et al., 1987, 1989). Studies of axonal injury in the peripheral nervous system show that Tα1 mRNA is rapidly reinduced, is maintained at high levels during the period of axonal outgrowth, and is subsequently down-regulated to control levels around the time of target contact (Miller et al., 1989).

To determine whether sprouting central mammalian neurons also recruit the major embryonic form of α-tubulin mRNA, we analyzed the expression of Tα1 mRNA in the rat hippocampus following unilateral electrolytic lesions of the entorhinal cortex. Using in situ hybridization, we found that one day following a lesion, there was a 68% increase over control levels of Tα1 mRNA in dentate granule cells in the ipsilateral hippocampus (Fig. 2A). Elevated Tα1 mRNA expression was also observed in polymorphic hilar neurons, in

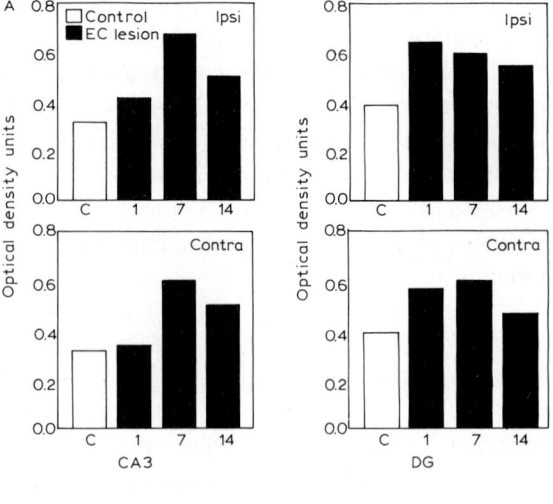

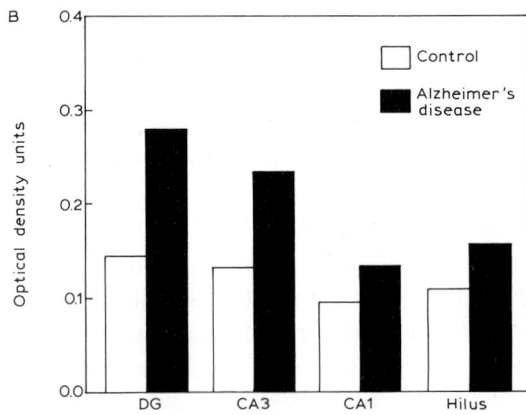

Fig. 2. Expression of Tα1 α-tubulin mRNA in the rat hippocampus at various times following unilateral electrolytic lesions of the entorhinal cortex (A) and in the human hippocampus obtained postmortem from 5 control patients and from 5 patients with AD (B). For measurement of relative mRNA abundance, optical density of the corresponding regions was determined using computer-assisted image analysis (MCID, St. Catherine's, Ontario, Canada) of the X-ray film autoradiogram. The image analyzer was calibrated to optical density units (Kodak) and the individual results represent the average of at least 5 measurements taken from across each region indicated. The human results represent the average obtained from 5 control and 5 AD cases. The results obtained in the dentate gyrus, CA3, and hilus were significantly different ($P < 0.05$) in the AD patients as compared to age-matched controls (see Geddes et al., 1990, for details). The rat results represent the results obtained from a single experiment but have been replicated in 3 separate experiments (Geddes et al., 1990; Geddes, Cotman, and Miller, unpublished results).

pyramidal neurons of the CA3 and CA1 regions, and in cortical neurons located near the site of the lesion. Concurrently, there was an increase in Tα1 mRNA expression in the contralateral hippocampus. Similar results were obtained following knife cut transections of the angular bundle. Tα1 mRNA was expressed at peak levels in the different neuronal populations at 3–5 days, and at lower levels two weeks following the lesion.

The rapid lesion-induced increase and subsequent decline in Tα1 mRNA correlated well with the pattern and time-course of sprouting and synapse turnover triggered by entorhinal cell loss (Cotman and Anderson, 1988). The neurons which exhibited increased Tα1 mRNA expression include those which are predicted to undergo extensive cytoskeletal reorganization following loss of entorhinal input. Specifically, the polymorphic hilar neurons and contralateral entorhinal neurons are expected to extend axon collaterals and the granule cells of the dentate gyrus and pyramidal cells in CA1 and CA3, which are expected to rebuild dendritic spines and postsynaptic densities. The change in Tα1 mRNA expression in the contralateral hippocampus is surprising in view of the selective ipsilateral increase in α-tubulin immunoreactivity (Kwak and Matus, 1988). It is, however, consistent with the synapse loss and replacement described in the contralateral dentate gyrus following unilateral lesions of the entorhinal cortex (Hoff et al., 1981).

Axon sprouting in Alzheimer's disease

One of the goals of research on animal models is to better understand human disease. A consistent feature of Alzheimer's disease (AD) is the degeneration of selected areas of the limbic system. AD is accompanied by a loss of large neurons in the entorhinal cortex (i.e. the layer II and III stellate and pyramidal cells) as well as loss of the pyramidal cells of the hippocampus (Hyman et al., 1984). These findings led to the suggestion that AD may be accompanied by a sprouting reaction

similar to that shown in rodent entorhinal lesion models.

In AD patients, cholinergic septal fibers sprout (as monitored by staining with AChE) in the dentate gyrus molecular layer when the cholinergic input to the hippocampus is still relatively intact (Geddes et al., 1985). This response is similar to the rodent brain AChE intensification in the outer molecular layer of the dentate gyrus in response to entorhinal lesions. The C/A fibers also appear to sprout in the AD brain, as evidenced by the expansion of KA receptor binding (Geddes et al., 1985; Geddes and Cotman, 1986) and other markers (Hamos et al., 1989).

To determine whether bα1 α-tubulin mRNA, the human homologue of Tα1 (Cowan et al., 1983), is also expressed at elevated levels in the hippocampus in AD, we performed in situ hybridization on sections of hippocampal tissues obtained from AD patients and age-matched controls. In the dentate gyrus and CA3 region of the AD hippocampus, analysis of X-ray film autoradiograms indicated a consistent elevation in bα1 mRNA levels (Fig. 2B). Analysis of the hybridized sections at higher resolution (emulsion autoradiography) revealed that the increase in bα1 mRNA was specifically localized to neurons. Neurons with increased numbers of grains in AD versus controls were located in the dentate gyrus, the hilus, and the CA3 regions. Grain counts, quantified in 2 of the 5 AD cases studied, demonstrated an average 3- to 4-fold relative increase in the amount of bα1 α-tubulin mRNA per CA3 neuron (Geddes et al., 1990).

Thus it appears that disease-induced neuronal loss in the entorhinal cortex may be a stimulus similar to entorhinal lesions in the rat brain. The selective loss of entorhinal neurons removes the perforant path input to the hippocampus, inducing a compensatory response in adjacent inputs. The observed sprouting responses in AD (e.g. increased AChE staining, increased synaptic reorganization) contrasts with the numerous decreases observed in transmitter-related markers in AD. That sprouting occurs in AD is consistent with the finding that spines on dentate granule cells are maintained in

AD despite the loss of input cells (Gertz et al., 1987).

Conclusion

Previously, we have hypothesized that sprouting in the early stages of select diseases such as AD may improve function, at least when cell loss is minor and pathology has not yet taken over. As cells are lost, new connections are made by the remaining healthy cells which may amplify weakened signals and assume similar functions of the fibers from the same or converging pathways (Cotman and Anderson, 1988). Although over a decade has passed since the cholinergic sprouting reaction was first described, its significance is still unknown. Following entorhinal damage, the increased cholinergic input may improve hippocampal function in the same way cholinergic transplants ameliorated behavior in aged animals (Gage and Björklund, 1986). It could enhance excitability, refine hippocampal theta rhythm, etc. In several ways the system may adjust the threshold at which behavioral impairments appear. This may delay functional loss relative to the integrity of neuronal circuits remaining so as to maintain functional stability despite neuronal loss. Clearly, however, there is much research yet to be done.

Previous cellular and new molecular data suggest that sprouting may involve in part a reinduction of developmental patterns of gene expression. In this context, the presence of some embryonic markers in AD may be a reflection of regenerative mechanisms. Other findings are also consistent with a replay of developmental events in AD. The presence of embryonic forms of cytoskeletal proteins, including tubulin, tau, and other microtubule-associated proteins (Nunez, 1988; Kosik et al., 1989), may impact on the polymerization, phosphorylation, and stability of the neuronal cytoskeleton in AD and even contribute to senile plaque formation. Thus, the inappropriate production of select developmentally regulated cytoskeletal proteins may contribute to the etiology of neuropathological disorders such as

Alzheimer's disease. An initially adaptive process may eventually become part of the pathological process. The high prevalence of AD in the elderly would indeed favor a rather general mechanism that is capable of being initiated from several points. As Blackstad predicted, the hippocampus has served to be an excellent system in which to define basic neurological phenomena and extend these to the study of disease states.

Acknowledgement

The authors are grateful to Dr. J. Ulas for her helpful comments on the manuscript.

References

Amaral, D.G. (1987) Memory: anatomical organization of candidate brain regions. In V.B. Mountcastle, F. Plum and S.R. Geiger (Eds.), *Handbook of Physiology – The Nervous System, V,* American Physiological Society, Bethesda, MD, pp. 211 – 294.

Blackstad, T.W. (1956) Commissural connections of the hippocampal region in the rat, with special reference to their mode of termination. *J. Comp. Neurol.,* 105: 417 – 537.

Blackstad, T.W. (1958) On the termination of some afferents to the hippocampus and fascia dentata. *Acta Anat.,* 35: 202 – 214.

Blackstad, T.W. (1963) Ultrastructural studies on the hippocampal region. *Prog. Brain Res.,* 3: 122 – 148.

Blackstad, T.W. and Kjaerheim, Å. (1961) Special axodendritic synapses in the hippocampal cortex: electron and light microscopic studies on the layer of mossy fibers. *J. Comp. Neurol.,* 117: 133 – 146.

Busciglio, J., Ferreira, A., Steward, O. and Caceres, A., (1987) An immunocytochemical and biochemical study of the microtubule-associated protein tau during post-lesion afferent reorganization in the hippocampus of adult rats. *Brain Res.,* 419: 244 – 252.

Cotman, C.W. and Anderson, K.J. (1988) Synaptic plasticity and functional stabilization in the hippocampal formation: possible role in Alzheimer's disease. In S. Waxman (Ed.), *Physiologic Basis for Functional Recovery in Neurological Disease,* Raven Press, New York, pp. 313 – 336.

Cotman, C.W. and Kelly, P. (1980) Macromolecular architecture of CNS synapses. In C.W. Cotman, G. Poste and G.L. Nicholson (Eds.), *Cell Surface Reviews,* 6: Elsevier/North Holland, Biomedical Press, Amsterdam, pp. 505 – 533.

Cotman, C.W. and Lynch, G.S., (1976) Reactive synaptogenesis in the adult nervous system: the effects of partial deafferentation on new synapse formation. In S. Barondes (Ed.), *Neuronal Recognition,* Plenum Press, New York, pp. 109 – 130.

Cotman, C.W., Matthews, D.A., Taylor, D. and Lynch, G.S. (1973) Synaptic rearrangement in the dentate gyrus: histochemical evidence of adjustments after lesions in immature and adult rats. *Proc. Natl. Acad. Sci. U.S.A.,* 70: 3473 – 3477.

Cotman, C.W., Monaghan, D.T., Ottersen, O.P. and Storm-Mathisen, J. (1987) Anatomical organization of excitatory amino acid receptors and their pathways. *Trends Neurosci.,* 10: 273 – 280.

Cotman, C.W. and Nieto-Sampedro, M. (1984) Cell biology of synaptic plasticity. *Science,* 255: 1287 – 1294.

Cowan, N.J., Dobner, P.R., Fuchs, E.V. and Cleveland D.W. (1983) Expression of human alpha-tubulin genes: interspecies conservation of 3' untranslated regions, *Mol. Cell Biol.,* 3: 1738 – 1745.

Gage, F.H. and Björklund, A. (1986) Cholinergic septal grafts into the hippocampal formation improve spatial learning and memory in aged rats by an atropine-sensitive mechanism. *J. Neurosci.,* 6: 2837 – 2847.

Geddes, J.W., Monaghan, D.T., Cotman, C.W., Lott, I.T., Kim, R.C. and Chui, H.C. (1985) Plasticity of hippocampal circuitry in Alzheimer's disease. *Science,* 230: 1179 – 1181.

Geddes, J.W. and Cotman, C.W. (1986) Plasticity in hippocampal excitatory amino acid receptors in Alzheimer's disease. *Neurosci. Res.,* 3: 672 – 678.

Geddes, J.W., Wong, J., Choi, B.H. Kim, R.C., Cotman, C.W. and Miller, F.D. (1990) Increased expression of the embryonic form of a developmentally regulated mRNA in Alzheimer's disease. *Neurosci. Lett.,* 109: 54 – 61.

Gertz, H.J., Cervos-Navarro, J. and Ewald, V. (1987) The septo-hippocampal pathway in patients suffering from senile dementia of Alzheimer's type. Evidence for neuronal plasticity? *Neurosci. Lett.,* 76: 228 – 232.

Gottlieb, D.I. and Cowan, W.M. (1973) Autoradiographic studies of the commissural and ipsilateral association connections of the hippocampus and dentate gyrus of the rat. *J. Comp. Neurol.,* 149: 393 – 422.

Hamos, J.E., DeGennaro, L.J. and Drachman, D.A. (1989) Synaptic loss in Alzheimer's disease and other dementias. *Neurology,* 39: 355 – 361.

Hoff, S.F., Scheff, S.W., Kwan, A.Y. and Cotman, C.W. (1981) A new type of lesion-induced synaptogenesis: I. Synaptic turnover in non-denervated zones of the dentate gyrus in young adult rats, *Brain Res.,* 222: 1 – 13.

Hoff, S.F., Scheff, S.W. and Cotman, C.W. (1982) Lesion-induced synaptogenesis in the dentate gyrus of aged rats: I. Loss and reacquisition of normal synaptic density. *J. Comp. Neurol.,* 205: 246 – 252.

Hyman, B.T., Van Hoesen, G.W., Damasio, A.R. and Barnes, C.L. (1984) Alzheimer's disease: cell-specific pathology isolates the hippocampal formation. *Science,* 225:

1168 – 1170.

Kosik, K.S., Orecchio, L.D., Bakalis, S. and Neve, R.L. (1989) Developmentally regulated expression of specific tau sequences. *Neuron,* 2: 1389 – 1397.

Kwak, S. and Matus, A. (1988) Denervation induces long-lasting changes in the distribution of microtubule proteins in hippocampal neurons. *J. Neurocytol.,* 17: 189 – 195.

Laurberg, S. (1979) Commissural and intrinsic connections of the rat hippocampus. *J. Comp. Neurol.,* 184: 685 – 708.

Lewis, S.A., Lee, M.G.-S. and Cowan, N.J. (1985) Five mouse tubulin isotypes and their regulated expression during development. *J. Cell Biol.,* 101: 852 – 861.

Lynch, G., Matthews, D., Mosko, S., Parks, T. and Cotman, C.W. (1972) Induced acetylcholinesterase-rich layer in rat dentate gyrus following entorhinal lesion. *Brain Res.,* 42: 311 – 318.

Matthews, D.A., Cotman, C.W. and Lynch, G.S. (1976) An electron microscopic study of lesion-induced synaptogenesis in the dentate gyrus of the adult rat. I. Magnitude and time course of degeneration. *Brain Res.,* 115: 1 – 21.

Miller, F.D., Naus, C.C.G., Durand, M., Bloom, F.E. and Milner, R.J. (1987) Isotypes of α-tubulin are differentially regulated during neuronal maturation. *J. Cell Biol.,* 105: 3065 – 3073.

Miller, F.D., Tetzlaff, W., Bisby, M.A., Fawcett, J.W. and Milner, R.J. (1989) Rapid induction of the major embryonic α-tubulin mRNA, Tα1, during nerve regeneration in adult rats. *J. Neurosci.,* 9: 1452 – 1463.

Mosko, S., Lynch, G.S. and Cotman, C.W. (1973) The distribution of septal projections to the hippocampus of the rat. *J. Comp. Neurol.,* 152: 163 – 174.

Nunez, J. (1988) Immature and mature variants of MAP2 and tau proteins and neuronal plasticity. *Trends Neurosci.,* 11: 477 – 479.

Reeves, T.M. and Steward, O. (1988) Changes in the firing properties of neurons in the dentate gyrus with denervation and reinnervation: implications for behavioral recovery. *Exp. Neurol.,* 102: 37 – 49.

Scheff, S.W. and Cotman, C.W. (1977) Recovery of spontaneous alternation following lesions of the entorhinal cortex in adult rats: possible correlation to axon sprouting. *Behav. Biol.,* 21: 286 – 293.

Steward, O. (1976) Topographic organization of the projections from the entorhinal area to the hippocampal formation of the rat. *J. Comp. Neurol.,* 167: 285 – 314.

Steward, O. and Vinsant, S.L. (1983) The process of reinnervation in the dentate gyrus of the adult rat: a quantitative electron microscopic analysis of terminal proliferation and reactive synaptogenesis. *J. Comp. Neurol.,* 214: 203 – 210.

Storm-Mathisen, J. and Blackstad, T.W. (1964) Cholinesterase in the hippocampal region. *Acta Anat.,* 56: 216 – 253.

Swanson, L.W. (1983) The hippocampus and the concept of the limbic system. In W. Seifert (Ed.), *Neurobiology of the Hippocampus,* Academic Press, New York, pp. 3 – 19.

434

Wainer, B.H., Levey, A.I., Rye, D.B., Mesulam, M.M. and Mufson, E.J. (1985) Cholinergic and non-cholinergic septohippocampal pathways. *Neurosci. Lett.,* 54: 45 – 52.

Ulas, J., Monaghan, D.T., and Cotman, C.W. (1990a) Plastic response of hippocampal excitatory amino acid receptors to deafferentation and reinnervation. *Neuroscience,* in press.

Ulas, J., Monaghan, D.T. and Cotman, C.W. (1990b) Kainate receptors in the rat hippocampus: a distribution and time course of changes in response to unilateral lesions of the entorhinal cortex. *J. Neurosci.,* in press.

Wolozin, B.L., Scicutella, A. and Davies, P. (1989) Re-expression of a developmentally regulated antigen in Down syndrome and Alzheimer disease. *Proc. Natl. Acad. Sci. U.S.A.,* 85: 6202 – 6206.

J. Storm-Mathisen, J. Zimmer and O.P. Ottersen (Eds.)
Progress in Brain Research, Vol. 83
© 1990 Elsevier Science Publishers B.V. (Biomedical Division)

CHAPTER 31

Hippocampal plasticity in normal aging and decreased plasticity in Alzheimer's disease

Dorothy G. Flood[1,2] and Paul D. Coleman[2]

Departments of [1]Neurology and [2]Neurobiology and Anatomy, School of Medicine and Dentistry, University of Rochester, 601 Elmwood Avenue, Rochester, NY 14642, U.S.A.

Different patterns of age-related dendritic change have been reported in different zones of the human hippocampal region in the normal and Alzheimer's disease (AD) brain. In normal aging there is an increase in average (net) dendritic extent (which we interpret as plasticity) in the parahippocampal gyrus and dentate gyrus. There is net stability of dendritic extent in CA2–3, CA1, and subiculum. In regions that show plasticity in normal aging, dendrites in AD show reduced or aberrant plasticity. In regions that show stability in normal aging, dendrites either are stable or regress in AD, depending upon how severely involved the region is with the pathology of AD.

Introduction

Age-related changes in dendritic extent in normal brain have been found to be quite variable, depending upon the region, species and age range studied (for a review see Coleman and Flood, 1987). All of the possible basic patterns of net dendritic change in normal aging have been observed: (1) growth (Buell and Coleman, 1979, 1981; Connor et al., 1980, 1981, 1982), (2) regression (Feldman, 1977; Vaughan, 1977; Hinds and McNelly, 1981; Leuba, 1983; Rogers et al., 1984; Nakamura et al., 1985; Levine et al., 1986), (3) stability (Coleman et al., 1986; Flood et al., 1987b), (4) regression followed by growth (Pentney, 1986), and (5) growth followed by regression (Hinds and McNelly, 1977; Cupp and Uemura, 1980; Uemura, 1985; Flood et al., 1985 and 1987a; Rafols et al., 1989). Most of the above studies quantified a static picture of dendrites in Golgi-stained postmortem tissue in subjects of varying ages, which evaluates *net* changes or stability of dendritic extent. However, net stability over time allows for considerable remodelling among the cells of the neuronal

population being studied, as long as growth and regression are equally balanced. Evidence for the simultaneous existence of these two processes in vivo is provided by electron microscopic study showing evidence of synaptic turnover (Adams and Jones, 1982) and by light microscopic study showing simultaneous growth and regression of dendritic processes (Purves and Hadley, 1985). Thus, subtle changes in dendrites are probably constantly occurring throughout the life span in response to internal and external environmental cues.

We interpret an age-related increase in dendritic extent as a plastic, compensatory response of neurons to the age-related death of their neighbors. As such, it is assumed that this is an adaptive process. It should, however, be noted that not all growth phenomena are necessarily adaptive. Growth may permit the formation of inappropriate connections among neurons that are more injurious to information processing than the original loss of connections. The plasticity described by us (Flood et al., 1987a) and others (Geddes et al., 1985; De Ruiter and Uylings, 1987; Gertz et al., 1987; Hyman et al., 1987) in Alzheimer's disease (AD) may be an example of this. Because the neuronal loss and transmitter deficits in the AD brain are more marked than in normal brain it is possible that the diseased nervous system is forced to reorganize in a deleterious manner.

Three of the 5 patterns of dendritic change found in normal aging, listed above, have been observed in the hippocampus and in the parahippocampal gyrus in the aging human. Age-related dendritic regression is the only pattern that has been absent among the cell types of the hippocampus. Thus, the hippocampus may be unique among cortical areas in not showing dendritic regression in normal aging since some of our preliminary data on middle frontal gyrus, as well as published data on primary motor cortex (Nakamura et al., 1985), suggest that dendritic regression does occur in some neocortical areas. Unlike the hippocampus, sufficient data do not exist for other cerebral cortical areas to describe the patterns of changes in detail.

A brief summary of hippocampal circuitry

Although other chapters in this volume more completely address hippocampal circuitry, especially in primates (Amaral, Chapter 1), it is appropriate to describe briefly the connections among the cell types that we have quantified in the hippocampus and its associated region, the parahippocampal gyrus. The parahippocampal gyrus integrates visual, auditory, and somatic inputs from sensory association areas of the temporal, occipital, and parietal lobes (Van Hoesen and Pandya, 1975a; Van Hoesen, 1982). It in turn projects to entorhinal cortex (area 28) (Van Hoesen and Pandya, 1975a; Insausti et al., 1987). The entorhinal cortex also receives neocortical afferents from orbitofrontal cortex, dorsolateral and medial frontal lobe, temporal lobe, cingulate gyrus, perirhinal cortex, olfactory cortex, and insular cortex (Van Hoesen and Pandya, 1975a; Van Hoesen et al., 1975; Insausti et al., 1987). Cortical input via the perforant path to the hippocampus proper is mainly from layer II and III neurons of entorhinal cortex and terminates on the dendrites of granule cells in the outer two-thirds of the molecular layer of the fascia dentata and in the stratum lacunosum-moleculare of CA1 (regio superior) and CA3 (regio inferior) (Van Hoesen and Pandya, 1975b; Witter et al., 1989). Granule cells also receive a largely uncrossed input (Demeter et al., 1985) from the hilus that synapses in the inner molecular layer (Laurberg, 1979). The mossy fiber axons of granule cells in turn project to the hilus (CA4) and to stratum lucidum and stratum pyramidale of CA3 (Blackstad et al., 1970; Rosene and Van Hoesen, 1977). Pyramidal neurons of CA3 project to stratum radiatum, stratum pyramidale, and stratum oriens of CA1 by the Schaffer collateral system of fibers; and pyramidal neurons of CA1 project to subiculum and entorhinal cortex (lower layers) (Rosene and Van Hoesen, 1977). Finally, the subiculum projects to pre- and parasubiculum and the lower layers of entorhinal cortex (Rosene and Van Hoesen, 1977; Kosel et al., 1982). The cortical projections of entorhinal cortex largely reciprocate its afferents (Kosel et al., 1982; Van Hoesen, 1982).

Hippocampal regions exhibiting net dendritic increase in normal human aging

We have examined 6 cell types in the hippocampal region. Two of these have shown age-related increases in dendritic extent, which we interpret as a compensatory, plastic response of surviving neurons to the death of their neighbors. The remaining 4 regions showed net stability of dendritic extent with increasing age. The two regions in which we found age-related increases in dendritic extent are the parahippocampal gyrus and dentate gyrus. In parahippocampal gyrus, Buell and Coleman (1979 and 1981) described an increase in dendritic extent of layer II pyramidal neurons between an "adult" group (mean age of 51.2 years) and an "aged" group (mean age of 79.6 years). In the apical dendritic trees the increase in total dendritic extent was the result of both an increase in the lengths of dendritic segments and in the numbers of segments (Buell and Coleman, 1981). However, in the basal trees the increase in dendritic extent was due only to the lengthening of segments, not to an increase in numbers of segments. In Fig. 1 the "aged" group has been subdivided into old-aged (OA, $n = 3$) and very old-aged (VOA, $n = 2$) groups (Buell and Coleman, 1980), for purposes of comparison with the data to be presented below from other hippocampal regions. The subdivision of the data shows that once the dendrites have increased in length in old age (seventies), they continue to be maintained at this increased, or only slightly reduced, length into very old age (nineties).

As in the parahippocampal gyrus, dendritic extent of the apical trees of dentate gyrus granule cells also increases significantly between middle age (MA, mean age = 52.3) and old age (mean age = 73.4) (Flood et al., 1985, 1987a). However

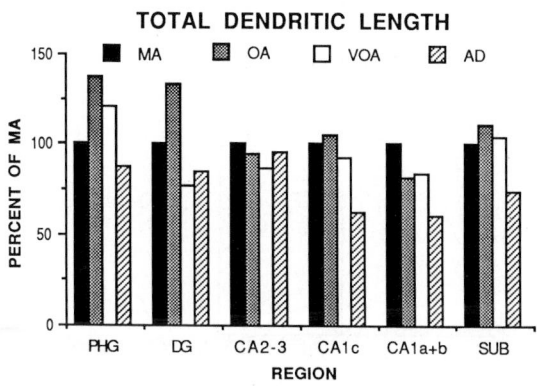

Fig. 1. Total dendritic length adjusted to a percent of that in the middle-aged group for each cell type studied in the hippocampal region. Age groups for neurologically and psychiatrically normal subjects are: middle-aged subjects (MA) with a mean age in the early fifties, old-aged subjects (OA) with a mean age in the early seventies, and very old-aged subjects (VOA) with a mean age in the early nineties. Subjects with clinically and neuropathologically verified Alzheimer's disease (AD) averaged in their mid-seventies. Data are shown for apical trees of parahippocampal gyrus (PHG) layer II pyramidal cells, apical trees of dentate gyrus (DG) granule cells, basal trees of CA2 – 3 pyramidal cells, basal trees of CA1c pyramidal cells, basal trees of CA1a + b pyramidal cells, and apical trees of subiculum (SUB) layer III pyramidal cells. See Lorente de Nó (1934) for a description of the subdivisions of CA1 and of the layers of the subiculum.

unlike the parahippocampal gyrus, the dentate gyrus granule cells were found to decrease significantly in total dendritic extent between old age and very old age (mean age = 90.2 years). The significant increases and decreases in total dendritic length were the result of concordant small, non-significant changes in both the numbers of segments and the lengths of segments. Thus, in granule cells the age-related pattern of dendritic change is that of an inverted U-shaped curve, in which dendritic growth in early old age is followed by regression in late old age (Fig. 1).

Two other studies have examined dendritic extent of dentate gyrus granule cells in a limited number of normal subjects over a wide range of ages. One examined dendrites from 13 cases aged 16 – 91 years and found a high degree of between subject variability in dendritic extent, with no statistically significant age-related change (Williams and Matthysse, 1986). However, their 4 oldest cases, aged 75 – 91 years, had the least extensive dendritic trees. The second study examined 5 cases aged 65 – 94 years old and found reduced dendritic extent in only their oldest subject (De Ruiter and Uylings, 1987). These studies are consistent with our data in suggesting dendritic regression in dentate gyrus granule cells of the very old cases. However, there are discrepancies among the studies with regard to the age at which the regression is first seen. The regression may begin as early as 75 years (youngest regressed subject) (Williams and Matthysse, 1986) or may be delayed until after 86 years (oldest non-regressed subject) (De Ruiter and Uylings, 1987).

Hippocampal regions exhibiting net dendritic stability in normal human aging

In contrast to findings of dendritic plasticity in normal aging in some structures in the hippocampal region (Buell and Coleman, 1979, 1981; Flood et al., 1987a), dendritic extent of pyramidal neurons in CA2 – 3 and CA1 of Ammon's horn and in layer III of subiculum is stable between middle age and very old age (Fig. 1). We have reported that dendrites of the apical and basal trees of CA2 – 3 pyramidal cells do not change significantly among normally aging groups (Flood et al., 1987b). We have also examined 2 subdivisions of CA1: (1) CA1c, the region adjacent to CA2 – 3; and (2) CA1a + b, the region adjacent to the subiculum in which the stratum pyramidale is wider than in CA1c (Lorente de Nó, 1934). Lastly, we have studied the layer III pyramidal neurons of the subiculum (Lorente de Nó, 1934). In all 3 of these regions there was no statistically significant change in dendritic extent of either the apical or basal tree in normal aging between the ages of 43 and 95.

Altered dendritic plasticity in Alzheimer's disease (AD) in regions which are plastic in normal aging

In the parahippocampal gyrus, an AD group (mean age = 76 years) showed significantly reduced dendritic extent of both the apical and basal trees compared with an age-matched control group, but was similar to a younger "adult" group (Fig. 1) (Buell and Coleman, 1979, 1981). Since the dendritic extent of the AD group was so similar to that of the "adult" group, the authors suggested that there may be a failure of the AD brain to undergo normal age-related dendritic proliferation, signifying a loss of dendritic plasticity. If neuroplasticity is impaired in AD, it is possible that the continuously occurring alterations in dendritic architecture described by Purves and Hadley (1985) are not taking place; and the absence of these alterations may be of greater importance than absolute dendritic extent.

Total dendritic extent of dentate gyrus granule cells was also significantly reduced in AD compared with the age-matched OA group (Flood et al., 1987a). However, unlike the parahippocampal gyrus, dentate gyrus granule cells in the AD group did appear to make some plastic alterations (Fig. 2). Although the lengths of dendritic segments were significantly reduced in the AD group compared with their age-matched control group, the

numbers of dendritic segments in the AD group were equivalent to that in their age-matched control group. These data indicate that dentate gyrus granule cells may mount a plastic response in the AD brain by branching. This plastic response is, however, not normal since this branching does not result in an increased total dendritic length, but rather in a shorter average segment length. These dentate gyrus granule cells are the only cell type in which an *average* increase has been found for any

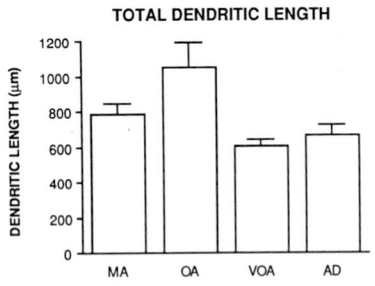

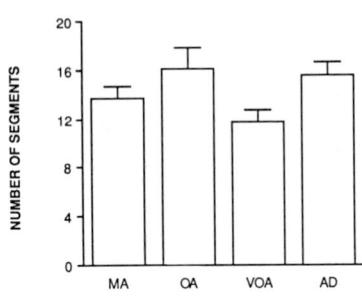

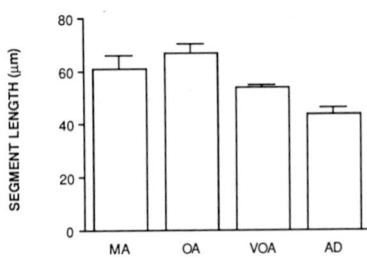

Fig. 2. Total dendritic length, numbers of segments, and average segment length for the apical dendritic trees of dentate gyrus granule cells. See Fig. 1 for a description of the subject groups. Error bars represent ± S.E.M. (From Flood and Coleman (1986). *Can. J. Neurol. Sci.,* 13: 475 – 479. Reprinted with permission).

dendritic parameter in AD. These findings have been confirmed by De Ruiter and Uylings (1987) who found significantly reduced dendritic length but maintenance of numbers of segments in dentate gyrus granule cells in AD. Thus, these data suggest that at least one part of the hippocampal region is capable of mounting a small, aberrant plastic response.

Dendritic extent in AD in brain regions which are stable in normal aging

The effect of AD on dendritic extent varies among regions showing stability in normal aging, depending upon their relative involvement in the disease process. CA2 – 3 is relatively spared the pathology of AD, while CA1 and subiculum are the most heavily involved with senile plaques, neurofibrillary tangles, granulovascular degeneration, and neuronal loss (e.g. Ball, 1978; Hyman et al., 1984; Doebler et al., 1987). Consequently, in AD dendritic extent of the apical and basal trees of CA2 – 3 pyramidal neurons is unchanged from that in normal subjects (Flood et al., 1987b). However, in CA1c, CA1a + b, and subiculum, dendritic extent in the AD cases is significantly reduced compared with control subjects. These data confirm a report of dendritic regression in the basal dendritic trees of CA1 pyramidal neurons in an older group of AD cases (80 – 90 years) (Yamada et al., 1988). The regression suggests that these regions are less functional in AD than is indicated by cell count studies alone.

Other findings of plasticity in Alzheimer's disease

Lesion studies in animals have for some time shown that the dentate gyrus granule cells and their afferents are plastic after lesions of the perforant path input. In particular, commissural-associational and cholinergic fibers have been found to invade the outer two-thirds of the molecular layer (e.g. Lynch et al., 1972, 1973; Stanfield and Cowan, 1982). With this invasion,

granule cell spines (Parnavelas et al., 1974; Caceres and Steward, 1983), synapses (e.g. Cotman et al., 1973; Hoff et al., 1982), and dendrites (Caceres and Steward, 1983) also regrow. Thus, when it was reported that the entorhinal cortical neurons forming the perforant path are lost in AD (Hyman et al., 1984), much attention was directed towards determining whether AD cases show similar plastic alterations to lesioned rats. Thus, in addition to quantifying regressive alterations in the granule cells and their afferents, an attempt has been made to quantify plastic changes, characterized as either maintenance or growth of structures in the dentate gyrus.

As in the perforant path lesioned rat, patients with AD have been found to show a substantial amount of afferent regrowth. When the cholinergic innervation of the hippocampus is intact in AD, there is an expansion of acetylcholinesterase staining into the outer molecular layer (Geddes et al., 1985; Hyman et al., 1987). Geddes et al. (1985) have also reported an expansion of the commissural-associational pathway, visualized with kainic acid receptor autoradiography. However, a recent report has failed to replicate this finding, and also claims that kainic acid binding is associated with mossy fiber endings (Represa et al., 1988). Although proof that the commissural-associational pathway is sprouting in AD may be questionable, there is good evidence that the cholinergic fibers are sprouting.

In addition to alterations suggestive of plasticity in the apical dendrites of granule cells described above, there are other reports that suggest that the granule cells are plastic. De Ruiter and Uylings (1987) have reported that a greater number of granule cells in the AD cases had basal dendritic trees than in the controls. This suggests either preferential survival of cells with basal dendrites or growth of basal dendrites on more cells in AD. The basal dendrites are, of course, in a position to contact the remaining commissural-associational innervation, even before it reaches the apical dendrites of the molecular layer. Although several groups have reported a reduction in spine density on granule cell apical dendrites in AD compared with age-matched controls (Williams and Matthysse, 1986; De Ruiter and Uylings, 1987; Gertz et al., 1987), the latter group has found a normal number of spines in the inner molecular layer where cholinergic and commissural-associational fibers end (Gertz et al., 1987).

The question of the role of plasticity in the etiology and/or pathophysiology of AD is a topic of much current interest. The specific alterations are probably more complicated than simply too little or too much plasticity because the outcome ultimately seen as neuronal growth and synapse formation involves complicated and unknown intercellular signaling mechanisms, production of one or more trophic factors, the neuron's ability to respond appropriately to the trophic factors and the functionality of the connections formed. In AD some types of neurons do seem to be able to show plastic responses. The dentate gyrus is particularly capable of plasticity in normal, as well as in diseased subjects (see above), and may therefore not be the most representative region in which to evaluate residual plasticity in the AD brain. In other regions of the AD brain neuritic sprouting has been described on cell bodies and dendrites (Scheibel and Tomiyasu, 1978; Arendt et al., 1986; Ihara, 1988; McKee et al., 1988) or on dendrites in association with neuritic plaques (Probst et al., 1983). We too have seen some examples of filopodial expansions from cell bodies and dendrites in our Golgi material, but there has not yet been a demonstration that these expansions are forming appropriate synapses. These outgrowths may be of little benefit or may be deleterious in the AD brain. In addition, the currently available quantitative data indicate that these expansions do not result in increased dendritic extent averaged over a randomly derived sample of cells.

Additionally, work is beginning to appear that suggests that there may be increased levels of trophic substances in AD (Birecree et al., 1988; Uchida et al., 1988) and that a portion of the amyloid precursor molecule itself may be neurotrophic (Whitson et al., 1989). Some trophic substances are present in the AD brain and some neurons appear to respond by neurite outgrowth. However, it remains to be determined whether neurons are responding in a normal manner but are overwhelmed by the pathology of AD or whether the neuronal plastic response is aberrant.

Conclusion

Regions involved in the early processing of information in the hippocampal circuitry (parahippocampal gyrus and dentate gyrus) exhibit plasticity in normal aging and reduced plasticity in AD. The dentate gyrus granule cells and their afferents in the AD brain maintain some plasticity that may not ultimately be beneficial. Regions involved with the later processing of information (Ammon's horn and subiculum) stand in marked contrast in showing dendritic stability in normal aging. In spite of neuronal loss in these regions, remaining neurons are capable of carrying on their function without resorting to major growth of the dendritic tree. In AD only those regions of Ammon's horn that are severely affected by the disease show dendritic regression. Thus, at least one region of Ammon's horn, CA2–3, is relatively well maintained in AD. There is little plasticity in CA1 and subiculum, regions severely affected in AD, and this may be so because these regions do not demonstrate dendritic plasticity in the normal aging human.

Acknowledgements

The authors received support from National Institute on Aging Grants AG 03644 (D.G.F. and P.D.C.) and AG 01121 (P.D.C.).

References

Adams, I. and Jones, D.G. (1982) Synaptic remodeling and astrocytic hypertrophy in rat cerebral cortex from early to late adulthood. *Neurobiol. Aging,* 3: 179–186.

Arendt, T., Zvegintseva, H.G. and Leontovich, T.A. (1986) Dendritic changes in the basal nucleus of Meynert and in the diagonal band nucleus in Alzheimer's disease – A quantitative Golgi investigation. *Neuroscience*, 19: 1265–1278.

Ball, M.J. (1978) Topographic distribution of neurofibrillary tangles and granulovascular degeneration in hippocampal cortex of aging and demented patients. A quantitative study. *Acta Neuropathol*, 42: 73–80.

Birecree, E., Whetsel Jr., W.O., Stoscheck, C., King Jr., L.E. and Nanney, L.B. (1988) Immunoreactive epidermal growth factor receptors in neuritic plaques from patients with Alzheimer's disease. *J. Neuropathol. Exp. Neurol.*, 47: 549–560.

Blackstad, T.W., Brink, K., Hem, J. and Jeune, B. (1970) Distribution of hippocampal mossy fibers in the rat. An experimental study with silver impregnation methods. *J. Comp. Neurol.*, 138: 433–450.

Buell, S.J. and Coleman, P.D. (1979) Dendritic growth in the aged human brain and failure of growth in senile dementia. *Science*, 206: 854–856.

Buell, S.J. and Coleman, P.D. (1980) Individual differences in dendritic growth in human aging and senile dementia. In D. Stein (Ed.), *The Psychobiology of Aging: Problems and Perspectives*, Elsevier, Amsterdam, pp. 283–296.

Buell, S.J. and Coleman, P.D. (1981) Quantitative evidence for selective dendritic growth in normal human aging but not in senile dementia. *Brain Res.*, 214: 23–41.

Caceres, A. and Steward, O. (1983) Dendritic reorganization in the denervated dentate gyrus of the rat following entorhinal cortical lesions: a Golgi and electron microscopic analysis. *J. Comp. Neurol.*, 214: 387–403.

Cotman, C.W., Matthews, D.A., Taylor, D. and Lynch, G. (1973) Synaptic rearrangement in the dentate gyrus: histochemical evidence of adjustments after lesions in immature and adult rats. *Proc. Natl. Acad. Sci. U.S.A.*, 70: 3473–3477.

Coleman, P.D. and Flood, D.G. (1987) Neuron numbers and dendritic extent in normal aging and Alzheimer's disease. *Neurobiol. Aging*, 8: 521–545.

Coleman, P.D., Buell, S.J., Magagna, L., Flood, D.G. and Curcio, C.A. (1986) Stability of dendrites in cortical barrels of C57Bl/6N mice between 4 and 45 months. *Neurobiol. Aging*, 7: 101–105.

Connor, Jr., J.R., Diamond, M.C. and Johnson, R.E. (1980) Occipital cortical morphology of the rat: alterations with age and environment. *Exp. Neurol.*, 68: 158–170.

Connor, Jr., J.R., Diamond, M.C., Connor, J.A. and Johnson, R.E. (1981) A Golgi study of dendritic morphology in the occipital cortex of socially reared aged rats. *Exp. Neurol.*, 73: 525–533.

Connor, Jr., J.R., Beban, S.E., Hopper, P.A., Hansen, B. and Diamond, M.C. (1982) A Golgi study of the superficial pyramidal cells in the somatosensory cortex of socially reared old adult rats. *Exp. Neurol.*, 76: 35–45.

Cupp, C.J. and Uemura, E. (1980) Age-related changes in prefrontal cortex of *Macaca mulatta*: quantitative analysis of dendritic branching patterns. *Exp. Neurol.*, 69: 143–163.

Demeter, S., Rosene, D.L. and Van Hoesen, G.W. (1985) Interhemispheric pathways of the hippocampal formation, presubiculum, and entorhinal and posterior parahippocampal cortices in the rhesus monkey: the structure and organization of the hippocampal commissures. *J. Comp. Neurol.*, 233: 30–47.

De Ruiter, J.P. and Uylings, H.B.M. (1987) Morphometric and dendritic analysis of fascia dentata granule cells in human aging and senile dementia. *Brain Res.*, 402: 217–229.

Doebler, J.A., Markesbery, W.R., Anthony, A. and Rhoads, R.E. (1987) Neuronal RNA in relation to neuronal loss and neurofibrillary pathology in the hippocampus in Alzheimer's disease. *J. Neuropathol. Exp. Neurol.*, 46: 28–39.

Feldman, M.L. (1977) Dendritic changes in aging rat brain: pyramidal cell dendrite length and ultrastructure. In K. Nandy and I. Sherwin (Eds.), *The Aging Brain and Senile Dementia*, Plenum Press, New York, pp. 23–37.

Flood, D.G. and Coleman, P.D. (1986) Failed compensatory dendritic growth as a pathophysiological process in Alzheimer's disease. *Can. J. Neurol. Sci.*, 13: 475–479.

Flood, D.G., Buell, S.J., DeFiore, C.H., Horwitz, G.J. and Coleman, P.D. (1985) Age-related dendritic growth in dentate gyrus of human brain is followed by regression in the "oldest old". *Brain Res.*, 345: 366–368.

Flood, D.G., Buell, S.J., Horwitz, G.J. and Coleman, P.D. (1987a) Dendritic extent in human dentate gyrus granule cells in normal aging and senile dementia. *Brain Res.*, 402: 205–216.

Flood, D.G., Guarnaccia, M. and Coleman, P.D. (1987b) Dendritic extent in human CA_{2-3} hippocampal pyramidal neurons in normal aging and senile dementia. *Brain Res.*, 409: 88–96.

Geddes, J.W., Monaghan, D.T., Cotman, C.W., Lott, I.T., Kim, R.C. and Chui, H.C. (1985) Plasticity of hippocampal circuitry in Alzheimer's disease. *Science*, 230: 1179–1181.

Gertz, H.J., Cervos-Navarro, J. and Ewald, V. (1987) The septo-hippocampal pathway in patients suffering from senile dementia of Alzheimer's type. Evidence for neuronal plasticity? *Neurosci. Lett.*, 76: 228–232.

Hinds, J.W. and McNelly, N.A. (1977) Aging of the rat olfactory bulb: growth and atrophy of constituent layers and changes in size and number of mitral cells. *J. Comp. Neurol.*, 171: 345–368.

Hinds, J.W. and McNelly, N.A. (1981) Aging in the rat olfactory system: correlation of changes in the olfactory epithelium and olfactory bulb. *J. Comp. Neurol.*, 203: 441–453.

Hoff, S.F., Scheff, S.W., Benardo, L.S. and Cotman, C.W. (1982) Lesion-induced synaptogenesis in the dentate gyrus of aged rats: I. Loss and reacquisition of normal synaptic density. *J. Comp. Neurol.*, 205: 246–252.

Hyman, B.T., Van Hoesen, G.W., Damasio, A.R. and Barnes, C.L. (1984) Alzheimer's disease: cell-specific pathology isolates the hippocampal formation. *Science*, 225:

1168 – 1170.

Hyman, B.T., Kromer, L.J. and Van Hoesen, G.W. (1987) Reinnervation of the hippocampal perforant pathway zone in Alzheimer's disease. *Ann. Neurol.,* 21: 259 – 267.

Ihara, Y. (1988) Massive somatodendritic sprouting of cortical neurons in Alzheimer's disease. *Brain Res.,* 459: 138 – 144.

Insausti, R., Amaral, D.G. and Cowan, W.M. (1987) The entorhinal cortex of the monkey: II. Cortical afferents. *J. Comp. Neurol.,* 264: 356 – 395.

Kosel, K.C., Van Hoesen, G.W. and Rosene, D.L. (1982) Non-hippocampal cortical projections from the entorhinal cortex in the rat and rhesus monkey. *Brain Res.,* 244: 201 – 213.

Laurberg, S. (1979) Commissural and intrinsic connections of the rat hippocampus. *J. Comp. Neurol.,* 184: 685 – 708.

Leuba, G. (1983) Aging of dendrites in the cerebral cortex of the mouse. *Neuropathol. Appl. Neurobiol.,* 9: 467 – 475.

Levine, M.S., Adinolfi, A.M., Fisher, R.S., Hull, C.D., Buchwald, N.A. and McAllister, J.P. (1986) Quantitative morphology of medium-sized caudate spiny neurons in aged cats. *Neurobiol. Aging,* 7: 277 – 286.

Lorente de Nó, R. (1934) Studies on the structure of the cerebral cortex. II. Continuation of the study of the ammonic system. *J. Psychol. Neurol.,* 46: 113 – 177.

Lynch, G.S., Matthews, D.A., Mosko, S., Parks, T. and Cotman, C.W. (1972) Induced acetylcholinesterase-rich layer in rat dentate gyrus following entorhinal lesions. *Brain Res.,* 42: 311 – 318.

Lynch, G.S., Mosko, S., Parks, T. and Cotman, C.W. (1973) Relocation and hyperdevelopment of the dentate gyrus commissural system after entorhinal lesions in immature rats. *Brain Res.,* 50: 174 – 178.

McKee, A.C., Kowall, N.W. and Kosik, K.S. (1988) Microtubule disorganization and growth cone formation characterize degeneration and regeneration in Alzheimer's disease. *Soc. Neurosci. Abstr.,* 14: 155.

Nakamura, S., Akiguchi, I., Kameyama, M. and Mizuno, N. (1985) Age-related changes of pyramidal cell basal dendrites in layers III and V of human motor cortex: a quantitative Golgi study. *Acta Neuropathol.,* 65: 281 – 284.

Parnavelas, J.G., Lynch, G.S., Brechna, N., Cotman, C.W. and Globus, A. (1974) Spine loss and regrowth in hippocampus following deafferentation. *Nature (Lond.),* 248: 71 – 73.

Pentney, R.J. (1986) Quantitative analysis of dendritic networks in Purkinje neurons during aging. *Neurobiol. Aging,* 7: 241 – 248.

Probst, A., Basler, V., Bron, B. and Ulrich, J. (1983) Neuritic plaques in senile dementia of Alzheimer type: a Golgi analysis in the hippocampal region. *Brain Res.,* 268: 249 – 254.

Purves, D. and Hadley, R.D. (1985) Changes in the dendritic branching of adult mammalian neurones revealed by repeated imaging *in situ. Nature (Lond.),* 315: 404 – 406.

Rafols, J.A., Cheng, H.W. and McNeill, T.H. (1989) Golgi study of the mouse striatum: age-related dendritic changes in different neuronal populations. *J. Comp. Neurol.,* 279: 212 – 227.

Represa, A., Duyckaerts, C., Tremblay, E., Hauw, J.J. and Ben-Ari, Y. (1988) Is senile dementia of the Alzheimer type associated with hippocampal plasticity? *Brain Res.,* 457: 355 – 359.

Rogers, J., Zornetzer, S.F., Bloom, F.E. and Mervis, R.E. (1984) Senescent microstructural changes in rat cerebellum. *Brain Res.,* 292: 23 – 32.

Rosene, D.L. and Van Hoesen, G.W. (1977) Hippocampal efferents reach widespread areas of cerebral cortex and amygdala in the rhesus monkey. *Science,* 198: 315 – 317.

Scheibel, A.B. and Tomiyasu, U. (1978) Dendritic sprouting in Alzheimer's presenile dementia. *Exp. Neurol.,* 60: 1 – 8.

Stanfield, B.B. and Cowan, W.M. (1982) The sprouting of septal afferents to the dentate gyrus after lesions of the entorhinal cortex in adult rats. *Brain Res.,* 232: 162 – 170.

Uchida, Y., Ihara, Y. and Tomonaga, M. (1988) Alzheimer's disease brain extract stimulates the survival of cerebral cortical neurons from neonatal rats. *Biochem. Biophys. Res. Commun.,* 150: 1263 – 1267.

Uemura, E. (1985) Age-related changes in the subiculum of *Macaca mulatta:* dendritic branching pattern. *Exp. Neurol.,* 87: 412 – 427.

Van Hoesen, G.W. (1982) The parahippocampal gyrus. New observations regarding its cortical connections in the monkey. *Trends Neurosci.,* 5: 345 – 350.

Van Hoesen, G.W. and Pandya, D.N. (1975a) Some connections of the entorhinal (area 28) and perirhinal (area 35) cortices of the rhesus monkey. I. Temporal lobe afferents. *Brain Res.,* 95: 1 – 24.

Van Hoesen, G.W. and Pandya, D.N. (1975b) Some connections of the entorhinal (area 28) and perirhinal (area 35) cortices of the rhesus monkey. III. Efferent connections. *Brain Res.,* 95: 39 – 59.

Van Hoesen, G.W., Pandya, D.N. and Butters, N. (1975) Some connections of the entorhinal (area 28) and perirhinal (area 35) cortices of the rhesus monkey. II. Frontal lobe afferents. *Brain Res.,* 95: 25 – 38.

Vaughan, D.W. (1977) Age-related deterioration of pyramidal cell basal dendrites in rat auditory cortex. *J. Comp. Neurol.,* 171: 501 – 516.

Whitson, J.S., Selkoe, D.J. and Cotman, C.W. (1989) Amyloid β protein enhances the survival of hippocampal neurons in vitro. *Science,* 243: 1488 – 1490.

Williams, R.S. and Matthysse, S. (1986) Age-related changes in Down syndrome brain and the cellular pathology of Alzheimer disease. In D.F. Swaab, E. Fliers, M. Mirmiran, W.A. Van Gool and F. Van Haaren (Eds.), *Aging of the Brain and Alzheimer's Disease. Progress in Brain Research, Vol. 70,* Elsevier Science Publishers, Amsterdam, pp. 49 – 67.

Witter, M.P., Van Hoesen, G.W. and Amaral, D.G. (1989) Topographical organization of the entorhinal projection to the dentate gyrus of the monkey. *J. Neurosci.,* 9: 216 – 228.

Yamada, M., Wada, Y., Tsukagoshi, H., Otomo, E.-I. and Hayakawa, M. (1988) A quantitative Golgi study of basal dendrites of hippocampal CA1 pyramidal cells in senile dementia of Alzheimer type. *J. Neurol., Neurosurg. Psychiatry,* 51: 1088 – 1090.

J. Storm-Mathisen, J. Zimmer and O.P. Ottersen (Eds.)
Progress in Brain Research, Vol. 83
© 1990 Elsevier Science Publishers B.V. (Biomedical Division)

CHAPTER 32

Hippocampal formation: anatomy and the patterns of pathology in Alzheimer's disease

Gary W. Van Hoesen[1,2] and Bradley T. Hyman[3]

Departments of [1] Anatomy and [2] Neurology, University of Iowa College of Medicine, Iowa City, IA 52242, U.S.A. and [3] Neurology Service, Harvard Medical School, Massachusetts General Hospital, Fruit Street, Boston, MA 02114, U.S.A.

Anatomical studies of the primate brain have shown that the subicular and CA1 allocortices give rise to hippocampal efferents that course to numerous telencephalic and diencephalic targets including other parts of the cortex. The hippocampal formation is damaged heavily in Alzheimer's disease, and is a focal point for pathology. We examined the anteroposterior extent of the hippocampal formation in 52 cases of Alzheimer's disease, 6 cases of other types of dementia and 10 age-compatible controls, to determine the patterns of pathology. We have observed that only certain subfields of the hippocampal formation are affected by cell loss, neurofibrillary tangles and neuritic plaques, while adjacent, anatomically distinct subfields are relatively spared. The portions of the hippocampal formation most crucial for both cortical and subcortical efferent projections are severely affected by Alzheimer pathological changes. Most notable are neurofibrillary tangles in the subicular and CA1 subfields. Layer IV of entorhinal cortex, which receives a large subicular projection and in turn projects to widespread limbic and association cortices, is also severely and specifically affected by neurofibrillary tangles. Hippocampal input is also compromised. For example, layer II of entorhinal cortex, which gives rise to perforant pathway hippocampal afferents, also undergoes severe neurofibrillary changes. Neuritic plaques appear in a distinct layer in the terminal zone of the perforant pathway, which carries the majority of corticohippocampal afferents. Plaques are also common in a zone that receives serotoninergic projections from the raphe complex, thus compromising another hippocampal afferent. In sum, these changes disrupt intrinsic and extrinsic hippocampal circuitry at multiple levels, and the pathological dissection deprives the hippocampal formation of many of its efferent and afferent connections with cortical and subcortical structures important in memory-related neural systems. These changes likely contribute to the memory impairment that characterizes Alzheimer's disease and the devastating intellectual decline that ensues.

Introduction

Alzheimer's disease presents typically with a memory impairment of varying severity that becomes more dense and global as the disease progresses. Forgetfulness of a name or a place may bring the patient to medical attention initially, but a global amnesia and agnosia, including the loss of self-identity, may characterize it at end stage. One would expect that this may be due, in part, to structural lesions and/or to neurochemical deficits that affect many neural systems important in normal memory (Coyle et al., 1983; Katzman, 1986). We have focused on pathological changes in the hippocampal formation and the relationship of such lesions to hippocampal neuroanatomy and the connections that link this structure with the parahippocampal gyrus, amygdala, certain thalamic nuclei, mammillary bodies, septum and the nucleus basalis of Meynert (Hyman et al., 1984, 1986; Van Hoesen and Damasio, 1987).

The hippocampal formation is known to be a central component of memory-related neural systems both from studies of patients with amnesia and from experimental studies in animals (Mishkin, 1982; Squire ande Zola-Morgan, 1983; Damasio, 1984). Its importance is exemplified by the profound amnesia that results in patients with bilateral hippocampal injury after surgery, herpes simplex encephalitis or anoxia (Scoville and Millner, 1957; Victor et al., 1962; McLardy, 1970; Volpe and Petito, 1985; Damasio et al., 1985; Zola-Morgan et al., 1986).

The hippocampal formation has long been known to be one of the brain areas most consistently affected by pathological changes in Alzheimer's disease. In fact, Fuller (1911) highlighted hippocampal involvement in his "review" article in 1911, only 4 years after Alzheimer's initial brief report describing the pathological changes of this disease. Since then, many investigations have noted the predisposition of the hippocampal region to neurofibrillary tangles, granulovascular degeneration and neuritic plaques (Goodman, 1953; Morel and Wildi, 1955; Hirano and Zimmerman, 1962; Jamada and Mehraein, 1968; Corsellis, 1970; Tomlinson and Kitchener, 1972; Ball, 1976; Brun and Gustafson, 1976; Tomlinson, 1977; Ball, 1978; Kemper, 1978; Burger, 1983; Gibson, 1983; Wilcock, 1983; Hyman et al., 1984; Ulrich and Stahelin, 1984). Many pathologists believe that hippocampal lesions are a *sine qua non* for Alzheimer's disease (Terry, 1985) and there is little reason to dispute this.

Despite these studies, the precise distribution of pathological changes within subfields of the hippocampal formation, and their relationship to its anatomy, has received little attention, although pioneering studies by Ball (1976, 1978) and Kemper (1978) provide an important start. Also, in the past decade a great deal has been learned about the detailed connectional anatomy of these regions in the non-human primate (Van Hoesen, 1982; Amaral, 1986, 1987), and more opportunities for a finer analysis now exist. As summarized by these authors, investigations have revealed that there is an intricate pattern of intrinsic and associational connections that link the hippocampal formation to widespread limbic, sensory-specific and multimodal association cortices. For example, anatomical studies in the primate have shown that the CA1 subfield and the subicular cortices of the

hippocampal formation give rise to efferents that end in the cerebral cortex, amygdala, basal forebrain and thalamus (Van Hoesen, 1982, 1985; Amaral, 1987). Such connections may provide the structural basis for the influence that the hippocampal formation has on widespread parts of the brain that play a role in memory. We have therefore re-examined the distribution of hippocampal formation pathology in a large series of brains of Alzheimer patients from the viewpoint of recent advances in experimental neuroanatomy in higher mammals and present a summary of our conclusions in this dedicated chapter.

Methods

Postmortem brain tissue from 68 patients was examined. Of these, 52 had dementia and the neuropathological alterations of Alzheimer's disease (ages 59 – 98). Six additional cases (ages 57 – 95) had a clinical history of dementia attributable to several causes: normal pressure hydrocephalus (1 case), multi-infarct (1 case), pseudodementia depression (1 case), Huntington's disease (1 case), and mixed infarcts plus Alzheimer changes (2 cases). There were 10 non-demented, neurologically normal controls (ages 58 – 83).

For our studies, the hippocampal formation and adjoining parahippocampal gyrus were dissected *en bloc* from the left hemisphere through their entire anteroposterior extent. The block was placed in a solution of 4% formalin, 10% glycerol and 10% sucrose at 4°C until saturated. Serial 50 μm thick sections were cut on a freezing microtome, and series were collected. These were mounted on acid-washed, gelatin-precoated microscope slides and stained with (a) thionin for Nissl substance, (b) thioflavin S for neurofibrillary tangles, neuritic plaques and amyloid, and (c) in 14 cases of Alzheimer's disease, 1 case of normal pressure hydrocephalus and 5 controls, two complete series of sections were each stained for acetylcholinesterase activity using the method of Geneser-Jensen and Blackstad (1971). In addition, selected sections were examined with Congo red (Stokes and

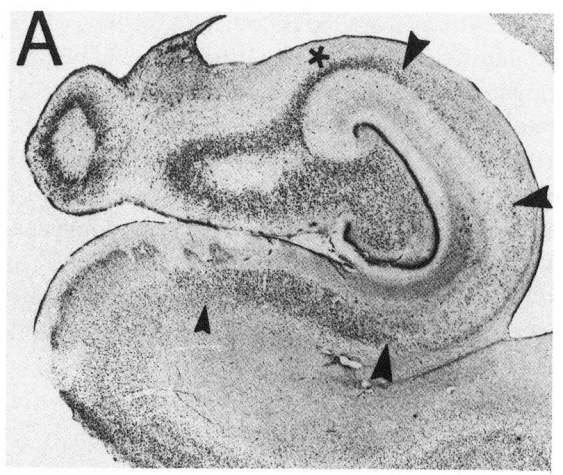

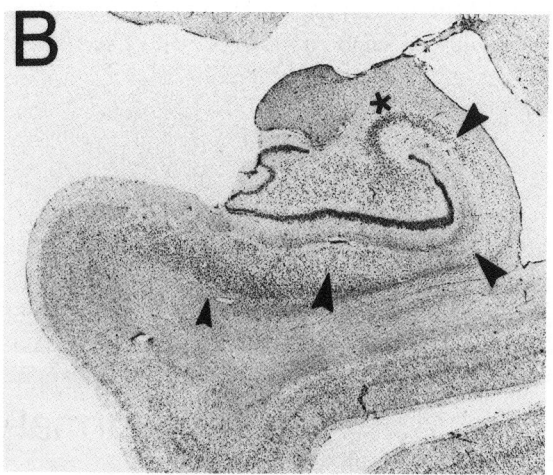

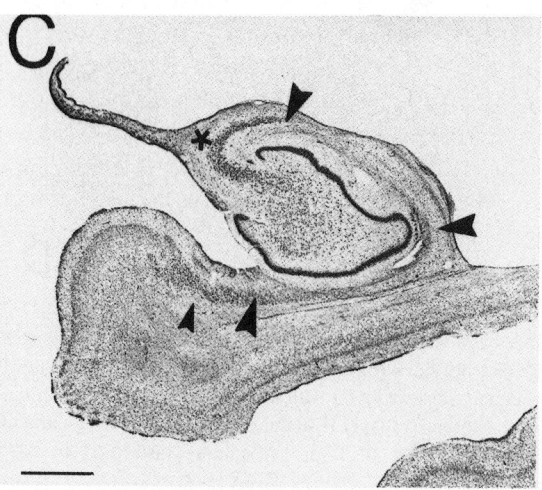

Trickey, 1973) and with a modified Bielschowsky silver procedure (Vogt, 1974). Finally, several sections were immunostained with Alz-50 (Hyman et al., 1988). Approximately 80 sections were generated from each brain. They were analyzed using brightfield, darkfield, cross-polarized light and fluorescent microscopy. The pattern of neuropathological alterations in representative sections was also mapped utilizing an X-Y recorder coupled electronically to the movements of the microscope stage, as well as by camera-lucida techniques.

Results

Cytoarchitecture of the hippocampal formation in Alzheimer's disease

Distinctive and consistent alterations in the normal cytoarchitecture of the hippocampal formation were observed in all cases of Alzheimer's disease, and in the cases of mixed Alzheimer changes plus infarcts. While the dentate gyrus, CA4 and CA3 regions were not grossly different from controls, a thinning of cortex with loss of pyramidal cell staining was apparent in the CA1/subicular area (Fig. 1). This was most pronounced in the prosubicular and parasubicular areas, while the most medial portion of the subiculum and presubiculum were affected to a much lesser degree. When viewed in terms of the longitudinal orientation of architectural subfields, this created the impression of alternating patterns of pathology in the hippocampal formation, i.e. pathology in parasubiculum, little pathology in presubiculum, pathology in the subicular/CA1 subfields and little pathology in the CA3 and CA4 subfields.

Fig. 1. A – C: Nissl-stained photomicrographs of the hippocampal formation in 3 severe cases of Alzheimer's disease demonstrating the pale and thin appearance of the subicular/CA1 zone (large arrowheads). Note that the presubiculum (small arrowheads) and CA3 zone (asterisks) are recognizable. Case A was 77 years, Case B was 87 years and Case C was 88 years of age at death and all had a 5 – 12 year history of dementia. Bar = 2 mm.

The 52 Alzheimer cases were not affected with uniform severity. For example, in some cases the subiculum was dramatically thinned with near total loss of pyramidal cells. Other cases had a cell-poor patchy appearance. Nevertheless, the pattern of subfield changes was observed in all cases in the pattern described above.

The adjacent anterior parts of the parahippocampal gyrus, Brodmann's area 28, or the entorhinal cortex, were consistently and heavily damaged in over 90% of our cases (Fig. 2). This was conspicuous in Nissl preparations in that the islands of large stellate neurons that form layer II were not present or greatly reduced in size and/or

numbers of neurons. Additionally, layer IV, which normally contains large modified pyramids, was irregular or incipient, creating the impression of an abnormally wide lamina dissecans and/or the presence of a lamina dissecans in parts of area 28 where it would not be expected (Fig. 3). Clearly, stainable ribosomes and rough endoplasmic reticulum were no longer present in these neurons; however, as discussed below, stainable neurofibrillary tangles marked the location of once viable neurons.

Pattern of neurofibrillary tangles in the hippocampal formation

Neurofibrillary tangles were visualized using thioflavin S, Congo red and Alz-50. The normal

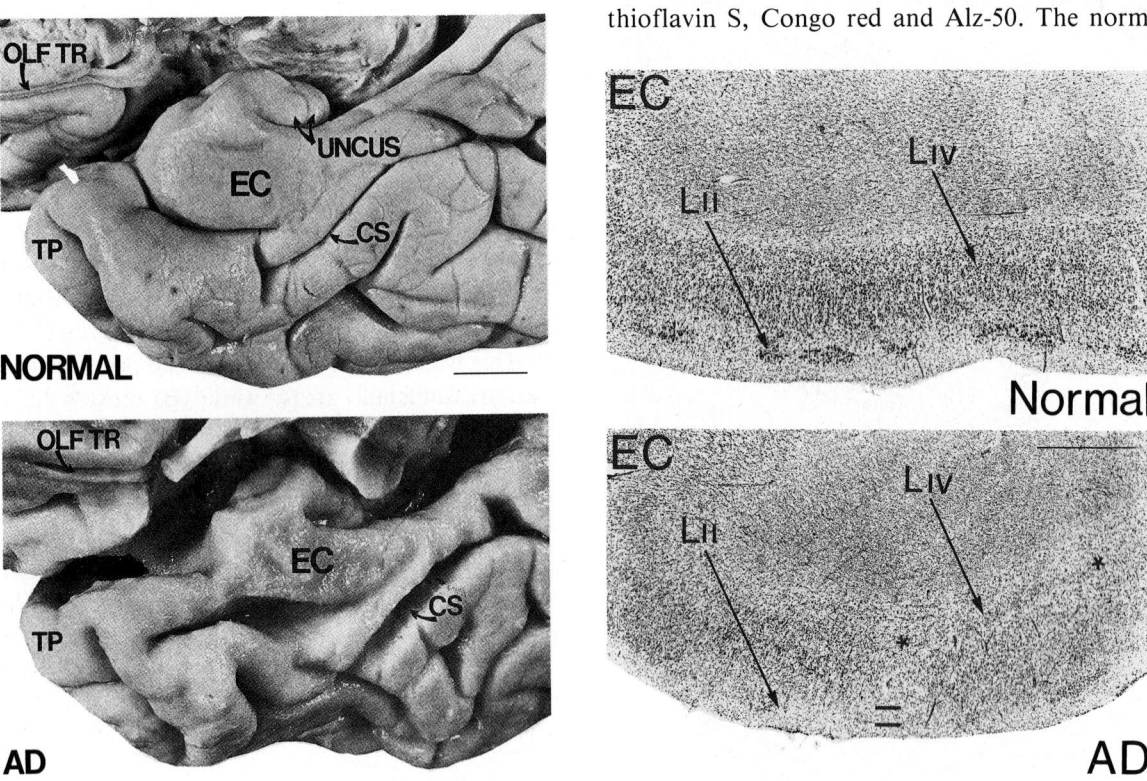

Fig. 2. Photographs of the ventromedial temporal lobe in humans showing the normal appearance of the entorhinal cortex (EC) in a 69-year-old normal with no history of dementia and a 67-year-old victim of Alzheimer's disease (AD). Note the atrophic and discolored appearance of the EC in AD. CS, collateral sulcus; OLF TR, olfactory tract; TP, temporal pole. Bar = 1 cm.

Fig. 3. Nissl-stained photomicrographs of the entorhinal cortex (EC) in a normal with no history of dementia and a victim of Alzheimer's disease (AD) with an 8-year history of dementia. Note the absence of layer II staining (bars) and the irregular and patchy appearance of layer IV staining (asterisks) in AD. Bar = 1 mm.

controls, and the cases of pseudodementia, Huntington's disease, normal pressure hydrocephalus and multi-infarct dementia, contained few or no neurofibrillary tangles. The Alzheimer cases and the mixed Alzheimer/infarct dementia cases contained a distinctive pattern of neurofibrillary tangles in the hippocampal formation which closely reflected the pattern of cell loss. Again, only certain subfields were primarily affected, with adjacent divisions relatively spared. The neurons of the subicular/CA1 area and, in particular, the pro-

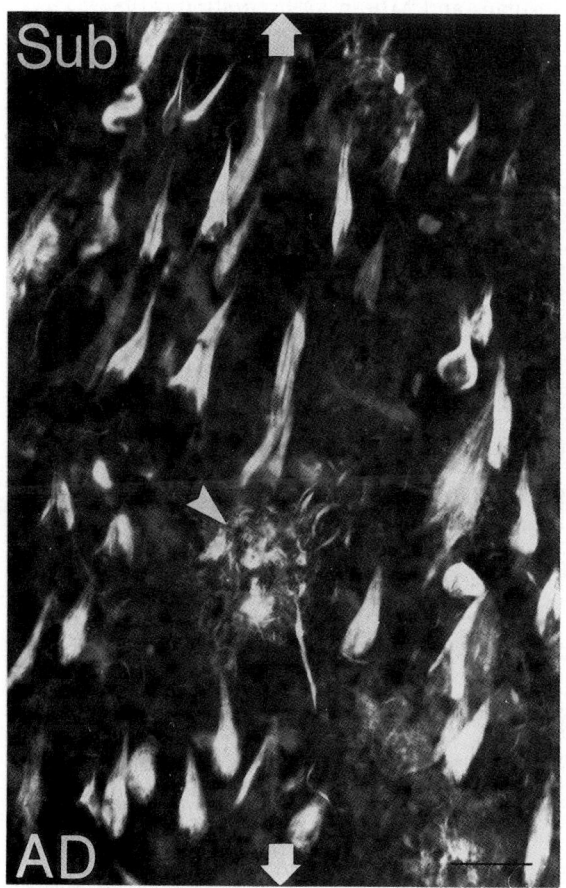

Fig. 4. Photomicrographs of thioflavin S stained tissue in the subiculum (Sub) in Alzheimer's disease (AD) demonstrating a dense number of neurofibrillary tangles. The arrowhead points to a large neuritic plaque. The white arrow at the top of the photomicrograph indicates the direction of the hippocampal fissure, while the arrow at the bottom of the photomicrograph denotes the direction of the alveus. Bar = 50 μm.

subiculum, were consistently the most affected by neurofibrillary tangles (Figs. 4 and 5). The granule cells of the dentate gyrus, the modified pyramidal cells of CA4 and the CA3 pyramids were largely uninvolved. In all cases the subicular-CA1 zone was more heavily affected than the more medial aspect of the subiculum proper and the medially adjacent presubiculum. The parasubiculum was consistently and severely affected. In the parahippocampal gyrus, layers II and IV of the entorhinal cortex (Brodmann's area 28) and layers III and V of the posterior parahippocampal cortex (Brodmann's areas 35 and 36) primarily contained neurofibrillary tangles (Figs. 6 and 7).

Pattern of neuritic plaques in the hippocampal formation

Neuritic plaques were visualized with thioflavin S and fluorescent microscopy, with confirmation by a modified Bielschowsky silver stain. The normal controls and non-Alzheimer cases of dementia had few or no neuritic plaques, whereas the Alzheimer cases and mixed Alzheimer/multi-infarct dementia cases all contained prominent numbers of neuritic plaques.

A general pattern of distribution of neuritic plaques was evident. Plaques were found prominently in a distinct line in the middle and outer portions of the molecular layer of the dentate gyrus, but rarely in the inner portion of the molecular layer or among the granule cells themselves. Plaques did occur in the hilum (CA4), CA3, CA2 and the adjacent portion of CA1, but the density in these regions was less than that observed in the prosubiculum and subiculum. In the latter areas plaques formed a distinct line in the deep part of the stratum moleculare (Fig. 8). Plaques were also found throughout the pyramidal cell layer of the prosubiculum and subiculum, especially in the superficial half of the pyramidal cell layer. The presubiculum rarely contained neuritic plaques.

In contrast to their consistent involvement by neurofibrillary tangles and neuronal loss, the parasubiculum and entorhinal cortex had a more variable number of plaques. When present in the parasubiculum they were aligned in columns spanning layers II and III. In the entorhinal cortex, approximately half of the cases examined contained a distinct band of plaques in layer III (Fig. 6). Other cases had plaques in the deep layers, or a few plaques without a distinct pattern. In comparison, adjacent temporal neocortex often contained more plaques than entorhinal cortex, but without a pattern of lamination or columnar alignment.

Many neuritic plaques stain for acetylcholinesterase (AChE) activity in the hippocampal formation. In the hippocampus and subiculum their distribution reflects that of neuritic plaques as revealed by thioflavin S staining. For example, AChE-positive plaques were located in the middle and outer portions of the molecular layer of the dentate gyrus, in the molecular layer of the parasubiculum and subiculum, and in the pyramidal cell layer of those cortices. They were located diffusely within CA4, and less frequently in the other subdivisions of the hippocampal formation, including the parasubiculum and entorhinal cortex. In addition, some neurofibrillary tangles were lightly AChE-positive, confirming Mesulam and Moran's observations (1987).

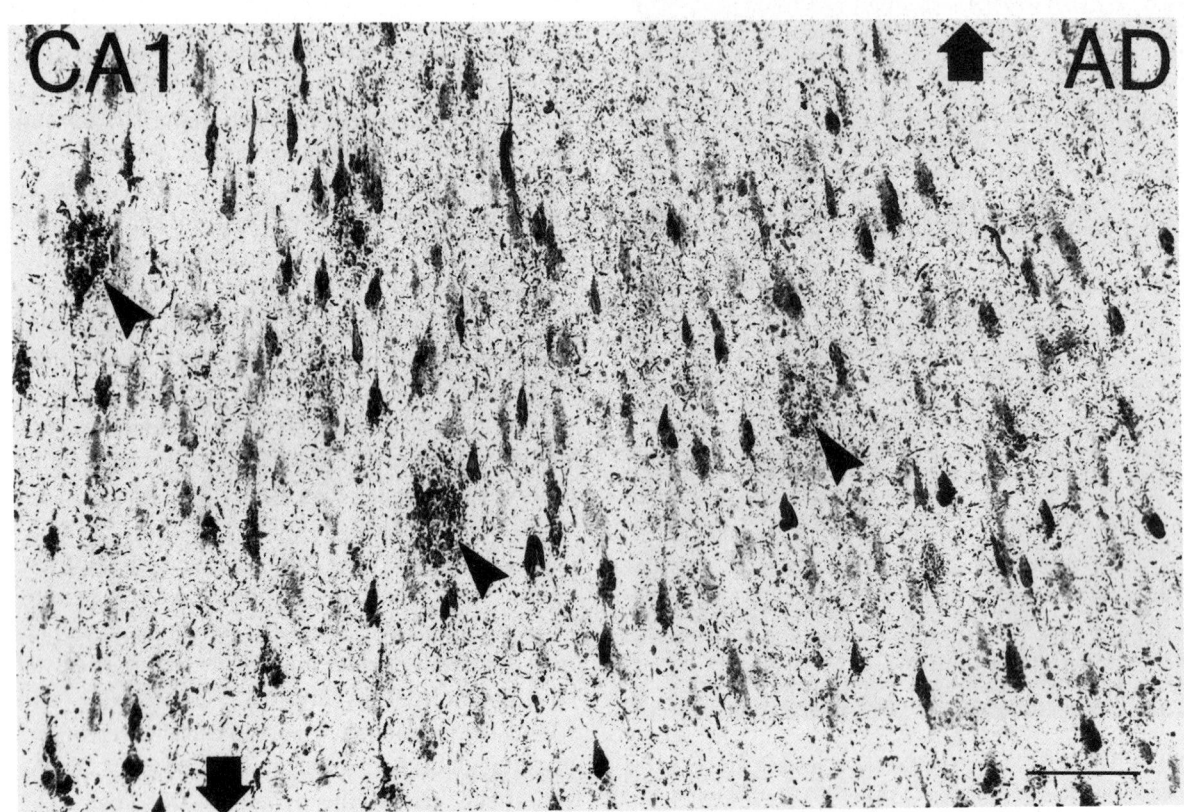

Fig. 5. Photomicrograph of Alz-50 immunoreactive neurons in the CA1 subfield of the hippocampal formation in Alzheimer's disease (AD). The arrowheads denote immunoreactive neuritic plaques. The black arrow along the top of the photomicrograph denotes the direction of the hippocampal fissure, while the one at the bottom denotes the direction of the alveus. The Alz-50 monoclonal antibody recognizes the A68 antigen which is found in high quantities in Alzheimer's disease. Bar = 100 μm.

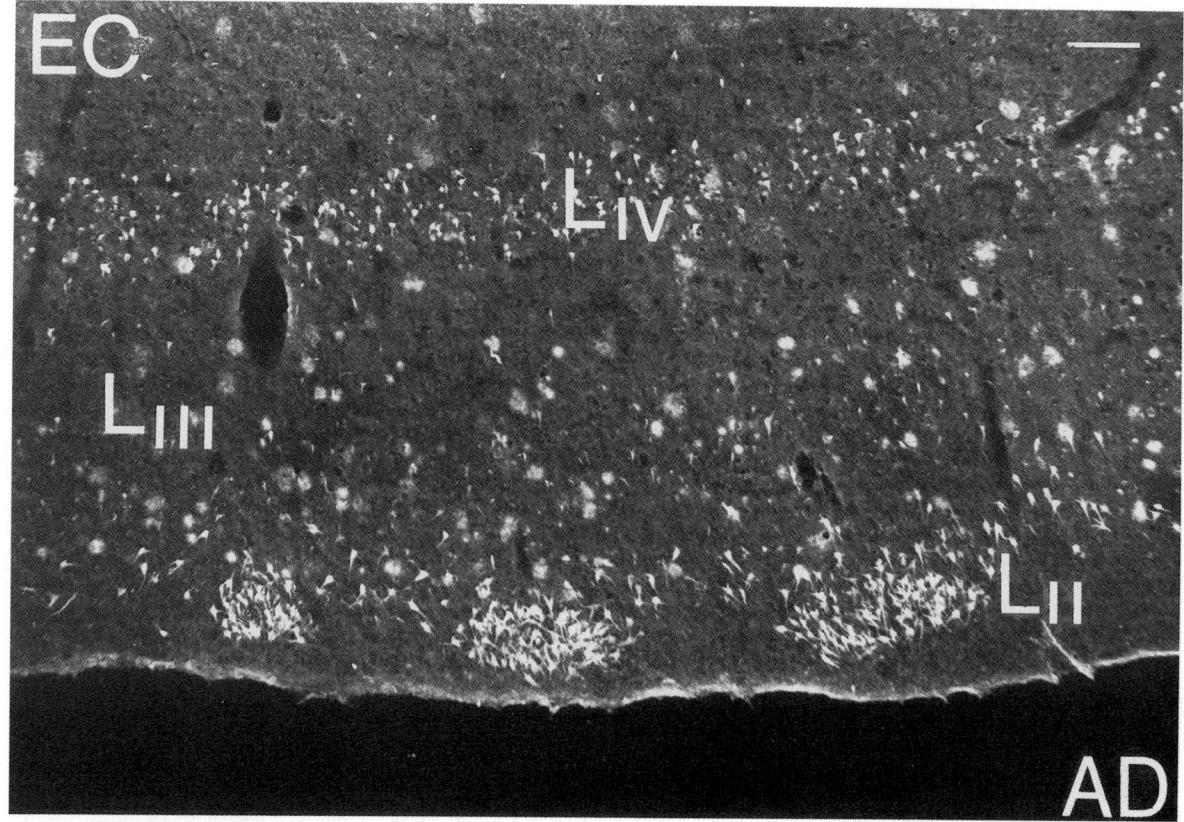

Fig. 6. The entorhinal cortex (EC) in Alzheimer's disease (AD) is shown with thioflavin S staining. Note the presence of neurofibrillary tangles in layer II and IV and neuritic plaques in layer III. In adjacent sections, layer II and parts of layer IV would not contain stainable Nissl substance, indicating that ribosomes and rough endoplasmic reticulum are no longer present. Bar = 250 μm.

Discussion

The distribution of cell loss in the hippocampal formation and that of neurofibrillary tangles and neuritic plaques in AD has been a subject of interest for many years (Goodman, 1953; Morel and Wildi, 1955; Hirano and Zimmerman, 1962; Jamada and Mehraein, 1968; Corsellis, 1970; Ball, 1976; Brun and Gustafson, 1976; Tomlinson, 1977; Ball, 1978; Burger, 1983; Gibson, 1983; Wilcock, 1983). Our observations reveal that specific areas within the hippocampal formation are affected severely while adjacent neurons are relatively spared. For instance, there is severe and consistent involvement of the prosubicular,

subicular and parasubicular cortices, but sparing of the presubicular cortices. In the hippocampus proper, the CA1 subfield is damaged heavily, but the CA2, CA3 and CA4 subfields are largely spared. Our results confirm and extend previous observations that certain specific areas are consistently at risk for Alzheimer pathological changes.

The significance of these patterns of pathology is relative to a consideration of the connectional anatomy of this region as understood from neuroanatomical studies. We will focus the discussion largely on experimental neuroanatomical results from non-human primate studies, although the general principles of hippocampal organization

452

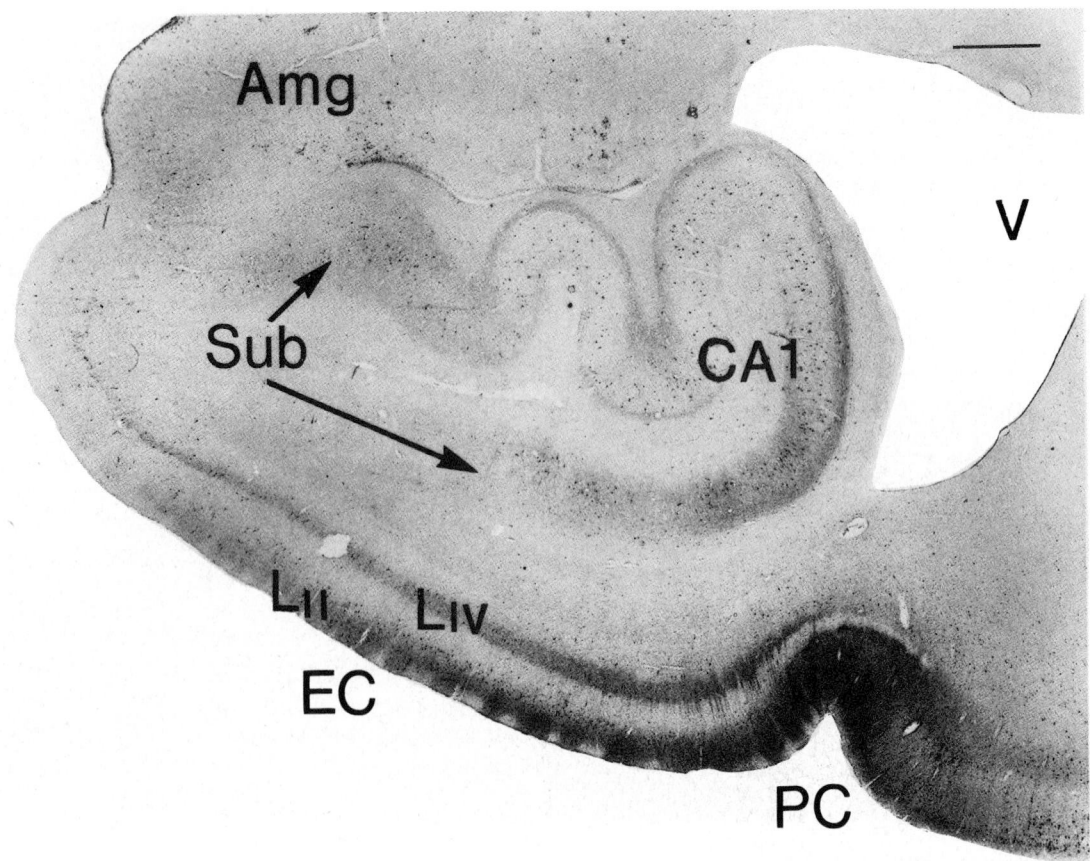

Fig. 7. Photograph of the entorhinal cortex (EC) and anterior hippocampal formation (Sub, subiculum) in Alzheimer's tissue immunostained with the monoclonal antibody Alz-50. Note the dense immunoreactivity in layers II and IV of the entorhinal cortex, in the perirhinal cortex (PC) and in the subicular (Sub)/CA1 parts of the hippocampal formation. Amg, amygdala; V, inferior horn of the lateral ventricle. Bar = 2 mm.

are similar in many mammals as demonstrated by the pioneering work of Blackstad (1956), his students (Hjorth-Simonsen, 1971, 1972, 1973; Hjorth-Simonsen and Jeune, 1972; Hjorth-Simonsen and Zimmer, 1975; Shipley, 1975; Shipley and Sørensen, 1975, 1976; Sørensen and Shipley, 1979; Sørensen, 1980, 1985), and his colleagues (Andersen et al., 1973; Andersen, 1975).

Hippocampal afferents from limbic and association cortices converge primarily on layers II and III of the entorhinal cortex and, via the perforant pathway, project to the dentate gyrus (Van Hoesen et al., 1972; Van Hoesen and Pandya, 1975a, b; Amaral et al., 1983; Insausti et al., 1987; Witter et

al., 1989). A set of intrinsic connections proceeds stepwise around Ammon's horn and leads eventually to the subiculum (Rosene and Van Hoesen, 1977). These begin with the mossy fibers, which project from the dentate gyrus granule cells to the CA3 pyramidal neurons. The Schaffer collaterals project from CA3 to CA1. The intrinsic system is completed by a large projection from CA1 to the subiculum.

The major efferent connections of the hippocampal formation to the cortex arise primarily from the subiculum and from the pyramidal cells of the CA1 zone (Rosene and Van Hoesen, 1977). In fact, it is the subiculum and CA1 zone that account for much of the diversity of hippocampal output to both subcortical and cortical targets (Rosene and Van Hoesen, 1977; Krayniak et al., 1979), either directly or through relays in adjacent limbic structures. For example, the subicular/CA1 zone provides strong direct connections to entorhinal, cingulate, posterior parahippocampal, perirhinal, prepiriform and prefrontal cortices. It also has major connections to subcortical structures such as the septum, mammillary bodies,

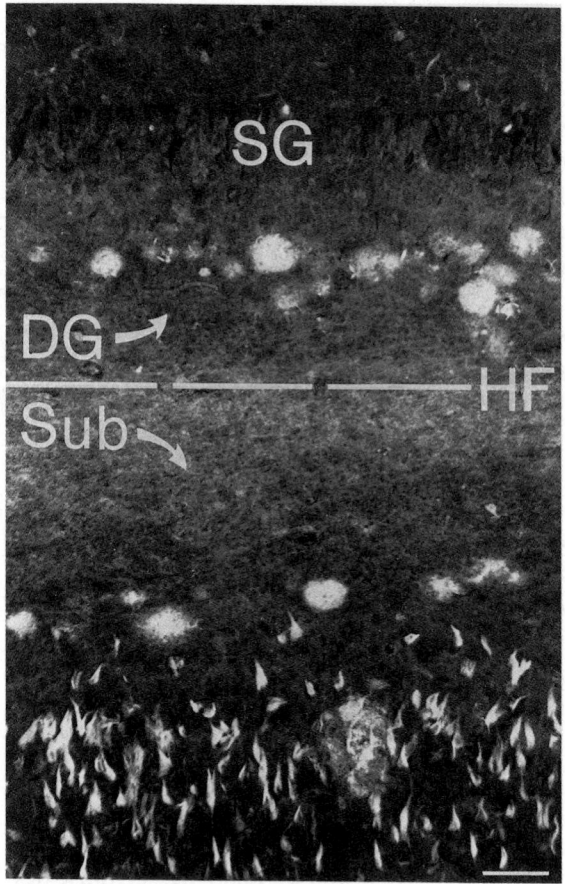

Fig. 8. A photomicrograph taken along the hippocampal fissure (HF) in Alzheimer's disease showing thioflavin S staining of neurofibrillary tangles and neuritic plaques in the subiculum (Sub) and dentate gyrus (DG) of the hippocampal formation. Note the distribution of neuritic plaques in the molecular layers, or dendritic zones, of both the dentate gyrus and the subiculum. SG indicates the location of the stratum granulosum, or layer of granule cell somata of the dentate gyrus. Bar = 100 μm.

nucleus accumbens, anteromedial and lateral dorsal thalamus, midline thalamic nuclei and the amygdala. By contrast, the CA3 zone projects primarily only to the septum. The devastating effect of subicular and CA1 pathology on hippocampal efferent connections is evident.

One of the strongest projections from the subiculum to the cortex is to layer IV of entorhinal cortex, which in turn projects and sends hippocampal output to widespread association and limbic areas (Kosel et al., 1982). In all of our cases, layer IV of entorhinal cortex also contained numerous neurofibrillary tangles. Thus, hippocampal efferent connections to the cortex are compromised at more than one level.

A close examination of the pattern of connections of the subicular cortices in the non-human primate is of further interest in view of the discrete areas of pathology in Alzheimer's disease. For example, the prosubiculum receives a major projection from CA1 and in turn projects strongly to the medial basal and accessory basal nuclei of the amygdala. In the hippocampal formation, the subicular region and, especially, prosubiculum are the major recipients of afferents from the lateral basal, accessory basal and medial basal amygdaloid nuclei (Amaral and Price, 1984; Amaral, 1986; Aggleton, 1986; Saunders and Rosene, 1988; Saunders et al., 1988). Neurofibrillary tangles and neuritic plaques in this region would thus interfere with a major direct connection between the hippocampal formation and the amygdala.

It is also of interest that this same region, i.e. the prosubiculum and subiculum, receives afferents from the prepiriform cortex (area 51), and has bidirectional connections with the entorhinal cortex (area 28), with the multimodal association cortices of the posterior parahippocampal gyrus and with the perirhinal cortex area 35 (Van Hoesen et al., 1979). The latter is a strip of proisocortex that is immediately adjacent to the entorhinal cortex, and is linked reciprocally with it. Each of these areas, including the perirhinal and prepiriform cortices, is heavily affected by pathological changes in Alzheimer's disease (Braak and Braak, 1985; Van Hoesen and Damasio, 1987).

Finally, input to the hippocampal formation in the rat from the raphe complex and the locus coeruleus is in part to CA1 and prosubiculum (Walaas, 1983). These presumably provide serotonergic and noradrenergic innervation to the hippocampal formation, both of which have been reported to be diminished in Alzheimer's disease (Hardy et al., 1985). In addition, both the raphe and the locus coeruleus are affected by neurofibrillary tangles and cell loss (Ishii, 1966; Forno, 1978; Mann et al., 1980; Bondareff, 1981).

The presubiculum appears largely spared of pathology in Alzheimer's disease, as judged by conventional pathological stains. However, recent observations suggest that it is a frequent site of diffuse A4 amyloid protein deposition (Hyman et al., 1989). The presubiculum receives input from the posterior parahippocampal gyrus and entorhinal cortex (Van Hoesen and Pandya, 1975a, b). It also receives direct cortical input from the inferior parietal lobule (Seltzer and Van Hoesen, 1979) and the dorsolateral prefrontal cortex (Goldman-Rakic et al., 1984). It has projections to the septum, anteroventral thalamus, mediobasal amygdala and prefrontal cortex. Its major influence on the hippocampus is indirect via a powerful projection to layer III of entorhinal cortex (Shipley 1975; Van Hoesen and Pandya, 1975a, b). Further study is obviously needed to fully characterize its alterations in Alzheimer's disease, but at this time there is little reason to believe that its cellular architecture is altered.

The pattern of neuritic plaques is also of interest from a connectional point of view. The line of plaques in the outer (but not the inner) portion of the molecular layer of the dentate gyrus partially occupies the terminal zone of the perforant pathway, which is the major source of cortical input to the hippocampal formation. A second line of neuritic plaques is often present in the molecular layer of the subiculum and prosubiculum. This zone receives input from the perirhinal cortex, temporal lobe association areas and ascending projections from the brainstem. The pattern of plaques in these areas raises the possibility that neuritic plaques disrupt the termination zones of important hippocampal afferents.

The distribution of AChE-positive plaques is also distinctive and of importance when examined in the perspective of the anatomy of cholinergic systems. It has been suggested that AChE-positive plaques represent degenerating terminals of projections from the cholinergic neurons of the basal forebrain (Price et al., 1982). The nucleus basalis of Meynert does not project primarily to the hippocampus or dentate gyrus, and instead the medial septum and cholinergic cells of the vertical limb of the diagonal band of Broca provide the source of subcortical cholinergic afferents to these structures (Mesulam et al., 1983). These terminate most heavily in the inner (plaque-free) portion of the molecular layer of the dentate gyrus. As assessed by AChE staining of the normal human brain, cholinergic terminations are very light or absent in the molecular layer of the subiculum. However, AChE plaques occur in large numbers in the outer portion of the molecular layer of the dentate gyrus and in the molecular layer of the CA1/subiculum subfields. Therefore our findings suggest that AChE-positive plaques are prominent in areas that are not normally termination zones of cholinergic afferents, and conversely, that the portion of the molecular layer of the dentate gyrus which receives the strongest cholinergic projection has few neuritic plaques. This would not seem to support the hypothesis that such plaques are degenerating cholinergic terminals. We have suggested previously that the AChE in these plaques may be related to a neuroplastic phenomenon, with sprouting of cholinergic fibers from remaining intact hippocampal afferents in adjacent zones or those normally present in sparse numbers in the deafferented zone (Geddes et al., 1985; Hyman et al., 1987).

Conclusions

Our observations reveal that specific areas of the

hippocampal formation, particularly the CA1 and subicular subfields, are heavily affected by Alzheimer pathology, while adjacent subfields are relatively spared. These regions respect a hierarchy of involvement as well as the cytoarchitectonic boundaries of the hippocampal formation. Moreover, the intricate and interlocking connections of the hippocampal formation itself are destroyed such that both sequential and parallel-processing pathways are affected at numerous points.

These changes in the hippocampus and the subiculum are clearly just a portion of the neuropathology of Alzheimer's disease, and do not account for all of the behavioral manifestations of this disorder, despite the fact that normal memory is an essential component of many cognitive abilities. From a neural systems viewpoint, these cell-specific changes deprive the hippocampal formation of its major input and output links to the cortex and to specific subcortical structures. Such changes are likely to be as disruptive functionally as hippocampectomy, and likely play a key role in many features of the memory impairment in Alzheimer's disease.

Acknowledgements

We thank Dr. M.N. Hart, Division of Neuropathology for consultation, P. Reimann, Department of Anatomy for photographic support, and L. Spence, Department of Anatomy for assistance in brain acquisition and preparation. Supported by NIH Grants NS14944, PO NS19632, AG08487, and a grant from the Mathers Foundation.

References

Aggleton, J.P. (1986) Description of the amygdalohippocampal interconnections in the macaque monkey. *Exp. Brain Res.,* 64: 515 – 526.

Amaral, D.G. (1986) Amygdalohippocampal and amygdalocortical projections in the primate brain. In Y. Ben-Ari and R. Schwarcz (Eds.), *Excitatory Amino Acids and Epilepsy,* Plenum, New York, pp. 3 – 17.

Amaral, D.G. (1987) Memory: anatomical organization of candidate brain regions. In F. Plum (Ed.), *Handbook of Physiology, Section 1: The Nervous System, Volume V. Higher Functions of the Brain, Part 1,* American Physiological Society, Bethesda, MD, pp. 211 – 294.

Amaral, D.G. and Price, J.L. (1984) Amygdalo-cortical projections in the monkey *(Macaca fascicularis). J. Comp. Neurol.,* 230: 465 – 496.

Amaral, D.G., Insausti, R. and Cowan, W.M. (1983) Evidence for a direct projection from the superior temporal gyrus to the entorhinal cortex in the monkey. *Brain Res.,* 275: 263 – 277.

Andersen, P. (1975) Organization of hippocampal neurons and their interconnections. In R.L. Isaacson and K.H. Pribram (Eds.), *The Hippocampus, Volume 1: Structure and Development,* Plenum Press, New York, pp. 155 – 175.

Andersen, P., Bland, B.H. and Dudar, J.D. (1973) Organization of the hippocampal output. *Exp. Brain Res.,* 17: 152 – 168.

Ball, M.J. (1976) Neurofibrillary tangles and the pathogenesis of dementia: a quantitative study. *Neuropathol. Appl. Neurobiol.,* 2: 395 – 410.

Ball, M.J. (1978) Topographic distribution of neurofibrillary tangles and granulovacuolar degeneration in hippocampal cortex of aging and demented patients. A quantitative study. *Acta Neuropathol.,* 42: 73 – 80.

Blackstad, T.W. (1956) Commissural connections of the hippocampal region in the rat, with special reference to their mode of termination. *J. Comp. Neurol.,* 105: 417 – 537.

Bondareff, W., Mountjoy, C.Q. and Roth, M. (1981) Selective loss of neurons of origin of adrenergic projection to cerebral cortex (nucleus locus coeruleus) in senile dementia. *Lancet,* 1: 783 – 784.

Braak, H. and Braak, E. (1985) On areas of transition between entorhinal allocortex and temporal isocortex in the human brain. Normal morphology and lamina-specific pathology in Alzheimer's disease. *Acta Neuropathol.,* 68: 325 – 332.

Brun, A. and Gustafson, L. (1976) Distribution of cerebral degeneration in Alzheimer's disease. *Arch. Psychiatr. Neurol. Sci.,* 233: 15 – 33.

Burger, P.C. (1983) The limbic system in Alzheimer's disease. In R. Katzman (Ed.), *Biological Aspects of Alzheimer's Disease,* Cold Spring Harbor, New York, pp. 37 – 44.

Corsellis, J.A.N. (1970) The limbic areas in Alzheimer's disease and in other conditions associated with dementia. In G.W.E. Wolstenholme and M. O'Connor (Eds.), *Alzheimer's Disease and Related Conditions,* J. & A. Churchill, London, pp. 37 – 45.

Coyle, J.T., Price, D.L. and DeLong, M.R. (1983) Alzheimer's disease: a disorder of cortical cholinergic innervation. *Science,* 219: 1184 – 1190.

Damasio, A.R. (1984) The anatomic basis of memory disorders. *Semin. Neurol.,* 4: 226 – 228.

Damasio, A.R., Eslinger, P.J., Damasio, H., Van Hoesen,

G.W. and Cornell, S. (1985) Multimodal amnesia syndrome following bilateral temporal and basal forebrain damage. *Arch. Neurol.,* 42: 252–259.

Forno, L.S. (1978) The locus coeruleus in Alzheimer's disease. *J. Neuropathol. Exp. Neurol.,* 37: 614.

Fuller, S.C. (1911) Alzheimer's disease (senium praecox): the report of a case and review of published cases. *J. Nerv. Mental Dis.,* 39: 440–455, 536–557.

Geddes, J.W., Monaghan, D.T., Cotman, C.W., Lott, I.T., Kim, R.C. and Chui, H.C. (1985) Plasticity of hippocampal circuitry in Alzheimer's disease. *Science,* 230: 1179–1181.

Geneser-Jensen, F.A. and Blackstad, T.W. (1971) Distribution of acetylcholinesterase in the hippocampal region of the guinea pig. I. Entorhinal area, parasubiculum and presubiculum. *Z. Zellforsch.,* 114: 460–481.

Gibson, P.H. (1983) Form and distribution of senile plaques seen in silver impregnated sections in the brains of intellectually normal elderly people and people with Alzheimer-type dementia. *Neuropathol. Appl. Neurobiol.,* 9: 379–389.

Goldman-Rakic, P.W., Selemon, L.D. and Schwartz, M.L. (1984) Dual pathways connecting the dorsolateral prefrontal cortex with the hippocampal formation and parahippocampal cortex in the rhesus monkey. *Neuroscience,* 12: 719–743.

Goodman, L. (1953) Alzheimer's disease: a clinico-pathologic analysis of twenty-three cases with a theory on pathogenesis. *J. Nerv. Mental Dis.,* 117: 97–130.

Hardy, J., Adolfsson, R., Alfuzoff, I., Bucht, G., Marcusson, J., Nyberg, P., Perdahl, E., Wester, P. and Winblad, B. (1985) Transmitter deficits in Alzheimer's disease. A review. *Neurochem. Int.,* 7: 545–563.

Hirano, A. and Zimmerman, H.M. (1962) Alzheimer's neurofibrillary changes. *Arch. Neurol.,* 7: 73–88.

Hjorth-Simonsen, A. (1971) Hippocampal efferents to the ipsilateral entorhinal area: an experimental study in the rat. *J. Comp. Neurol.,* 142: 417–438.

Hjorth-Simonsen, A. (1972) Projection of the lateral part of the entorhinal area to the hippocampus and fascia dentata. *J. Comp. Neurol.,* 146: 219–232.

Hjorth-Simonsen, A. (1973) Some intrinsic connections of the hippocampus in the rat: an experimental analysis. *J. Comp. Neurol.,* 147: 145–161.

Hjorth-Simonsen, A. and Jeune, B. (1972) Origin and termination of the hippocampal perforant path in the rat studied by silver impregnation. *J. Comp. Neurol.,* 144: 215–231.

Hjorth-Simonsen, A. and Zimmer, J. (1975) Crossed pathways from the entorhinal area to the fascia dentata. *J. Comp. Neurol.,* 161: 57–70.

Hyman, B.T., Van Hoesen, G.W., Damasio, A.R. and Barnes, C.L. (1984) Alzheimer's disease: cell-specific pathology isolates the hippocampal formation. *Science,* 225: 1168–1170.

Hyman, B.T., Van Hoesen, G.W., Kromer, L.J. and Damasio, A.R. (1986) Perforant pathway changes and the memory impairment of Alzheimer's disease. *Ann. Neurol.,* 20: 472–481.

Hyman, B.T., Kromer, L.J. and Van Hoesen, G.W. (1987) Reinnervation of the hippocampal perforant pathway zone in Alzheimer's disease. *Ann. Neurol.,* 21: 259–267.

Hyman, B.T., Van Hoesen, G.W., Wolozin, B.L., Davies, P., Kromer, L.J. and Damasio, A.R. (1988) Alz-50 antibody recognizes Alzheimer-related neuronal changes. *Ann. Neurol.,* 23: 371–379.

Hyman, B.T., Van Hoesen, G.W., Masters, C.L. and Beyreuther, K. (1989) A4 amyloid protein immunoreactivity is present in Alzheimer's disease neurofibrillary tangles. *Neurosci. Lett.,* 101: 352–355.

Insausti, R., Amaral, D.G. and Cowan, W.M. (1987) The entorhinal cortex of the monkey. II. Cortical afferents. *J. Comp. Neurol.,* 264: 356–395.

Ishii, T. (1966) Distribution of Alzheimer's neurofibrillary changes in the brainstem and the hypothalamus of senile dementia. *Acta Neuropathol.,* 6: 181–187.

Jamada, M. and Mehraein, P. (1968) Verteilungsmust der senilen Veraenderungen im Gehirn. *Arch. Psychiatr. Zeitsch. Neurol.,* 211: 211–308.

Katzman, R. (1986) Alzheimer's disease. *New Engl. J. Med.,* 314: 964–973.

Kemper, T.L. (1978) Senile dementia: a focal disease in the temporal lobe. In K. Nandy (Ed.), *Senile Dementia: A Biomedical Approach,* Elsevier, Amsterdam, pp. 105–113.

Kosel, K.C., Van Hoesen, G.W. and Rosene, D.L. (1982) Nonhippocampal cortical projections from the entorhinal cortex in the rat and rhesus monkey. *Brain Res.,* 244: 201–213.

Krayniak, P.F., Siegel, A., Meibach, R.C., Fruchtman, D. and Scrimenti, M. (1979) Origin of the fornix system in the squirrel monkey. *Brain Res.,* 160: 401–411.

Mann, D.M.A., Lincoln, J., Yates, P.O., Stamp, J.E. and Toper, S. (1980) Changes in the monoamine containing neurons of the human CNS in senile dementia. *Br. J. Psychiatry,* 136: 533–541.

McLardy, T. (1970) Memory function in hippocampal gyri but not hippocampi. *Int. J. Neurosci.,* 1: 113–118.

Mesulam, M.-M. and Moran, A. (1987) Cholinesterases with neurofibrillary tangles related to age and Alzheimer's disease. *Ann. Neurol.,* 22: 223–228.

Mesulam, M.-M., Mufson, E.J., Levey, A.I. and Wainer, B.H. (1983) Cholinergic innervation of cortex by the basal forebrain: cytochemistry and cortical connections of the septal area, diagonal band nucleus basalis (substantia innominata), and hypothalamus in the rhesus monkey. *J. Comp. Neurol.,* 214: 170–197.

Mishkin, M. (1982) A memory system in the monkey. *Phil. Trans. R. Soc. Lond. (B),* 298: 83–95.

Morel, F. and Wildi, E. (1955) Contribution à la connaissance des differentes alterations cérébrales du grand age. *Schweiz. Arch. Neurol. Psychiat.,* 76: 195–222.

Price, D.L., Whitehouse, P.J., Struble, R.G., Clark, A.W., Coyle, J.T., DeLong, M.R. and Hedreen, J.C. (1982) Basal forebrain cholinergic systems in Alzheimer's disease and related dementia. *Neurosci. Comment.,* 1: 84 – 92.

Rosene, D.L. and Van Hoesen, G.W. (1977) Hippocampal efferent reach widespread areas of cerebral cortex and amygdala in the rhesus monkey. *Science,* 198: 315 – 317.

Saunders, R.C. and Rosene, D.L. (1988) A comparison of the efferents of the amygdala and the hippocampal formation in the rhesus monkey: I. Convergence in the entorhinal, prorhinal, and perirhinal cortices. *J. Comp. Neurol.,* 271: 153 – 184.

Saunders, R.C., Rosene, D.L. and Van Hoesen, G.W. (1988) Comparison of the efferents of the amygdala and the hippocampal formation in the rhesus monkey: II. Reciprocal and non-reciprocal connections. *J. Comp. Neurol.,* 271: 185 – 207.

Scoville, W.B. and Milner, B. (1957) Loss of recent memory after bilateral hippocampal lesions. *J. Neurol. Neurosurg. Psychiatry,* 20: 11 – 21.

Seltzer, B. and Van Hoesen, G.W. (1979) A direct inferior parietal lobule projection to the presubiculum in the rhesus monkey. *Brain Res.,* 197: 157 – 161.

Shipley, M.T. (1975) The topographic and laminar organization of presubiculum's projection to the ipsi- and contralateral entorhinal cortex in the guinea pig. *J. Comp. Neurol.,* 160: 127 – 146.

Shipley, M.T. and Sørensen, K.E. (1975) On the laminar organization of the anterior thalamus projections to the presubiculum in the guinea pig. *Brain Res.,* 86: 473 – 477.

Shipley, M.T. and Sørensen, K.E. (1976) Some afferent and intrinsic connections in the guinea pig hippocampal region and a new pathway from subiculum feeding back to parahippocampal cortex. *Exp. Brain Res.,* Suppl. 1: 188 – 190.

Sørensen, K.E. (1980) Ipsilateral projection from the subiculum to the retrosplenial cortex in the guinea pig. *J. Comp. Neurol.,* 193: 893 – 911.

Sørensen, K.E. (1985) Projections of the entorhinal area to the striatum, nucleus accumbens, and cerebral cortex in the guinea pig. *J. Comp. Neurol.,* 238: 308 – 322.

Sørensen, K.E. and Shipley, M.T. (1979) Projections from the subiculum to the deep layers of the ipsilateral presubicular and entorhinal cortices in the guinea pig. *J. Comp. Neurol.,* 188: 313 – 334.

Squire, L.R. and Zola-Morgan, S. (1983) The neurology of memory: the case for correspondence between the findings for human and nonhuman primate. In J.A. Deutsch (Ed.), *The Physiological Basis of Memory,* Academic Press, New York, pp. 200 – 268.

Stokes, M.I. and Trickey, R.J. (1973) Screening for neurofibrillary tangles and argyrophilic plaques with Congo red and polarized light. *J. Clin. Pathol.,* 26: 241 – 242.

Terry, R.D. (1985) Some unanswered questions about the mechanisms and etiology of Alzheimer's disease. *Dan. Med. Bull.,* 32, Suppl. 1: 22 – 24.

Tomlinson, B.E. (1977) Morphological changes and dementia in old age. In W.L. Smith and M. Kinsbourne (Eds.), *Aging and Dementia,* Spectrum, New York, pp. 25 – 86.

Tomlinson, B.E. and Kitchener, D. (1972) Granulovacuolar degeneration of hippocampal pyramidal cells. *J. Pathol.,* 106: 165 – 185.

Ulrich, J. and Stahelin, H.B. (1984) The variable topography of Alzheimer type changes in senile dementia and normal old age. *Gerontology,* 30: 210 – 214.

Van Hoesen, G.W. (1982) The parahippocampal gyrus. New observations regarding its cortical connections in the monkey. *Trends Neurosci.,* 5: 345 – 350.

Van Hoesen, G.W. (1985) Neural systems of the non-human primate forebrain implicated in memory. *Ann. N.Y. Acad. Sci.,* 444: 97 – 112.

Van Hoesen, G.W. and Damasio, A.R. (1987) Neural correlates of cognitive impairment in Alzheimer's disease. In F. Plum (Ed.), *Higher Functions of the Nervous System, The Handbook of Physiology,* Williams and Wilkins, Baltimore, MD, pp. 871 – 898.

Van Hoesen, G.W. and Pandya, D.N. (1975a) Some connections of the entorhinal (area 28) and perirhinal (area 35) cortices of the rhesus monkey. I. Temporal lobe afferents. *Brain Res.,* 95: 1 – 24.

Van Hoesen, G.W. and Pandya, D.N. (1975b) Some connections of the entorhinal (area 28) and perirhinal (area 35) cortices in the rhesus monkey. III. Efferent connections. *Brain Res.,* 95: 39 – 59.

Van Hoesen, G.W., Pandya, D.N. and Butters, N. (1972) Cortical afferents to the entorhinal cortex of the rhesus monkey. *Science,* 175: 1471 – 1473.

Van Hoesen, G.W., Rosene, D.L. and Mesulam, M.-M. (1979) Subicular input from temporal cortex in the rhesus monkey. *Science,* 205: 608 – 610.

Victor, M., Argevine Jr., J.B., Mancoll, E.T. and Fisher, C.M. (1961) Memory loss with lesions of hippocampal formation. *Arch. Neurol.,* 5: 244 – 263.

Vogt, B.A. (1974) A reduced silver stain for normal axons in the central nervous system. *Physiol. Behav.,* 13: 837 – 840.

Volpe, B.T. and Petito, C.K. (1985) Dementia with bilateral medial temporal lobe ischemia. *Neurology,* 35: 1793 – 1797.

Walaas, I. (1983) The hippocampus. In P.C. Emson (Ed.), *Chemical Neuroanatomy,* Raven Press, New York, pp. 337 – 358.

Wilcock, G.K. (1983) The temporal lobe in dementia of Alzheimer's type. *Gerontology,* 29: 320 – 324.

Witter, M.P., Van Hoesen, G.W. and Amaral, D.G. (1989) Topographical organization of the entorhinal projection to the dentate gyrus of the monkey. *J. Neurosci.,* 9: 216 – 228.

Zola-Morgan, S., Squire, L.R. and Amaral, D.G. (1986) Human amnesia and the medial temporal region: enduring memory impairment following a bilateral lesion limited to field CA1 of the hippocampus. *J. Neurosci.,* 6: 2950 – 2967.

Subject Index